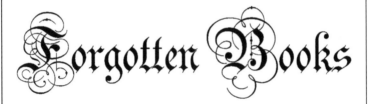
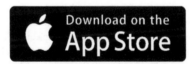
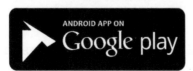

ISBN 978-1-334-52236-9
PIBN 10727177

1 MONTH OF
FREE
READING

at

www.ForgottenBooks.com

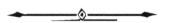

By purchasing this book you are eligible for one month membership to ForgottenBooks.com, giving you unlimited access to our entire collection of over 700,000 titles via our web site and mobile apps.

To claim your free month visit:

www.forgottenbooks.com/free727177

English
Français
Deutsche
Italiano
Español
Português

www.forgottenbooks.com

Mythology Photography **Fiction**
Fishing Christianity **Art** Cooking
Essays Buddhism Freemasonry
Medicine **Biology** Music **Ancient**
Egypt Evolution Carpentry Physics
Dance Geology **Mathematics** Fitness
Shakespeare **Folklore** Yoga Marketing
Confidence Immortality Biographies
Poetry **Psychology** Witchcraft
Electronics Chemistry History **Law**
Accounting **Philosophy** Anthropology
Alchemy Drama Quantum Mechanics
Atheism Sexual Health **Ancient History**
Entrepreneurship Languages Sport
Paleontology Needlework Islam
Metaphysics Investment Archaeology
Parenting Statistics Criminology
Motivational

AMERICAN JOURNAL

OF THE

MEDICAL SCIENCES.

EDITED BY

EDWARD P. DAVIS, A.M., M.D.

NEW SERIES.

VOL. CII.

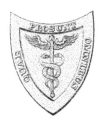

PHILADELPHIA:

FER   9 1966

1056237

DORNAN, PRINTER,
100 North Seventh Street, Philadelphia.

CONTENTS.

ORIGINAL COMMUNICATIONS.

REVIEWS.

PROGRESS OF MEDICAL SCIENCE.

THERAPEUTICS.

MEDICINE.

VOL. 102, NO. 1.—JULY, 1891.

SURGERY.

OBSTETRICS.

GYNECOLOGY.

PÆDIATRICS.

THE

AMERICAN JOURNAL

OF THE MEDICAL SCIENCES.

JULY, 1891.

SOME RESULTS OF THE TREATMENT OF TUBERCULOSIS WITH KOCH'S LYMPH, OR TUBERCULIN.

BY R. H. CHITTENDEN, PH.D.,
PROFESSOR OF PHYSIOLOGICAL CHEMISTRY IN YALE UNIVERSITY,

AND

J. P. C. FOSTER, M.D.

THE discovery of a remedy offering such possibilities in the way of curative action as Koch's tuberculin has naturally led to a widespread trial of its efficacy in all forms of tuberculosis. Considering the nature of the disease in its several varieties, it is obvious that a true estimate of the power of the remedy can be formed only after long and repeated trials. It is only too plainly evident, however, from the tenor of the reports already published, that the remedy has failed to accomplish all that was at first hoped for. On the other hand, it is equally certain that when used with due precautions it may have, in some cases at least, a decidedly beneficial and curative action, the extent and permanency of which time alone can determine. Hence, all cases of treatment with the new remedy, if properly watched and the results recorded, cannot fail to afford data of more or less value in determining its limitations and the conditions under which beneficial results may be looked for.

The following report is a statement of the results obtained in a somewhat long-continued treatment of one case of pulmonary tuberculosis, one case of tubercular laryngitis, and three cases of lupus:

Case of Pulmonary Tuberculosis.—Male, aged twenty-eight years; occupation, electrical engineer. No known hereditary predisposition to consumption. This case first came under the observation of one of us on

November 30, 1889. The appearance of the patient at that time was markedly anæmic, and he was troubled by a frequent dry cough. Pulse, 120; temperature, 102.5° F. Physical examination showed the following signs: Right lung sound; over left lung considerable loss of resonance on percussion; from the upper border of the fourth rib to the sixth rib there was marked dulness extending round under the angle of the scapula; on auscultation the vesicular murmur was found weakened throughout the whole lung and completely absent over the area of dulness previously mentioned. The patient admitted that for some months he had been suffering from pain in the left lung at the point indicated, and that he had had profuse hemorrhages every month since the preceding May. At this time, November 30, 1889, there was no expectoration. There were no moist râles or any other evidence of disease than already stated. On December 4th, the patient had a very profuse hemorrhage, and was compelled to remain in bed. From this date there was a gradual improvement, the temperature and pulse became normal, and on February 12, 1890, the patient was able to go to Florida. Up to this date there was practically no expectoration and consequently no microscopic examinations were made for bacilli. The patient remained in Florida and the Southern resorts until June, during which period he gained in weight and strength and "felt able and ready to resume work." On his way North, after very severe exercise, he was attacked by a violent hemorrhage, and this was quickly followed by another of still greater severity at Asheville, N. C. After he had regained sufficient strength he was examined by Dr. J. H. Williams, of Asheville, who wrote the following report, June 11, 1890:

"Examination of Mr. — shows exaggerated bronchial respiration on right side, which is compensatory. Percussion note good throughout. On left side there is supra-clavicular dulness, decreasing as you pass downward to fourth intercostal space, where the note is amphoric, which again fades away till the lower border of upper lobe is reached, where it is dull. Coarse râles in upper part and crepitant râles in lower. On posterior surface, left side, amphoric note clearly marked just below spine of scapula. Indication of cavity in lower part of upper lobe near the posterior surface."

The patient returned to New Haven in the middle of June, and has been under close observation ever since. On August 4th there was another serious hemorrhagic attack, and again during the first week in October. The loss of blood during this latter attack was quite remarkable. There were hemorrhages every three hours, night and day, from October 4th to October 10th, in which from one to three ounces of bright blood were expectorated each time. The progress of the disease in the left lung went steadily on up to December 3d. For some months there had been regular purulent expectorations. The cavity had increased in size and moist râles could be heard all through the portion of the lung remaining. The patient was extremely weak and anæmic, the loss of blood in October having left him bedridden. The digestive powers were so impaired that only milk and liquid foods could be used. The general depression was greatly out of proportion to the extent of the disease.

This somewhat lengthy history of the case up to December 3d shows a gradual progress of the disease in the left lung from initial consolidation up to the formation of a large cavity, with a possible distribution of the disease throughout the greater part, if not the whole, of this lung. On the other hand, the right lung was perfectly sound, and possibly some portion of the left lung may have been in fair order. The weakness, however, was extreme, and this, together with the enfeebled digestive powers, rendered the moving of the patient to a more favorable climate impossible.

At the urgent request of the relatives of the patient, treatment with Koch's lymph was decided upon, with a clear understanding of the fact that the case did not belong to the class of incipient cases in which complete recovery could be looked for with certainty, but as one where at least some benefit might be expected, assuming the lymph to have the virtues ascribed to it.

The first injection was made on December 3d.[1] At this time the coughing was severe; the expectoration, however, was slight, not exceeding in quantity one ounce during the twenty-four hours, and the sputum contained only a few tubercle bacilli. A short time prior to the injection the pulse was 72, respiration 16, and temperature 98.8°. At 4.20 P.M. 0.5 milligramme of lymph was injected, temperature, pulse, etc., being recorded every hour. Four hours after the injection, the patient complained of a peculiar burning sensation at the seat of the disease in the left lung. This was followed two hours after by stiffness, soreness of the joints and a slight rise in temperature, 99.6°.

On the following day the injection was omitted, the only thing noted being a continued soreness in all the joints.

December 5. A second injection of 0.5 milligramme of lymph. This, like the first, was followed by a slight rise in temperature four hours after the injection, and the same sensation in the chest and soreness of the joints, together with a general feeling of chilliness.

6*th.* Injection of 0.5 milligramme without noticeable change in temperature, pulse, or respiration.

7*th.* Injection of 1 milligramme. Eight hours after injection, slight rise in temperature (1°), stiffness of the joints, severe attacks of coughing, with labored breathing.

8*th.* Injection of 1 milligramme. No noticeable reaction aside from increased coughing and the general feeling of malaise and soreness of the joints, which was very marked after these initial injections. There was almost no expectoration during the last three days.

9*th.* No injection, on account of the general depression and lassitude of the patient.

10*th.* Injection of 1 milligramme. Slight rise in temperature, pain over the left lung, same soreness of joints, shortness of breath.

11*th.* Injection of 1 milligramme. No reaction; a very quiet and restful day. Patient ate a little steak for the first time without disturbance of digestion.

12*th.* Injection of 2 milligrammes. At the time of injection the pulse was 86; temperature, 98.6°; respiration, 19. Ten hours after, pulse was 92; temperature, 100°; respiration, 23, with labored breathing.

13*th.* No injection; severe coughing during day and night. General malaise very pronounced.

1 For this early receipt of the lymph the writer is indebted to the kindness of his friend, Professor Kühne, of Heidelberg. Later samples were received directly from Dr. Libbertz, R. H. C.

14th. Injection of 2 milligrammes. This was followed by a comparatively strong reaction with considerable disturbance, as indicated by the following table:

Time.		Pulse.	Temp.	Resp.	
14th. 11	A.M.	84	98.9°	19	
11.15	"	Injection of 2 mg.			
12	M.	82	98.5	19	
1	P.M.	91	99.1	25	
4	"	70	98.2	23	
8	"	95	101.1	16	Extremities cold;
11	"	114	101.1	22	[vomiting.
15th. 8	A.M.	95	100.0	26	
10	"	97	99.8	23	
12	M.	88	99.8	20	
4	P.M.	80	98.6	19	

16th. No injection; patient depressed; profuse sweating and general malaise.

17th and 18th. No injection; increased appetite; restful sleep. Expectoration very slight, mostly mucus with only a few tubercle bacilli.

19th. Injection of 1 milligramme. No reaction.

20th. No injection.

21st. Injection of 2 milligrammes. This was followed by much the same reaction as on the 14th, without, however, the nausea and vomiting.

Time.		Pulse.	Temp.	Resp.
21st. 10.30 A.M.		84	98.2°	16
11	"	Injection.		
1	P.M.	85	98.8	14
2	"	83	99.6	16
4	"	80	98.6	14
5		103	99.0	16
6		96	100.0	23
8		104	101.0	20
10	"	102	100.0	20
22d. 8	A.M.	83	98.6	16

23d. Injection of 2 milligrammes. This gave rise to a reaction similar to the preceding, but less severe, the temperature rising only to 100°.

24th to 26th. No injection. Up to this date there was certainly in many ways decided evidence of gain in the condition of the patient. The appetite had improved, likewise the digestive powers, so that solid food could be taken with comfort. Furthermore, after the depressing effects of the injection had worn away, the strength of the patient appeared to be increased; in other words, the remedy, even in the small quantities employed, appears to have had a general stimulating effect. In a general way, the expectoration seems to have been somewhat increased by the action of the remedy, although at no time excessive. On one or two days the increased expectoration was accompanied by a change in the character of the sputum, more pus conglomerations appearing, together with more mucus. The number of bacilli, however, remained essentially the same; in fact, this case has been characterized throughout by the small number of bacilli, both tubercular and other varieties, in the sputum.

27th. A slight hemorrhage, the first since October 8th, with attendant weakness and depression.

28th to 31st. No further hemorrhage. On the 30th, an attack of labored breathing, relieved by strophanthus ; no coughing or expectoration ; pulse and temperature normal.

January 1, 1891. An egg for breakfast, the first solid food taken at breakfast for two months. Patient sleeps well, feels stronger, and is able to be dressed and up for several hours during the day.

2d to 9th. Injection of 1 milligramme of lymph each day. More or less of reaction following each injection, the temperature, however, never rising above 100°. On one day, accompanying the maximum temperature there was a slight chill with profuse perspiration. As in the preceding injections, even these small quantities of lymph produced a general reaction out of all proportion to the slight rise of temperature ; soreness and stiffness of the joints, malaise, and a general feeling of discomfort being the prominent features. Although the fever reaction was slight, we deemed it injudicious to increase the amount of lymph while the general reaction was so pronounced. At the end of these eight successive injections, the weariness of the patient was so marked that the injections were discontinued until February 30th. During this period the temperature remained perfectly normal throughout, but the general weakness was so pronounced that it seemed unwise to add to it the fatigue incidental to the reaction of the lymph. During the last ten days of the resting period, the patient became stronger and felt decidedly better.

February 4. Injection of 2 milligrammes. No reaction.

5th. Injection of 2 milligrammes. Pronounced reaction ; temperature rising to 100.2°, pulse 105, with stiffness of the joints.

6th and 7th. Injection of 3 milligrammes each day. On the 6th, the reaction was pronounced, the temperature rising to 100.3°, pulse 108. Considerable pain was felt in the left lung ; considerable coughing ; slight increase in expectoration ; one or two periods of shortness of breath. On the 7th, the reaction was less pronounced.

8th and 9th. Injection of 4 milligrammes each day. No rise of temperature on either day. Malaise less pronounced than with previous injections. Good appetite, patient eating a hearty dinner without distress. The only noticeable feature was a profuse perspiration at several periods during the two days.

10th and 11th. Injection of 5 milligrammes each day. On the 10th, there was a rise of temperature to 100.2°. On the 11th, no rise in temperature. Sweating less profuse. Considerable coughing, but expectoration not over 10 cubic centimetres per day. Sputum, however, thick and purulent.

12th to 13th. Injection of 7.5 milligrammes each day. On the 12th, rise of temperature to 100.3°. No rise of temperature on the 13th. Almost no sweating ; considerable dry coughing ; no increased expectoration. Two very comfortable days, free from all malaise or pain in joints, etc.

14th. Injection of 10 milligrammes. No reaction.

Injections of lymph were then suspended until March 10th.

We were led to this by the fact that the evening temperature showed a tendency to rise to 100°, something unusual in this case, except under the influence of the lymph, and as the expectoration had diminished, and at the same time had become more purulent, it seemed probable that in some portion of the left lung there was going on a partial breaking down of necrotic tissue, which, if unduly excited by further injections of lymph, might, from the inability of the patient to remove the necrotic matter, lead to an uncontrollable septic fever.

This temporary discontinuance in the use of the lymph was finally followed by the gradual lowering of the evening temperatures, until at last the temperature remained approximately normal during the entire twenty-four hours.

On March 10th and 11th, injections of 2 and 4 milligrammes respectively were made, without reaction.

13*th*. Injection of 6 milligrammes. Reaction very marked, temperature gradually rising, until eight hours after the injection it reached 104°, where it remained for two hours or more. No other unusual indications.

14*th*. Temperature normal, but patient still uncomfortable and languid from the reaction of the preceding day.

15*th*. Temperature and pulse normal. Restless night, great difficulty in breathing, and constant faintness, requiring stimulants and open windows to revive him. At mid-day, the patient had a fairly free hemorrhage of dark and more or less clotted blood, quite different in nature from his previous hemorrhages. In fact, the peculiar appearance of the material discharged, together with its marked putrid odor, was strongly suggestive of the hemorrhage having been caused by the breaking away of semi-necrotic tissue. It seems quite probable that this hemorrhage was at least indirectly connected with the very pronounced reaction induced by the injection of the 6 milligrammes of lymph on the 13th, and the effect on the patient was beneficial rather than harmful. At first, there was naturally considerable weakness, but the patient rallied after this hemorrhage as never before after a hemorrhage of like extent. Indeed, the removal from the lungs of such putrid matter as accompanied the blood discharged could not be other than ultimately helpful.

16*th*. Expectoration of a moderate amount of blood, of the same character as on the 15th, at intervals during the day. Pulse, full and of fair strength, 80.

17*th*. Temperature 99°; pulse 81; respiration 20. No bleeding.

18*th to* 21*st*. Patient quite comfortable with good pulse and normal temperature; apparently far less prostration than after an ordinary hemorrhage.

22*d*. There was another slight hemorrhage, followed on the 27th by several more profuse ones.

23*d to April* 5*th*. No injections. The patient gradually gaining strength and recovering the lost ground.

On April 6th, injections were again commenced, beginning with 1 milligramme and continued with gradually increasing doses up to the date of writing, without any pronounced reaction being obtained until 6 milligrammes of lymph were given, when the temperature rose to 102°.

In this case the treatment, so far as it has progressed, has not resulted in any radical improvement in the condition of the patient's lung. There has been a ready response to the remedy, and the reactions produced have agreed essentially with the descriptions given by Dr. Koch.

As already stated, however, the general reaction produced by the tuber-culin has been, in most instances, out of all proportion to the rise of temperature; in other words, general malaise, pain in the joints, etc., have been more pronounced with the small quantities of the remedy employed than the rise of temperature.

In one respect the reagent has produced a very marked effect. It has certainly had a decidedly stimulating action, this being manifest not during the period of injections, but in the after-periods, or periods of rest. It is to be remembered that the treatment was commenced at a time when the patient's strength appeared nearly gone; there was a lack of appetite and weakened digestion. After the use of the lymph, however, this condition was greatly improved; the appetite was stimu-lated, the patient's digestion responded to the increased tax upon it, until, finally, even more than the full complement of nutritive food was taken and assimilated each day. Coincident with this gain, the patient's strength was increased, and he was able to move about his apartments with greater ease than for some time past. The patient himself fully recognized the stimulating action of the remedy, and when the injections were discontinued for lengthy periods frequently remarked that he felt the need of more lymph.

On the other hand, the course of the disease in the lung has not appa-rently been materially modified by the use of the lymph.

During the later injections, the general or constitutional reaction pro-duced has been less pronounced—that is, no marked soreness of the joints, malaise, or feeling of lassitude.

Further, in the later injections the sputum has tended to diminish in quantity, and at the same time to grow thicker and more muco-purulent.

Case of Tubercular Laryngitis.—Male, aged twenty-seven years. Body weight 136 pounds. Family history shows several cases of laryngitis. This patient was kindly submitted for treatment by Dr. Henry L. Swain, of New Haven, who has given us the early history of the case, as far as it came under his observation. Patient had been out of health for a period of five years, during which time he had had more or less continu-ous cough. For a year back he had been hoarse continuously, sometimes able to talk only in whispers. He had had several hemorrhages, the last occurring in May, 1889. In February, 1890, soreness was felt in swallowing on the left side. His throat was first examined by Dr. Swain on the 2d of June, 1890, at which time the condition of both throat and lungs was essentially the same as on December 4, 1890. On the latter date, lesions in the throat were as follows: Swelling of the epiglottis and redness confined to the left edge and the ary-epiglottic fold. The mucous membrane covering the left arytenoid and false vocal cord was swollen very considerably, and the upper surface of the arytenoid, as also a portion of the ary-epiglottic fold, presented decided erosions of the epithelium, but no very marked ulceration. On the false vocal cord there was an ulceration decidedly gray and unhealthy in appearance, and the cord itself was so swollen as to entirely conceal the true vocal cord of that side. The right vocal cord was visible and apparently free from ulceration. The arytenoid of the left side was half again as thick antero-posteriorly as the right, the latter being one-half thicker than what might be considered normal for this case. The patient could swallow only on the right side.

The condition of the patient's lungs at this date was as follows: Consolidation of the right lung down to the third rib in front and half way between the spine of the scapula and lower angle behind. Over this entire region, large and small moist râles were very abundant. A few moist râles could be heard through the entire lung. On the left side, in the mammary region, was a spot slightly tympanitic. At the same level behind, the breathing appeared slightly bronchial. Infrequent râles were scattered through the entire lung.

From this it is plainly evident that the case was one of exaggerated laryngeal tuberculosis, complicated, as is usually found, with a seriously diseased condition of the lungs. Treatment with Koch's lymph was decided upon at the urgent request of the patient and his family, in the hope that some relief might be afforded the exceedingly dangerous laryngitis.

Prior to the injection of lymph, and for some time thereafter, the expectoration was quite abundant, the sputum being more or less watery, with lumps of mucus and pus. It was found exceedingly rich in the ordinary forms of mouth bacteria, and contained in addition a fairly large number of tubercle bacilli.

The patient was fairly strong, with good digestion and a fair appetite.

The first injection of lymph was made on December 4th. Temperature, pulse, and respiration were noted every hour, and the larynx was examined, as a rule, each day. All of the laryngeal examinations were made by Dr. Swain, to whom we are greatly indebted for his careful observation of the changes occurring in the larynx during the progress of the case. At the first injection, 1 milligramme of lymph was used. The temperature rose from 99.4° to 101° in three hours, and remained above 100° for two hours, after which it went down to 99.2°. There was a slight chilliness of the extremities at the time of fever, and an unusual feeling of dryness in the naso-pharynx and larynx.

5th. Injection of 1 milligramme. No noticeable rise in temperature. Several severe attacks of coughing with increased expectoration. Examination of the larynx showed a slight additional swelling in most of the infiltrated tissue of the already thickened parts, especially noticeable on the arytenoids and on the edge of the epiglottis.

6th. Injection of 2 milligrammes. Temperature did not rise above 99.9°. Hands and feet were chilly at times, and covered with cold perspiration. The left arytenoid appeared less swollen than on the previous day, and the ulcer upon the left false vocal cord had commenced to assume a slightly cleaner appearance. It is to be observed that on these first days of treatment hourly observations of temperature, continued up to midnight, and sometimes beyond that hour, failed to show any rise of temperature beyond 99.9°, except on the days when the lymph was injected.

7th. Injection of 3 milligrammes. Eight hours after the injection the temperature rose to 100.8°, accompanied by a chill which lasted for half an hour, followed by profuse sweating. A slight trace of blood was observed, tingeing the lumps of mucus in the sputum. There was a severe fit of coughing, with gagging, which finally terminated in vomiting. Throat felt constricted and sorer than usual.

8th. Injection of 3 milligrammes. Six hours after injection, the temperature rose to 101.2°, without the accompanying chill. Coughing was quite severe through the day.

9th. No injection was given on this day, as the temperature remained above 100°. Patient furthermore complained of soreness in the joints and of some pain in the right lung. There was also more or less depression. Examination of the larynx showed less swelling of the arytenoids and a cleaner appearance of the ulcers.

10th. Injection of 3 milligrammes. Maximum temperature 102.1° ten hours after the injection, accompanied by more or less oppression in breathing. Patient reports greater ease in swallowing than for a long time previously. Vomited once during the day; pain in the left side; stiffness of the phalangeal articulates; urine dark-colored, very thick, and of high specific gravity. Slept quietly all night without any spells of coughing.

11th. Injection of 3 milligrammes. Rise of temperature from 99.5° to 102 8°, ten hours after the injection. Soreness in all the joints; severe headache; face flushed; feeling of constriction in the lungs; extremities cold; back covered at times with perspiration; peculiar rattling in the left side of the chest near the nipple. This latter phenomenon continued with greater or less intensity for several hours. When first noticed it was not very marked, but rapidly increased so as to be very evident and alarming to the patient himself, and could be heard distinctly by any one standing near him. This peculiar rattling or gurgling sound was synchronous with the impulse of the heart, continuing when the breath was held, but was heard only when the patient was lying on his left side. It was probably due to an accumulation of liquid in one or more of the cavities of the left lung, the splashing being naturally produced through the agitation of the cavity by the cardiac movements. The heart-sounds were entirely normal and distinct through it all. No intermittence. Coincident with this apparent exudation, the urine was much diminished in volume. The twenty-four hours' quantity amounted to only 320 c.c, with a specific gravity of 1025.5. It was entirely free from albumin, sugar, etc., and contained 14.2 grammes of urea and 0.63 gramme of phosphoric acid (P_2O_5). This condition was relieved by treatment. On this date the larynx showed considerable improvement. Owing to the diminished swelling of the left ary-epiglottidean ligament, the epiglottis was more erect than formerly. The ulcers in the interior of the larynx were quite free from gray necrotic tissue, and showed some little color. The left vocal cord, which, up to this time, had not been visible, could now be distinctly seen, ulcerated on its free border. The left edge of the epiglottis was distinctly thinner.

12th. Temperature during the day oscillated between 100.1° and 102.4°. No injection was given. The urine was increased in volume to the normal quantity, and the patient appeared much more comfortable. No disturbance in the chest. Examination of the larynx showed the right vocal cord of paler color, and the ulcer on the right false vocal cord very superficial.

13th. Early morning temperature (7 A. M.) 98.8°. During the remainder of the day, the temperature varied between 100° and 102°, with a tendency to rise in the afternoon. Pain still persisted in the joints, together with periods of chilliness during the day. There was likewise a feeling of constriction in the upper part of the chest with severe coughing spells and increased raising of thick masses, in which no great increase of tubercle bacilli could be detected. There was likewise some vomiting, presumably caused by the use of digitalis, which had been prescribed a few days previous. A very clear view of the larynx was obtained, showing the ulcer on the left side of the epiglottis very red, but not as deeply colored as formerly. One portion of its edge presented a translucent appearance, as if either œdematous or covered with a thin layer of false membrane. Right vocal cord was visible its entire length. False vocal cord not swollen. Left vocal cord very plainly visible, with the ulceration less extensive, and the false vocal cord of the same side less swollen.

14th. Injection resumed, with 1 milligramme of lymph, although the body temperature was higher than normal. The only thing peculiar noted during the day was more or less "tickling" and pain in the throat, most marked eight hours after the injection, with temperature 102.2°, and long attacks of coughing and raising. Patient could not lie down comfortably owing to the condition of the throat.

15th. Early morning temperature 98.8°. Patient feeling quite weak. Highest temperature recorded, 101.2° at 9 P.M. No injection given. Observation of the larynx showed on the inner surface of the epiglottis, left side, a mass of tissue at the median border of the old ulcer, which appeared about to detach itself. Otherwise, the larynx appeared the same as on the previous examination.

16th. Morning temperature 98.5°. Injection of 2 milligrammes at 10 A.M. Highest temperature 101.2° at 8 P.M. Some sweating during the day, with a hard coughing spell of nearly an hour's duration, six hours after the injection

17th and 18th. Morning temperature 98.7°. Highest evening temperature 101.6°. No injections. It is to be observed now, in distinction from what was stated under December 6, that even when no lymph is injected there is a decided tendency towards an evening rise of temperature.

19th. Injection of 2 milligrammes. Maximum temperature 102.3° nine hours after injection. Great difficulty in swallowing.

20th. Patient could scarcely swallow anything save a glass of milk. Solids only go down in very small quantities after repeated attempts; liquids pass down more readily, but are apt to be regurgitated. Swallowing, within the last few days, has been gradually growing more difficult, and the last injection of lymph appears to have produced an increased swelling, especially on the left side, with considerable pain. Examination of the larynx showed marked swelling of the arytenoid posteriorly, with redness of the ligamentum ary-epiglottici leading sideways to the palate. Local application was made to relieve pain in swallowing.

Maximum temperature to-day, without injection of lymph, 101.5°.

21st. Injection of 2 milligrammes. Maximum rise of temperature 102.6° eight hours after the injection. Swallowing somewhat easier.

22d. No injection. Maximum temperature 101.3° at 6 P.M. It is thus plainly evident that at this date the rise in evening temperature is always greater by one degree or more on those days when lymph is injected than when it is omitted, showing that the small doses of lymph still used continue to produce a slight fever reaction. Examination of the larynx showed the ulcer on the edge of the epiglottis to be graun-lating nicely, while the swelling of the left arytenoid was somewhat less, and its erosions disappearing.

23d and 24th. Injections of 1 milligramme each day. Maximum temperature 101.8° and 102.2° respectively. Throat still very sore, with great difficulty in swallowing. Sputum more purulent, and show-ing some increase in the numbers of tubercle bacilli.

The edge of ulcer on the left side of the interior of the epiglottis was found filled with bright-red granulations, and showed a tendency to encroach upon the margins of the epiglottis. Erosions were to be seen upon the palato-epiglottic fold. Vocal cords were clear, except the free edge of the left one. All ulcers in the interior of the larynx appeared clean and granulating. The lump of tissue mentioned a few days ago as on the epiglottis had almost entirely come away.

No more injections of lymph were given in this case. The morning temperature each day now reached 100°, and rose gradually during the day to 102°–103,° in spite of treatment with acetanilid, phenacetin, etc. There was, likewise, more or less vomiting and great weakness. On the 29th, there was considerable pain on the right side of the chest, about the third intercostal space. The moist râles over the lungs had almost entirely disappeared. Respiration was full and easy. By January 2d the patient was able to swallow much more comfortably. The condi-tion of the larynx at this date was as follows: The ulcer on the edge of the epiglottis was less reddened than formerly, and the entire edge of the epiglottis was thinner. The erosions on the palato-epiglottic fold had entirely disappeared. The swelling on the left false-vocal band appeared to be growing steadily less. In the centre of the false vocal cord of the right side a new ulceration was to be seen, very red, with ragged edges.

January 3, 1891. The same high range of temperature. Quite a mass of necrotic tissue was thrown off from the throat, irregular in shape, and consisting of thoroughly disorganized tissue, mixed with mucus and slightly tinged with blood. It came from the median border of the left interior ulcer of the epiglottis. The left border of the epiglottis, where it is ulcerating, showed signs of cicatrizing.

4th. The evening temperature reached 103.6°; the sputum was very thick and purulent.

9th. The bacilli in the sputum appeared much more numerous. The bacilli likewise seemed somewhat smaller and thicker at the ends, as if forming spores. Temperature was not quite as high during the last four days. The extreme edge of the epiglottis had healed, but the ulceration appeared to be advancing to the median line. Patient swallowed as easily as before the injections.

12th. At 8 P.M. the body temperature reached 103.9°. The ulcer on the right false vocal cord, which had steadily been growing less, appeared now to be entirely filled up and about to heal.

During the next week the patient's condition remained much the same except that he was steadily growing weaker. Maximum evening tem-perature ranged frequently between 103°–104°.

18th. Maximum evening temperature 104.2° Some difficulty in swallowing on the right side. The right side of epiglottis and the ary-epiglottic fold were found slightly thickened, but not reddened. This was the only thing observed that could account for the difficulty. At this date, the patient began to use the left side in swallowing, succeeding very well with fluids, aside from a little smarting—something which he had not been able to do for over a year. In the left fossa sigmoidea there was found a small swelling not previously seen. The ulcer on the left side of the epiglottis was plainly healing, as also that on the left false vocal cord.

19th. Maximum evening temperature 105°. On auscultation, at the lower border of the third rib, on the right side, very loud coarse râles were noticed. This was attributed to the breaking down of the tissue at this point. It was likewise observed that the moist râles over the left lung were much more persistent than formerly. In fact, there was every indication of a serious breaking down of both lungs. Coincident with this the sputum became much thicker, being filled with cheesy masses, and accompanied by an enormous increase in the numbers of tubercle bacilli.

20th to 22d. Same high fever temperatures in spite of treatment. Severe coughing followed by expectoration of very large dark-green masses, so large indeed as to produce gagging. The thick sputum contained an immense number of tubercle bacilli, the general outlines of which were not apparently different from the usual form.

23d to 25th. Maximum evening temperature 103°–104°. Expectoration had rapidly diminished in quantity. Prior to January 19th, the average amount of sputum for the twenty-four hours varied from half a pint to one pint, now it did not exceed three to four ounces.

26th. Fever less severe, the maximum temperature being 102° at 8 P.M. Patient was extremely exhausted and much emaciated. Swallowing, however, in the last few days had grown very much easier. The swelling on the right side of the larynx had entirely disappeared. The left side of the epiglottis was now quite healed and the median border of the ulceration appeared ready to heal. This was likewise true of the ulceration on the left false vocal cord. Further, the swelling of this latter cord had so far disappeared that the true vocal cord could be seen through its entire length. The two vocal cords appeared of about the same color and of the same width, but the free edge of the left was somewhat irregular, although no actual ulceration could be observed. The left vocal cord did not move quite as easily as its fellow. Moreover, the arytenoid of this side was only a trifle larger than the right arytenoid, the latter being almost normal in thickness.

During the next few days the temperature did not rise as high as formerly, but it was plainly evident that the patient's strength was nearly exhausted. The sputum retained its same thick purulent character and was full of tubercle bacilli. The larynx was seen daily, but on account of the weakened condition of the patient only hurried glimpses were obtained, This much, however, is certain, that up to twelve hours before death no swelling or ulceration occurred to alter the good condition of the various parts of the larynx above described.

For some time prior to this date the patient had been able to take a full amount of fluid nourishment, and on the evening before his death (February 2) had taken his normal complement of food. Indeed, two minutes before his death he drank easily, swallowing without difficulty.

His voice was clearer than it had been for some time past and possessed none of the elements due to mucus and ulceration, which had previously been so evident. His death occurred on the morning of February 2d, from the natural progress of the disease in the lungs, and was entirely free from the agony and terrible struggling for breath so characteristic of death from tubercular laryngitis.

We have, then, in this case very decided evidence of the healing and curative action of the remedy on tuberculous tissue in the larynx. It is further evident that this action is a very strong one, for it is to be remembered that the amount of lymph injected in this case at any one time never exceeded three milligrammes, and moreover that the process of healing was a continuous one, up even to the time of death and in spite of the extreme weakness of the patient. Moreover, the general character of the reactions induced by the remedy was, as seen from the foregoing report, essentially the same as described by Dr. Koch in his several communications, and its great power is likewise manifest from the intensity of the reactions induced by the small quantities employed. So far as it is proper to draw conclusions from this single case, the results would seem to suggest the advisability of continuing the use of the remedy in small quantities as long as favorable action can be obtained, and this would apply as well to cases of laryngitis not complicated with pulmonary trouble, from the evident tendency of the diseased portions of the larynx to become œdematous under the influence of the remedy and thus perhaps necessitate a tracheotomy to save the patient's life. This indeed may happen even with small quantities and with the exercise of the greatest care, and will doubtless always constitute one of the great dangers to be apprehended in the use of the remedy in laryngeal tuberculosis. Fortunately, in this case there was at no time any serious œdema; although such as was produced would probably have been increased to a dangerous extent by large doses of the remedy.

Although the patient died from the natural course of the tubercular disease in the lungs, the process was apparently accelerated by the use of the lymph, as was evidenced by the character of the expectoration, the physical signs which clearly indicated rapid breaking down of the lung tissue at the points previously noted as the most active seat of the disease, and the continuous high temperature which had not existed previons to the lymph treatment.

We are greatly indebted to Drs. T. G. Lee, L. S. De Forrest, C. A. Tuttle, and G. W. Lawrence for their continued assistance in watching the above case.

Case of Lupus.—A., male, aged sixty years, in good general health. This case, kindly submitted for treatment by Dr. Francis Bacon, was an ordinary case of lupus vulgaris of eight years' standing. The lupus was confined to a small area on the left side of the face closely adjacent to the eye, and extending a short distance upward on to the temple.

The active portions at the time the treatment was commenced consisted of an irregular shaped ulcer in the locality indicated, about one inch in its longer diameter, while close to it, directly under the eyebrow, was a hard nodule as large as a good-sized pea. The eyelid was somewhat involved and there was a scarred appearance to the surrounding tissue extending into the hair, showing where the sore had been successfully combatted. During the first five years the patient was not under treatment, as the process of ulceration was not rapid. During the last three years the usual forms of treatment had been followed very thoroughly with only temporary relief. When apparently under control, it had broken out afresh each time either in the same or in a closely adjacent locality, until at the time the treatment with lymph was commenced it occupied the area above indicated.

The first injection of lymph was made on December 4th, the amount injected being 5 milligrammes. The patient was closely watched, the temperature, pulse, and respiration being taken every hour during the twenty-four hours following the injection and at varying intervals thereafter. No reaction followed this first injection. The temperature remained constant at 98°–98.5°, and there were no perceptible changes in the appearance of the lupous swelling or surface, either on the day or night of the injection, or on the following day.

On December 6th, 10 milligrammes of lymph were injected. The temperature did not rise above 99.3°, and there were no noticeable changes in the appearance of the sore, either on this or the following day. The only thing noted was a darting pain around the edges of the sore, felt several times during the day, which the patient stated he had never noticed before.

The next injection, of 15 milligrammes, was made on December 12th. This gave rise to a decided reaction as indicated in the following table:

Time.		Temp.	Pulse.	Resp.	
3.15	P.M.	98.8°	86	20	
	Injection.				
4.00	"	98.8	84	28	
5.00	'	98.3	72	18	
6.00	'	98.9	72	18	
7.00	'	98.9	88	18	
8.00	'	98.6	80	18	
9.00	'	99.0	78	18	Pain over left eye.
10.00		99.6	76	18	Slight chill, headache.
11.00		100.6	86	20	Edge of ulcer swollen.
11.30	"	100.4	86	20	Decided chill.
12.30	A.M.	100.3	88	20	Surface of old scars red.
2.30	"	101.0	98	22	
4.30	"	100.6	86	20	
7.45	'	99.0	84	18	
8.45		99.2	84	18	
10.35	"	98.3	76	17	

Some evidence of this reaction remained until the evening of the 14th, in the form of a redness noticeable here and there on the affected surface.

19th. Another injection of 15 milligrammes was given, without any fever reaction whatever. Six hours after the injection the edges of the ulcer became slightly reddened and swollen, the scab appearing puffed out. This condition persisted for some hours, then disappeared.

The injections were repeated on an average of once a week up to the date of visiting, with gradually increasing amounts of lymph, the last dose consisting of 100 milligrammes. With this last dose there was a slight reaction, the temperature rising to 100.6°, and a more or less pronounced reddening of the entire face. Aside from the reaction of December 12, and the one just noted, no rise of temperature whatever followed these injections. Neither was there any very pronounced local change on or about the surface of the sore, such as has been described by Dr. Koch, or such as we have witnessed in a case of lupus to be described later. There was, however, after some injections, as in the two cases mentioned, a slight reddening of the lupous surface, accompanied it may be by a slight swelling. Other minor symptoms indicative of some action on the part of the lymph were noted from time to time, such as an irritation and inflammation of the eye adjoining the ulcer, with considerable conjunctivitis. Further, removal of the scab from the ulcer several times revealed indications of healthy granulation, but at this writing it is difficult to see any marked improvement either in the condition of the sore or of the nodule above the eye. There has been all though the treatment just enough of a suggestion of improvement to warrant the hope of some ultimate gain, in spite of the utter lack of any very marked constitutional reaction. During the treatment, the general health of the patient has been better than usual, so that, at all events, no apparent ill effects have resulted from the continued use of the lymph.

We have been greatly assisted by Drs. W. G. Daggett and J. H. Townsend in our observations of the above case.

Case of Lupus.—B., male, aged fifty years, in good general health. The lupus was confined to a spot on the side of the face extending from the left ear about two inches forward. It was of seven years' standing, and had never been very active. At the time of treatment it had a hard, elevated border, with smaller ulcerating spots scabbed over. Most of the surface was well cicatrized, but red and inflamed in appearance. The size of the whole sore was about two inches in diameter each way.

The first injection was made on February 1st with 5 milligrammes of lymph. This was not followed by any reaction whatever.

Injections were continued at the rate of one a week with gradually increasing doses of lymph up to March 8th, on which date 40 milligrammes of lymph were injected. On the 15th of March, a second injection of 40 milligrammes was made, after which the treatment was discontinued. None of these injections were followed by any elevation of temperature, or any other constitutional reaction. Further, there was during the treatment no change in the appearance of the lupous spot, except in one instance, in which the changes noted .occurred two days after the injection. Thus, on February 22d, 20 milligrammes of lymph were injected without reaction. On the 24th the whole diseased surface assumed a deep-red color, felt "puffy," was decidedly swollen, and painful to the touch. This continued for forty-eight hours. At the same time a red papule appeared at the end of the nose, brilliantly colored and prominently elevated. During this period there was no change in temperature or other constitutional reaction.

The treatment was discontinued, as it was plainly evident that the lymph, owing possibly to the quiescent state of the lupus, was yielding essentially negative results.

We are greatly indebted to Drs. Jackson and C. J. Foote for their assistance in watching the above case.

Case of Lupus.—C., female, aged thirty-three years. This was a case of very active lupus vulgaris of six years' standing. During this time it had been constantly under treatment. The original ulcer was situated on the right cheek near the nose, but was finally healed by the use of caustics. At the time the treatment with lymph was commenced the condition of the diseased parts was as follows: There was an ulcer just beginning on the right side of the nose; a second ulcer extended from the right nostril on to the lip; there was likewise an ulcer on the septum in the left nostril of the size of a five cent piece; the skin of the nose was generally reddened and apparently diseased; the outer wall of both nostrils was partially destroyed by previous ulcerations.

The first injection was made on February 6th, at 11 A.M., with 10 milligrammes of lymph. Temperature 99.5°, pulse 94. At 3 P.M. the patient complained of a palpitation all over the body; the nose appeared much swollen, very hard, of a deep-red color, and very hot; the eyes were watery and the old scar much congested; a reddish papule likewise appeared on the cheek about four inches from the nose. At 5.30 P.M. the patient had a very pronounced chill; the nasal passages were greatly swollen, rendering breathing laborious; small red spots appeared on the left cheek, fifteen or twenty in number; there was pain in all the joints and the general malaise was extreme. At 7 P.M. the temperature was 103°; at 9 P.M. 101.5°, with a pulse of 104; at 10 P.M. the temperature was 102°, with a pulse of 106; all of the symptoms previously noted were greatly increased, while the nose was fully three times as large as before the injection.

7th. At 10.30 A.M. the temperature was 100.6°, the nose still swollen and the old scars deeply congested; there were likewise small spots of congestion over both cheeks; the throat was somewhat sore, while the pain in the joints still continued. The temperature oscillated during the day between 100° and 101°.

8th. Temperature 99° to 99.5°. There was a general feeling of improvement; the pain in the joints was less, the nose less swollen, the cheeks no longer congested, and crusts had begun to form over the ulcerated spots. The general redness of the parts was less pronounced, and there was an apparent scaling on the lips and nose where no ulcers existed.

9th and 10th. Still evidence of the reaction. The temperature had fallen to normal, but the nose was still swollen; the crusts were decidedly thicker, especially on the upper lip. Portions of the skin of the nose and lip appeared white and waxy, while other portions had a deep-red and even purple color.

11th. The scabs on the outside of the nose and lip had fallen off, leaving good, clean surfaces. The scabs on the inside of the nose were still prominent, obstructing the breathing. The redness and swelling of the parts were considerably reduced, but there was a constant and more or less intense pain in the nose, referred by the patient to the outer walls of each nostril. The skin over the greater portion of the nose had a scaly appearance. The old scars had resumed their usual appearance, and the spots on the cheek had entirely disappeared.

12th and 13th. Feeling of malaise nearly gone, although there were occasional pains in the back. Pain in the nose was less severe, the evidences of inflammation were disappearing, and the nose was assuming its usual appearance. Breathing through the nostrils was freer, although the passages were still obstructed somewhat by scabs.

15th. All signs of the reaction having disappeared, a second injection of 10 milligrammes of lymph was given at 11 A.M., with the temperature prior to the injection 98.2°. At 3 P.M. the patient was attacked by a severe coughing spell which continued intermittently for several hours. This was followed by a chill, and at the same time there appeared a white line entirely surrounding the diseased spots and the old scar on the cheek. At 5 P.M. the temperature had risen to 102.8° and the pulse to 108. The temperature remained at 102° to 103°, and the pulse at 110 to 118, until after 9 P.M., when both began to fall. The nose became swollen to two or three times its natural size, taking on at the same time a dusky red or even purplish color; the scar on the cheek was likewise much reddened. No spots made their appearance on the cheek as in the first reaction, but the general symptoms were fully as severe as on the preceding week.

16th. The reaction still continued quite severe, the whole diseased area being greatly swollen and congested. The temperature at 8 P.M. was 101.8°. The coughing had stopped, but the throat was very dry. There was a decided exudation and crusting over of the spots similarly affected last week, but the crusts were not as thick.

17th and 18th. Temperature normal. On the 17th the swelling was rapidly disappearing, and the patient appeared comfortable except on sitting up or moving, when the coughing was incessant and exhausting. There was considerable palpitation of the heart. The pulse was full and of fairly good tone. On the 18th there was less cough and the patient was able to sit up with comfort, although feeling quite weak. The appetite, which had failed after the injection, was returning. The throat appeared very sore; the entire pharynx was reddened, and on the base of the tongue was a white spot, and also on the soft palate, the latter spot being as large as a quarter of a dollar. These were apparently exudations similar to what had appeared on the skin.

19th. The general symptoms were all better; the throat, however, remained the same, and the weakness was so pronounced that a tonic was prescribed.

20th. The throat was nearly clear and the patient appeared much better. The nose has returned to its normal size and the crusts on the skin had fallen off; the ulceration spots within the nose, however, were still crusted over.

In view of the intensity of the reactions following these two injections, the patient was given a rest of two weeks.

March 6. A third injection was given, this time with only 5 milligrammes of lymph. There resulted, however, a reaction of the same order as the preceding, only of less severity and without the cough and sore-throat. The throat showed no signs of inflammation or white spots. The maximum temperature was 102.6° ten hours after the injection. The temperature remained slightly above 100° during the whole of the following day. There was great pain all over the body, which persisted for some time, and the surface was painful on pressure. There was the same swelling and congestion of the diseased parts as previously noticed, which, however, subsided more rapidly than with the preceding injections.

11th. 10 milligrammes of lymph were injected at 9.30 A.M. At 3 P.M. the temperature was 101.4°, the nose swollen and the diseased surfaces reddened. At 7 P.M. the temperature was 103.4°, at which point it remained until after 10 P.M. The general symptoms were less marked than on any preceding injection. The patient was able to sleep at night and there was an entire absence of cough, sore-throat, etc. On the following day the temperature was normal, while the congestion and swelling of the diseased surfaces were rapidly subsiding, thus showing a more rapid passing off of the reaction than on any preceding occasion.

29th. 10 milligrammes of lymph injected. Maximum rise of temperature, nine hours after the injection, 103.6°. The reaction, both locally and constitutionally, was far less intense than the preceding ones.

No further injection was given until April 18th. At this date, the change in the patient's condition was truly marvellous. Every vestige of the original ulcerations, which before the treatment were so conspicuous, had disappeared except one little point hardly larger than a pin's head, situated externally on the edge of the septum. The inner walls of the nostrils were perfectly clean and free from every trace of ulceration. New tissue had commenced to fill in at one or two points, and the entire external surface had a clean, natural look (although naturally scarified), aside from a possible exudation at one point on the right side of the nose very limited in extent.

An injection of 10 milligrammes of lymph on this date was followed by only a slight reaction. The temperature rose to 100.2°, while the local and general reaction was very slight as compared with those induced by previous injections.

In this case, then, so far as the treatment has progressed, we have a complete fulfilment of Dr. Koch's statements regarding the action of the lymph on lupus. What the final outcome will be time alone can determine, but at present there is every indication of a speedy and complete cure.

Why the remedy failed to bring about correspondingly pronounced reactions in the two preceding cases of lupus is difficult to determine. There can be no doubt that they were true cases of lupus vulgaris, although evidently in a more quiescent state than the case just described. Furthermore, the lymph used was the same in all three cases; in fact, in the case of lupus first described injections were made with five distinct samples of lymph without any noticeable difference in the result (April 30, 1891).

Obviously, any general conclusions regarding the efficacy of the remedy, to be of value, must be founded upon a larger number of observations than we have to offer. In view of this fact we refrain from drawing any deductions from the above results, but present them as a contribution which may aid in the formation of a true estimate of the value of the remedy.

THE TREATMENT OF LEPROSY, AS OBSERVED IN KASHMIR, BY NERVE-STRETCHING.

BY A. MITRA, L R C.P., L.R.C.S. (EDIN.).

CHIEF MEDICAL OFFICER, KASHMIR.

BEFORE proceeding with the subject-matter of this article, I have thought it proper to give a short description of the Valley of Kashmir, the beauties of which have been so often celebrated in prose and verse. The Valley of Kashmir, surrounded by snowy and lofty mountain ranges, is imbedded like a gem in the great Himalayan chain, stretching between latitude 33° 15′ and 34° 35′ N., and longitude 74° 10′ and 75° 40′ E. In form it is irregularly oblong, lying northwest and southeast, about 100 miles in length, with an average width of 20 miles. Its area is about 4500 square miles, and its average height is 5200 feet above the level of the sea. Its population is nearly 760,815. To Vigne a cursory view of the physical features of the valley gave an idea of its having been originally formed by the falling in of an exhausted volcanic region ; but on detailed examination he agreed with the popular tradition that the valley was originally a large mountain lake. Whether the desiccation was due to volcanic action or otherwise, and whether it was gradual or sudden, are still moot questions. The mountains in and around Kashmir are chiefly basaltic in character, their usual formation being in some places composed of gray compact mountain limestone, in which marine fossils and shells are often found imbedded. That volcanic action is still at work beneath the surface of the valley is evidenced by the frequent shocks of earthquake. The soil of Kashmir is a very rich and fertile alluvium. Rice, cereals, and fruit trees grow luxuriantly. Numerous medicinal plants grow wild in the valley, such as ophelia chiretta, papaver somniferum, cannabis sativa, rheum palmatum, artemesia absinthum, aconitum ferox, and anthemis nobilis. This extensive alluvial tract is intersected by the river Jhelum and its numerous tributaries. There are also three large lakes in the valley. In the rivers and lakes fish are found in abundance. There are several mineral springs scattered over different parts of the valley, chalybeate and sulphurous.

The climate of the valley is very similar to that of the south of Europe. It is therefore well suited as a health resort to those whose constitution has been broken by the heat of the plains of India. To phthisical patients the climate is also admirably suited. The hottest months are July and August, and the coldest months are December and January, when heavy snow usually falls. There is a most lamentable want of ordinary sanitation in Srinagar, the capital of Kashmir. The Kashmirees are notoriously filthy and negligent of even personal cleanliness. The soil of Srinagar is saturated with the filth of ages. The people have a scrupulous respect for all old and insanitary practices, and any innovation is looked upon as an oppressive measure. Cholera is not endemic, but frequently pays visits in epidemic form, during which violated Nature wreaks its full vengeance. The inhabitants of the valley speak a distinct language. They are either Mohammedans or Hindoos, the former predominating. The Kashmirees are a fine race—strong, muscular, generally fair-complexioned, and with true Aryan features. Rice forms their staple food, which they eat twice daily with boiled vegetables. Meat is also eaten. Fish is freely used, either fresh or dried.

Syphilitic diseases are the scourge of Kashmir. The rate of infant mortality is very high on account of syphilitic diseases. The disease is so widespread among all classes of people that it has almost assumed the magnitude of a national calamity. Tuberculosis and rickets are very rare. Leprosy is by no means common. It is certainly met with, but the proportion of lepers to the general population is infinitesimal. During the last six years I have not met with more than fifteen real Kashmiree lepers, of which only two were Hindoos.

In the beginning of 1890 a census of lepers was taken in Kashmir. The revenue officers took it unassisted by medical officers, consequently it could not be very correct. It has no doubt included many cases of other diseases than leprosy and might have overlooked many cases in the incipient stage. The following was the result of the census:

Estimated population, 602,184. Total lepers, 202—male, 168; female, 34. Hindoos, 4; Mohammedans, 198.

The slopes of the hills between the flat ground and the limits of forests are a mixture of cultivating and grazing grounds and forests of cedar and pine, etc. These slopes are inhabited by a class of people called Goojurs, or cowherds, who keep buffaloes and cows. In winter these Goojurs live at the foot of the hills, and in summer in temporary huts on the mountains. The Goojurs are darker in complexion than Kashmirees. They speak a different language and their habits of life are different. Their food is Indian corn, or maize, and wheat. They eat buffalo meat. Living in the territories of the Maharajah of Kashmir, within which cow-killing is a heinous crime, they are not at all beef-eaters. They seldom get fish, as they pass the greater part of the year on the mountains. Among these Goojurs leprosy is a common disease. Lepers are looked down upon and not allowed to mix freely in society in the Goojur country. The lepers therefore usually come to Kashmir or go to adjoining British districts in the Punjaub for means of livelihood. The Punjaub is very hot in summer, and Punjabi lepers find that during the hot season eruptions frequently break into ulcers, which heal in the temperate climate of Kashmir. So, annually a large number of Punjabi lepers flock into Kashmir during summer and live on the charity of the Kashmirees. Thus, though Kashmir itself is comparatively free from leprosy, opportunities for treating lepers are by no means rare in Kashmir.

During the last five years I have treated nearly 500 cases of leprosy, a larger portion of them having been treated as outdoor patients at the Maharajah's Hospital in Srinagar. I now proceed to give my opinion on some points connected with the disease which will, perhaps, be found different from that given by several eminent members of the profession. In the republic of the medical profession, however, even its humblest member has a right to record his observations; nay, it is his duty.

HEREDITY.—Heredity is no doubt an important factor in the causation of leprosy. Such is the opinion I have formed after careful inquiry among Goojur lepers. I have seen a family with three generations of lepers. I have not seen acquired leprosy in children. Of course, in many cases heredity could not be easily traced, but in all such cases unsatisfactory answers were elicited. To the question, "Was your grandfather a leper?" the answer was, "I cannot say, as he died before I was born;" or some such answer. There are no doubt cases of acquisition, but among the Goojurs inheritance plays a more important part than acquisition.

IS LEPROSY CONTAGIOUS?—I saw one instance of a wife acquiring leprosy from an affected husband. Five years after marriage, the husband showed symptoms of leprosy; after another five years the wife became affected. When I saw the couple they had no children. I have seen in a family the grandmother, an old woman, suffering from a very bad type of ulcerative leprosy, attended with fetid discharge and sloughing. The affectionate daughters and granddaughters nursed her without the slightest thought of themselves. The old woman died two years ago. None in the family was affected. From my experience I can cite no instance in which the disease was transmitted from a leper to any member of his family, with whom he lived together and mixed closely in social life, except the one in which the wife was affected. The Leper Asylum in Calcutta is situated in the midst of a populous part of the city, and—if it be not the case now—fifteen years ago I saw lepers coming out of the asylum and begging at the adjoining houses, especially at a public school in that locality, but no one ever heard of special prevalence of leprosy in that quarter of the town. I know of several houses in Calcutta in which among old household servants there are lepers. Though leprosy is not common among the Kashmirees, still Kashmir is resorted to by a large number of lepers for its climate and means of livelihood. These lepers freely mix with the people, sit, eat, and pray with them (lepers are usually found at the doors of Moslem prayer-houses), and no precaution against contagion is thought of, still the disease does not spread among the Kashmirees. In India and in the northern hilly countries we find lepers freely mixing with their relatives, walking about in public streets; leprous husbands having progeny from their unaffected wives; in short, the public is exposed to the disease in every conceivable way. Does it extend in the proportion it ought if contagion by contact be admitted?

Of course, contagion by inoculation is possible, and often takes place in various ways.· All the different ways by which syphilis can be passed from one individual to another extra-genitally hold good for leprosy. In India people usually have their feet and skin bare, and therefore there is every likelihood of inoculation. The question of compulsory segregation can only come where it is finally proved that leprosy is contagious by contact. It is no doubt a loathsome disease, with public feeling strongly against it. The word "leper" is synonymous with everything that is abhorrent. Whether this public opinion is right or wrong, we as scientific observers should lay aside our prepossessions, and steer clear of preconceived notions and prejudices. Then, again, it is difficult to conceive how segregation can be complete, even if it were tried for experimental purpose. Is it always easy to recognize the disease in its early stages? Is it not very common that early stages continue for a prolonged period, during which the contagion, if any, will be equally communicable as in later stages? Does it not sometimes baffle even experienced physicians to recognize and distinguish the disease from several forms of skin diseases and neuroses? Will not the rich try to evade, and the poor be submitted to unnecessary hardships?

It is not easy to conceive how isolation can be humanely carried out, and how it can be complete, regular, and perfect; and unless it is so its very object is defeated. I think, however, that, unless proved by fresh observations and experience, our present knowledge of the disease does not justify belief in contagion by contact.

HUTCHINSON'S FISH THEORY.—The Goojurs do not get fish. Since this theory first came to my notice in the pages of the *Lancet* I have always asked lepers if they have been fish-eating, and in the large majority of instances the reply was in the negative. The theory is untenable in India, where we do not find the disease more prevalent among fish-eating people than among abstainers from such food, as *vaisnabs*. The Kashmirees, among whom leprosy is rare, are fish-eating, both fresh, dried, and salted. In India European sportsmen, planters, etc., use largely preserved fish, but there are no facts to show that fish-eating ever produced leprosy among them. High-class Hindoo widows are strictly prohibited from taking fish, but I have seen several cases of leprosy among them. But the fact that leprosy is common among Goojurs completely disproves the fish theory.

VARIETIES.—By far the majority of cases among Goojurs are of the anæsthetic type, characterized by diminution or complete loss of sensation of one or both extremities, with characteristic flush in the face and thickening of the skin. The eyelashes usually drop off. In many cases trifling symptoms continue for a prolonged period; in others anæsthesia becomes general, and ulcers of a trophic kind break out, sloughing takes place, gangrene may follow, and natural amputation of phalanges, fingers, or toes occurs. Wasting of muscle takes place. In cases of anæsthetic variety nodules form in groups, which, as a rule, remain long as such. In the hot climate of India these nodules ulcerate more quickly. These nodules are pathologically analogous to lupus, and that is the reason, I believe, that Koch's fluid is said to have done some good in certain cases of leprosy. Perhaps the bacilli are not affected, but the large lepra-cells are.

BACILLI LEPRÆ.—I have on three occasions searched for bacilli. In one instance I found them from lymph in a vaccinated leper. No doubt the bacilli are always present; my method of staining, etc., was perhaps not accurate. Methylene-blue was the staining reagent used. The figure in Green's *Pathology*, page 378, 7th edition, very faithfully depicts the bacilli.

TREATMENT.—In the treatment of lepers, chalmugra oil, gurjon oil, both internally and locally, neem (azadirachta Indica), and arsenic have been given trial. In the ulcerative stages of both tubercular and anæsthetic varieties local applications of gurjon oil or neem oil prove of some value in healing and checking fetor. Creolin does the same. These, however, have little or no power in arresting the progress of the disease.

In the anæsthetic variety I have practised nerve-stretching in fifty-seven cases. I am of the opinion that in the early stage nerve-stretching produces very satisfactory results in a large majority of cases. The result, however, I regret to say, is not lasting. Still the patient feels very much better after the operation, and leaves the hospital in an improved condition. It often happens that the ulcers heal rapidly, the general health of the patient improves. This treatment can, therefore, be safely called a palliative treatment. The following is an abstract of cases treated by me:

Abstract of Cases of Nerve-stretching for Leprosy at the Maharajah's Hospital, Kashmir.

No.	Sex	Age	Variety.	Duration.	Period under treatment.	Nerve stretched.	Result.	Remarks.
1	M.	40	Anæsthetic	5 years.	2 weeks	Sciatic.	No improvement.	
2	M.	35	"	2 "	1 week.	"	"	
3	M.	30	"	2 "	1 "	"	"	Gives history of heredity.
4	M.	33	"	1 year.	2 weeks.	"	Decided improvement.	
5	M.	40	Anæsthetic with tubercles.	2 years.	1 month.	"	Slight improvement.	
6	M.	40	Anæsthetic.	6 "	1 week.	"	No improvement.	} Brothers.
7	M.	36	"	5 "	4 days.	"	Slight improvement.	
8	M.	30	"	5 "	1 week.	Both.	"	
9	M.	35	"	3 "	2 weeks.	Sciatic.	No improvement.	
10	M	35	"	2 "	2 "	"	"	
11	M.	36	"	4 months.	1 week.	"	Decided improvement.	Patient left the hospital very well satisfied with the result of treatment.
12	M.	30	"	2 years.	6 days.	"	Improved.	
13	M.	33	"	9 "	5 "	"	No improvement.	
14	M.	19	Mixed.	8 "	1 week.	"	"	
15	M.	40	Anæsthetic.	7 "	2 weeks.	"	"	
16	F.	27	"	1 year.	1 week.	"	Improved.	
17	M.	35	Mixed.	6 years.	1 "	"	No improvement.	
18	M.	29	Anæsthetic.	4 "	4 days.	"	"	
19	M.	30	Tubercular.	3 "	5 "	"	Improved.	
20	M.	55	Slight anæsthesia.	2 "	1 week.	"	"	
21	M.	40	Mixed.	2 "	1 "	"	"	
22	M.	33	Anæsthetic.	4 "	5 days.	"	"	
23	M	35	"	5 "	2 "	"	No improvement.	
24	M.	37	"	1 year.	1 week.	"	Very satisfactory.	Anæsthesia disappeared.
25	M	30	"	4 years.	1 "	"	Slight improvement	
26	M.	26	"	7 months.	1 "	"	"	
27	M	29	"	1 year.	2 weeks.	"	"	
28	M.	40	"	8 years.	3 days.	"	No improvement.	
29	M	40	"	10 "	5 weeks.	"	"	
30	M.	37	"	7 "	1 week.	"	"	
31	M.	45	"	3 "	2 weeks.	"	"	Nodules present.
32	M.	47	"	2 "	2 "	"	Slight improvement.	
33	M.	30	"	9 "	1 week.	"	No improvement.	
34	M.	35	"	7 "	1 "	Ulnar.	"	Ulcers breaking.
35	M.	35	"	10 "	4 days.	"	"	
36	M.	47	"	5 "	5 "	"	"	
37	M.	50	"	3 "	7 weeks.	"	Improved.	
38	M.	54	"	2 "	2 "	"	"	
39	M.	50	"	2 "	4 days.	"	"	
40	M.	47	"	1 year.	5 "	"	No improvement.	
41	M.	32	"	4 years.	3 "	"	"	
42	M.	33	"	7 "	2 "	"	Improved.	
43	M.	25	"	2 "	2 weeks.	"	Left hospital in same state as he came.	Ulcers all over foot and hand.
44	M	40	"	15 "	2 months.	"	Slight improvement.	
45	M.	35	"	3 "	1 month.	"	No improvement.	
46	M.	36	"	7 "	1 week.	"		

Total number of cases, 45. Improved, 14. Slightly improved, 8. No improvement, 23.

LAMNECTOMY: A REVIEW OF ONE HUNDRED AND THREE CASES OF SPINAL SURGERY.[1]

BY SAMUEL LLOYD, M.D.,

INSTRUCTOR IN CLINICAL SURGERY IN THE NEW YORK POST-GRADUATE MEDICAL SCHOOL
AND HOSPITAL.

IT seems not out of place to enter a protest against the further use of the term trephining in connection with the spine. As a matter of fact, at the present time the trephine is seldom used for the removal of the posterior arches of the vertebræ, having given place to the mallet and chisel, or preferably to the rongeur forceps. I should prefer to speak simply of operations upon the spine, resection of the laminæ, or perhaps lamnectomy (Λαμνια, a plate, a lamina; ἐκτεμνω, to cut out), instead of laminectomy,[2] which has been employed lately. This term has the advantage of being derived from two Greek words, instead of a Latin word and a Greek ending. The claim advanced by some recent authors that the first operation upon the spine was performed by Louis[3] in 1762 may be correct in part; he may deserve the credit of having first cut down upon the spine and of removing comminuted fragments of bone, but Louis[4] himself says that his patient suffered a fracture of the spine from a gunshot wound, and consequently had a compound fracture. In the present condition of surgery there can be no question of the advisability of operative interference in such cases as this, and therefore it is hardly necessary to consider Louis's case further; and as we shall have no reason to refer to compound fractures of the spine again, this case, together with the large number of others that might be collated, is passed over.

There can be no doubt that the credit of having first operated upon the spine (in 1814) belongs to Mr. Henry Cline,[5] although the operation had been suggested by Heister[6] and others. Between that date and 1882, when Maydl,[7] of Vienna, attempted to remove some of the dorsal arches and unite the severed ends of the spinal cord, operations upon the spine were undertaken a number of times with little encouragement. In 1885 R. T. Morris,[8] of New York, made a similar attempt to reunite

1 Read before the Medical Society of the State of New York, February 4, 1891.

2 Lane: London Lancet, July 5, 1890, p. 11.

3 Chipault: Gaz. des Hôp., September 13, 1890, p. 809.

4 "Remarques et Observations sur la Fracture et la Luxation des Vertèbres," Arch. Gén. de Med., 2d series, vol. xi. p 397.

5 South's Chelius, London, 1847, vol. i. p. 539.

6 A General System of Surgery. Seventh edition, Book I., chap. vi, p. 143. London, 1745.

7 Albert: Lehrbuch der Chirurgie, Vienna, 1884, vol. ii. p. 55.

8 Annals of Surgery, vol. iii. p. 490.

the separated portions of the cord, but both these operators found the procedure impracticable. In 1889, Abbe,[1] acting upon a suggestion of Dana's, opened the spine with the same idea, or if failing in this, intending to make an attempt to unite some of the nerve-roots of the inferior detached portion of the cord to the posterior nerve-roots of the superior portion, hoping thus to furnish a means of communication between the severed sections. The difficulties of the operation proved too great to be overcome in this particular case, and the attempt had to be abandoned. Duncan,[2] in 1889, drew the sheath above and below a crushed portion of the cord together and stitched them there, thus relaxing the injured portion, but no improvement followed.

In spite of the sweeping denunciations of the earlier surgeons, and the bitterness with which its opponents have striven to prove the operation unjustifiable, we now have a sufficient amount of material at hand from which to deduce conclusions. Successful results are recorded not only in cases of traumatic injury, but in Pott's disease, tumors, and intra-dural section of the posterior nerve-roots for intractable neuralgias. We have tabulated all the cases up to date (February 28, 1891) whose records we have been able to find. Several of our cases have not yet been reported, and I am indebted to Drs. A. G. Gerster, J. A. Wyeth, C. K. Bridden, A. McCosh, C. McBurney, J. E. Kelly, R. T. Morris, and F. A. Manning, of New York; Geo. Ryerson Fowler and D. Myerle, of Brooklyn, and C. B. Stemen, of Indiana, for kindly placing the records of their unpublished cases at my disposal. I am also indebted to Dr. Southgate Leigh, of Mt. Sinai Hospital; Dr. Frank Le Moyne Hupp, of the Presbyterian Hospital; Dr. A. M. Newman, of Charity Hospital; and Dr. O. A. Schultze, of Roosevelt Hospital, for assistance in completing some of the histories. In this table we find one hundred and three traumatic cases, with fifty-eight deaths, of which thirty have occurred since the introduction of Listerism, and the other twenty-eight prior to that period. An analysis of these thirty cases shows that those of Halsted,[3] both of Morris's,[4] Hardie,[5] Duncan,[6] Allingham,[7] Bell,[8] Pilcher,[9] Jaboulay,[10] and McCosh,[11] either died after the lapse of considerable time, or had other injuries which rendered a favorable result impossible. This leaves, therefore, only twenty cases where the operation could have had any effect upon

[1] New York Medical Record. July 26, 1889, p. 85.
[2] Edinburgh Medical Journal, March, 1889, p. 830.
[3] Philadelphia Medical News, January 3, 1885.
[4] Annals of Surgery, loc. cit., and personal communication.
[5] Thorburn: A Contribution to the Surgery of the Spine, p. 20.   [6] Loc. cit.
[7] Brit. Med. Journ., 1889, vol. i. p. 838.
[8] English Monthly Med. Journ., June, 1890.
[9] Annals of Surgery, vol. xi. p. 186.
[10] Lyon Médical, June 22, 1890, vol. lxiv. p. 265.   [11] Personal communication.

the ultimate result. In these last, one of Jones's[1] was found to have suffered a crush of the cord opposite the 4th, 5th, and 6th cervical vertebræ, and would probably have died, even without the operation, from the traumatic inflammation of the cord involving the point of origin of the phrenic nerve. The same condition of phrenic disturbance existed in one of Jaboulay's, one of Bridden's, one of Bell's and Manning's, and Keetley's[2] cases.

Of the twenty-eight not treated antiseptically: Tyrrell's,[3] Holscher's,[4] Rogers's,[5] Laugier's,[6] Hutchinson's,[7] Potter's second case, McDonnell's,[8] and all three of Nunneley's[9] had other injuries to which the fatal issue could be traced, making eight of the twenty-eight that can be attributed to other causes than the operation.

If now we consider all the deaths due to the operation, we find that in the antiseptic class, 50 per cent. survived; but if we exclude those enumerated the mortality would be only 25 per cent. In the non-antiseptic series, including all the cases, we have 63 per cent. of deaths, or excluding those due to other injuries, 45 per cent. In this latter series we have one cure, 2 per cent.; seven partial recoveries, 16 per cent.; two results unknown, 4 per cent.; and five showing no improvement, 11 per cent. In the first series, however, there are four cures, 6 per cent.; fifteen partial recoveries, 25 per cent.; one unknown, 1 per cent.; and eleven no improvement, 18 per cent. This is a more favorable showing than Ashhurst was able to make from his table of forty-three cases.[10] He had 72 per cent. of deaths, 9 per cent. not benefited, 9 per cent. improved, and 9 per cent. whose results were unknown, and no cures. Thorburn's[11] statistics of 61 cases did not include those of Goldsmith,[12] Boyer,[13] Massoneuve,[14] Eve,[15] Halsted,[16] Pinkerton, Morris,[17] nor any later than June 29, 1889.

It is interesting in this connection to compare the statistics of the antiseptic class with those of fractures treated conservatively. Thus, Gurlt[18] reports 217 deaths out of 270 fractures, over 80 per cent.; while

[1] Thorburn, loc. cit., p. 26.   [2] Brit. Med. Journ., 1888, vol. ii. p. 421.
[3] Tyrrell: Cooper's Lectures on Surgery, 1825, vol ii. p. 20.
[4] Hannov. Annal f. d. ges. Heilk., Bd. iv. 1839, p. 330.
[5] Amer. Journ. Med. Sciences, O. S., vol. xvi. p. 91, 1835.
[6] Bull. Chir., vol. i. p. 401.   [7] Amer. Med Times, 1861.
[8] Dublin Journ. Med. Sci., vol. xl.   [9] Med. Times and Gaz., August, 1869.
[10] International Encyclopædia of Surgery, vol. iv. p. 890.
[11] Surgery of the Spinal Cord, 1889, p. 144.
[12] Gross's System of Surgery. Second edition.
[13] Heyfelder: Traité des Resections (trans. by Boeckel), p. 244.
[14] Chipault: Gaz. des Hôp., September 13, 1890, p. 809.
[15] Philadelphia Medical News, January 3, 1885.
[16] International Encyclopædia of Surgery, vol. iv.   [17] Loc. cit.
[18] Handbuch der Lehre v. d. Knochenbruchen, 1864, vol. ii. p. 172.

Burrill, from the tables of the Boston City Hospital,[1] has compiled 82 cases with 64 deaths, 79 per cent. Of the 22 per cent. of recoveries, only 11 per cent. were satisfactory, the other 11 per cent. being completely disabled. Of the fatal cases the greater number died within a few days.

In addition to the one hundred and three traumatic cases we have tabulated thirty-nine of Pott's disease, eleven tumors, and five intra-dural nerve-sections, making a total of one hundred and fifty-five operations upon the posterior arches of the spine.

We have found that the percentage of deaths in all the cases operated upon for the relief of symptoms due to traumatism was 56 per cent.; but the percentage of all the other classes taken together is but 26 per cent., showing that the mortality is 30 per cent. higher in the former than in the latter series. The mortality of traumatic cases operated upon prior to Listerism was 63 per cent., since Listerism 50 per cent.

In the cervical region there are in the non-antiseptic class ten cases. Seven died; five from the spinal injury, and two from other causes; two, one of resection of the sixth and the other of the fifth and sixth arches, made partial recoveries, while one recovered from the operation, but having sustained a complete crush of the cord, showed no improvement in symptoms.

In the antiseptic series of eighteen there were fifteen deaths; one of these, however (Morris's), survived ten months, and should be included among the unimproved. In addition to this, one of Hardie's, one of Jones's, one of Bell's, one of McCosh's, and Manning's were practically hopeless at the time of the operation, while in Bell's first case the author says " the operation did not seem to complicate the case in any way." Including in the statistics all these cases except Bell's, in which there were other injuries that would probably have proved fatal, we still have thirteen deaths due to the operative manipulation, 72 per cent. Excluding all those enumerated, the percentage is only 44. In this series there is one cure, 5 per cent.; one improved, 5 per cent.; and two unimproved, 11 per cent.

In the dorsal region there were seventeen cases operated upon prior to the introduction of antisepsis, with twelve deaths; two of the latter should not be included, one having died of general œdema after fifteen weeks, and the other of fractured ribs and pyo-pneumothorax, making 58 per cent. of deaths due to spinal injury. Two cases, 12 per cent., show incomplete recovery, and three, 18 per cent., no improvement.

In the second series (antiseptic) there are twenty-eight cases, with eight, 28 per cent., deaths. One other death occurred at seven months, and another at five months after the operation, and consequently they

[1] Medical Publications of the Harvard Medical School. 1887.

are included in the unimproved class. Of the remaining cases, nine, 32 per cent., including the two cases that died after some months, were unimproved. Nine cases were improved, and of this number, one (McBurney's) is still under treatment and improving. Two, 7 per cent., are reported as cured.

In the antiseptic class there are four dorso-lumbar cases, two of which were fracture-dislocations in which reduction was almost impossible ; in one as soon as the traction was removed the deformity was reproduced. Three of the cases died, both dislocation cases, one of which had other injuries that would alone have proven fatal ; the third case lived four months and should consequently be included among the unimproved cases. The fourth case was not improved.

In the lumbar region, out of four cases in the old series, three, 75 per cent., died, and one made an incomplete recovery.

There are five cases in the antiseptic class in this region, and of these two died. In one the cause of compression was not found at the operation, and the second died of other injuries and should not be included in the death-rate, leaving only four cases to be considered, with 25 per cent. fatal. One case was improved, one was cured, and one showed no improvement. In this series I have to report the following case :

Man, aged twenty-nine years, Swede, engineer. On April 20, 1889, while on his hands and knees removing a block from under a gas generator weighing about two tons, the machine toppled over, the flange striking him in the back and pressing him down until it was arrested by an upright pipe which was fixed in the floor. He was unable to move from this position until the machine was raised. When he was pulled out he was laid on his back and "felt a queer sensation in his feet, which were numb." In a few minutes he began to have severe pain in the back, which was increased by motion, and had no control over his right leg. He was taken to Roosevelt Hospital. For the following notes of the case during his stay in the hospital I am indebted to Dr. Charles McBurney, who kindly placed them at my disposal. "On admission the spines of the upper lumbar vertebræ have a feeling of retrocession and there is also obscure crepitus, obscured by blood-clot beneath the skin."

During the next few days he lay on his side and retention of urine and of feces was a prominent symptom ; the urine showed a large number of hyaline casts and albumin.

On the 27th, seven days after his admission, his bowels responded copiously to medicine, and it was found that he had no control over his rectum ; the casts had disappeared from the urine.

"May 4. There seems to be paralysis of the extensors of the right foot. The patellar reflexes are responsive and apparently diminished.

"10th. The bedsore over the sacrum (due to feces irritating), which started ten days ago, is looking better.

"20th. Condition unchanged. Still catheterized. Movements of bowels are involuntary but conscious. Semi-paralysis of right foot. Temperature not taken. No pain except when patient attempts to roll

on his side. The extensive ecchymosis is fading, but the parts are very
sensitive to pressure.

"*June 2.* Still catheterized. Discharged, improved, June 3d."

On July 29, 1889, I first saw the patient at his home. He was confined to his bed, his right thigh slightly drawn up and the leg flexed.
There was little or no atrophy, but loss of sensation and paralysis with
incontinence of feces and of urine. A bedsore a little larger than a
silver dollar existed over the sacrum. As he was suffering with a severe
diarrhœa, it was impossible to make a careful examination for several
days, but on August 7th he had recovered sufficient strength for me to
examine him thoroughly. There was then a tumor of some size over
the lumbar vertebræ, and consequently no depression or other sign of
fracture could be discovered. I suppose this thickening was due to the
hæmatoma that existed at the time of the accident. He had pain running down the right leg and in the toes of the foot on that side, and still
had incontinence of urine and feces. He was able to stand by holding
on to the furniture, but could not stand erect. His right leg was flexed
on the thigh and his body bent at about 20° from the perpendicular.
Anæsthesia was present over the region indicated in the figure.

Electrical reactions are shown in the following table :

Left galvanic.	Left faradic.		Right faradic.	Right galvanic.
KCC>AnCC	50	Peronei	Lost	Total loss 8 m.amp.
KCC>AnCC	52	Anterior tibial	Lost	" " 10 "
" "	54	Posterior tibial	Lost	" " 8 "
	Lost	Glutei	Lost	
	Preserved	Tensor vaginæ femoris	Preserved	
	Diminished	Posterior thigh muscles	Diminished	
	40	Adductor	69	
	70	Biceps	72	

Reversals at 10 milliampères ; no reaction.

Is able to have sexual intercourse, without emission or sensation, but
occasionally has an emission during sleep with the usual sensations. Has
some voluntary control over the muscles of the thigh, but practically
complete paralysis of the leg. Atrophy very slight. Knee-jerks present
and about normal; superficial reflexes over paralyzed areas wanting;
no ankle clonus; temperature of right leg lower than left and skin
quite dry. Being convinced that there was compression in the lumbar
region, I advised operation at this time, but the patient refused. He
was, therefore, put upon a course of massage and electricity. In November, 1889, he complained that the pain in the lumbar region running down the back of the right leg and foot was increasing, although
his condition otherwise remained much the same.

In May, 1890, he concluded to be operated upon. At this time the
thickening over the lumbar region had disappeared, and it was possible
to make out a very slight depression at the third lumbar vertebra.

With a view to having my examination and conclusion corroborated,

I requested Dr. M. Allen Starr to see the case with me. The following is his report:

Examined by Dr. Starr, May 21, 1890. The man walks with much difficulty, dragging the right foot and being unable to raise it from the

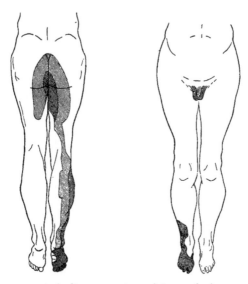

Dark shading—area of complete anæsthesia.
Light shading—area of partial anæsthesia.

ground. The entire pelvis appears to be so displaced that the right hip is higher than the left. He has considerable voluntary power over the muscles above the knee, but those below the knee are almost completely paralyzed. He cannot turn or move his ankle or flex or extend his toes. The entire right extremity is smaller than the left, the difference being half an inch in the middle of the thigh and one inch in the middle of the leg. In the paralyzed muscles there is a complete loss of faradic reaction, and no response to interruptions of a galvanic current of ten milliampères in strength. There is a loss of tone in the muscles paralyzed, they are flabby and have lost their mechanical excitability to percussion. The muscles are nowhere rigid or contractured.

Reflex action.—The knee-jerks are equal on both sides and normal in degree. There is no ankle clonus. Plantar reflex to tickling is absent.

Sensation.—There is complete anæsthesia of the penis, perineum, anus, and of a saddle-shaped area over both buttocks reaching down to within two inches of the popliteal fossa. On the right side the anæsthetic area extends downward over the back of the leg and over its outer side, and includes the entire foot, sole and front, excepting along the inner side, as determined by tests with cotton and with needles. The same area is insensitive to heat and cold. He complains of severe pain over the lower sacral region, and in this area there is a bedsore. The temperature of the right leg is perceptibly cooler than that of the left.

Automatic action.—There is imperfect control of the bladder and rectum. He has erections and has had connection since his injury, but there is no emission during the act.

Diagnosis.—Injury and compression of the cauda equina at the level of the lower lumbar vertebræ.

He was also examined at this time by Dr. Robert Abbe, who concurred with the opinion expressed by Dr. Starr. On July 5th, assisted by Drs. Abbe, T. Halsted Myers, and C. E. Denison, he was etherized and the operation performed. An incision about seven inches in length, having the third lumbar vertebra as its centre, was made along the right margin and close to the spinous processes; the incision was carried rapidly down to the laminæ, where it became evident that there was an ununited fracture of the spinous process of the third lumbar vertebra. The spines of the second and fourth were cut off close to the laminæ with Liston's bayonet forceps, and the muscles were dissected back from the arches on both sides by means of a periosteotome. The severed spines were left attached to the flaps of the left side. The posterior arches of the three vertebræ were then removed by gnawing them off piece by piece with rongeur forceps, and we were able to make out a slightly depressed fracture of the right lamina of the third lumbar vertebra, which was surrounded by considerable callus, especially on the anterior surface. This somewhat diminished the size of the vertebral canal. A probe was passed in both directions in the canal to make sure no further compression existed either above or below the point of operation. A slight laceration in the dura, which was healthy and otherwise not opened, allowed the escape of some cerebro-spinal fluid. The hemorrhage, quite severe in the first two or three minutes of the operation, was controlled by compression with sponges and retractors. The wound was closed by means of deep and superficial catgut sutures, a drainage-tube being inserted at the lowest point of the incision, and the spinous processes were left attached to the left flap. The etherization occupied one hour and twenty minutes. There was practically no shock. The next day all pain had disappeared, and the dressing, which was soaked through, was removed and the drainage-tube withdrawn. There was some irritation in the bladder with retention of urine, and a bedsore below the original one, which had been threatening for some time, became fully developed. Five days later, however, the wound was healed and I was able to make a test of the anæsthetic area, which was slightly improved. The bedsores were better and he had less cystitis. On July 19th he was allowed to sit up. The subsequent course of the case showed simply a progressive improvement, until, at the present time, although still suffering from some paralysis and anæsthesia, he is able to remain at work for the usual number of hours, either running his engine or in the bottling-room of a soda-water establishment in New York. He has never worn any retentive apparatus and has never suffered inconvenience from the condition of his spine.

In seventeen of the cases the dura was opened and cerebro-spinal fluid escaped; six of these died. Of these six, one had a ruptured diaphragm with hernia of the stomach, etc.; another lived seven months, but the wound healed in about two weeks; one lived eighteen days ; and in one the cause of the compression was not removed. Three of the cases may be thrown out of consideration—leaving three, and one of these doubtful, that might possibly have been fatal in consequence of the escape of the cerebro-spinal fluid. Several cases, notably Duncan's[1] and Horsley's,[2] of spinal tumor, have illustrated the fact that the escape of this fluid may continue for a considerable time yet offer no obstacle to favorable progress. It has drained away in considerable quantities in cases of spina bifida that have been subjected to operation, and in several cases of tumor of the spine and of intra-dural section of the posterior nerve-roots.

Two conditions present themselves for consideration in deciding whether the operation should be done early or whether some time should be allowed to elapse. If undertaken at once, there is danger of interference where a spontaneous cure would result if the patient were left alone, or where a complete destruction of the cord renders any operative interference useless. If, however, operation be delayed too long and compression allowed to continue, a degeneration may result which would be as serious as though the functions of the cord had been destroyed by the original injury. This question of the selection of the proper time for operation is, therefore, a most important one. Lauenstein[3] says : " If after the lapse of six or ten weeks there is incontinence of urine with cystitis or incontinence of feces, and especially if there is also the development and spreading of bedsores, but little is to be hoped from the unaided efforts of Nature." And Thorburn advances practically the same proposition in injuries to the cauda equina.[4]

In determining the influence of time upon the operation, there are fifty-one antiseptic cases where the time that elapsed between the injury and the operation is stated. Out of this number twenty-four died and twenty-seven recovered from the operation. Within the first eight days after the injury twenty-four of these were operated upon, with a mortality of twenty-one (all but three of the deaths) against three recoveries. In the non-operative cases it is also true that the greatest number of deaths occur within the first few days. In one of the cases the cause of death is given as myelitis reëstablished by the operative manipulation.[5] It is impossible to draw any conclusion with regard to the effect of myelitis in the delayed cases from the histories I have been able to study.

From the result of my study of these cases I am inclined to agree with Horsley,[6] that operation should be undertaken at once " in all cases

[1] Loc. cit.   [2] Trans. Med.-Chir. Soc., vol. lxxi. p. 377.
[3] Centralblatt für Chir., 1886, No. 51, p. 888.
[4] Surgery of the Spinal Cord, p. 162.
[5] Pinkerton : Phila. Med. News, January 3, 1885.
[6] Brit. Med. Journ., Dec. 6, 1890. -

where displacement or crepitus indicates compression, and where extension directly after the accident clearly fails to reduce the deformity,"
provided there are symptoms present which indicate interference with
the functions of the cord.   In other cases I should wait until the shock
following the injury had been overcome.   During this time, however, the
patient's condition should be most carefully watched, and at the first
indication of any symptoms pointing to an extension of the interference
with the action of the spinal cord, whether that interference be due to
hemorrhage or to myelitis from compression, to callus, or to the exudation of lymph, the patient should be subjected to operation at once.   It
is of course unnecessary to say that no interference would be considered
in any case where there was or seemed to be any amelioration of the
patient's condition so long as that improvement continued.

Hutchinson,[1] in his conclusions based upon twenty post-mortem
examinations, says : " Permanent compression of the cord or of any part
of it is very rare, not more than one in ten, and as most fractures in this
region are due to bends, fractures of the laminæ are of little consequence
and never cause compression.   Instances of great displacement sometimes occur and can rarely be benefited by operation, while cases in
which during life there is the greatest displacement are not always the
most serious."   He, in common with Legros Clark,[2] considers pyæmia
and spinal meningitis the principal reasons for non-interference.   " To
weaken still further the remaining connection of a broken spine," says
the latter, " to convert a simple into a compound fracture, to expose the
sheath and possibly the cord itself to the risks attending the period of
repair, cannot be regarded as matters of indifference."   White[3] sums up
the possible dangers as follows :

1st. Disturbance of the cord is more or less involved in almost every
form of operative procedure, and its exact importance is as yet unknown.

2d. The hemorrhage from the external and internal spinal plexus of
veins.

3d. Laceration of the membranes, the risk of which accident would,
of course, be increased if they were adherent to the bony walls of the
vertebral canal.

4th. The danger from etherization, which is much increased by the
prone position of the patient and by the paralysis of the abdominal walls.

Horsley considers sepsis the only real danger.

Chipault, as a result of a further experimental study of the points
advanced by Hutchinson, comes to the same conclusion, but from a

[1] Clinical Record and Reports of London Hospital.
[2] British Medical Journal, vol. ii. pp. 49–52.
[3] Annals of Surgery, 1889, vol. x. pp. 1–39.

clinical point of view we find that the cases of Cline, Laugier, Tillaux,[1] Maydl, Horsley, both of Jones's cases, Abbe, Jaboulay, Pilcher, and McCosh, apparently fulfil these conditions, while those of Mayer,[2] McDonnell, Maunder,[3] Lucke,[4] Halsted, Lauenstein, Hardie, Duncan, Péan,[5] Abbe, Jaboulay, Dawbarn,[6] Wyeth, and my own, show that the bone either did not spring back to place, or that the depressed laminæ were the compressing factors. It is clear, from a clinical standpoint at least, that the statement made by Hutchinson, with regard to the bone as the compressing agent, is too radical; for out of thirty-five cases, fifteen more than Hutchinson reported, in which the cause of compression is given, we find eleven due to temporary, and thirteen to continued bony displacement.

In four cases the compressing cause is stated as extravasation of blood (Oldknow,[7] G. W. Jones,[8] Stephen Smith,[9] and Willett[10]), and Pilcher's, in addition to the crush of the cord, had two extra-dural hemorrhages, a condition which Hutchinson said he had never seen "to the extent of possible compression, and in the majority of cases little or none."

Of the objections of Legros Clark little need be said. Antisepsis, with its improved technique and more careful observation and treatment of operative wounds, has swept away the dread of septic infection; we have already proven that a free incision of the dura mater has little or no effect upon the result, and so far there are only two cases in which it has been necessary to apply a plaster-of-Paris jacket at any length of time after the injury. In my case with the posterior arches of three lumbar vertebræ removed, the man has returned to his work and is able to do an ordinary day's labor. Morris's case, too, which died ten months after the operation, was found to have a dense mass of fibrous tissue filling in the place from which the bone had been removed; and Page,[11] in a case operated upon for Pott's disease, reports that the site of the removed arches was apparently filled with solid bone.

There can be no doubt that disturbance of the cord is more or less necessary in all operative cases. How much effect this has upon the

---

[1] Bull. Gén. de Thérap. Méd. et Chir., 1866, p. 202.

[2] v. Walther and v. Ammon: Journ. der Chir., Bd. xxxviii.

[3] Lancet, 1867, vol. i.

[4] Werner: Die Trepanation der Werbelsäule, Strassburg, 1879; Rev. des Sci. Méd., April, 1880.

[5] Brit. Med. Journ., 1888, vol. i. p. 672.

[6] N. Y. Med. Journ., June 29, 1889, p. 711.

[7] Cooper's Fractures and Dislocations, 1822.

[8] Med. Times and Gaz., 1856, vol. ii. p. 86; Brown-Séquard: Dis. Central Nervous System, p. 255.

[9] Phelps: N. Y. Journ. Med , vol. vi. p. 87.

[10] St. Barthol Hosp. Reports, vol. ii. p. 242.

[11] London Lancet, Dec. 1890, p. 1210.

subsequent course of the case cannot be told from existing data. In one of McBurney's cases, in Page's case of Pott's disease, and in my case, the symptoms were increased for a few hours, and yet it is impossible to say how much of this was due to shock after the operation, and how much to disturbance of the cord. In Page's it is probable that it was due to concussion from the use of the mallet and chisel in removing the bone.

It is also probably true that the dangers of etherization are somewhat increased in cases where there is paralysis of any portion of the respiratory apparatus, but the only case reported in which this seemed to affect the result was Pilcher's, where the injury was practically hopeless.

Thorburn[1] in his *résumé* of the indications for operative treatment founded upon his sixty-one cases of fracture, says: "The operation of trephining the spine for traumatic lesions, as compared with the lesion it is intended to relieve, does not present any very great dangers and appears unlikely to increase the gravity of the prognosis, but as both *a priori* argument and the results of published cases show that it is unlikely to be of service, it should be abandoned, except in cases of injury to the cauda equina, and that in the latter, on the other hand, it will probably prove to be an eminently justifiable and serviceable procedure."

Adopting these views, we should condemn the 30 per cent. or more of cases that have been shown to be relieved under the present methods of operating, as compared with the statistics of Gurlt[2] and Burrell,[3] to death, or to a miserable existence, without hope of relief. If, on the other hand, we do undertake an operation we increase the number of those improved 20 per cent., and add to the unimproved only 13 per cent. Horsley[4] reports only one death out of nineteen cases of lamnectomy. We must conclude, then, that the procedure is not only justifiable, but eminently proper.

The operation is evidently contra-indicated in all cases where the patient has not recovered from the direct shock of the injury; where the cord is completely crushed or severed, whether by a simple blow from the displaced bone, which has sprung back to its place, or from direct and continued compression; in all cases where improvement has appeared early and is progressing; and, where a severe traumatic myelitis is still present or but just controlled. It is indicated, on the other hand, in all cases where improvement has ceased and the patient is still helpless, and where there is reason to think that the disability is due to compression rather than to complete degeneration.

It is essential in discussing this subject to fully appreciate the symptoms indicating compression or destruction of any part of the spinal cord. Interference with the voluntary action of the muscles places them

---

[1] Spinal Surgery, p. 161.   [2] Loc. cit.   [3] Loc. cit   [4] Loc. cit.

entirely under the control of the reflex centres in the cord, causing the affected limbs, owing to the difference in strength of the various groups of muscles, to take certain well-defined positions.

In regard to position, Starr[1] says: "If the lesion is near to and below the third lumbar segment and irritates it, but does not destroy it, the patient is likely to lie with the thighs drawn up and the legs flexed. If the lesion is above the third lumbar segment he will lie with the thighs and legs extended, unless the lesion produces great irritation, as in the last stages of lateral sclerosis, when the thighs and legs are flexed and adducted. If the lesion is about the two lower cervical segments and irritates the fifth and sixth, he will lie with his arms abducted about at a right angle, his forearms flexed on the arms, and hands supinated or their position dependent upon gravitation, and fingers flexed. If the lesion is about the middle cervical segment as high as the fourth, the arms will lie at the sides and cannot be moved." Bowlby[2] has observed the condition of the reflexes in twenty-one cases of cervico-dorsal fracture, all but one confirmed by autopsy; in the other twenty cases, where there was a complete transverse destruction of the cord, there were no reflexes nor rigidity of the muscles. The superficial reflexes were also generally lost immediately after the accident, although this was not always true. Unlike the deep reflexes, too, the superficial reflexes may return. "On the other hand, when the cord has been injured and when it is compressed, but when its continuity has not been entirely interrupted, the reflexes are not only preserved, but may be, and generally are, exaggerated." Bastian first made this observation as early as 1882, and again in a recent paper.[3]

As a result of this investigation Bowlby says: "Where there is a complete loss of deep reflexes there is probably a total transverse lesion; but when these reflexes are present the cord is certainly not completely crushed." "If the exaltation of the reflex power," says Tillaux, "has been considered as a sign of destruction of the dorsal or cervical cord, I think that the absolute abolition of these reflexes in the cases of fractures in the lumbar region would be generally an indication of the destruction of the medullary substance. I consider, therefore, that the persistence of the reflex action in lumbar fractures would be a favorable sign and its abolition an unfavorable one."

Starr says: "Examine for an area of anæsthesia corresponding to the sensory nerve, along which the impulse is carried to the segment, or for a condition of paralysis with atrophy and reaction of degeneration in the muscles supplied by the nerve which conveys the impulse from

[1] Familiar Forms of Nervous Disease.
[2] Med.-Chir. Trans., 1890, vol lxxiii. p. 313.
[3] Ibid., p. 151.

the segment. If neither of them is found alone the segment is probably diseased. In crushed injuries the limbs are flaccid, the tendon reflexes abolished, and there is ankle clonus and rigidity."

In all cases the motor paralysis and anæsthesia will vary with the location and extent of the spinal lesion, but, as a rule, both are present to a greater or less degree. If, now, we have a complete motor and sensory paraplegia below the distribution of the nerves arising in the segment above that involved in the injury, with paralysis of the rectum and bladder, abolition of the reflexes whose centres are below the level of the injury, with rapid atrophy of the muscles, which are also flabby and relaxed, and which give the reaction of degeneration, the probabilities are that there is a total destruction of the cord. If the reflexes are present and controlled or exaggerated ; if the atrophy is gradual and not very great, due to lack of muscular exercise, even though there is more or less trophic disturbance, anæsthesia and paralysis, and the reaction to the electric current is arrested in the paralyzed areas, the probabilities are that there is compression, rather than destruction, of the cord.

The methods of operating have varied with different surgeons. Cline, in the first case, made two parallel incisions on either side of the spinous processes, and then, having retracted the muscles, removed the spines before attempting to cut through the arch. Horsley makes a similar use of the double incision and then makes a cut at right angles to the first through the lumbar aponeurosis and muscles. This subcutaneous incision is placed about the centre of the field of operation and is employed to increase the retraction of the flaps. Bullard and Burrell and Dawbarn have employed an H incision, placing the two arms of the H in the vertebral grooves perpendicular to an incision carried across the median line at the point of greatest deformity. Demons used a V-shaped incision, the arms of the V passing on either side of the vertebral column. Morris employs a crucial incision, but the majority of the operators have employed the two parallel incisions. Abbe uses a single incision on one side and close to the spinous processes, cutting them free from the laminæ and leaving them attached to one of the flaps. I prefer this method of operating because it occupies less time, causes less hemorrhage, and can be completed without disturbing the interspinous ligaments. The hemorrhage must be a matter of careful consideration, since it is for a few minutes usually copious and very general. The incision should be carried at once and very rapidly down to the laminæ, and then the wound should be packed firmly for a minute or two. This will arrest the bleeding in great part and will enable the operator to see and ligate any arterial branches that may continue to spurt. The flap on the side of the spinous processes with the incision can then be dissected away from the arch until the articular and transverse processes are in full view. The spinous processes can then be cut away at their bases with Liston's forceps, and the flap on the opposite side, including the spinous processes, can be dissected away in the same manner as the first.

The methods of removing the laminæ have differed very materially. Bullard and Burrell used a surgical engine, which, with the usual facility of most of these labor-saving inventions in surgery, broke down at the critical moment, and the removal was completed by means of an osteotome. The trephine and Hey's saw are also used. The reason given for the employment of these devices is that buttons of bone can be preserved and replaced. In Page's case of Pott's disease, where the mallet and chisel were employed, every blow of the mallet caused involuntary muscular twitchings in the limbs, and consequently may have been the cause of the increased symptoms exhibited by the patient after the operation. So far as the replacing of the bone is concerned, I do not think it has any important bearing on the subsequent course of the case. In fact, so far, only two cases—Thompson's and McBurney's, unless we also include Page's—in which the tubercular disease in the body of the vertebra was not removed, have required the application of any apparatus to strengthen the spine. In the latter the site of the operation is reported to have filled in with bone. It seems to me much more satisfactory, both as regards time and the saving of concussion, to employ the rongeur forceps to remove the laminæ; and for this purpose several different pairs should be provided, a straight pair being especially useful. It is best in every case where the cause ot the compression is not found to be extra-dural, to open the membranes and ascertain if there is any difficulty between them and the cord. When this is done, Mr. Horsley says, "the anæsthesia should be very profound, because the dura is extremely sensitive, and any motion at this time might prove fatal to the operation." There can be no doubt but that the anæsthesia should be complete. The danger of causing involuntary muscular action has been proven, by Abbe's case of nerve-section, where the dura was opened without any anæsthetic, to be due rather to irritation of the posterior columns of the cord than to the sensitiveness of the dura.

When the membranes are opened they should be closed very carefully by means of fine catgut. Some operators have not stitched the dura, but in view of the irritating qualities of the cerebro-spinal fluid this precaution to prevent a fistula should be taken.

Care should be had to ascertain at the time of the operation that the cause of the compression has been found and removed, and for this reason I believe it is best to explore the canal above and below the opening with a probe, being careful not to injure the dura. It may be best to remove more laminæ in some cases, in order that one may be convinced that this end has been attained. In three cases—in one of Bridden's and in Demons' and in Kraske's—of Pott's disease, the compression was found at the autopsy to have been under other laminæ than those resected.

Chipault advocates the omission of a drainage-tube in every case where the dura has been opened, but I prefer even in these cases to drain away the considerable quantities of serous fluid that are exuded during the first few hours, placing a suture in position, however, to bring together the portions of the flap separated by the tube when it is removed. Deep and superficial sutures should be used in approximating the flaps.

In case a sinus occurs, or it is necessary to continue the use of the drainage-tube, and there is an escape of cerebro-spinal fluid, the skin about the orifice should be kept greased to prevent the contact of the escaping fluid, for it has been observed in every case where this fluid has drained away for any period it has caused excoriation of the skin.

In operating in the cervical region, particularly about or above the level of the fourth vertebra, care should be exercised not to puncture the cord. In Deaver's[1] case this precaution was not observed, and the patient died from inhibition of the phrenic nerve.

Eve[2] says that the operation, if not almost impracticable, is certainly one of the most difficult in surgery, but this is not borne out by present experience. The operation in itself is neither tedious nor difficult.

THE ETIOLOGY OF EMPYEMA IN CHILDREN:

AN EXPERIMENTAL AND CLINICAL STUDY.

By Henry Koplik, M.D.,

ATTENDING PHYSICIAN FOR DISEASES OF WOMEN AND CHILDREN TO THE EASTERN DISPENSARY, NEW YORK.

THE first aspiration and exploratory puncture of the pleural cavity was performed by Bowditch, the American physiologist, and from this bold innovation upon the former methods in vogue may be traced our decided advances in the treatment and proper understanding clinically of the pathological conditions of the pleura. In his address before the Tenth International Medical Congress, Sir Joseph Lister in speaking upon empyema said: "There are few more beautiful things in antiseptic

---

[1] Internat. Journ. Med. Sci., Dec., 1888.   [2] Ashhurst, Int. Ency. Surgery.

surgery, as contrasted with the results of former practice, than to see the abundant purulent contents of the pleural cavity give place at once to a serous effusion, rapidly diminishing from day to day." Surgery has therefore been in advance of pathology, and it was reserved to a very recent period for some enlightenment upon the nature of empyema and pleurisy to appear, and supplement the surgical advance in this department of medical learning.

This advance has been made through the avenues of modern bacteriological methods. I am certain that with the light thus thrown upon the nature of empyema in the adult, the diagnosis and understanding of this disease will have received incalculable aid, and the future treatment in both surgical and medical directions will be based upon more certain data than hitherto. I think we have passed that stage which justifies the general grouping of all suppurating pleural processes as empyema without modifying this term so as to point out at once the etiology. If the above is true of the adult, we would naturally expect the same phase of this question when applied to children. Though we have many of us taken for granted that what was true of the adult might be equally so of the infant and child, it has been the object of the author of this paper to make such an inquiry in exact channels, as had been done by others concerning the adult. The literature upon the etiology of empyema in the adult is not so very extensive, if we regard those works only which are really systematic, and therefore of satisfactory merit. The first complete contribution, an attempt to formulate the different varieties of empyema from a bacteriological standpoint, was that of A. Fränkel.[1] This paper contains the result of a series of studies extending back as far as 1886. The author divides empyema into the following groups:

Those in which the etiology is still a matter of speculation. In these we cannot point to anything positive, because both the clinical history and bacterioscopic examination of the purulent exudate give no support to any definite theory. In these cases the exudate upon examination fails to yield anything but a microörganism which is found in processes of diverse nature in the body. From the chain-coccus, or streptococcus pyogenes, we could with much justice presuppose an antecedent pneumonia; we might follow this chain-coccus in its migrations through the lymph-channels of the pulmonary pleura; but, on the other hand, there are authors who, like Fraentzel, believe in the occurrence of a " pleuritis acutissima." Unfortunately, this disease described by Fraentzel is of most rare occurrence and doubtful etiology. Traumatism or cold have been invoked in these cases as predisposing causes which allow such microörganisms as streptococci to act upon the economy by reducing its resistant vitality. We must here presuppose the continued presence of

---

[1] " Ueber die bakterioscopische Untersuchung eitrige Ergüsse,'' Charité Annalen, 1888, p. 147.

microörganisms in the subpleural tissue, even in subjects who clinically cannot be said to be suffering from any active disease. In the course of investigations upon empyema, the question has arisen whether an effusion into the pleural cavity might from the very onset be purulent; those of experience answer in the affirmative. In children especially we are apt to think that an effusion is serous, or rather non-purulent, if the exploratory needle gives what to the eye appears a clear, not turbid fluid. The inquiries into the pathology of these cases show that those acute cases showing a serous exudate which subsequently becomes purulent are really at the time purulent (from the beginning, in the most modern acceptation). To return to our first premise, though Weichselbaum has distinctly shown, in lobar and lobular pneumonia of the adult, that the streptococcus pyogenes and also the staphylococcus are present as so-called mixed infections, yet when we come to consider the exclusive presence in the exudate of empyema of these microörganisms there is a gap to be explained which, as far as we know, has not yet been clearly elucidated.

In another group of cases Fränkel found the exclusive presence of the pneumococcus or diplococcus pneumoniæ; this microörganism was found in pure culture in the exudate derived from the pleural cavity. The pus was of a thick, adhesive character, and the cases of this group are classed as post-pneumonic or concomitant with pneumonia (lobar pneumonia). Fränkel maintains that in these cases suppuration is maintained in the presence of a closed pleural cavity by the presence of bloodvessels with the existence of a different nutritive medium than in the artificial structures.

The third group of empyemas are those whose nature is tubercular. In all these cases he could not establish the presence of tubercle bacilli, for some baffled all the aids to diagnosis of this microörganism, both in plain stain, culture, and experiment. Fränkel has come to the conclusion that the absence of any result as far as stain and culture were concerned, in the study of exudates, pointed very strongly toward a tubercular element in the etiology of the empyema. Garré and Rosenbach in experimenting with the pus of cold abscesses had a similar result. Fränkel found tubercle bacilli by staining methods in only one case of four investigated ; in the others the results were negative.

There is, according to this author, a fourth group of cases, in which we can find a focus of infection situated outside of the pleural cavity. He had two such cases, in both of which the chain-coccus was found, and one of which followed a perforating peritonitis, the other a retro-pharyngeal abscess. The conclusions of this author relating to empyémas are that the presence of the chain-coccus or streptococci, or staphylococcus pyogenes is not diagnostic. The presence of the diplococcus pneumoniæ points to a preceding pneumonia or complicating pneumonia. An exudate which fails to yield any positive result either by stain or culture is in all probability tubercular.

Weichselbaum's name is also indissolubly connected with much good work in this field. He examined eleven cases of pleuritis.[1] Two of these cases were of a purulent and one of a sero-purulent nature, the remaining eight were serous. In the empyemas he found the streptococcus pneumoniæ, or what we may call streptococcus pyogenes, and in another case, which proved fatal, the diplococcus pneumoniæ was found. About this time, Fränkel published[2] two cases of empyema following pneumonia, in which he found the diplococcus pneumoniæ.

The above historical review would be incomplete without the mention of the important work of Ehrlich in the study of pleurisies.[3] He investigated by staining methods the bacterial character of fluids obtained from the pleural cavity in forty-five cases of pleurisy ; of these, nine were tubercular, twenty simple pleurisy, six carcinomatous, and nine empyemas of various kinds. Of nine tubercular cases in which the sputa of the patients contained tubercle bacilli this microörganism was found in only two. The negative result in the remaining seven does not by any means prove the absence of tuberculosis of the pleura.

The work upon empyema in children is, in contrast to what has been recorded of the adult, limited to a few scattered notices in the literature. The most important is found in the work of Rosenbach, who examined the exudate of a case of empyema and found the micrococcus tenuis (pyogenes), or what is now thought might have been the diplococcus pneumoniæ, present.

The recent articles of Von Ziemssen (" Vorträge ") and Liebermeister are simple literary *résumés* upon the subject.

ORIGINAL INVESTIGATION.—My own work upon empyema was framed upon the lines outlined in the above review. An attempt was made to see how far the results in children, from a bacteriological standpoint, would correspond to those attained in the adult, or whether they would differ. In June of last year, I reported in brief my results in twelve cases ; there are three additional cases to report, in one of which at least some interesting points will arise. The work done was upon material which at the time, for the most part, was in a hospital ward, evidently an advantage. The mode of bacterial study was in accord with what is practised by the Koch school of investigators. Some of my cases were taken from my dispensary class ; others from private practice or those of my friends. It being established both

---

[1] " Ueber die Etiologie der acuten Lungen- und Rippenfellentzündungen," Medizin. Jahrbücher, 1886, Heft 8, p. 483.

[2] Zeitschr. für klin. Med., 1886.

[3] Beiträge zur Ætiologie pleurit. Ergüsse," Charité Annalen, 1882, p. 207.

from the clinical history and physical signs that there was a probable existence of empyema, the chest of the patient was carefully cleansed with soap and water, and then with sublimate; the excess of antiseptic fluid having been removed, a clean and sterilized hypodermic needle was introduced into the chest. To avoid contamination, a new syringe was used for each case, for it is very difficult to be certain as to the cleanliness of a syringe which has been once used for pus. The ordinary hypodermic syringe was used after being cleansed with sublimate, alcohol and ether, and then sterilized distilled water. The needle was sterilized with heat in the dry oven at a temperature of 160 to 170° C., kept in a sterile test-tube and only put upon the syringe at the last moment. A specimen of the contents of the pleural cavity once withdrawn was placed in an empty sterilized test-tube and taken as soon as possible to the laboratory and examined. The examination included not only the study of the gross specimen, the preparation of crude pus upon cover-glasses in the ordinary way, and then stainings of the crude pus, but plates and cultures were made upon media to establish the bacteriological character of the fluids withdrawn. The media used for culture experiments were bouillons, gelatin, glycerin agar, agar-agar, Weichselbaum's agar;[1] blood-serum and potato plates were first made to obtain colonies, as also test-tubes prepared by rubbing the fluid to be examined upon the obliquely solidified media, as agar (Weichselbaum); and pure cultures were also obtained from the plates, and if growth occurred in the tubes, plates were made to test the purity of the growths. Re-inoculations upon other media were made; when pure cultures were obtained, these were injected into animals for experiment. The animals used were rabbits, guinea-pigs, rats and mice. The most uniform results were attained from the rabbit experiments. The microörganisms were taken from a pure culture from an agar tube and suspended in sterilized distilled water, or, mostly, a pure bouillon culture was directly injected. The injections upon animals and autopsies were performed with the ordinary precautions followed in the bacteriological laboratory.

The characters of the crude pus withdrawn from the various cases are of interest when considered in relation to one series of cases, namely, those in which the diplococcus pneumoniæ of Fränkel and Weichselbaum was present. In some of this set of cases, the pus seemed of a rather glutinous adhesive nature; it would adhere to the sides of the test-tube when the same was inclined; this pus was either creamy-white in color, or greenish, or greenish-yellow. In these cases the chest was sometimes filled with enormous clots of fibrin, which were expelled from the opening

---

[1] By Weichselbaum's agar is meant the agar recommended by this author, containing 1½ per cent. of agar, peptone, and grape sugar, with ½ per cent. of salt.

made by resection of the rib. The pus also in some cases separated in a serous and opaque greenish layer upon standing; in other cases, as in greenish pus, the same had no adhesiveness. I mention these facts, because Fränkel has pointed out the adhesive or glutinous nature of the pus withdrawn from the adult cases, and the same characters in similar cases were easily established in children. In none was a fœtid odor perceptible, either in the pus derived from the cases in which the diplococcus pneumoniæ was present, or in those in which the streptococcus or staphylococcus pyogenes was found. Primarily, none in the series I have examined were fetid. In two cases the pus became fetid after the chest had been opened, and these cases, both of diverse nature, I will attempt to explain later. In all cases the crude pus was spread upon cover-glasses and stains made both for tubercle bacilli, diplococcus pneumoniæ, and other microörganisms; care was taken to follow out a routine in each case by which tubercle bacilli (Ehrlich's stain) could be excluded. In those cases in which the capsule cocci were found by simple stains with methyl or gentian-violet, the resistance to Gram's discolorization was tested.

For the sake of simplicity, we can formulate results in the following manner: In the pus of the fourteen recorded cases, I found the following microörganisms:

> The streptococcus pyogenes.
> The staphylococcus pyogenes aureus.
> The diplococcus pneumoniæ (Fränkel and Weichselbaum).
> The tubercle bacillus (Koch).

In few of the cases did I find these microörganisms associated, but usually existing alone in a specimen of pus. The tubercle bacilli were found associated with the streptococcus, as I shall later explain. It was certainly striking, at least in my series of cases, that the organism found existed in the fluid withdrawn from the chest in so-called pure state. The pus was really equivalent to a pure culture of one of the microörganisms. It would be tiresome and of little value to go into detailed description of the staphylococcus pyogenes aureus and streptococcus pyogenes found in my cases, and it will suffice to say that they are in culture media, and when injected experimentally acted in a way exactly corresponding to all that is known of these microörganisms.

THE DIPLOCOCCUS PNEUMONIÆ (Fränkel and Weichselbaum).— When the pus from an empyema is rubbed upon the surface of an obliquely solidified tube of agar-agar of Weichselbaum, and placed in a temperature of 35° to 37° C., there appears within about six hours a thin, almost imperceptible coating very much like dew on the surface of the agar; within twenty-four hours this is more marked, though it is still very delicate and veil-like, and does not seem to grow vigorously. In the depth of the agar, if the same has been inoculated, there is a delicate veil-

like reticulum. If such a surface culture be examined after successive
re-inoculations, it is made up of very minute transparent punctate areas
or colonies; as a whole, the growth does not attract the eye by any particular hue. If a puncture culture, as it is called, is made on agar, the
area around the top of the puncture is very minute and scarcely perceptible. Colonies from pus sown upon agar-agar plates are at first so
small as to be discovered only by the aid of a lens; they never attain
a very large size, and are situated in the depth of the medium, and
inoculated by means of the platinum point only with the greatest difficulty. The reason of this seems to be that the microörganism is so
delicate that not enough adheres to the platinum tip to favor growth in
the test-tube. The colonies after forty-eight hours are round, granular,
with a darker centre, some of them, than periphery; they are of a
transparent very light grayish tint or straw color by transmitted light;
when the plate with colonies is held against a dark background, the
reflected impression is that the colonies have a whitish tint. Unless this
microörganism is transferred very early during the first few days to
other tubes, it stops at a certain point and ceases growing—in other
words, it may be lost. The colonies, especially in four or five days,
begin to die out, becoming fainter to the lens and taking on the color
more and more of the surrounding agar. The above applies to the
diplococcus in pure culture derived from pleuritic fluid. After inoculation into animals, the growth, though the same in all essentials, seems
to have attained a greater vigor, though even here, if not saved by
repeated re-inoculations upon media, it dies out quickly.

Gelatin.—In gelatin, at the ordinary room temperature, there is no
growth; at the temperature of 23° or 24° C. there is a very delicate
growth which never becomes vigorous; along the puncture there is a
granular minute beaded structure, but of the greatest delicacy, and the
gelatin is not fluidified.

Blood-serum.—The growth here is much the same as on agar-agar of
Weichselbaum, though the colonies making up the surface culture may
be said to be more grayish in tint, or slightly more perceptible than upon
the agar.

Bouillon.—Here there is first a general clouding of the medium, and
then a deposit of flocculi along the sides of the tube, and finally a small
deposit in the bottom of the test-tube, leaving the fluid or bouillon above
finally clear. When shaken, there is great turbidity and abundance of
fine flocculi.

Potato.—There is here no perceptible growth.

Ordinary agar.—It is certainly a waste of energy to attempt to cultivate the diplococcus successfully upon ordinary agar, for failure will be
the most frequent reward. In other words, much valuable time has

been wasted by others as by myself in making such attempts. The least variation in moisture or reaction will compromise the growth, so that I have worked mostly with the agar-agar of Weichselbaum, rather than with that made up by the old formula.

Glycerin agar—six per cent. to eight per cent.—did not seem to present any advantages. The growth was very slow and difficult of re-inoculation, and capricious.

Stainings.—The crude pus shows us the diplococcus with its capsule. I have had no difficulty in establishing the presence of the capsule coccus by means of the simple methyl-violet or gentian-violet and aniline water stain, taking care not to over-stain. If the specimen should have been over-stained, it can be easily decolorized (but this very lightly) with dilute alcohol. The pure culture shows the diplococcus from agar very beautifully, as oval or round diplococcus forms of apparently the size seen in the crude specimen without any capsule; the diplococci may be single or in chains of two or three pairs. By the Gram stain there are also seen both in the crude pus and crude culture some of the peculiar lancet-shaped forms; while I could find here and there a beautiful lancet form, there were many which upon analysis appeared peculiarly crenated, perhaps due to either unequal decolorization or overheating. The capsules in the crude specimens are decolorized by the Gram method, though the light decolorized zone of their presence may be seen by strong and favorable illumination in some cases.

THE STAPHYLOCOCCUS PYOGENES AUREUS which was met in these empyema cases could in no way be distinguished from the staphylococcus which I separated and cultivated for comparison from the ordinary furuncle of the skin. It reacted in the same manner in the various culture media. In the gelatin it grew at the ordinary room temperature along the puncture and had the same yellow-gray or straw-color beaded look. The gelatin, after the third or fourth day, became liquefied; this began at the top and proceeded along the puncture in length and breadth. After a time the liquefied gelatin showed the finely granular suspended colonies, and the sediment at the bottom of the liquefied gelatin took on the same orange-yellow color.

Agar-agar.—Upon obliquely solidified agar there was at a raised temperature a very vigorous growth on the surface, and in the depth, which, at first whitish-yellow, after a time assumed a rich orange-yellow tint; the surface of the growth was moist, and its edges sinuous and raised very perceptibly above the surface.

Potato.—The well-known orange-yellow moist growth was perceptible within twenty-four hours, increasing in vigor and luxuriance; it was at first golden-yellow, then deeper orange-yellow, having the peculiar odor of the ordinary culture of staphylococcus.

THE STREPTOCOCCUS which I have isolated from cases of empyema reacts in media exactly similarly to the ordinary streptococcus pyogenes. In agar-agar plates the colonies remain small but some large, some irregularly round, others oval of a brownish-olive tint and granular appearance. In punctures the finely beaded dots and zone surrounding the top of the puncture exhibit no tendency to spread to any extent; on the surface of obliquely solidified agar a pearly-gray growth is seen (Weichselbaum's agar) made up of drop-like masses in the depth; the same beaded appearance in either a band or puncture that is seen in ordinary agar.

Gelatin.—Small finely granular colonies, at first straw-tint and sharply round, later more brownish with an olive tendency. At border, through gelatin, they appear straw-color, on surface of gelatin they have a distinct cupola (raised); they grow in depths also. In punctures, finely granular, no liquefaction of gelatin.

Bouillon.—In twenty-four hours we have a cloudy appearance, and deposit of masses on sides of test-tube, finely granular in the centre. Stainings show exquisite chains.

Potato.—Nothing characteristic or perceptible.

EXPERIMENTAL.—The experimental part of my work was laid out upon very simple lines, and is intended merely to add confirmatory evidence upon the nature of the microörganisms which I have isolated from the various cases of empyema reported. The results attained, it will be seen, are almost identical with those obtained by other observers (Fränkel and Weichselbaum).

My method consisted first, in isolating microörganisms so as to obtain a pure culture of each variety, and then injecting this pure culture into the animal to be experimented upon. The animals used were mostly rabbits, but a few scattering experiments were performed with guinea-pigs, rats, and mice. The injections were made with sterilized hypodermic needles underneath the skin and into the pleural cavity or lung. There were no inhalation experiments. A pure culture of any microörganism having been injected into the animal, the same was observed, and if the animal survived, it was, after a sufficient period had elapsed, killed and pathological effects noted. If the animal died from the effects, the blood, and the pleuritic, pericardial and peritoneal fluids were examined, and the nature of the contained microörganisms established in exactly the same manner as had been done with the original pus obtained from the empyema. Re-injections of these pure cultures from animals were made, as also injection of pleuritic and peritoneal fluids from animal to animal. Pus in crude state from empyemas was also injected into animals, and the microörganisms cultivated from the blood and fluids of such animals.

The most interesting series of experiments in their results were those performed with the pure cultures of the diplococcus pneumoniæ. In every case the isolated microörganism was injected into a set of animals, and the results have been noted.   After the first effects of the injection had passed off (chest injections into pleura), the animal in some cases seemed to be as well as ever, but after a few days, varying in different cases, the animals in most cases died.   Death was, as a rule, preceded by a short period of dyspnœa, or again the animals may have appeared ill through the whole experimental life.   The autopsies revealed in most cases pleurisy single or double, even though injection was made into one side of the chest.   The lungs in no case were the seat of complete hepatization (pneumonia) lobar in distribution ; but in rabbits 1, 3, 6, 9, and 11 there was a condition of the lung not dissimilar to an engorgement in areas to smaller or greater extent.   In rabbit 6 this approached closest the type of hepatization in the upper lobe of the left lung.   Pericarditis was present in most and also very marked peritonitis.   Care was in all cases exerted to inject the fluid containing the microörganism just beneath the rib into the pleural space, though it was often impossible to say that it had not penetrated the lung ; at least care was taken that it should not do so.

In most of the cases the spleen was enlarged to palpably twice or thrice its original size.   Cultures made of the blood and pleuritic or pericardial fluids of such animals also yielded a uniformly certain growth of a diplococcus which in every way and reaction corresponded to the diplococcus pneumoniæ of Fränkel and Weichselbaum.   Its growth was at first quite vigorous on the Weichselbaum agar, but it died out and was soon lost if not re-inoculated, just as the original pure culture obtained from the empyema pus.   Animals injected with the pleuritic or peritoneal fluid of other animals that had died of injection of pneumococcus also died certainly and even rapidly.   The lung and spleen fluids (obtained by expression) with cover-glass stain also showed myriads of these diplococci.   By the injection of pure cultures of diplococcus underneath the skin, the results were not so certain, though in some the animals died with the above features.   The pus from empyemas known to contain nothing but diplococcus pneumoniæ also killed the animals with unfailing certainty ; cultures made from these animals revealed the diplococcus only, and injections of peritoneal fluids from these animals into others proved fatal with results showing pneumonia, pleuritis, pericarditis, and peritonitis, and in all the fluids of such animals, inclusive of the blood, the diplococcus was found.   In some cases the animals would seem to have had vitality enough to have resisted this organism, and completely recovered from the effects of their injections and consequent inflammatory disturbances.   Such animals were killed after a sufficient period had elapsed, and in most cases there could be seen adhesions of the pulmonary to the costal pleura, and adhesions of the pericardial surfaces.   Some guinea-pigs injected gave results much the same as those seen in rabbits.   In other cases the animals seemed to have successfully resisted the effects of the micro-organisms, for upon autopsy nothing was revealed that could be traced to any pathological process.

Experiments with the streptococcus which was isolated from the pus of the empyemas recorded in this paper, and which appears to be identical with the streptococcus pyogenes, though positive in some features were yet not so distinctive. The results seemed to vary, for while in some cases streptococci did not prove fatal, in another the effects seemed most virulent and rapidly lethal. In some, injection of streptococci into rabbits had no effect, the animals survived, and being killed after weeks had elapsed, absolutely nothing abnormal was found. In other cases streptococci (from the same empyema) caused marked disturbances ; the animal appeared quite ill, but recovered and was for weeks apparently in good health ; when killed, a few pleuritic adhesions only were found.

In other cases, an injection of a pure bouillon culture of streptococci, notably in rabbit 15, taken from Case XI., caused the death of the animal in two days, and autopsy revealed nothing but an enormous spleen (the largest I have seen in my experiments) with kidneys palpably swollen ; cultures of the blood revealed streptococci. Thus, in this case, we have the symptoms of a pure septic effect, a septicæmia without inflammatory lesions. Again, this same bouillon culture, which was pure in every way and repeatedly tested as to purity by plate methods, was injected at the same time into another animal in the same amounts, though not in the same manner, and there resulted the unusually virulent effects seen in rabbit 16, in which small metastatic abscesses appeared in different organs of the body, and general jaundice. The spleen also was notably enlarged. The results, though corresponding in certain ways, do not give anything not characteristic of streptococci isolated from other inflammatory processes in the body, and the experiments upon rabbits 15 and 16 agree closely with what is recorded of experiments made with streptococci pyogenes isolated from cases of pyæmia, and notably that of the kind recorded by Baumgarten.

I did not make any experiments with staphylococci isolated in my cases, the reactions of the microörganisms being so familiar in every laboratory. It appeared to me sufficient to establish its biological identity.

The experiments with the pus obtained from the cases of tuberculous empyema were negative. The pus was contaminated at first with streptococcus pyogenes and later with putrefactive microörganisms, and this clouded the reliability of the experiments. Injections into the eyes and pleuræ of animals gave no results that were of scientific value.

(To be continued.)

THE TREATMENT OF ERYSIPELAS.

A PERSONAL EXPERIENCE IN FIFTY CASES.

By CHARLES W. ALLEN, M.D.,

SURGEON TO CHARITY HOSPITAL, NEW YORK

I HAVE prepared for consideration four series of tabulated cases : No. 1 being the cases admitted to Charity Hospital in 1888; No. 2, those in 1889; No. 3, those received up to June 1, 1890; and No. 4, the cases treated by myself outside the hospital. For the opportunity of observing cases in the wards, and for the privilege of publishing them, I am indebted to my colleagues of the surgical staff of the hospital.

The cases in the hospital tables for the two and a half years number 419, and my own cases since January 1, 1889, 47 ; making a total of 466 cases available for study.

While not bearing directly upon the question of treatment, I may be pardoned if I speak of some points made prominent in the tables before me. Thus of the 300 cases which were received at the hospital during 1888–89, the greater number by far occurred in the winter and spring months, as follows :

December	.	. 18	June	. .	. 13
January .	.	. 28	July .	. .	. 4
February	.	. 49	August	. .	. 8
March	.	. 37	September	.	. 12
April	.	. 64	October .	.	. 11
May	.	. 47	November	.	. 9
Total .	.	. 243	As against	.	. 57

There is no doubt that more patients seek hospital treatment during the cold and damp seasons than during the pleasant months ; still, there must be something beside this fact to account for the marked increase of the one over the other season, because the same thing is found in private. practice, though in a less marked degree. My experience in town practice corresponds, in a great measure, with the showing of the hospital tables, and I find that the number of cases by months was as follows :

December .	.	. 2	June .	. .	. 6
January .	.	. 7	July .	. .	. 0
February .	.	. 9	August	. .	. 2
March	.	. 5	September .	.	. 1
April	.	. 3	October	.	. 2
May	.	. 8	November .	.	. 2
Total .	.	. 34	As against	.	. 13

This demonstration of the greater prevalence of erysipelas in New York during the cold and moist seasons of the year agrees with the results obtained by the majority of investigators who have given attention to the subject in other countries. Carl Haller's statistics, based upon ten years' study of erysipelas at the Vienna Hospital, show the greatest number of cases in April, May, October, and November. Kaposi's observations, carried out over a period of two years and published in 1887, show the largest numbers in March, May, November, and December of one year, and January, February, April, May, and December of the other.

To quote a recent observer, Linden, of Finland, whose study of the question extended over a period of eight years and embraced over 5000 cases, found 27.1 per cent. in the winter, and 20.4 per cent. in the summer months for Stockholm, and 29.2 per cent. in winter with only 18.8 per cent. in summer for Helsingsfors: an appreciable difference, though not so marked as that shown in the Charity Hospital record.

The most plausible explanation seems to be the sudden and decided variations in the temperature and moisture of the atmosphere in these seasons, but whether these factors influence the outbreak of the disease by weakening the patient's powers of resistance to the erysipelas coccus or by favoring an increased production or increased activity of the microörganisms outside of the human body is a question which must remain for future solution.

The relative frequency of facial erysipelas is another point made prominent in my tables. Thus of the 419 cases at Charity Hospital 267 were of the facial variety, or 63.7 per cent.

It is quite remarkable to note that of the 531 cases in Kaposi's statistics 336 were facial, or 63.27 per cent., almost an identical percentage.

The table of my personal cases shows, out of a total of 47 cases, 24 instances of facial erysipelas, or about 50 per cent. Of these 18 were so-called genuine facial cases, and 4 were consecutive to trauma or skin disease. Erysipelas of the extremities gives 23 cases, 19 of which followed trauma or skin lesions. There were no deaths from the facial erysipelas, and only 3 from other forms, or 6.4 per cent. The deaths all occurred in infants; one at five months following varicella, and the two others at three weeks of age respectively, both the result of ritual circumcision done in a bungling manner. Forty-two cases were cured after an average length of treatment or duration of the erysipelatous process of 7.57 days. Two cases passed from observation.

The tables of the Charity Hospital cases show 21 deaths, or 5 per cent., and in the 267 instances of facial erysipelas, 10 deaths, or 3.7 per cent. The average stay in hospital for 56 cases in 1888 was 21 days; for 190 cases in 1889 was 24.3 days; for 116 cases in 1890 was 20.4 days, or a general average of 22 days. Having digressed to this extent, I will now briefly outline the various methods of treatment which I have employed, first, however, giving the course of treatment which has been applied in the Charity Hospital cases.

1. In idiopathic facial erysipelas, as well as in non-traumatic cases elsewhere located, a paint having the following composition is applied over the affected region:

R.—Tinct. benzoin. comp.　.　.　.　.　.　.　.　ʒij.
　　Collodion flex.　.　.　.　.　.　.　.　.　ʒj.
　　Glycerin.　.　.　.　.　.　.　.　.　ʒj.

Occasionally, acid. salicylic. ʒi has been added to the above. Internally, the tincture of the chloride of iron, 20 minims three times daily, is given in a routine manner to nearly all cases.

2. In consecutive cases, *i. e.*, of traumatic origin, where the inflammation is not deep-seated and there is not much tension, this protective and antiseptic paint is likewise employed, and a bichloride solution 1 : 5000 or 1 : 6000 is applied hot to the wound or raw surface. Iron is given as above in these cases.

3. In cases where there is much tension and the integument has been broken by bullæ or otherwise, hot bichloride 1 : 6000 is applied and several coats of the paint are used as a limiting strip above the affected part if upon the extremity, or surrounding it if practicable. The same dose of iron is likewise given in these cases.

The tables show that quinine enters largely into the treatment of the hospital cases, especially those in which a high temperature is present. Other drugs mentioned as being occasionally employed are calomel, digitalis, aconite, belladonna, antifebrin, antipyrine, and bromide for the delirium.

At times the above line of treatment has been deviated from by the trial of spirits of turpentine internally instead of iron, in dose of 10 drops three times daily. This appeared to do as well as the iron in some cases until about the third or fourth day of treatment, when it ceased to be tolerated by the stomach. Occasionally, too, iron has been omitted because it was thought to disagree in some way with the patient, but, as I have said, in the great majority of cases it was given as a matter of course.

Baths of a 2 per cent. solution of creolin have been tried, but without good results. Injections of iodoform in solution have been practised in some cases about the margin of patches with the idea of limiting the progress of the erysipelas, but no appreciable benefit has followed. Tincture of iodine used with the same object in view has resulted not more favorably.

Although my belief is that erysipelas is a disease of more or less definite course, tending, when uncomplicated, to terminate favorably— excepting in the very young, when death almost invariably results—still I believe that by judicious treatment this course can be very materially lessened and in some cases brought to an abrupt termination; and for this reason I cannot agree with those who put faith in no treatment at all, and argue that because erysipelas is one of the diseases in which so great a number of diverse drugs and methods have been advocated, that none is good; nor yet can I accept the dictum of those who take a *laisser aller* view of the matter, thinking that the cases will do well enough if left to themselves.

Since Fehleisen's discovery of the streptococcus erysipelatus and the demonstrations of Hueter and others, which go to show that it is truly an infectious disease in all probability due to the presence and multiplication in the skin and subcutaneous tissues of a micrococcus, methods of treatment have in a measure changed, and the therapy of to-day is based largely upon antiseptic, anti-bacterial, mechanical and surgical procedures.

I presume that all have accepted Fehleisen's experiments with pure cultures in 1882 and the subsequent investigations of others as showing the contagious nature of the disease, and I believe that the future treatment of erysipelas must, in a measure at least, conform to bacteriological findings. Thus it has been found that the streptococcus grows more rapidly in parts well supplied with oxygen, and nothing seems to me more rational than to endeavor in treatment to shut off this supply so far as possible.

In twenty-two of my cases I have endeavored to accomplish this purpose by the application of an occlusive dressing having collodion as a base. In nineteen of them I have incorporated with the collodion ichthyol, and in three cases aristol. In four instances I have employed white-lead paint, as recommended by Lewis for the same purpose; in two I have used an ichthyol ointment; in two a resorcin ointment; in five a strong solution of permanganate of potassium; in seven a solution of the hyposulphite of sodium; in one case a bichloride solution; in one lead and opium; in one a saturated solution of boric acid; and in one the application of the tincture of the chloride of iron. In two instances I have performed scarification, and in two others have applied a tight adhesive strip above the affected area upon an extremity.

I will take up the more interesting cases one by one and speak of the treatment, and its effects as we proceed. First for the "genuine" facial cases.

CASE I.—Female, aged eighteen years. Erysipelas of face, involving first one side and spreading to the other, with formation of large bullæ.

Treatment.—Internal: Tr. ferri chlor. m xx every three hours. External: The same locally applied.

Result.—Recovery at end of ten days. The application of iron is not an agreeable dressing, and as it appeared to do no good I have not since tried it.

Case II.—Female, aged forty-five years. Erysipelas involving whole face and subsequently the scalp.

Treatment.—White-lead paint to cover the whole face. When extension took place to the scalp the hair was cut short and the whole scalp painted. The general symptoms were very severe, and convalescence was not established until the twenty-third day. The paint was removed slowly and with difficulty from the scalp, and I would not advise its application to hairy parts.

In this case the use of the paint did not make a very favorable impression upon me, though the patient and friends appeared well enough satisfied with the result.

Case III.—Male, aged thirty-four years. Erysipelas of one side of face. White-lead paint. Improvement till seventh day, when extension took place to opposite side of face and patient entered hospital. I saw patient about a week later, when recovery had taken place.

Case IV.—Male, aged fifty-eight years. Treated with a very weak solution of hyposulphite of soda (ʒij to Oj) and internal symptomatic remedies (antipyrine, bromide). He was convalescent on the eighth day.

Case VI.—Male, aged fifty years. Erysipelas of face. The same external treatment and iron internally (gtt. x every hour part of the time). The scalp became involved and the disease ran its course in fifteen days. Decided alopecia followed.

Case VII.—Male, aged fifty-three years. Erysipelas began simultaneously in both ears and extended to the right side of the face. Same external applications. Although extension to cheeks, forehead, and scalp occurred, and large bullæ formed, after seven days the patient was practically well.

Case VIII.—Female, aged forty-five years. Had previously suffered from erysipelas of face seventeen years before. Present attack began after exposure to cold and wet. After two days of hyposulphite solution locally, iron was given internally. On the seventh day desquamation had begun, there was no longer any fever, and convalescence was rapid.

Case X.—Female, aged thirty-seven years. Whole face involved and great headache, not relieved by a drachm of antipyrine in divided doses. Great delirium at night. Here I used resorcin ointment in strength of ʒj to ʒj for the face, and a wash of ʒj to Oj for the scalp. Convalescence after eighth day, when wine and iron were given. The daughter of this patient had been a daily visitor at the house of Case VI., often being in patient's room during his illness, and probably in some unknown way brought the cocci home to her mother.

Case XIX.—Male, aged eleven years. Erysipelas began at back of neck and extended over scalp. A younger brother of this patient was sick in the same room with migratory erysipelas of the body and extremities (Case XVIII. of table).

Treatment.—Ichthyol ointment ʒij to ʒj. In three days the boy was entirely well.

Case XXIX.—Female, aged forty-four years. Erysipelas of a week's duration, starting from a lachrymal fistula. Involvement of both cheeks and ears and severe general symptoms.

Treatment.—Ichthyol ointment, ꝫij to ʒj. Antipyrine and whiskey internally.

Result.—Erysipelas at a standstill in two days. Recurrence after four days which lasted for five days, after which patient remained well.

Case XXX.—Male, aged twenty-three years. Patient has rosacea. The day before my visit erysipelas had begun upon the left cheek. I painted the area over with a solution of permanganate of potassium, gr. xx. to ʒj. This had the effect of aborting the process within two or three days. Some three days later, however, the opposite cheek became affected, and under the same external treatment was well in four days without having spread to scalp or ear.

Case XXXI.—Male, aged twenty-three years, son of Case No. VIII., which I attended in the same room one year ago. Three days before my visit there had been a decided chill, followed on the next day by a bright-red spot upon the bridge of the nose. There had been no injury or preceding lesion upon the face. When I saw the patient both cheeks, the lower eyelids, and the middle of the forehead half way to the margin of the hair were involved, and extension to the upper lids was just beginning. On the left side the redness extended quite to the ear, while on the right there was an inch and a half of apparently unaffected skin intervening. The usual general symptoms were present. This appeared to me a most suitable case for treatment by scarification. Securing the patient's consent, I placed a circle of criss-cross cuts about the patch upon the forehead midway between its margin and the hair line, extending them down over the side of the forehead and between the border of the erysipelas on tne cheek and the right ear. As the disease had already reached as far as the left ear, no cuts were made on this side. I also laid a series of quadrilateral cuts just at the lower margin of the patch on a line with the angle of the mouth upon the right side, the cuts being made equally in the diseased and sound skin, according to the Riedel method, not over half to three-quarters of an inch in length, but quite close together.

Permanganate of potassium, gr. xxx to ʒj, was now applied over the whole surface, including the scarified portion. By the following day the disease had spread beyond the barrier, for about an inch upon the forehead, slightly beyond it on the right side as far as the ear, and not at all in a downward direction either upon the scarified or non scarified side. Neither ear as yet involved. Bullæ over cheeks and forehead. Redness and swelling diminished in region of nose and lower lids. The following day both ears swelled and were included in the painting with permanganate. Two days later there was no pain or tenderness, the face appeared well, appetite good, tongue clearing, bowels regular. The next day the permanganate-blackened crusts were peeling off, and patient regarded himself as well and I so regarded him. No internal treatment had been used.

Case XXXII.—Female, aged thirty-two years. (Wife of Case XXIV., who had twelve days before recovered from an erysipelas of the leg and thigh.) Chill on February 7th, erysipelas beginning in centre of left cheek February 8th and extending by February 11th to the whole face, causing closure of both eyes and almost occluding the nares.

Treatment.—Internally. Whiskey and antipyrine; locally, permanganate of potassium, gr. xxx to ʒj.

On the 26th the erysipelas was well, after having extended over the entire scalp.

CASE XXXIV.—Female, aged twenty years. Patient has had two previous attacks; last one a year ago in same room. First seen March 26th, with history pointing to primary erysipelas of the larynx two weeks before. Aphonia still present.

The skin erysipelas began three days previously upon the bridge of the nose, and now involves the whole face and scalp. Eyes cannot be opened, delirium pronounced. Temperature 104° +. Had been treated. Ordered hair cut short, ice-bag to scalp, stimulants at frequent intervals, antipyrine to reduce the temperature. Locally, ichthyol collodion ʒij to ʒj (ichthyol ʒij, ether ʒj, collodion ʒj).

Next day, February 27th, great improvement. Menses occurred. No headache or delirium, less fever. Eyes can be slightly opened. Scalp covered with a 1 : 3000 bichloride wash. Iron internally. Four days later bullæ on face and scalp had dried into crusts and patient was up.

A month later patient came to me with a stye on the right upper lid, and six days later with a second one, and upon the cheek below was an erythematous spot strongly suggestive of a return of the erysipelas. I incised the styes, washed out with a bichloride solution, and prescribed a zinc oxide ointment for the erythematous blush, under which it entirely disappeared. Three days later, however, a bright-red, tender spot appeared just in front of the ear and upon the cheek on the left side. I now ordered to be applied twice daily a solution of permanganate, gr. xxx to ʒj. By the following day the whole face was again covered by erysipelas and the eyes closed by swelling. There was some pain from the strong permanganate, so I substituted a 1 : 1000 solution of same to be applied hot. Three days later patient was up, the face free from swelling and beginning to desquamate. Patient remained well for three days, when a recurrence took place in one cheek. Ichthyol ʒj to water ʒj was applied, and iron was given in 15-drop doses every three hours. In two days symptoms were all absent, and no further recurrence took place.

CASE XXXV. occurred in a German woman, aged sixty-eight years, who had a hemiplegia of six years' standing, and was otherwise dehilitated. Whole face and scalp were affected and there were severe general symptoms. Low muttering delirium day and night; dry, glazed tongue, sordes, etc.

Locally, permanganate gr. x to ʒj, abundant supply of alcohol, and iron ♏xx every three hours.

Thirteen days later patient was up attending to household duties. Fifteen days subsequent to this date a recurrence took place, but under the same treatment she was entirely well in four days.

CASE XXXIX.—A pregnant woman, aged thirty-seven years, had four weeks previously recovered from an erysipelas of the face treated with lead and opium wash, under the care of another physician. I saw patient the day after a recurrence had taken place, and ordered ichthyol collodion and iron ♏xv every two hours. Case terminated favorably six days later.

CASE XL.—Female, aged twenty-five years. Erysipelas of whole upper portion of face, and eyes nearly closed. Treatment by ichthyol collodion ʒj to ʒj. Cure in three days.

CASE XLIII.—Female, aged seventeen years. Patient had just recovered from a tonsillitis. Erysipelas of left cheek, treated with ichthyol collodion and entirely well in three days, without extending.

Six other cases of facial erysipelas were subsequent to trauma or skin diseases, but presented all the features of the other cases. One started in an unhealed varicella pustule upon the ear of a girl of seven years and spread to the face and scalp. It was treated with ichthyol collodion and was well in five days. Another developed upon a scalp the seat of an impetigo, and was well under the same treatment in four days.

CASE XLI.—Female, aged twenty-three years. Six days after a scalp wound, in which several stitches were taken, erysipelas began upon the opposite side of the scalp at some distance from the wound and extended down over the forehead and cheek. I cleansed the wound, which was still discharging pus, and dressed it with aristol powder. To the erysipelas of the scalp I applied a 10 per cent. solution of ichthyol in water, and to the face ichthyol in collodion. In eight days patient was entirely well and wound had healed. At no time had there been any evidence of erysipelas very near the wound, although both sides of the face became affected.

CASE XLIV.—Female, aged sixty years, who had the most extensive gummous ulceration of the entire scalp which I have ever seen. There was an open ulcer the size of a half-dollar just within the hair line, and it was undoubtedly through this that inoculation took place. The whole face and both ears participated in the erysipelatous process, but the scalp remained free.

Treatment.—Solution of aristol in collodion, 5 per cent., and aristol powder freely applied to the open ulcers upon the scalp. The erysipelas was well upon the eighth day, when I made my last visit.

This case of neglected and untreated syphilis subsequently showed most rapid improvement under antisyphilitic remedies, with aristol applied locally to the ulcers.

CASE XVII.—Female, aged twenty-six years. Erysipelas of hand and arm. The special interest in the case is that the patient is the subject of marked elephantiasis of the legs, the right being much enlarged. Until this attack, it was not known that the upper extremity was affected with elephantiasis as I subsequently found it to be. There have been two previous attacks of erysipelas of the legs. I saw patient the day after erysipelas had begun in the hand, and painted the hand and arm with white-lead paint, and ordered some anodyne and antipyretic remedies. The heat and pain were so great in the night that the paint was removed and ice-cold cloths applied by the advice of another. These proved so soothing that the patient placed her hand upon the cake of ice which was kept at the bedside to cool the cloths, and went to sleep. At my next visit the fingers were icy cold, insensible, and presented a bluish, frozen appearance. I refused to give patient further advice excepting that she enter the hospital. This she did, and there had removed the distal phalanges of three fingers and the thumb.

CASE XXXVI. refers to this same patient. About a year after the unfortunate occurrence above narrated, I was called to attend her for an erysipelas of the left leg and foot, which had begun two days before in the region of the knee and had rapidly extended to the foot. The leg appeared enormously enlarged in consequence of the elephantiasis from which she suffered. I at once painted the whole area with ichthyol ʒij, ether ʒj, collodion ʒj, and gave internally:

R.—Quin. sulph. . . . . ʒss.
    Tinct. fer. chlor. . . . . . . ʒij.
    Aq. dest. . . . . ad ʒij.—M.
S.—One drachm every two hours.

In four days the patient was well and out of bed.

These attacks of erysipelas in elephantiasis have not been looked upon by some dermatologists as identical with the true erysipelas, but rather regarded as a species of lymphangitis. I must say, however, that I cannot take this view of the case in point. The appearances and symptoms entirely resembled those of other cases of erysipelas of the extremities, and I never saw a more typical instance of the disease than that presented by this patient's hand and arm the year before. There was in the case of the hand, as in that of the leg, marked striæ and cords of lymphangitic inflammation extending to the glands in the axilla and groin, attended with great tenderness and pain; but the same thing is often observed in ordinary erysipelas of the extremities without elephantiasis. This was true of Case XXIV. An erysipelas of the leg in a man aged forty-five years, not attributable to trauma, was attended with very decided lymphatic involvement causing painful red cords to extend from the patch to the groin, where the glands became very greatly enlarged. The usual ichthyol paint was applied over the whole extent of inflamed tissue in this case as well, and the iron and quinine mixture above mentioned was given internally. Patient was well in six days, though gland in groin remained tender for some days afterward.

As illustrating in a graphic manner the identity of this form of erysipelas and genuine facial erysipelas, the wife of this patient, who had carefully nursed him during his illness, was taken down with facial erysipelas twelve days after the latter's recovery, and hers is Case No. XXXII. of the present report and has already been referred to under the non-traumatic series of cases. One case developed from vaccination in a child of ten months, and four started in a varicella lesion.

One of these (Case XXVIII.), in a five-months' girl baby, proved fatal on the thirteenth day of the disease and five days after I first saw it. This was one of the cases in which I employed scarification. The erysipelas, which had begun in a varicella pustule upon the leg eight days before, had now extended up the back to the shoulders, over the thorax in front, to the ankle on the left side, and to below the knee on the right. The prognosis was most unfavorable, but I thought scarification offered a chance of checking the upward spreading. I made crossed incisions deep enough to draw blood about an inch above the margin of disease, according to Lauenstein's method, entirely surrounding the

chest. On the right leg I made the incisions just in the border, extending equally into the patch and the healthy skin. On the opposite leg the same was done just above the ankle. The whole was then washed with a bichloride solution 1 : 1000, and this was also used as a dressing for the whole affected area. By the following day the margin of redness had extended slightly beyond the scarification upon both legs. On the right side of the chest it had gone about half an inch beyond both behind and in front, but on the left side the erysipelas had stopped exactly at the boundary line. General appearance of child improved. Brandy in frequent doses.

On the following day child began to cough and was very restless and weak, with faint moaning cry. Left leg and genital region much swollen and œdematous. No further extension beyond the scarified barriers excepting upon the right side of thorax, where the pink line has advanced about half an inch. The physician who had attended the child during the first days of its illness now again took charge of the case, which terminated fatally three days later.

CASE XXVII.—Brother of last case, aged one and a half years. Varicella had begun at same time fourteen days before, and erysipelas had shown itself coincidentally in both children eight days before I saw them. Here the dorsum of the foot was first affected in the neighborhood of a varicella lesion. Great prostration, complete anorexia, very weak pulse. Treatment up to this time had been iron internally and cold-water dressings. Ordered iron continued and brandy in frequent doses. Milk, etc. The affected areas and healthy skin beyond were thickly covered with ichthyol collodion.

Next day, no extension, slight improvement in general symptoms. Following day, extension to scrotum and pubic region, with great swelling. Ichthyol continued to the whole.

For three days both cases were in care of another physician. I now resumed charge and continued the ichthyol locally to leg, scrotum, and penis, which were enormously enlarged. One week later the boy was convalescent.

CASE XXXVIII.—Male, aged four months. Erysipelas of right leg and thigh, beginning in a varicella pock and rapidly extending. Patient had lived till recently with the grandmother, whom I had treated the preceeding year for a severe erysipelas of the face (Case No. II.).

Treatment.—Ichthyol collodion, and internally iron, quinine, and brandy.

Following day, extension to groin. Fifth day, patient well.

CASE XX.—Male, aged three weeks. Erysipelas migrans gradually extending over the whole body, the head alone escaping. Disease began upon the genitals about a week after circumcision so badly done that the skin had been removed from the whole under surface of the penis down to the peno scrotal junction. In this case the erysipelas wandered for a second time over regions where recovery had apparently taken place. Finally, the day before death the bullæ became hemorrhagic, œdema of the skin in the region of the throat occurred, the breathing became much oppressed and the child sank rapidly.

Treatment had consisted in ichthyol collodion and ichthyol ointment to the wound upon the penis.

CASE XLVI.—Male infant aged three weeks. This child had been circumcised upon the eighth day, and when I saw him presented an extensive triangular wound left by the moël, who had removed the frænum and a large portion of the skin from the under surface of the penis just as in the preceding case.

Seven days later and two days before my visit a redness and swelling had appeared in the left groin. This was regarded by the physician who first saw the case as a beginning bubo. By the time of my examination, however, the erythema had extended to the scrotum, pubic region, and the inner and posterior surface of the thigh. Up to this time lead and opium wash had been employed without apparent benefit. Prognosis extremely unfavorable.

Having had what appeared to be a very favorable result from aristol in a case already related, I painted the whole surface over with a 5 per cent. solution in collodion of this new preparation, extending it beyond the margins of the disease. I also applied aristol powder to the wound. Internally, brandy.

Extension by next day to middle of back and over buttocks, downward to upper third of right thigh and to middle of left, entirely surrounding both limbs. I did not see child again, but was notified by the physician in charge that it died some three days later.

Another case in which aristol was used with good results is Case XLV., first seen on June 11th, one day after an erysipelas had shown itself near a lesion of ecthyma upon the leg of a boy aged nineteen months. At that time it extended from the middle of the thigh to the ankle. I applied a tight adhesive strip of plaster above the patch, as well as about the ankle below it, and painted the intervening space with a 5 per cent. aristol collodion. Brandy internally. The following day large bullæ had formed beneath the plaster bands and an erythematous blush extended for a slight distance beyond. The adhesive strips were removed and the whole surface was again painted with aristol collodion. Two days later erysipelas had extended above the rim of the pelvis. I now applied ichthyol ʒj to ʒj of collodion, as I could not obtain aristol. Extension next day to middle of back. Aristol collodion was now used again, and no further extension took place; the bullæ dried into crusts, and improvement rapidly followed.

The last case is in some ways the most satisfactory. It occurred on August 7th of the present year in the person of a three-year-old boy at a seaside hotel. Following a chill and high fever, erysipelas began simultaneously at both legs at about an inch distant from a pustule of unknown nature situated upon the anterior portion of either shin. When I examined the child I found a patch upon the left leg two inches in width almost surrounding the limb, and upon the opposite side a smaller patch. I at once bound up both legs in a solution of hyposulphite of soda in strength of ʒj to ʒj. Temperature was then 103¼° F. The same evening, in consultation with the family physician, Dr. Stub, of Brooklyn, a solution of iodine in collodion gr. x to ʒj was applied to the patches and about an inch beyond them. Later in the night the rectal temperature was 107° and there were some convulsive movements and delirium. Antifebrin gr. v. was now given with whiskey and repeated every three hours. Several slight chills occurred and there was extension of the process about an inch beyond the painted margin on the left side.

The following morning temperature 105°, and gradual creeping of disease toward the knee. Application was made an inch beyond erysipelas margin as often as spreading was noticed. By evening the temperature was 106°, and the patch had nearly reached the knee. I now applied several coatings of the paint one above the other just below the knee, and going above it I surrounded the lower third of the thigh with a tight band of adhesive plaster one inch wide. By the morning of the 9th the erysipelas had extended over the knee and the whole leg was now tensely swollen, painful and tender, with bullæ forming posteriorly. I found the plaster had just been removed because of complaint of tightness, but I at once reapplied it and forbade its being disturbed. During the day the. disease extended to the lower border of the adhesive band, where it stopped abruptly. The temperature fell and convalescence began. The erysipelas was at an end in three days, but where the iodine had been applied in several coats below the knee there was a burning of the skin which took ten days to heal. The erysipelas had gone beyond the thick coating of iodine, but had been arrested so suddenly at the plaster that the family physician and friends were convinced equally with myself of the efficacy of this method, first proposed, I believe, by Wölffler, and recently recommended by Dr. Weber, of this city.

Other attempts at formation of a barrier have failed in my hands, excepting the partial success following scarification. I had previously tried iodine and strong solutions of silver, but do not remember a successful case. It has seemed to me that the power of the cocci to penetrate deeply into the tissues and their mode of travelling through the lymph channels rendered any method dealing with the surface alone as unlikely to check the spread. I can understand, however, how pretty firm compression of all the tissues of a limb, as by a tight band, might act in checking the onward march of the microörganisms. It is at least a rational proceedure.

Scarification has had much said in its favor, and I have no doubt proves and will prove beneficial in some cases. To be successful, however, it must be repeated on successive days and one line of cuts after another be made as the spreading oversteps the attempted barrier. It is not an entirely new method, as many suppose. Leuroth proposed a method of treatment in the *Gazette Medical de Strasbourg* in 1870 which consisted in superficial linear scarification over the patch with others made so as to circumscribe it. Should the disease overstride this boundary, it was to be tried again.

Dobson is said to have proposed much the same process as early as 1828. Kraske, of Freiburg, operated first by scarification in 1886. After making crossed incisions he applied a five per cent. solution of carbolic.

Riedel in 1887 did the same thing in a number of cases, employing a 1 : 1000 sublimate instead of carbolic, and Lauenstein modified this in 1889 by cutting only in the sound skin. The latter is the process which strikes me most favorably.

Among other recently advocated modes of treatment (and new ones are being daily added, a fact which shows rather that anything may appear to do good in uncomplicated cases running their natural course), is that of Behrend,[1] consisting of the application of absolute alcohol; that of Hueter, who advises injections of a 3 per cent. carbolic solution to encircle the patch. If a case is thus treated in an early stage, it is said to be possible to stop the whole process within twenty-four to forty-eight hours. J. Koch paints the diseased parts once daily with an ointment of

R.—Creolin . . . . 1 part.
      Lanolin . . . . 10 parts.
      Iodoform . . . . 4 parts.

and over this applies gutta-percha tissue. Kroell advises a band of gutta-percha in place of Wölffler's adhesive strip.

Calvelli uses a 1 per cent. solution of picric acid to paint over the erysipelas. Pirogoff, it will be remembered, treated a large series of cases by camphor, I believe in the army, with excellent results. (His paper is not now accessible to me.) Rosenthal[2] has employed with marked success a combination of the Pirogoff and Hueter methods, giving 2½ grains of camphor at a dose.

Levy proposes[3] a spray of corrosive sublimate in ether 1 : 100, to be applied for a few minutes twice daily. Under this the fever in his cases lasted but three and a half days, while other methods showed eight days of fever.

With the most of these latter suggestions I have had no experience. In view of what I have learned from those cases which have fallen under my observation, I think the plan of treatment which offers the best results is about as follows:

First, internally, such symptomatic treatment as the nature of the case seems to require. Antipyretics only in case of high or persistent fever (over 103½° to 104°). Then antipyrine in dose of at least gr. xv–xx, for an adult, guarded by alcohol. Cooling drinks. Calomel or saline aperients in full dose if constipation. If much weakness, alcoholic drinks given freely, especially at critical periods, and iron or iron and quinine; digitalis if much fever and prostration; bromides for delirium; antipyrine or phenacetin for headache, with cold applications to head, and as concentrated and nutritious a diet as possible.

Second, locally, I would paint the patch and surrounding margin of healthy skin thickly with ichthyol in collodion, ʒj–ʒij to ʒj. If the scalp is the region affected, a watery solution or ointment of ichthyol can be employed. To arrest the spread I should in every case make an attempt either with the band of adhesive plaster or by scarification, or both, the latter to follow the former, in case the disease spreads beyond the

---

[1] Berlin klin. Wochenschrift, 1889.   [2] Ibid., No. 42, 1889.
[3] Médecine Moderne, No. 20.

adhesive strips. In erysipelas of the face which had not yet reached the forehead, or at least its upper part, I would apply a band tightly about the forehead and just above the ears, cutting the hair in a strip around if necessary to secure firm pressure. The chances of arresting the process here should be at least equal to those of checking the spread upon an extremity, for we have a hard bony base over which to make our compression. If the boundary is passed, then I should at once have the scalp shaved and apply another band higher up. The hair should be cut in any case in which the scalp is invaded or threatened. Then the same application of ichthyol in collodion can be made, as to the face or other part. If there be much tension, swelling, heat, and discomfort, (which is not apt to be the case under collodion), any oily substance can be applied over it.

In treating erysipelas the uncertainty of *prognosis* must always be kept in mind. Cases to all appearances mild in the beginning may become severe and prove fatal, while formidable appearing areas may suddenly cease spreading spontaneously. It is scarcely more safe to say a case will progress favorably (though the great majority do) than to claim that the particular line of treatment instituted has prevented an unfavorable termination, or proven abortive, unless a whole series of cases under a given method have terminated in a shorter than the average time.

Naturally, when the erysipelatous process has its sources in a pus collection such as an abscess, pustule, ulcer, foul wound, carious tooth, diseased duct, etc., the first care must be to secure as prompt and thorough disinfection and cleansing as possible. Pus must be destroyed and purity maintained. A solution of the peroxide of hydrogen will often be found useful in effecting this purpose. In such case a spontaneous halt may be hoped for. In the same way a diseased mucous membrane must be cared for ; excoriations, ulcerations, rhinitis or other disease of the nasal mucous membrane or affection of the throat must be looked after. It is probable that every case of facial erysipelas starts from some local solution of continuity either upon the skin or adjacent mucous membranes, and we simply call some cases " idiopathic ' or " genuine " when we fail to find the point where the micrococci have entered. I further believe it is because of this close proximity of various mucous membranes that erysipelas of the face is so comparatively frequent. That so-called idiopathic erysipelas of the face is identical with the traumatic variety I think is shown by the clinical history, course, and identity of the skin lesions in both processes, as is illustrated by Cases XXIV. and XXXII., where the husband's recovery from erysipelas of the leg was coincident with an outbreak of facial erysipelas in the wife. Since instances of direct contagion are not often seen, I would call attention to the frequency with which two cases occurred in the same family—no less than six times in the 47 cases. Twice husband and wife, twice in brothers, once mother and son, and once grandmother and grandchild. It will be noted in the histories given that internal treatment played a very unimportant part, and I am convinced that cases do quite as well without the large doses of iron so habitually given in this country.

As a prophylactic measure in those predisposed to repeated attacks, great care should be taken to discover and cure affections of mucous membranes, carious teeth, ulcerations, or other disease processes or conditions which I have mentioned as possible means of maintaining the tendency. Recurrences after apparent cure must be kept in mind and treatment continued sufficiently long to prevent them.

Since this paper was written I have applied the adhesive strip in three cases. Two were in erysipelas confined to the lower extremity. In the third it had already extended over the buttocks to the lumbar region before I saw the case. In the latter I applied a strip nearly two inches wide tightly about the abdomen, and painted the patch with 10 per cent. of aristol in collodion. No spreading occurred, and convalescence began at once. In one of the other cases the same treatment was successful, but failed in the second to arrest extension of the disease.

696 MADISON AVENUE.

REVIEWS.

INFLUENZA, OR EPIDEMIC CATARRHAL FEVER. AN HISTORICAL SURVEY
OF PAST EPIDEMICS IN GREAT BRITAIN FROM 1510 TO 1890. Being a
new and revised edition of *Annals of Influenza*, by THEOPHILUS THOMPSON,
M.D., F.R.C.P., F.R.S. By E. SYMES THOMPSON, M.D, F.R.C.P.,
Gresham Professor of Medicine and Consulting Physician to the Hospital
for Consumptives and Diseases of the Chest, Brompton. 8vo. pp. 490.
London : Percival & Co., 1890.

THE interest of this book, as indicated by its title, is chiefly
historical, but this is far from saying that it is not also of decided practical value. One fact which stands out prominently before the eye of
the discriminating reader shows the fallacy of any system of medicine
which prescribes for the disease rather than for the patient. The fact
to which we refer is the variation of epidemic type, which is perhaps
more marked in influenza than in any other affection. Regarding mankind as an individual, and supposing, as everyone does, the causes of
disease to retain their identity, it must be admitted either that both
suffer marked alterations with age, or that both undergo temporary
modifications from transient external influences. The fact that much
can be said in favor of each of these propositions might be regarded by
the unreflecting as proof of greatly increased knowledge, but the ability
to discuss does not necessarily imply wisdom. As regards influenza, the
rays, so to speak, of which our knowledge is composed, instead of all
uniting in a common focus, are, many of them, widely divergent. Indeed, little has been learned from the various epidemics beyond the fact
that the disease is infectious, and this is nothing new. As our author
pithily remarks: "The nomenclature of the disease, now definitely
known as influenza, is not of the clearest. It is said that the word was
originally introduced by the Italians, at a time when less was understood of its nature and origin than at present, if, indeed, this be possible."

It was an excellent idea to embody the writings of our professional
forefathers in a modern treatise, if only that they might serve as studies
of English style of a time when, as many hold, English was at its best.
In this statement we refer particularly to the accounts of Willis, Short,
and Sydenham, of which the quaint phraseology, instead of impairing
their scientific value, rather serves to give them zest and flavor.

It is superfluous to say that this work will take a permanent place in
the literature of influenza, for it is largely made up of writings recognized
as classic. Dr. Thompson has brought it down to the present time by
adding an account of the epidemic of 1889–90, which we can heartily
recommend to all interested in this medical topic of the day.

F. P. H.

KOCH'S REMEDY IN RELATION SPECIALLY TO THROAT CONSUMPTION. By
LENNOX BROWNE, F.R.C.S. Ed. Illustrated by 31 cases and by 50 origi-
nal engravings and diagrams. 8vo. pp. 114. London and Philadelphia:
Lea Bros. & Co., 1891.

THAT a considerable monograph, based upon personal observations of
31 patients—14 seen under Gerhardt's care and 8 under Krause's in
Berlin, and 9 under his own care—and copiously illustrated by laryngoscopic drawings and temperature charts, should have appeared as early
as January, is an evidence of great assiduity on the part of the author,
and, whatever be the outcome of the treatment, the effort will command
appreciation for all time, for the accuracy with which the changes noted
have been described and illustrated.

Beginning with a review of the author's previously published opinions
on tuberculous laryngitis, in which he contended for the possibility of its
existence as a primary lesion long before the fact had been demonstrated,
Mr. Browne adds, as corollary to Virchow's statement, that the larynx
is the most appropriate organ for the study of true tubercle, that it is
also the most appropriate and convenient site for accurate observation
of the various stages of its development toward reparation which takes
place under Koch's treatment. He endeavors to show, step by step,
that every stage in the life-history of the disease, which may extend over
many months, or even years, can, under Koch's treatment, be developed
and be compressed into a space of a few days, or, at most, of a few weeks,
Not only this, but that reparation of ulcers and necroses may take place
with amazing rapidity as recognizable in a series of laryngoscopic images
observed from day to day.

While points of similarity occur in the natural evolution of the disease
and in the evolution induced by the Koch treatment, there are a number
of differences, the knowledge of which is important. Instead of the
pallor peculiar to the natural form of the disease, reddening of the
surface is produced under the injections, sometimes to an intense degree, and in some cases to such an extent as would lead to error in diagnosis by one ignorant of the treatment. Interarytenoid tumefaction,
pyriform infiltration of the arytenoid regions, and the horseshoe and
turban-shaped tumefactions of the epiglottis take place in the modified
or induced laryngeal tuberculosis of the injection treatment, as they do
in the natural evolution of the disease. In addition, infiltration often
occurs lower down the larynx, not only in the ventricular bands, in the
vocal bands, or directly beneath, leading to constriction of the lumen of
the larynx as in the natural form, but with a levelling, as it were, of the
horizontal planes of the larynx, so that the swollen ventricular band is
almost on a line with the ary-epiglottic fold; while there is obscuration
of the natural lines of definition and contour of the various component
intra-laryngeal structures. These conditions lead to a stenosis which is
one of the dangers to be apprehended as an immediate reactionary result
of an injection, not always to be avoided even by very small or by slowly
increased quantities of the remedy, or by its infrequent repetition. The
gravity of this condition, however, is stated to have been grossly exaggerated. Ulcerations occurring under Koch treatment in the process of
elimination of the necrotic tissues are rarely active at more than one or

two points. Their color is at first white or whitish-gray with intensely red areolas, changing to pale yellow in a day, not unlike the appearance of the lenticular ulcer seen in connection with the exanthemata as well as with tuberculosis. Ulcerations in progress when the treatment is instituted become redder and are bathed in liquid pus for a day or two, after which they become cleaner and show a tendency to repair, though cicatrization is less rapid than is the case with erosions induced by the treatment. The rapidity of the process seems to account for the fact that perichondrial inflammation does not appear to progress to death of the cartilage. On the other hand, ulceration of the epiglottis at least has been seen to undergo arrest, and has been known to have undergone partial repair. Occasionally an area of disease has been aroused in the trachea.

The subjective symptoms, hoarseness, loss of voice, dysphagia, and suffocative dyspnœa may each and all be induced and subside with impressively distinctive rapidity. Extreme sensibility to laryngoscopic examination diminishes under the Koch treatment as does pain attending glutition. Mr. Lennox Browne would select those cases for treatment in which the pulmonary lesions were as chronic or limited as possible. He alludes to the risk of developing severe pulmonary complications, to arousing a latent pulmonary infiltration or the recrudescence of a lesion believed to have been healed. The existence of fibroid changes in the lungs would contra-indicate the treatment, or at least indicate great care in its employment.

The cases which form the basis of the observations recorded are described with more or less detail, and are largely illustrated by laryngoscopic pictures. It can hardly be conceded, however, that the results are encouraging enough to justify the conclusions of the author that they warrant perseverance in pursuing the treatment, even provided that due caution be exercised in the selection of patients and in every detail of administration.

There is much argumentative and instructive matter of general interest in connection with tuberculosis and its reaction under the tuberculin, the subject-matter of which must now be so familiar to our readers as to render further allusion to it superfluous.			J. S. C.

THE PROCLIVITY OF WOMEN TO CANCEROUS DISEASES AND TO CERTAIN BENIGN TUMORS, WITH AN APPENDIX ON HEREDITY AS A CAUSE OF CANCER. By HERBERT SNOW, M.D. Lond., etc. Pp. 58. London: J. & A. Churchill, 1891.

THIS little brochure is a lecture delivered at the London Cancer Hospital by one of the attending surgeons. The facts presented, while not especially new, are interesting and suggestive. Statistics form a prominent feature of the argument, and medical statistics, as Billings has conclusively shown, are only reliable when employed in a scientific manner.

The author's deductions are not all equally sound, since they may be divided into two classes: those resting upon a basis of fact, and those founded upon premises which are purely theoretical. We cannot deny that the greater number of cases of cancer occur in women, and that the disease affects most frequently the breasts or uterus; but the statement that fibrous tumors of these organs are due to imperfect nutrition or perverted functional activity in civilized, as compared with savage, races is one not supported by such evidence as the scientific student demands. Is it a fact that carcinoma is "almost absent in the savage, while rapidly increasing in prevalence among the civilized?"

An ingenious attempt is made to show that the neurotic factor holds a position in the etiology of cancer hardly secondary to that of traumatism. "We never (?) see," the author remarks, "malignant disease of the pathological species in question (except as the result of injury) developed in the mamma of a woman leading a healthy, happy, well-balanced life."

The connection which he seeks to establish between chronic invalidism (which he attributes to the powerful causes, constipation, corsets, overstudy and tea-drinking) and malignant disease is somewhat obscure, though the argument is by no means unfamiliar.

More interesting to the reader than the lecture itself will be the short appendix on heredity, in which, after carefully weighing the statistical evidence pro and con, the author arrives at these conclusions:

"1. That belief in heredity is derived merely from popular tradition, and is wanting in any sound basis of scientific proof.

"2. That extremely practical issues are involved, and that the views now prevalent often lead to disastrous results."   H. C. C.

ESSENTIALS OF SURGERY, TOGETHER WITH A FULL DESCRIPTION OF THE HANDKERCHIEF AND ROLLER BANDAGE. Arranged in the form of Questions and Answers. Prepared especially for Students of Medicine. By EDWARD MARTIN, A.M., M.D., Instructor in Operative Surgery, University of Pennsylvania; Surgeon to the Howard Hospital; Assistant Surgeon to the University Hospital. Illustrated. Fourth Edition. Revised and enlarged by an Appendix. Philadelphia: W. B. Saunders, 1891.

THE development of special departments in modern medicine, and the consequent overcrowding of the student's time, have made necessary some measures of relief. While it is easy to say that a student should not be helped to a parrot-like method of acquiring knowledge by putting in his hands an epitome arranged in the form of question and answer, there are two sides to the question from the student's point of view. The wisdom of so planning a course in medicine that the work of five years is attempted in three may be questioned, but where such a plan is in force the student must accommodate himself.

Doubly unfortunate is it when, as is too often the case, fundamental subjects like general surgery are submitted to a scaling process. While such a book as that under consideration is, without doubt, abused by the indolent, it has still a limited field in helping the better student under pressure to crystallize information obtained in other ways. The question whether this epitome fills the place well is partially answered by the fact that four editions have been called for in a little more than two years.

The author has at command good English, and has, moreover, a happy
way of saying definite things directly. There is a freedom from provincial or personal teaching which is very commendable. The treatment advocated, while it represents fairly that which is taught at the
University of Pennsylvania, is in general decisive, but safe, and such as
would, with a few exceptions, be accepted anywhere as sound. The
plan of giving constantly definite suggestions for a typical treatment might be adopted with advantage by many systematic authors.
It is not alone the beginner who sometimes searches in vain for a working method among the generalities of a text-book.

For such value as they may have, the appendix contains formulas
with brief directions for the medical treatment of many surgical affections. Here, also, may be found explicit directions for the preparation
of the usual antiseptic materials, including Lister's double-cyanide gauze.
The book is one of the best of its class.   G. E. S.

RECENT WORKS ON DIAGNOSIS:

LEHRBUCH DER AUSCULTATION UND PERCUSSION, MIT BESONDERER
BERÜCKSICHTIGUNG DER BESICHTIGUNG, BETASTUNG, UND MESSUNG
DER BRUST UND DES UNTERLIEBES ZUR DIAGNOSTISCHEN ZWECKEN.
Von DR. C. GERHARDT. Fünfte, vermehrte und verbesserte Auflage.
Pp. 363. Tübingen, 1890.

(HANDBOOK OF AUSCULTATION AND PERCUSSION, WITH SPECIAL CONSID-
ERATION OF INSPECTION, PALPATION, AND MENSURATION OF THE
CHEST AND ABDOMEN FOR DIAGNOSTIC PURPOSES. By DR. C. GER-
HARDT. Fifth, improved and corrected edition.)

AUSCULTATION AND PERCUSSION. By FREDERICK C. SHATTUCK, M.D.,
Professor of Clinical Medicine in Harvard University. Pp. 121. Detroit:
George S. Davis, 1890.

THE PHYSICAL DIAGNOSIS OF THE DISEASES OF THE HEART AND LUNGS
AND THORACIC ANEURISM. By D. W. CAMMANN, B.S. Oxon., M.D.
Pp. 178. New York and London: G. P. Putnam's Sons, 1891.

A GUIDE TO THE PRACTICAL EXAMINATION OF URINE. FOR THE USE
OF STUDENTS AND PHYSICIANS. By JAMES TYSON, M.D., Professor of
Clinical Medicine in the University of Pennsylvania, etc. Seventh edi-
tion. Pp. 255. Philadelphia: P. Blakiston, Son & Co., 1891.

NOTES ON TYPHOID FEVER; TROPICAL LIFE AND ITS SEQUELÆ. By
JEFFERY A. MARSTON, M.D., C.B., M.R.C.P., F.R.C.S., Surgeon-General
Medical Staff (retired). Pp. 165. London: H. K. Lewis, 1890.

DIFFERENTIATION IN RHEUMATIC DISEASES (SO CALLED). Read before
the Bristol Medico-Chirurgical Association. By HUGH LANE, L.R.C.P.,
etc. Pp. 27. London: J. & A. Churchill, 1890.

LITTLE need be said regarding a work so well and favorably known
to the reader of German interested in methods of medical diagnosis as
that of Gerhardt, beyond a brief mention of the appearance of a new

edition after the lapse of a number of years. This edition has been brought fully up to date in the various departments of physical diagnosis, of which it so ably deals. We know of no manual so complete without superfluous details. It is to be regretted that no English translation exists for the use of those who cannot readily read it in the original.

Dr. Shattuck's *Auscultation and Percussion* is one of the "Physician's Leisure Library," an excellent and popular series, issued in attractive form in neat paper cover for the modest sum of twenty-five cents. It covers a similar field to that of Gerhardt, though much less completely. It furnishes, however, an excellent *résumé*, in small compass, of the essentials of auscultation and percussion, and, so far as it goes, is quite beyond other criticism than that applicable to all more recent books on this subject—that the necessity for them does not exist. But since none has before been brought so within the reach of the most impecunious, its publication may not be amiss.

We cannot speak in very favorable terms of Dr. Cammann's manual, regarding it in the light of what he states he has endeavored to make it —a text-book on the Physical Diagnosis of Diseases of the Heart and Lungs. In addition to the criticism just applied to Dr. Shattuck's book, this one merits censure because of its inaccuracies and of the extreme views expressed on debatable points, the result of which cannot but be misleading to the student who looks to it for guidance. Not being satisfied with the generally accepted explanation of the origin and cause of crepitant and subcrepitant rāles, and believing that identical rhonchi may be produced in the pleura, the author holds, as regards crepitant rāles at least, that they are always of pleural production. There is no doubt that occasionally pleural friction may so closely resemble true crepitant and subcrepitant intra-pulmonary rhonchi that it is impossible to indubitably differentiate their site of production without attention to accompanying signs; but there are few who will accept, with this author, that these rāles are always intra-pleural. According to this view, which Dr. Cammann devotes considerable space and ingenious argument to prove, the crepitant rāle is indicative not of pneumonia but of pleurisy, and when encountered in the first stage of pneumonia indicates an accompanying pleuritis; so that in uncomplicated pneumonia the crepitant rāle would not be present. Dr. Cammann neglects to explain why crepitation disappears with the onset of solidification and reappears with resolution. According to his view crepitus should be decided in the second stage of pneumonia; for he states that, to produce a shower of crepitant rāles, an abundance of pleural exudation is necessary, and the accompanying pleuritis is more likely to furnish an abundance of exudate in the stage of consolidation than in that of engorgement.

It is very evident, however, that Dr. Cammann does not make a very nice distinction between crepitant and other forms of rāles, for we find he states that crepitant rāles are *usually* heard with inspiration, occasionally throughout it, and *sometimes* only at its close; indicating that they also occur with expiration. This may reasonably account for his ultra position. It is elsewhere, we believe, pretty well accepted that the true vesicular rāles are heard only with the *end* of inspiration and never with expiration, while fine subcrepitant rāles and friction-sounds resembling these and the crepitant rāle occur with both *in-* and *expiration*.

Under the caption, Respiration in Health, it is stated that the duration of inspiration is three or four times longer than that of expiration. This, of course, applies to the *time* that the two signs are audible to the auscultator, but this is not made clear, and the ratio might be supposed to apply to the relative duration of inspiration and expiration, which of course is very different from this.

Dr. Cammann fails to grasp the difference between puerile respiration and harsh or vesiculo-bronchial, using these terms synonymously. Flint long ago pointed out the distinction, which, if not recognized, might readily lead to error. Puerile respiration has as its distinctive feature *increase in intensity without alteration in pitch;* whereas, harsh or vesiculo-bronchial breathing has alone *elevation in pitch.* Harsh respiration is a mingling of the bronchial and vesicular elements in varying proportions, while puerile respiration is simply an increased vesicular murmur.

The curious statement appears on page 157 that basic anæmic murmurs are usually heard in the aortic area and less commonly over the pulmonary.

We fear Dr. Cammann is somewhat over-sanguine as to the possibilities of auscultatory percussion. There is no doubt as to the great value of this much-neglected and little-understood method in the differentiation of organs and in outlining their boundaries, but that it ever can be of much practical use in detecting morbid changes in the viscera, especially the kidneys, through alteration in their percussion-note, is very problematical.

Little opportunity has been afforded Dr. Tyson to materially revise this edition of his very popular *Practical Examination of Urine,* because of few changes of importance in urine-testing occurring since the preceding issue of this book. The excellent albumimeter of Esbach is described; the newer tests for sugar are given, and a half-page is devoted to the description of phosphatic diabetes, an ailment which has recently attracted some attention abroad through the writings of Teissier and Ralfe.

Dr. Marston has prepared some very interesting notes, based on a large experience with enteric fever occurring among British troops in India. As is well known, enteric fever always has been very prevalent among these in that country, while it is exceptionally rare among the native population. Two powerful factors combine to enormously increase the susceptibility of the recruit to enteric fever—early manhood and recent arrival in a new, hot climate. So that no better opportunity could be afforded of studying the natural history of the disease than is presented in India.

Clinical features and anatomical characters of typhoid fever are the same in India as elsewhere, but whether the etiological factors are always similar Dr. Marston regards as somewhat doubtful. His remarks on causation are of great interest, based as they are on wide experience and accurate judgment. He finds himself unable to account for the origin of all cases of Indian enteric fever by the view of Budd (specific infection), or even by that of Murchison, and seems inclined to look with some favor on the doctrine that under certain conditions (chiefly climatic) this fever may originate unfathered by a specific bacillus or a pythogenic cause. He cannot well understand otherwise the development of certain cases in which all the evidence points against specific infection or spontaneous origin through filth. He, however, regards it as more difficult, in a country like India, to exclude a pythogenic source than a bacillary one. He does not commit himself positively to either the autogenic or to Murchison's view, evidently feeling that the evidence in either direction is of a negative nature, which may be invalidated by more thorough methods of investigation. In this connection it may be of interest to recall the opinion of Rodet as to the relationship which he believes exists between the bacillus coli communis and the bacillus of Eberth; that under certain conditions the former bacillus, which when cultivated at a temperature of 44° to 46° C. becomes morphologically similar to Eberth's, may acquire pathogenic properties and induce enteric fever. An acceptance of Rodet's views would explain the pathogenic origin of typhoid fever and might throw light on the supposed autogenic cases of Dr. Marston. The altered condition of life of the newly arrived soldier in India, entailing increased physiological activity of the lymphatic and glandular system, especially of those of the intestines, might tend to furnish the suitable conditions for the transformation of the benign bacillus coli communis into the virulent bacillus of Eberth.

The chapters devoted to Tropical Life and its Sequelæ are not the least interesting in the book. They deal with the immediate and remote effect produced on Europeans who have resided in hot climates without having undergone thorough "acclimatization."

Differentiation in Rheumatic Diseases is a graphically illustrated reprint of a paper which appeared in the *Lancet*, October, 1890, by one who has had a large experience with this class of affections. It deals with the diagnosis and treatment of rheumatoid and rheumatic arthritis. The author believes that in most cases of the former a strumous taint exists which is very likely the underlying cause of the rheumatoid condition. It is, however, difficult to understand what he means by struma, since he uses the terms scrofula, struma, and tuberculosis as if they were quite unrelated. But the so-called theory advanced by Mr. Lane as to the association existing between struma, phthisis, and rheumatoid arthritis is not, as he seems to suppose, new. Dr. Garrod long ago stated his belief that the subjects of the tubercular diathesis— which nowadays we are to understand includes struma or scrofulosis —are especially susceptible to it.   D. D. S.

THE BARBARITY OF CIRCUMCISION AS A REMEDY FOR CONGENITAL ABNORMALITY. By HERBERT SNOW, M.D. Lond., etc., Surgeon to the Cancer Hospital. London: J. & A. Churchill, 1890.

THE author hopes to "contribute in some small measure toward the abolition of an antiquated practice, involving the infliction of very considerable suffering upon helpless infants."

Circumcision as a religious rite is traced from its first historical employment by Abraham to the present day. It is stated to have been long before that time widely observed among Ethiopians, Egyptians, Phœnicians, and other peoples; while at present the list of those who practise it includes many widely separated nations in Asia, Polynesia,

South America and Africa. It is considered to be "simply and solely a relic of barbarism," long antedating historical record ; and as probably associated with a primitive sacrificial idea, the devotion of a part for the whole body to some demon or deity. The practice has no real relation to hygiene as a motive.

The relative frequency of congenital phimosis and its causal relation to many important reflex conditions are admitted. From various eminent surgical writers opinions are quoted in favor of the wide extension of the operation of circumcision. It is admitted also that among uncleanly peoples cleanliness is favored by it, but shaving of the head might be universally advised with as much reason. The argument that it promotes chastity is considered of doubtful value. The evils of possible hemorrhage or sepsis, of unwritten suffering from exposure of highly sensitive surface, of premature excitement in children, of contracted meatus when the operation is early, are thought to weigh against the cutting method of treatment. Separation of adhesions and rapid dilatation of the prepuce under anæsthesia with some simple instrument, such as dressing forceps, will be found, in the author's opinion, to render cutting unnecessary in the large majority of cases.

In this neat little book no claim to originality of thought is made. The subject is simply reviewed, and the above conclusion drawn, with copious reference to a literature which is already sufficiently exhaustive.

G. E. S.

ESSAY ON MEDICAL PNEUMATOLOGY: A PHYSIOLOGICAL, CLINICAL AND THERAPEUTIC INVESTIGATION OF THE GASES. By J. N. DEMARQUAY, Surgeon to the Municipal Hospital, Paris, and of the Council of State, etc. Translated with Notes, Additions, and Omissions, by SAMUEL S. WALLIAN, A.M., M.D. 8vo., pp. xvi. 300. Philadelphia and London : F. A. Davis, 1890.

THE work before us is a translation of portions of the original of Demarquay, reported to the Academy of Medicine of Paris and published in 1866. The section on emphysema, and the chapters devoted to experiments with carbonic acid, in the original, are omitted in the translation ; while at the conclusion of the work the translator has introduced notes, comments and additions. The subject of the gases in the blood is first taken up ; then oxygen is discussed from an historical point of view, as to its physiological action, its mode of preparation and administration, and its therapeutic application ; finally, some consideration is devoted to nitrogen, nitrogen monoxide and hydrogen. The subject of pneumatology has not, perhaps, received the attention, nor its principles the general application, which their importance deserves. Within the past few years, however, a fair amount of work in this department of therapeutics has been done, and the current literature contains numerous papers in evidence of the growing interest in the subject of the use of oxygen as a therapeutic agent. The translator's statement that Demarquay's work had been ignored in this country is erroneous. As long ago as 1867, it and the whole subject of pneumatotherapy received full attention at the hands of J. Solis-Cohen in his work on *Inhalation in the Treatment of Diseases*. Dr. Wallian by his labors has contributed materially to disseminate the principles of pneumatology, and to indicate the lines of their practical application. A. A. E.

PROGRESS

OF

MEDICAL SCIENCE.

THERAPEUTICS.

UNDER THE CHARGE OF
FRANCIS H. WILLIAMS, M.D.,
ASSISTANT PROFESSOR OF THERAPEUTICS IN HARVARD UNIVERSITY.

Corrosive Sublimate as a Disinfectant.

Experiments published by Dr. A. C. Abbott, made in the pathological laboratory of the Johns Hopkins Hospital, have a very practical bearing upon the value of corrosive sublimate as a germicide, and the results of these experiments lessen the high estimation in which this agent has been held by most investigators.

Dr. Abbott selected the staphylococcus pyogenes aureus for a series of experiments as to germicide power in consequence of the importance of this subject to the surgeon.

The tests hitherto made upon corrosive sublimate as a disinfectant have agreed in giving to it the first place in the list of these agents.

One method commonly employed in testing the value of any chemical substance as a disinfectant is to expose organisms dried upon bits of silk thread to its action for different lengths of time, and then, after removing and carefully washing the threads in water and alcohol, to place them in nutrient media at a favorable temperature and notice if any growth results from them. If no growth appears, the disinfection was presumably successful. Another common method is to mix fluid cultures of organisms with the disinfectant, and, after different intervals of time, a portion is taken from the mixture and placed in nutrient media just as in the other method.

Now, in both of these methods it is easy to see that unless special precautions are taken a minute portion of sublimate may be carried along with the thread or drop into the medium which is to determine whether or not the organisms on the thread or in the drop still possess the power of growth. For organisms in their normal condition—that is, those which have never been exposed to the action of a disinfectant—the amount necessary to restrain growth, for certain disinfecting agents, is very small indeed; and for those organisms which have previously been exposed for a time to such agents, Geppert shows it is very much less.

In the case of the organism we are considering, Dr. Abbott finds the amount of sublimate necessary to prevent the growth of perfectly normal staphylococci to be 1 part of sublimate in 75,000 parts of the ordinary peptone bouillon, or 200,000 parts of bouillon without peptones. So that, if organisms which have been once exposed to stronger solutions of this salt (1 to 1000) require less than these amounts to inhibit their growth, it is plain that special precautions must be taken to prevent transportation of this minute trace into the nutrient medium which is to demonstrate whether or not the organisms are capable of development.

The author gives in detail a series of experiments, and draws the following conclusions :

That, under the most favorable conditions, a given amount of sublimate has the property of rendering inert only a certain number of individual organisms —that is to say, the process is a definite chemical one taking place between the protoplasm of the individual bacteria and the sublimate in the solution.

The disinfecting activity of the sublimate against organisms is profoundly influenced by the proportion of albuminous material contained in the medium in which the bacteria are present. It was found that the relation between the golden pyogenic staphylococci and sublimate is not a constant one, organisms from different sources and of different ages behaving differently when exposed to the same amount of the disinfectant for the same length of time.

Many of the results of previous experimenters, who have assigned to corrosive sublimate more powerful disinfectant properties against the staphylococcus pyogenes aureus in cultures than the observations reported in this paper indicate, are attributable to the neglect of certain precautions now recognized as essential to the proper conduct of such experiments.

At the present stage of our knowledge in this direction it is plain that for use in surgical practice the solutions of corrosive sublimate do not possess all the advantages hitherto attributed to them.

In regard to the employment of sublimate solutions upon wound-surfaces, it is plain that there exist at least two serious objections : First, the albumin of the tissues and fluids of the body tends to diminish the strength of, or, indeed, renders entirely inert, the solution employed ; and, second, the integrity of the tissues is materially injured by the application of this salt. The first objection cannot be met with certainty, for the surgeon possesses no means by which he can determine the amount of albuminous material with which his solutions are to come in contact, and in any case this large amount of albuminous material is an almost insuperable obstacle to complete disinfection with sublimate. He is, therefore, never in a position to say, a priori, that his efforts at disinfection of the wound are or are not successful.

During the past two years we have had sufficient evidence to lead us to believe that the normal tissues and fluids of the body possess the power of rendering inert many kinds of organisms which may have gained access to them. This function is therefore diminished, or, indeed, may be quite destroyed, by any agent which brings about alterations in the constitution of these tissues. We know that just such changes as those to which we refer are known to follow the application of sublimate solutions. It is plain, then, if we bring about in these tissues a condition of superficial necrosis—the condition following upon the application of sublimate—they are much less able to resist the inroads of infectious organisms than they would have been had they been left in their natural condition.

As a disinfectant, in the strict sense of the word, there are, perhaps, few substances which possess the property in a higher degree than does corrosive sublimate, but at the same time there is nothing which is employed for this purpose that requires greater care in its manipulation, in order to obtain its best results, than does this salt. In practice its action is influenced by a number of conditions which it is difficult, if not quite impossible, to control.

For these reasons we seem hardly justified in continuing to give to it the first place in the list of substances which may be employed practically for the purpose of rendering harmless materials containing the germs of infectious maladies.—*Johns Hopkins Bulletins*, No. 12.

OINTMENT FOR HEMORRHOIDS.

Hydrochlorate of cocaine	grs. xvj.
Sulphate of morphine	grs. v.
Sulphate of atropine	grs. iv.
Powdered tannin	grs. xvj.
Vaseline	℥j.
Essence of rose	q. s.

Make an ointment and apply to the affected parts after each movement from the bowels.

It is necessary to have the discharges of soft consistence.—*Journ. American Med. Assoc.*, 1891.

ANTISEPTIC TREATMENT OF TYPHOID FEVER.

In a lecture on this subject, at King's College Hospital, DR. YEO has called attention to the progress that the idea of an antiseptic treatment of typhoid fever is making amongst physicians in all parts of the world. He is unwilling, in the present stage of our knowledge, to put too much stress upon any particular manner of carrying out this idea, as we have probably not yet arrived at the very best means for doing so. What he says about the application of the idea of antisepsis in typhoid fever by various practitioners is of interest.

PROFESSOR PETRESCO, of Bucharest, has borne valuable testimony to the efficacy of naphthol. He had previously experimented with carbolic acid, salicylic acid, turpentine, benzoic acid, kairin, calomel, corrosive sublimate, and boric acid without any very favorable results. He then tried a saturated solution of sulphide of carbon, with which he was much better pleased; and lastly he tried naphthol, 15 grains three times a day, and had results more favorable than with any other remedy: the rate of mortality was reduced, and the course of the disease favorably modified.

DR. CLARKE, of Bristol, used hydronaphthol in five cases of typhoid fever, and all did well. It soon stopped the diarrhœa, and the stools lost their

offensive odor.   He gave from 3 to 4 grains every two hours until the diarrhœa was checked, and then every three hours so long as there was fever.

DR. TEISSIER, of Lyons, prefers a-naphthol for producing intestinal antisepsis in typhoid fever. He gives it in 6-grain doses, combined with salicylate
of bismuth, and he at the same time promotes free diuresis by cold-water
enemata.   He also gives enemata of quinine and cinchona as an "antithermic
tonic." He observed that as soon as intestinal antisepsis was established the
urine became green, the temperature fell, the albuminuria disappeared, the
spleen diminished in size, and the tongue became remarkably moist.   Convalescence was very rapid. He considers that naphthol acts by sterilizing
the bacterial products in the intestine.

DR. SCHWARTZ has demonstrated that naphthalene administered internally
diminishes the number of bacilli in fecal matter in the proportion of one-
third to one-fourth. When its administration is discontinued, this proportion increases again. But naphthalene is not so safe or suitable an intestinal
antiseptic as β-naphthol or a-naphthol.

DR. W. H. THOMPSON, of the Roosevelt Hospital, New York, is an advocate
of intestinal antisepsis in typhoid fever. He looks carefully after the food
administered ; he never gives milk undiluted, but always mixed with an equal
quantity of lime-water. He objects to beef-tea as setting up gastro-intestinal
fermentation. He gives, also, 10 grains of saccharated pepsin with 10 minims
of dilute hydrochloric acid every three hours. He also gives 10 grains of
subcarbonate of bismuth every three hours ; sometimes both medicines every
two hours. He regards these as the best agents for the purposes of intestinal
antisepsis.

Many physicians have recorded their approval of an initial laxative, and
no doubt it is well, if there is no diarrhœa, to begin with one ; we shall then
have less hesitation in keeping the bowels quiet afterward. Indeed, it has
been said that "purgation and antisepsis are, to some extent, interchangeable
terms."   An aperient expels the poisonous ptomaines and other decomposing
substances from the intestinal canal, and, if given in the early stages, may
actually prevent subsequent serious diarrhœa. But the use of aperients, to
be perfectly safe, must be limited to the first ten or twelve days of the fever,
the great risk attending their use in the later stages is the possibility of the
existence of deep ulceration in the ileum, and, in that case, an aperient may
mean the difference between life and death to the patient. At that period
of the disease intestinal antisepsis can only be safely secured by the use of
intestinal antiseptics.—*Lancet*, No. 3529, 1891.

DIAGNOSTIC VALUE.

Before the Niederrheinische Gesellschaft für Natur und Heilkunde,
SCHULTZE (*Deutsche med. Wochenschr.*, March 26, 1891) stated that he did not
consider the occurrence of reaction following injection of the Koch fluid, in
cases in which tuberculosis was not suspected, as diagnostic of latent tuberculosis, as he had seen reaction take place in cases not tuberculous.   In
seventy-two cases of pulmonary and laryngeal tuberculosis treated with
tuberculin, he found, by comparison, that the results did not materially differ
from those obtained in previous years with other methods of treatment.

An Alkaloid from Tubercle Bacilli.

By treating the contents of tubes containing agar-agar cultures of the tubercle bacillus with hot water acidulated with hydrochloric acid, filtering, evaporating, precipitating with platinum chloride, separating the double salt with hydrogen sulphide, filtering, and evaporating to dryness, ZUELZER (*Berliner klin. Wochenschrift*, 1891) was able to obtain a chloride of an alkaloid, 0.01 of which, injected into rabbits and guinea-pigs, caused, in from three to five minutes, increased frequency of respiration, elevation of temperature and protrusion of the eyeballs. The eyes were brilliant, the pupils slightly dilated and the conjunctiva injected. The protrusion was the more marked on the side on which the injection was made. The symptoms lasted for from fifteen to twenty minutes. Three rabbits died after injections of 0.02 or 0.03. The muscles into which the injections were made were reddened and the seat of hemorrhages; there were also hemorrhages in the mucous membrane of the stomach and of the upper portion of the duodenum. In two cases there was ascites. Similar results followed introduction of the substance into the conjunctival sac.

The Chemistry and Toxicology of the Tubercle Bacillus.

WEYL (*Deutsche med. Wochenschrift*, 1891) examined, at the Hygienic Institute at Berlin, the product obtained by treating with dilute sodic hydrate, the scrapings from 600 glycerin-agar cultures of the tubercle bacillus. The yellowish turbid mixture coagulated, by gradual cooling, into two layers—an upper, resembling coagulated agar, and a lower, containing small, white shreds. The lower layer, after treatment with warm dilute sodic hydrate, consisted, microscopically, of folded membranes, and at irregular intervals of apparent, inflated tubes. It contained carbon, hydrogen, sulphur and nitrogen. Special interest attached to it because it displayed the specific staining qualities of the tubercle bacillus. This " white substance " probably represents the capsule of the bacillus, while the gelatinous substance of the upper layer represents the protoplasm of the organism. Analysis of this gelatinous substance places it among the mucins. Solutions of it were prepared and injected subcutaneously into rabbits, guinea-pigs and mice. In the guinea-pigs and mice, at the end of three or four days, local necrosis took place at the site of injection and a crust formed, which fell off in four or five days. From these experiments Weyl concludes that from cultures of tubercle bacilli a toxomucin can be obtained, which he does not believe to exist preformed in the bacilli.

Hydrochlorate of Phenocoll—a New Antipyretic and Anti-rheumatic.

This substance appears in the form of a white powder soluble in water. It is a compound of phenetidine and seems to be similar in action to antipyrine. Fifteen grains of phenocoll reduces the temperature about as much as would be accomplished by 22 to 30 grains of antipyrine or about 15 grains

of phenacetine. It has analgesic properties in doses of 7 to 15 grains.—
Deutsche med. Wochenschrift, No. 15, 1891.

VEGETATIONS ON THE GENITALS.

R.—Acid. salicylic. .   .   .   .   grs. viij.
    Acid. acetic.   .   .   .   .   ℨij.

Apply to the warts with a camel's-hair brush once or twice a day.—*Médecine
Moderne*, 1891.

PIPERAZIN.

This substance has the property of dissolving a large proportion of uric
acid. One part of the urate of this substance is soluble in about 50 parts of
water. Urate of lithia requires 368 parts of water to dissolve it; the piperazin salt is, therefore, seven times more soluble than the lithia salt. Piperazin
is not toxic and not caustic, and it appears to have advantages over other
substances which may be used to act as solvents for uric acid. It seems to
be worthy of trial in suitable cases.—*Berliner klinische Wochenschrift*, No. 14,
1891.

METHODS FOR THE ADMINISTRATION OF AMYL-HYDRATE.

A teaspoonful of amyl-hydrate may be taken at night in a small glass of
beer. It should be stirred for seven minutes to insure solution. Or, of the
following, one-half may be taken at night :

Hydrate of amyl   .   .   .   .   ℨi.
Water   }
Orange-flower water }   .   .   .   .   .   āā   ℥ij.
Syrup of bitter orange   .   .   .   .   .   .   ℥j.

It is necessary to remember that amyl-hydrate dissolves slowly in water and
beer (one part to eight).

Amyl-hydrate may also be given in capsules, each one containing one-
quarter of a drachm ; three or four of these may be used for a dose.—*Nou
veaux Remèdes*, No. 2, 1891.

DEATH DURING CHLOROFORM ADMINISTRATION.

The patient was a bright, perfectly healthy little girl, about eleven years of
age. The operation was for the removal of a large mole, covering the greater
portion of the surface of the cheek. There was nothing in the appearance
of the child upon examination that would contra-indicate the use of an
anæsthetic in any way, and chloroform was chosen.

The operation was done by Dr. C. T. PARKES, surgeon to the Presbyterian
Hospital, Chicago, and the chloroform was administered by internes of that
hospital.

The operation required about twenty-five minutes, and as it was about
the face, the hands of the surgeon prevented the continuous administration
of the anæsthetic; very little chloroform was given to the child. The instrument used for giving the anæsthetic was Esmarch's inhaler, a wire frame

covered with flannel, with which it is impossible to absolutely prevent the entrance of air. The child made no demonstration of any kind that would attract attention. The operation was practically completed; the pigmented nævus was removed, and pieces of skin taken from the thigh for tranplantation, to cover the defects and diminish the amount of sear, were being put in position; when, without any warning, without the administration of any chloroform for at least five minutes, the child was seized with general convulsions; she ceased to breathe, her heart ceased to beat, she gave a few gasps, and was dead.

Every effort was made for an hour and a half to restore circulation and respiration, by artificial respiration, injection of ether and whiskey and nitrite of amyl, and the use of electricity, but all efforts failed.—*Journal of the American Medical Association*, No. 7, 1891.

IODOFORM AND ARISTOL.

DR. RICHTMANN recommends that iodoform should in all cases be replaced by aristol; the latter has the advantages of iodine and of thymol without their drawbacks. It is not irritating, its absorption is not followed by toxic symptoms, and its odor is not disagreeable. Unfortunately, it is insoluble in water.

The following are some of the ways in which it may be used:

In the form of powder, externally, or one part dissolved in ten parts of ether for external use.

A mixture containing 3 per cent. of aristol, in 20 of olive oil and 77 of lanolin, is a good application for burns.—*Nouveaux Remèdes*, No. 4, 1891.

MEDICINE.

UNDER THE CHARGE OF

W. PASTEUR, M.D. LOND., M.R.C.P.,

ASSISTANT PHYSICIAN TO THE MIDDLESEX HOSPITAL; PHYSICIAN TO THE NORTHWESTERN HOSPITAL FOR CHILDREN;

AND

SOLOMON SOLIS-COHEN, A.M., M.D.,

PROFESSOR OF CLINICAL MEDICINE AND APPLIED THERAPEUTICS IN THE PHILADELPHIA POLYCLINIC; PHYSICIAN TO THE PHILADELPHIA HOSPITAL.

TUBERCULIN: PRODUCTION OF DISSEMINATED MILIARY TUBERCULOSIS.

VIRCHOW (*Deutsche med. Wochenschr.*, 1891), before the Berlin Medical Society, opposed the view of B. Fränkel, that a period of three weeks must necessarily elapse between the invasion of the bacillus and the appearance of symptoms of miliary tuberculosis in man as in guinea-pigs. He then presented specimens from a case in which miliary tuberculosis appeared more than three weeks after injection of tuberculin, and which, therefore, escaped criticism. The subject had enjoyed good health until a year previously. In August he had pleurisy, from which he recovered and was well for two months. In mid-December he had another attack, with cough, anorexia, debility, and sharp pain posteriorly on the right side of the chest. Examination, January 16th, revealed a large pleuritic effusion on the right. At the right apex the resonance was slightly impaired, the vesicular murmur enfeebled, and ill-defined râles were heard. The spleen was enlarged. Exploratory puncture brought clear serous fluid. There was slight fever, but no expectoration. The first injection, of 0.02, was made January 19th, and was followed by the usual reaction. January 20th, the effusion, which had reaccumulated, was again withdrawn; the fluid was serous. January 25th, the night-sweats increased; the dulness on the right rose above the angle of the scapula; headache and dry cough set in. February 5th, the seventh injection, of 0.02, was followed by shortness of breath, dryness of the throat, and pain in the right side. February 7th, rusty sputum appeared for the first time, in small quantity. February 8th, the expectoration was mixed with blood; there was pain in the throat. February 9th, the epiglottis was swollen and reddened, with small hemorrhages at its margin; the adjacent wall of the pharynx was swollen, reddened, and the seat of small hemorrhages; its surface was uneven from irregularities which were not typical tubercles; the right ary-epiglottic ligament was swollen, the interior of the larynx only reddened. February 10th, the temperature rose to 104°, and, with remissions, remained at about this level; the expectoration was at no time abundant. February 15th, it was bloody and purulent; for the first time bacilli were found; dyspnœa and cough increased. February 17th, grayish-yellow nodules were for the first time seen on the epiglottis. February 19th, a little more than four weeks after the first injection, coma, pulmonary œdema, cyanosis and death occurred.

The autopsy disclosed a general miliary or submiliary tuberculosis of unusually wide distribution. The lungs were large, inelastic, intensely reddened and slightly œdematous, with slate-colored induration at the apices; on the right there was a bronchiectatic cavity; otherwise the lungs were studded with small and large nodules, mostly miliary tubercles and some miliary areas of inflammation. The spleen was enlarged and pulpy and contained large numbers of delicate, translucent, light-gray submiliary tubercles. The liver, the cortex of the kidney, and the mucous membrane of the larynx and pharynx also contained many tubercles. The thyroid gland contained a small number. The eruption was profuse in the medulla of the upper third of the epiphysis of the femur. Beginning eruption and fibrinous exudate were present in circumscribed areas of the peritoneum and the recto-vesical cul-de-sac.

OESTREICH, for Virchow, showed specimens from a female patient, thirty-six years old, admitted to the hospital with involvement of the apices and signs of peritonitis, thought to be tuberculous. Twenty injections were given in the course of six weeks and a half. Each injection was followed by typical reaction, but fever existed also in the intervals. The condition of the patient became worse and death occurred. The apices of the lungs were destroyed by the phthisical process. The upper portion of the lower lobes presented caseous bronchitis at several points. The peritoneum was studded with innumerable tubercles, from a size scarcely visible to that of a poppy-seed, gray, translucent, microscopically showing no sign of caseation, macroscopically showing retrograde changes. The development of a portion of the tubercles occurred during the time the injections were being given. Between the liver, stomach, spleen, and lung, an abscess had originated from an ulcer of the stomach. The mucous membrane of the intestine had undergone amyloid degeneration.

PRODUCTION OF ACUTE TUBERCULOUS MENINGITIS.

RÜTIMEYER (*Berliner klin. Wochenschrift*, 1891) reports a fatal case of acute tuberculous meningitis arising subsequently to treatment of a case of incipient phthisis with injections of the Koch fluid. Following an attack of influenza, the patient had cough, night-sweats, and a sense of oppression of the chest. There was some impairment of resonance on the right side of the chest, over the apex, anteriorly and posteriorly, with enfeebled vesicular murmur, harsh inspiration and bronchial expiration, and some fine râles. The sputum contained a small number of tubercle bacilli. Thirteen injections, in gradually increasing doses up to 0.03, were given in the course of sixteen days. There was the usual reaction ; râles were, for the first time, heard at the left apex; the expectoration was increased; the sputum contained an increased number of bacilli. The patient lost eleven pounds in weight. The injections were withdrawn. Headache and vomiting set in. There were anorexia, weakness, and malaise. The sense of prostration became marked ; there were pains in the limbs, mental unrest, and irritability, with a clear sensorium. Sopor, rigidity of the neck, immobility of the pupils, Cheyne-Stokes breathing, tracheal râles and death followed. In addition to miliary tubercles, lobular pneumonia and cavities in the lungs, the pia mater was cloudy and infiltrated, the posterior cranial fossa contained an ounce of reddish fluid, the ventricles were dilated, a small, cheesy nodule was found in the right occipital lobe, another at the base of the cerebellum, and submiliary tubercles at various parts of the brain.

BACILLI IN THE BLOOD.

LIEBMANN, of Trieste, reports (*Berliner klin. Wochenschr.*, 1891) nine cases, in which, after one or several injections of the Koch fluid, tubercle bacilli were found in the blood. In a note, the editor of the *Wochenschrift* disclaims all responsibility for the accuracy of the observations.

BACILLI IN THE FLUID.

MEYER (*Deutsche med. Wochenschr.*, 1891) found tubercle bacilli in each of five vials of the Koch fluid. To determine if these bacilli possessed activity, he injected portions from three into the anterior chamber of three rabbits, subcutaneously in two rabbits and one guinea-pig and into a vein of the ear of one rabbit. No reaction, either local or general, had occurred at the end of five or six weeks.

LIBBERTZ (*Deutsche med. Wochenschr.*, 1891) makes the following announcement: In the preparation of tuberculin an occasional tubercle bacillus may find its way into the fluid. No harm results, because the bacilli have been killed by the long-continued action of boiling. Koch states that dead tubercle bacilli introduced beneath the skin cause suppuration. This is true of infusions of cultures containing large numbers of bacilli. Single bacilli give rise to neither local nor general reaction. They cannot gain entrance to the blood-current from the subcutaneous connective tissue if not injected directly into a bloodvessel. Tuberculin is prepared from pure cultures of tubercle bacilli, and in its original condition can contain no other bacteria. Atmospheric germs may subsequently gain entrance, but these are usually not pathogenic and cannot multiply, on account of the large proportion of glycerin which the fluid contains. Tuberculin always has an alkaline reaction.

Histological Changes.

Nauwerck (*Deutsche med. Wochenschr.*, 1891) presented to the Verein für Wissenschaftliche Heilkunde, at Königsberg, a report of the results of examinations in twenty-one fatal cases and of fifteen specimens removed by operation from patients treated with tuberculin. The injections were followed by hyperæmia and exudative inflammation; not rarely with hemorrhage around the tubercle, which was often infiltrated with polynuclear round cells. In the base of tuberculous ulcers of the bowel, after prolonged treatment, a peculiar isolation of the tubercle was repeatedly observed, the cellular infiltration being limited to the surrounding structure. In a fatal case of gonitis, the appearances were such as to create the impression that acute necrosis and exfoliation had taken place; the surfaces of the exposed bone seemed to have been curetted. The loose structures in the joint presented the microscopic appearances of caseous necrosis. Tubercle bacilli were found in them as well as on the joint-surfaces. The walls of an abscess in connection with caries of the vertebra contained a large number of bacilli, as if, as a result of the injections, an enormous multiplication had taken place. In a fatal case of uro-genital tuberculosis, injections of tuberculin were followed by cough and an increase in the number of bacilli in the urine. The autopsy disclosed cheesy cystitis, ureteritis, old tuberculous pyelo-nephritis on the right, florid pyelo-nephritis on the left, with an eruption of fresh miliary tubercles in the mucous membrane of the pelvis of the kidney. The lungs contained small cavities, groups of gray or yellow nodules and miliary or submiliary tubercles. The spleen and liver contained miliary tubercles. In a fatal case of advanced phthisis, the autopsy revealed a general miliary tuberculosis, with tuberculous meningitis. In the case of a girl, three years old, with an ulcer of one cornea and purulent infiltration of the other, terminating fatally, a croupous exudation was found in the pharynx and larynx, together with a miliary tuberculosis. New nodules developed, in some cases, around older foci of disease. Tuberculous ulceration of the stomach was observed in two cases. Perforation of the pleura and pneumothorax were observed once. In numerous cases pulmonary cavities and intestinal ulcers presented evidences of a tendency to heal.

Untoward Effects in Tuberculosis of Bones.

Braun (*Deutsche med. Wochenschrift*, 1891), before the Verein für Wissenschaftliche Heilkunde, at Königsberg, reported the results of treatment in surgical cases by means of the Koch fluid, covering a period of ten weeks. Adults, with external tuberculosis, in whom pulmonary involvement could not be detected, were given 0.01, children 0.005. Subsequently, the quantity was reduced to 0.005 and 0.003 respectively. Injections were repeated at intervals of two days. Other than transient redness or swelling, there were no local complications. Of 198 injections, in 92 the ascent of the fever-curve began in from five to seven hours; in 49 during the first four hours; in 43 between the seventh and tenth hour; and in only 7, later. The elevation of temperature in all cases was decided. Its duration varied from two to fifty-two hours. The pulse was usually accelerated. In the case of two children, the pulse was slowed and the temperature became subnormal. Headache was a pretty constant phenomenon. Chills occurred after eighty injections out of seven hundred. Cough and shortness of breath were present even when no pulmonary lesion existed. Vomiting, abdominal pain and diarrhœa were occasionally noted. Of 56 patients, 7 had herpes of the lips and cheek; in 10, other exanthemata appeared. In 4 cases an erysipelatoid eruption developed. Constitutional phenomena did not manifest themselves in all cases. Alarming collapse took place in one patient. The local manifestations were not constant. The swelling of an affected joint usually increased; occasionally it diminished. Existing sinuses sometimes closed rapidly. At times secretion was diminished, at others increased. To determine the diagnostic value of the remedy, injections of 0.01 were made in 33 patients in whom tuberculosis could not be detected, and thermometric observations made at intervals of two hours. Fever appeared in 10, but in slight degree. In exceptionally rare cases of tuberculosis injection was not followed by fever. This was demonstrated in a child with inflammation of the knee-joints, the tuberculous nature of which was proved by microscopical examination after an operation performed subsequently. It may be stated that, when local changes occur in a sinus or other evidence of bone or joint disease of doubtful character, following injection of 0.005 or of 0.01 of the Koch fluid, the disease may be considered to be tuberculous; while the absence of local changes, notwithstanding the possible occurrence of slight fever, excludes tuberculosis.

Of 7 cases of lupus treated, complete recovery took place in but one. In a second, recovery appeared to have taken place, but the cicatrix reopened. In two others there was decided improvement. One case obstinately resisted treatment. The results in 5 cases of tuberculosis of the vertebræ and of the pelvis were not good. In one, a latent osteo-myelitis was stimulated into activity. Four cases of hip-joint disease, without sinuses, improved. To prevent contractures the patients were kept in bed and extension employed. In cases of tuberculosis of the knee-joint, the swelling was usually aggravated, in one case to such a degree as to render incision necessary. The results were more favorable when sinuses existed. The sinuses closed speedily and the joints became relaxed and more mobile. In some instances the cure was facilitated by scraping. In one case, an anal fistule, the result of tuberculous ulceration of the rectum, was uninfluenced by the injections. In another, of tuberculosis of the epididymis, improvement at first appeared to take place, the enlargement diminishing, subsequently, however, becoming greater than it previously had been. The injections were discontinued because headache and vertigo raised the suspicion of tubercles in the brain or membranes. In cases in which resection had been performed some little time previously, early injections were followed by fever without local reaction. In the case of a boy, however, in whom a coxitis had been cured by resection two years previously, two injections were followed by fever and by redness and swelling at the site of operation. In a case of multiple osteomyelitis, with swelling of one hand, gangrene of the tips of the fingers of the same hand took place. In another case, in which resection of the knee-joint was performed, gangrene of the foot ensued.

ABSCESS; GLANDULAR ENLARGEMENTS; REMITTENT FEVER.

KIRCHHEIM (*Deutsche medicinische Wochenschrift*, 1891) presented to the Medical Society of Frankfort the results of his experience with the Koch fluid, and discussed certain questions related to the treatment. In one case, notwithstanding most careful asepsis, an abscess formed at the site of injection. The injections were made in cases in all stages of tuberculosis, except when death was imminent. With a single exception, febrile patients were not subjected to the treatment. In the case with hectic fever, after injections of from 0.003 to 0.005, with decided elevation of temperature, infiltrations of hitherto uninvaded pulmonary tissue, with consonating râles, could be detected, which phenomena disappeared in from twenty-four to forty-eight hours. In almost all other cases increase in weight was noted. This was especially marked in a man seventy years of age, who, during seven weeks, living under unchanged conditions, gained sixteen pounds in weight. In several cases of slight apical involvement, mostly in young persons, small doses early in the treatment, were followed by enlargement of the glands in various parts of the body, especially in the axillary and inguinal regions, occasionally in the submaxillary region. In one case, in spite of withdrawal of the injections, a mild, remittent fever continued for eight days, corresponding to so-called glandular fever. The swellings disappeared in the course of the treatment. In two cases, herpes of the cornea, without injection of the conjunctiva, developed and disappeared without local treatment. Kirchheim believes the reaction following injection a direct result of the action of the fluid, rather than an evidence of absorption of breaking-down tuberculous tissue. By a gradual increase in dosage, tolerance is established — the system accommodates itself to the action of the remedy. If a long interval be permitted to elapse between injections, treatment must be renewed with smaller doses. Even healthy individuals react to large doses. A tendency to cumulative action has not yet been demonstrated. The part which the reactionary fever plays in the curative effect is interesting. Fever is thought to be the means provided by nature for recovery from infectious diseases. Applying the principle to treatment by the Koch fluid, the intervals between injections would be made longer and the doses rapidly increased. Such a course, however, would be too dangerous to be maintained.

In the case of lupus or accessible surgical tuberculosis, the injections may be continued in increasing doses as long as local reaction or improvement takes place. In case of pulmonary tuberculosis, treatment may be withdrawn when the subjective condition has become good, cough and expectoration have almost entirely ceased, bacilli are no longer present in the urine and a dose of 0.05 has been reached. In febrile pulmonary cases, in which, though a dose of 0.05 has been reached, no improvement in the objective condition has taken place and the sputum and presence of bacilli are variable, Kirchheim would rapidly run the dose up to 0.01, until further experience demonstrates the unwisdom of such a course.

ENCOURAGING RESULT IN LUPUS OF THE NOSE AND THROAT.

KRAUSE (*Deutsche medicinische Wochenschrift*, 1891), before the Verein für Innere Medicin, at Berlin, presented a case of lupus of the nose, gums, tongue and hard and soft palate, of four years' standing, in a woman, twenty-two years of age. Previous treatment had been only partially successful. On January 12th, treatment was begun with injections of the Koch fluid, the initial dose being 0.005. The reaction was intense, the affected parts becoming greatly swollen and new ulcers forming. The temperature rose to 104° after each of four subsequent injections. After the sixth, the temperature reached only 99.1°, and subsequently never more than 100.4°. At the end of the fifth week fourteen injections had been given and the dose reached was 0.06. The changes in the diseased areas were characteristic. Infiltrated nodules, however, remained, which may require surgical interference. Twelve pounds in weight were lost in three weeks, of which four pounds had since been regained. The loss of weight was due not only to the fever but also to the difficulty of swallowing in consequence of the great swelling of the parts. The result, while not complete or perfect, was encouraging.

BATCH OF GOOD AND BAD RESULTS.

Before the Berlin Medical Society, LASSAR (*Deutsche med. Wochenschr.*, 1891) presented a girl, thirteen years of age, who, for two years, had had a tuberculous ulcer, as large as the palm of the hand, on the extensor surface of the left thigh, which, in the course of about four weeks, after a number of injections of small quantities of the Koch fluid, cleared up and closed completely.

FLATAU presented a case of tuberculosis of the larynx, in which, after the eighteenth injection of 0.06, an eruption of acute miliary and submiliary tubercles developed in the larynx.

VIRCHOW presented the lungs of a man who had received twelve injections in the course of six weeks. At the end of this time there was continuous fever, and death occurred seventeen days subsequently. The lungs presented the picture of "black phthisis." There was extensive carnification, discolored by deposits of coal-dust, the interlobular septa presenting a grayish network. Two-thirds of one lung and somewhat less of the other were involved in the process. Within this tissue what would be called a dissecting pneumonia had developed. Large suppurating fissures had formed, while the adjacent tissue was transformed into masses almost cheesy. Microscopically, these masses were found to contain tubercle bacilli and to consist principally of amorphous matter. Nowhere could the beginning of a cheesy hepatization be found. The only appearances indicative of such a beginning were found in small areas at the periphery of the lobules, where the alveoli were filled with epithelial cells undergoing fatty metamorphosis. In a second case, which illustrated the transition from simple hepatization to gangrene, thirty injections were given in the course of twelve weeks. Death took place after a large cavity with pleural adhesions had formed. To this was added fresh hepatization in the lower lobe, in which unusually rapid and extensive breaking down of tissue, with the formation of cavities, was going on. In the intestine beyond the ileo-cæcal valve were an extraordinarily large number of ulcers, in the cæcum and ascending colon in part confluent, and all, Virchow expressed his satisfaction in saying, clearing up and in process of healing. A third case presented a combination of syphilis, phthisis and amyloid degeneration. But two injections, of 0.001 and 0.005 respectively, had been given. In addition to extensive florid phthisis, there was an exquisitely healed syphilis of the larynx, with extensive destruction of the margins of the epiglottis and the formation of deep cicatrices; the tonsils were also atrophied. In a child with tuberculous caries of the right hip, no signs of pulmonary disease were at first detected. Resection of the head of the femur was followed by an apparently good result. Subsequently, fifteen injections of the Koch fluid were made in the course of fourteen days. The autopsy disclosed an intense miliary tuberculosis, especially well marked in the medulla of the right femur, in the lungs and in the liver. In the region of the arytenoid cartilages, on either side, were deep perichondritic ulcers, the rest of the larynx being intact.

GRABOWER stated that his experience led him to believe that the development of gray miliary tubercles in places hitherto uninvaded was not a contra-indication for the continuance of the treatment. He presented two cases in which such nodules had appeared in the hitherto healthy larynx. In one, they disappeared in the course of treatment; in the other they were in process of disappearance. Transference of diseased tissue is to be expected in a curative process completed by absorption, but the process ought to exercise the greatest influence upon these new formations, as has been demonstrated in the larynx. The occurrence of new nodules becomes thus not a contra-indication, but an urgent indication for the continuance of the treatment.

JOLLY discussed the psychoses caused by the fever resulting from the injections, and reported three illustrative cases. In one, the injections had been made for two weeks, with considerable febrile reaction and delirium, following which a psychosis, lasting two weeks, developed. This is a so-called "fever-psychosis," of the variety which occurs after the decline of fevers, and known as collapse-delirium or delirium of defervescence, or epicritic or post-critic delirium. Such conditions are occasionally observed after all fevers e. g., after prolonged fever occurring in the course of tuberculosis. The predisposing cause in the case in question was the mental depression in connection with the disease. The second case was in a feeble-minded individual, who stuttered and was hard of hearing. Relatively mild febrile reaction induced the psychosis in his case, which took a melancholic-hypochondriac type. The third case illustrated the correspondence of the action of the artificial fever with that of natural fever. The patient had formerly had hysterical attacks. Following an abortion, a rapid phthisis developed. During and following the fever there was delirium, which ceased with the fever. Then, when the injections produced fever the delirium returned. Such conditions do not counter-indicate the treatment, but they admonish caution.

HENOCH expressed himself as disappointed with- the results of the treatment. Of twenty children, including only two or three in an advanced stage, but without fever, many became worse; hectic fever developed in those who previously had no fever; the children wasted. Great care was exercised and the smallest doses were used. In a single case, in which the disease was checked and apparent improvement resulted, the condition subsequently became worse than it originally had been. The bad results are probably ascribable to anatomical conditions. In children, tuberculosis, as a rule, has a wider distribution than in adults; the glands, especially the bronchial glands, are rarely uninvolved.

PARACENTESIS OF THE THECA VERTEBRALIS IN TUBERCULAR MENINGITIS FOR THE RELIEF OF FLUID PRESSURE.

DR. W. ESSEX WYNTER (*Lancet*, No. 3531) has performed this operation on four occasions at the Middlesex Hospital, in cases where coma supervened with great rapidity, in the hope of relieving cerebral pressure by draining away cerebro-spinal fluid continuously by the theca vertebralis.

Case I. Boy aged five years. Coma on eighth day. A fine Southey's trocar and canula inserted close to the spine of the second lumbar vertebra, until the point touched the lamina, when it was diverted downward and inward through the ligamentum sub-flavum and theca. Clear fluid welled up at once on withdrawing the trocar, and more than four drachms of fluid escaped during the next twenty-four hours. The Cheyne-Stokes rhythm gave place to regular breathing, the color improved, and the child was enabled to swallow. The improvement was not maintained; the fluid ceased to run, and the case terminated fatally. Post-mortem there was considerable tubercle at the base, with opaque lymph, but no excess of fluid. The prick in the theca was not discoverable, and there was no evidence of damage to the cauda equina.

Case II. Girl aged eleven years. Coma on ninth day. The theca was punctured with a fine knife at the level of the second lumbar spine. Clear fluid escaped with some force, and a small drainage-tube was inserted and an antiseptic dressing applied. Next day the temperature had fallen to normal and the child could be roused. The dressings were saturated with fluid and changed. On the third day the fluid ceased to escape and death occurred next day from coma. After death the aperture in the theca was found to have closed, and when the membrane was incised fluid spurted out in quantity. There was very little meningeal tubercle.

Case III. Boy aged two years and four months. Coma on fourteenth day. Theca opened at level of first lumbar vertebra, when several drachms of fluid escaped, the flow being increased with each inspiration. A drainage-tube was inserted. On the escape of the fluid the pupils, formerly dilated and inactive, contracted and regained their reflex activity at once. Twelve drachms of clear alkaline fluid were obtained, having a specific gravity of 1004, containing a large quantity of chlorides, but giving no reaction to tests for albumin and sugar. The child died five hours after the operation.

Case IV. Girl aged thirteen months. Ailing fourteen days. Semi-conscious on admission, with irregular breathing, sunken fontanelle, and well-marked *tache cérébrale*. Two days later convulsions occurred. Four ounces of cerebro-spinal fluid were withdrawn by a Southey's tube between two lumbar spines, the last two ounces being blood-stained. Death occurred the same day. The prick in the theca was not visible, but there was slight extravasation of blood on its outer surface. The cauda equina was unhurt. There was extensive general tuberculosis.

Though none of the cases were successful, no harm in any one resulted from interference. To some there was temporary relief of the symptoms, and the necropsy in each case showed ample reason for the fatal termination.

SURGERY.

UNDER THE CHARGE OF

J. WILLIAM WHITE, M.D.,

PROFESSOR OF CLINICAL SURGERY IN THE UNIVERSITY OF PENNSYLVANIA; SURGEON TO THE
UNIVERSITY AND GERMAN HOSPITALS;

ASSISTED BY

EDWARD MARTIN, M.D.,

CLINICAL PROFESSOR OF GENITO-URINARY SURGERY IN THE UNIVERSITY OF PENNSYLVANIA; SURGEON
TO THE HOWARD HOSPITAL AND ASSISTANT SURGEON TO THE UNIVERSITY HOSPITAL.

SPONGES AND THEIR USES IN SURGERY.

After a careful consideration of the methods of preparing sponges in commerce, MAYLAND (*Annals of Surgery*, vol. xiii., No. 5), incited thereto by two cases of septic poisoning occurring in his practice, carefully considers the best methods of rendering sponges absolutely sterile.

He finds that sponges of close texture, even if soaked in a solution of carbolic acid up to the strength of 1 to 40, are not rendered sterile throughout. The central portions of such sponges, if planted upon nutrient gelatin, show abundant growths of putrefactive microbes. Again, the ordinary surgical sponge, impregnated with foul discharges and thoroughly cleansed with a solution of carbolic acid, likewise exhibits, when implanted upon nutrient gelatin, abundant growths. If, however, a solution of 1 to 2000 bichloride of mercury is employed, such sponges remain entirely sterile. He considers the small cut Turkey sponges the best, because, though their texture is close, their shape prevents them from being anywhere so thick as to prevent the thorough penetration of the antiseptic solutions.

The question of the proper manner to store sponges is one of extreme importance. A number of sponges were kept for nine months, some in a solution of 1 to 20 carbolic, others in a solution of 1 to 500 bichloride. Both sets were darkened, but neither suffered in consistence, and even by microscopical examination no changes in texture could be detected. The sponges will in time darken, not from being actually dirty, but from the process of pigmentation. It would seem, then, that after the sponges have been thoroughly cleansed, storing in 1 to 500 bichloride solution renders them absolutely sterile and does not impair their useful qualities.

The author has usually employed the hyposulphite process in preparing sponges; that is, the sponges are first steeped in a hydrochloric acid solution, 1 to 10, then immersed in a bath composed of hyposulphite of soda one part, hydrochloric acid two parts, water twelve parts. This solution is then pressed out, and the sponges are well washed in cold water. They are finally placed in a bath containing half an ounce of carbonate of potash.

Objection is raised to using the sponges more than once, since while it is quite possible to render a septic sponge aseptic, there is no means of knowing whether or not ptomaines or toxic albumoses may be present, and there is no known agent which can be relied on to counteract the possible toxic effect of such substances.

RESECTION OF THE APPENDIX VERMIFORMIS DURING THE QUIESCENT STAGE OF CHRONIC RELAPSING APPENDICITIS.

WEIR (*Annals of Surgery*, vol. xiii., No. 5), after a careful study of the reported cases of operation upon the appendix vermiformis during the intervals of attack, sums up his ideas upon the subject as follows:

1. That the final outcome of the review of these cases has been that the large majority of recurrent attacks are due to catarrhal appendicitis, which, though to an unknown degree capable of producing explosive and serious peritoneal inflammation, yet generally, from the lumen of the tube being previously shut off from the cæcum, limits correspondingly the chances of fecal or severe infection of the peritoneum.

2. That the simple catarrhal appendicitis can be suspected when the recurrences are frequent—that is to say, more than four or five times, as in the acute processes this is seldom exceeded—and when such attacks are not of a severe type, nor of greater duration than a week, and particularly so if there be no appearance of a distinct tumor.

3. In such cases delay in operating may be encouraged to a reasonable extent, at least until it is indubitably proven that the invalidism is a confirmed one. Out of five cases seen by Weir in the last year for recurrent attacks of appendicitis, in three, of the above-described simple form, it was advised to wait till the next acute attack presented itself as a further justification of surgical interference; but this did not occur in any of these. In the two others, from the persistent invalidism or the severity of some of the attacks, an operation was advised.

4. Where a tumor is present in the quiescent stage, or has been decidedly felt after the acuteness of the attack has passed off, more urgency is present, as it indicates, it is believed, either an accumulation of noxious contents or

of ulceration within the appendix, or an already present small perforation. It is in such cases that Mackenzie says that we can expect, if an acute process is subsequently set up, that it will be a circumscribed rather than a general suppurative peritonitis. The frequent conjunction, in the collected cases, of adhesions with the severer forms of the catarrhal appendicitis with retained secretions or with minute perforations, seems to corroborate this view.

5. That as the diagnosis of the separate condition of simple catarrhal appendicitis and its complications of distention from retained fluids and of ulceration, are not at present to be differentially diagnosticated, and as it has been shown that each case can give rise to dangerous conditions, recurrences of severity and frequency should hereafter mean that an exploratory laparotomy should be resorted to, on the general principle of this being of less risk than the disease itself.

———

THE TREATMENT OF HYDATID DISEASE BY INCISION AND EVACUATION OF THE CYST WITHOUT DRAINAGE.

BOND (*British Medical Journal*, No. 1580), while conceding that all hydatid cysts in which suppuration has taken place should be treated by incision and drainage, believes that for cysts which are still living and growing, and which contain clear fluid with or without daughter cysts, incision and evacuation of the cyst contents without any subsequent drainage, or with only temporary drainage for a few hours after the operation, is a procedure which deserves prominence in the minds of surgeons. He reports a case in point. There was a large cyst situated between the bladder and rectum beneath the peritoneum; this had grown upward, filling the pelvis and blocking the bladder and the urethra. The bladder was dragged up till its fundus reached to within two inches of the umbilicus.

The cyst was at first aspirated. Three weeks later it was treated by incision. The elastic cyst proper had separated from the outer cyst wall and lay loose in the cavity, together with much pus and several smaller daughter cysts. The elastic membrane and contents were removed entirely. The cavity was sponged out and a large drainage-tube was inserted. On exploring the general peritoneal cavity, a small cyst about the size of an orange was found in the reflection of the peritoneum in the right iliac fossa. This was incised, and the elastic membrane and clear fluid were removed. The remains of the cyst were then returned into the peritoneal cavity. At a subsequent operation no trace of this cyst could be found. A third large cyst was noticed in the epigastric region, but was left for subsequent treatment.

Five months later, on examination, the cyst in the epigastrium was the size of a fœtal head, and there was another cyst in the lower part and to the left of the abdominal cavity. The abdomen was opened by median incision, passing through the umbilicus, and three cysts were discovered; these were incised. As a result of this the white elastic cyst proper shrunk somewhat away from the walls or ectocyst, and lay, together with daughter cysts, in the cavity. It was easily withdrawn with ring forceps, although, from its brittleness, in several pieces. One omental cyst was removed entire, after tapping, by ligaturing that portion of the omentum to which it grew. The two cysts treated by removal of the walls were drained for sixteen hours.

As a result of experience in these cases, Bond concludes that when there is difficulty in bringing the cyst wall to the surface of the body, provided due care be taken to evacuate the cavity of all the fluid and elastic contents, the inverted edges of the incision into the cyst may be sutured, and the whole may be returned into the abdominal cavity. Hemorrhage will probably not occur unless it is occasioned by interference with the outer wall or ectocyst. Sutures should be applied to the inverted opening to prevent the entrance of a coil of intestine. Cysts of the liver and other organs are apparently amenable to the same treatment. The elastic lining shrinks on withdrawing the fluid, and can be drawn out by means of gentle traction with forceps. Even in suppurating cysts in which drainage is necessary, it is important to remove the solid contents at the time of incision.

The Operative Treatment of Rectal Cancer.

In a brief but very excellent résumé of this subject, THORNDIKE (*Boston Medical and Surgical Journal,* vol. cxxiv., No 19) reviews the methods of operation for malignant disease of the rectum. From the study of a large number of statistics he finds that excision of the rectum from below gives a mortality of about 15 per cent., and that about 10 per cent. of the cases which survive the operation are permanently cured. Only those cases in which the examining finger in the rectum easily reaches the upper limit of the disease are subject to operation from below.

Kraske, by approaching the seat of disease from behind, instead of from below, has greatly extended the possibilities of complete extirpation of cancerous disease, even when the bowel is involved high up. By enucleation of . the coccyx and the removal of a small portion of the lower part of the sacrum, he secures a large opening which affords ample opportunity to view the rectum and to work upon it. If the anal portion of the bowel is involved, and the disease is not very extensive, a resection is readily performed. The two ends of the bowel may then be brought together in front, the posterior opening being left to be closed by secondary operation. Or the following plan, devised by Hochenegg, may be adopted: The upper segment of the bowel may be telescoped through the lower, and may be held in this position by a double row of sutures, one row above the anus and the second row about the margin of the anus. If the anal portion of the gut has been removed, an artificial anus must be formed. In this case the bowel involved is brought out through the sacral opening, the wound being allowed to heal with a drainage-tube packed into it. The sacral anus is provided with a pad made by Leiter, which does its work so thoroughly that patients are exceedingly comfortable while wearing it.

Ligation of the Saphena Magna for Varicose Veins of the Lower Extremity.

TRENDELENBURG (*Beitr. zur klin. Chir.,* Bd. vii., Heft 1, and *Rundschau,* 32 Jahr., Heft 5) recommends as an exceedingly efficient treatment in certain cases of varicose dilatation of the veins of the leg, where this dilatation affects not only the branches of the vein but the main trunk also, ligature of the saphena magna. Before operating the surgeon must assure himself that the dilated trunk is the only one which carries the blood from the parts below, since very frequently there are two principal branches of the saphena, which, if both are so widely dilated that the valves are incompetent, must both be tied before any amelioration can be expected. The best place to perform this ligation is about the middle of the thigh. An incision an inch long is made in this region; the vein is exposed, a double ligature is applied, and the vessel is divided between. As a result, the blood is carried from the superficial portions of the limb by the deep communicating veins. The improvement is immediate and permanent. Long lasting varicose ulcers heal quickly after this operation. Frequently the varices do not entirely disappear, but the condition is always greatly improved. Of course, this method of operating requires the most careful application of antisepsis.

EXTIRPATION OF THE LARYNX.

TAUBER (*Archiv f. klin. Chir.*, Bd. xli., Heft 3) has tabulated 163 cases of extirpation of the larynx, and has analyzed his tables with typical German minuteness. As a general result he finds that the operation is followed by death in 69.9 per cent. of all cases. Permanent cure—that is, failure of the disease to return for three years after operation—is noted in 7.9 per cent. of the cured cases. It is a well-known fact that in Spencer Wells's hands ovariotomy gave a mortality of 70 per cent., and that by improvement in technique this mortality has fallen to less than 4 per cent. There is little hope held out by Tauber that a similar improvement in the results of laryngectomy may be expected, since the percentage of death is the same now as it was ten years ago.

It would seem from this study that laryngectomy is an operation which should not be performed, since even when from mechanical interference a tumor of the larynx threatens to produce a fatal result, tracheotomy will afford immediate relief, and there is about as much assurance against recidivity as is afforded by complete extirpation of the larynx, at least in such cases as are far advanced.

BARDENHEUER (*Ibid.*) takes quite an opposite view of this operation. He believes that he has so improved the technique that the mortality will be greatly lowered, and instances, in proof of this fact, that while his first four patients died immediately following the operation, the last four, treated by a different method, all recovered. He found that the patients died not immediately after the removal of the tumor, but in from eight to four days, and that the mortality was due to septic inflammation, usually beginning in the deepest portion of the wound, in the space between the trachea and the surrounding muscular tissues. From this position inflammation extended along the loose cellular tissue of the neck into the mediastinum, and death usually resulted from septicæmia and pneumonia. The cause of infection was usually penetration of the liquid food and of the secretions of the mouth into the deeper portions of the wound. Bardenheuer modified his laryngectomies by attempting to sterilize the mouth for several days before operation.

The teeth were subjected to repeated frictions with antiseptic solutions, and the mucous membrane was dried with salicylic cotton. His next modification consisted in so placing the patient after operation that secretions of the mouth could not drain into the wound. The mattress was so arranged that the head was extended backward, and the pharynx was on a lower level than the cavity made by extirpating the diseased trachea; hence fluids gravitated to the mouth, and not away from it. His final modification consisted in carefully respecting the anterior wall of the œsophagus and the mucous membrane of the trachea immediately below the epiglottis, so far as it was healthy. After removal of all the diseased portions, the anterior wall of the œsophagus was brought forward and stitched to the mucous membrane of the trachea, thus forming a septum between the mouth and the wound cavity. Further, the free edge of the epiglottis was freshened and stitched back to the anterior wall of the œsophagus. The cavity of the wound was then firmly packed with sterilized gauze, and the dressing was changed in from two to eight days, depending upon the length of time the stitches held. Frequently the patient was able to swallow, thus relieving the operator of the necessity of passing an œsophageal tube. The sutures shutting the mouth from the wound cavity need not be left longer than fourteen days, since this is a sufficient time to allow of protective granulations being formed.

PALLIATIVE OPERATIONS IN CASES OF ENLARGED PROSTATE.

VIGNARD (*Annal des Malad. des Org. Génito-urin.*, vol. x., 1891; *Centralbl. f. Chir.*, No. 10, 1891) believes that in the very great majority of cases of hypertrophy of the prostate, bloodless therapeutic measures are sufficient. He would recommend surgical intervention—that is, puncture of the bladder or supra-pubic cystotomy, or the boutonnière operation—only in cases of retention where catheterization is impossible, and where septic urine absolutely requires evacuation; in cases where great difficulty in passing the catheter is not relieved by permanent catheterization; and in cases of cystitis not relieved by careful and long-continued medication. In the first two instances the boutonnière operation is indicated, whilst where cystitis is present supra-pubic cystotomy should be practised.

OBSTETRICS.

UNDER THE CHARGE OF

EDWARD P. DAVIS, A.M., M.D.,

PROFESSOR OF OBSTETRICS AND DISEASES OF CHILDREN IN THE PHILADELPHIA POLYCLINIC;
CLINICAL LECTURER ON OBSTETRICS IN THE JEFFERSON MEDICAL COLLEGE;
VISITING OBSTETRICIAN TO THE PHILADELPHIA HOSPITAL, ETC

THE RELATION OF THE WEIGHT OF THE PLACENTA TO THE WEIGHT OF THE CHILD.

J. H. SMITH, Assistant in the Frauen-klinik, Munich, took the opportunity of searching the records of five hundred births to obtain statistics regarding

the relative weight of the child and the placenta: the results have been incorporated in a series of elaborate tables, from which he draws the following
conclusions:

The placenta being completed at the sixteenth week, a study of its relative
size may begin appropriately at the seventeenth week. In the cases observed,
the average weight of the placenta to that of the child was one-third from
the seventeenth to the thirty-second week. Between the thirty-second and
thirty-third week the placenta attained its acme of weight, and remained stationary at this point unless influenced by derangements of the fœtal ciren-
lation, until birth at the fortieth week. Thus, during the thirty-third and
thirty-fourth week the ratio remains one-third ; during the thirty-fifth, thirty-
sixth, and thirty-seventh weeks, it is one-fourth; in the thirty-eighth and
thirty-ninth, one-fifth ; and at the end of the thirty-ninth, two-ninths. From
the end of the thirty-ninth week until birth, whether labor occurs at the
fortieth week or is delayed until the forty-fourth, the ratio remains one-fifth.
After the fortieth week, the placenta seems to grow rapidly in multiparæ, or
with women having large children, thereby raising the average from one-fifth
to one-fourth.

A Case of Retro-peritoneal Pregnancy.

JAGGARD (*American Journal of Obstetrics*, April, 1891) describes a case of
retro-peritoneal pregnancy in the seventh month as follows: The pregnancy was the first, the patient suffering during the entire time from pain
and weakness. The size and shape of the abdomen were suggestive of twin
pregnancy; the uterus did not exhibit the usual signs of pregnancy, and the
woman's condition was so serious as to render operation impossible. Transfusion of twenty ounces of salt solution was performed, and it was determined
to wait, hoping for an increase in the strength of the patient; she became
able to leave her bed and seemed to be gaining ; on the ninth day symptoms
of septic infection manifested themselves and the tumor became emphysematous. It was determined to dilate the cervix and version was performed,
with the extraction of a macerated fœtus. The placenta was half adherent
and half detached ; death followed soon after the operation. A post-mortem
examination was immediately made; it was then discovered that the pregnancy originally developed in the right broad ligament, the ovum passed up
into the abdomen behind the peritoneum. Death of the fœtus, with placental hemorrhage, was caused by exertion. The dilator employed to dilate
the cervix had ruptured the posterior wall of the lower uterine segment and
opened into the fœtal sac.

Intra- and Extra-uterine Pregnancy occurring Coincidently in the Same Patient.

The unusual coincidence of normal and ectopic pregnancy is illustrated in a
case reported by WORRALL, in the *Medical Press*, page 296, 1891. The patient
was a multipara who was awakened at night by severe abdominal pain, followed by slight hemorrhage ; she recovered her health, the abdomen enlarged,
and she was told that she was pregnant; the tumor gradually decreased in
size and menstruation returned ; when examined, the abdominal tumor was

found composed of two parts, one the uterus with a living fœtus, the other, probably, an ectopic fœtus. Upon laparotomy, a dead fœtus was found in the abdomen, which had developed in the posterior layer of the broad ligament; it was removed and the sac stitched to the abdominal incision. The next day labor came on and the intra-uterine fœtus was delivered; the patient recovered, the sac being drained and irrigated by an antiseptic fluid. The case is of an especial interest, as one in which intra- and extra-uterine pregnancy occurred concurrently.

THE TREATMENT OF PREMATURE DETACHMENT OF THE NORMALLY SITUATED PLACENTA.

FOUR cases of this abnormality are reported by MEYER (*Correspondenzblatt für Schweizer Aerzte*, No. 7, 1891). His experience leads him to believe that these cases are best treated by avoiding the rupture of the membranes, thereby maintaining the tension of the uterine muscle and preventing bleeding, while the physician should watch his patient until dilatation is so far advanced that speedy labor is possible. These cases demand close attention. When the mouth of the uterus is as large as a dollar, and the cervix is obliterated, the membranes may be ruptured if the condition of the patient justifies it; active measures may be taken to terminate labor after delivery. Special precaution should be taken to empty the uterus of all its contents, and to bring about firm uterine contraction.

PERNICIOUS VOMITING AND PTYALISM OF PREGNANCY AS HYSTERO-NEUROSES.

AHLFELD advances the theory, in the *Centralblatt für Gynäkologie*, No. 17, 1891, that pernicious vomiting and ptyalism of pregnancy are hystero-neuroses of reflex nature. He has treated such cases successfully by measures adapted for the cure of neuroses, removing all possible irritants from the patient, and using sedatives addressed to the nervous system.

stage in which exact diagnosis as to the degree and probable severity of th infection is difficult; during this stage the sharp curette is the most inappro priate of instruments, antiseptic injections being much more suitable an efficient.

GOTTSCHALK discussed the question from the standpoint of bacteriology remarking that Braun, who introduced the curette in obstetric practice, ad vised its use in sapræmia and not in septicæmia and pyæmia.

He recognized the difficulty of making a differential diagnosis in a give case between these conditions, and, furthermore, when such a diagnosis made, the abrasion of tissue produced by the curette was extremely injuriou. In the unmolested uterus the conditions are not favorable for septic absorp tion; saprophytic products are not injurious to living cells, and are safel removed by the lochia. At the placental site but little mucous membrane left to harbor bacteria.

Curetting removes thrombi from sinuses and favors the absorption of cor

FIVE HUNDRED LABORS WITHOUT INTERNAL DISINFECTION.

MERMANN completes his account of a series of 500 labors without an internal disinfection, in the *Centralblatt für Gynäkologie*, No. 20, 1891. In the 500 cases there occurred no death from sepsis or its complications. In the last 200 cases a vaginal douche was given once, in a case of placenta prævia which had been tamponed before admission to the hospital. The complications of pregnancy and labor are all fairly represented in the series, and with surprisingly good results. The only precaution taken against ophthalmia was irrigating the eyes with distilled water; but one case, and that a mild one, occurred.

Mermann employs scrupulous cleanliness and antisepsis externally. but none internally, and limits vaginal examinations to the least possible number.

————

HEMORRHAGE FROM THE MEMBRANES DURING LABOR.

BALLANTYNE (*Edinburgh Medical Journal*, No. 581, p. 1006, 1891) reports the case of a primipara who had uterine hemorrhage during the first stage of labor; examination failed to reveal any cause for the hemorrhage; labor proceeding, slight hemorrhage occurred and the patient was delivered spontaneously of a small and feebly developed fœtus. A slight amount of hemorrhage followed the birth of the child, but no unusual bleeding occurred after' the delivery of the placenta; the child perished of heart failure soon after birth. During the lying-in state slight fever occurred on the second and third day, with an attack of urticaria and painful swelling of the breasts.

When the placenta and membranes were examined the placenta showed a small apoplexy with areas of fibroid thickening; around the aperture where the membranes ruptured there was a vascular zone varying in breadth from three-quarters of an inch to two inches; the bloodvessels of this zone were situated either in the chorion or in the shreds of the decidua attached to its surface. Two primitive villi were found in this zone; an intra-mural fibroid was found in the lower segment of the uterus, which may have favored the hemorrhage by maintaining a vascular condition of the parts.

examination was immediately made, it was that——————
nancy originally developed in the right broad ligament, the ovum passed up into the abdomen behind the peritoneum. Death of the fœtus, with placental hemorrhage, was caused by exertion. The dilator employed to dilate the cervix had ruptured the posterior wall of the lower uterine segment and opened into the fœtal sac.

————

INTRA- AND EXTRA-UTERINE PREGNANCY OCCURRING COINCIDENTLY IN THE SAME PATIENT.

The unusual coincidence of normal and ectopic pregnancy is illustrated in a case reported by WORRALL, in the *Medical Press*, page 296, 1891. The patient was a multipara who was awakened at night by severe abdominal pain, followed by slight hemorrhage; she recovered her health, the abdomen enlarged, and she was told that she was pregnant; the tumor gradually decreased in size and menstruation returned; when examined, the abdominal tumor was cm. at eight months, with 7½ cm. at seven and a half months, and with 7 cm. at seven months.

He has found the balloon dilator employed extensively by Tarnier most useful. He endeavors in induced labor to secure, if possible, a vertex presentation and a spontaneous labor, and where these conditions were present he lost no mothers and but one child in twenty-four cases. In cases where delivery was accompanied by forceps, breech extraction or version, nearly one-half of the children perished.

CURETTING THE PUERPERAL UTERUS.

The subject of the advisability of the use of the curette after labor at term was discussed in a recent meeting of the Obstetrical Society of Berlin (*Centralblatt für Gynäkologie*, No. 18, 1891). FRITSCH had given the method of treatment by curetting a fair trial, but was convinced of the danger and injury accompanying the practice. He believed that recovery in cases of puerperal sepsis depended largely upon the encapsulation of the focus of infection, and this was prevented by the interference of the curette. The advocates of curetting consider it indicated in sapræmic cases, but the diagnosis of sapræmia is often impossible during the life of the patient.

OLSHAUSEN did not favor curetting the puerperal uterus on account of the danger of rupturing the uterus, which is greatly thinned after labor.

He considered the danger of accidents when the puerperal uterus is curetted with a sharp curette to be very great.

He also believed that in most cases septic infection gains entrance to the uterus through lesions in the cervix. Portions of the endometrium become involved at a time, rarely the whole. It is impossible with the curette to select the affected portion, and hence more harm than benefit may result from curetting.

VEIT narrated his observations with four cases where he had seen injury and a bad result follow curetting. He considered the proposition to treat the uterus in puerperal sepsis like an abscess cavity a distinct step backward, not an advance.

After the period of incubation there is in puerperal sepsis an indifferent stage in which exact diagnosis as to the degree and probable severity of the infection is difficult; during this stage the sharp curette is the most inappropriate of instruments, antiseptic injections being much more suitable and efficient.

GOTTSCHALK discussed the question from the standpoint of bacteriology, remarking that Braun, who introduced the curette in obstetric practice, advised its use in sapræmia and not in septicæmia and pyæmia.

He recognized the difficulty of making a differential diagnosis in a given case between these conditions, and, furthermore, when such a diagnosis is made, the abrasion of tissue produced by the curette was extremely injurious. In the unmolested uterus the conditions are not favorable for septic absorption; saprophytic products are not injurious to living cells, and are safely removed by the lochia. At the placental site but little mucous membrane is left to harbor bacteria.

Curetting removes thrombi from sinuses and favors the absorption of concentrated solutions of ptomaines, which are highly poisonous. Most rational and safe is the treatment of this condition by irrigating the uterus with sterilized water at 104° F. The heat stimulates the uterus to contract and expel poisonous materials, while the water dilutes the ptomaine solutions until they are innocuous.

GYNECOLOGY.

UNDER THE CHARGE OF
HENRY C. COE, M.D., M.R.C.S.,
OF NEW YORK.

THE ACTION OF ANTISEPTICS UPON THE PERITONEUM.

DELBET, GRANDMAISON, and BRESSET (*Annales de Gynécologie et d' Obstétrique*, 1891) as a result of their united experiments and observations, arrive at the following conclusions :

1. The strong antiseptics, such as carbolic and salicylic acids, corrosive sublimate and biniodide of mercury, present more disadvantages than advantages, since they irritate a healthy peritoneum and thus favor the formation of adhesions.

2. The most useful solutions to be employed in laparotomy are one of sodium chloride (six or seven parts to one thousand), and of boric acid (three parts to one hundred).

3. Iodoform and salol exert but little action upon the peritoneum, and it is a question if they have any antiseptic effect.

URETERO-VAGINAL FISTULA.

ALTHEN (Inaugural-dissertation, Munich, 1889; abstract in *Centralblatt für Gynäkologie*, 1890) analyzes thirty-five cases, the histories of three of which were recorded at Winckel's clinic, and finds that in the majority the condition could be traced to a previous severe instrumental delivery or operation, especially vaginal hysterectomy and the opening of pelvic abscesses. Ureteral fistulæ are to be distinguished etiologically as congenital, traumatic, and spontaneous. In twenty cases an operation was performed, only ten of which were successful.

TORSION OF THE PEDICLE IN OVARIAN CYSTS.

KÜSTNER (*Centralblatt für Gynäkologie*, 1891) has made a number of observations bearing on this interesting subject, and differs from other authors in his explanation of the etiology. In his last thirty-six ovariotomies he found in fourteen cases (38.8 per cent.) torsion of the pedicle up to at least 180°. Rokitansky records 13 per cent., Thornton 9.5 per cent., Olshausen 6.3 per cent., and Horwitz 23.2 per cent. He explains the greater frequency of this complication in the Dorpat clinic by the fact that in most of the cases inflammatory adhesions existed. In the majority of the cysts of the right ovary the torsion was toward the *left*, in those of the left ovary toward the *right*. His explanation is as follows: As soon as the tumor rises out of the pelvis and comes in contact with the abdominal wall it tends to fall forward, displacing the uterus backward. The ovarian ligament is now put on the stretch and crosses the tube, so that when the tumor lies in contact with the abdominal wall there is really a torsion of its pedicle to the extent of 90°, which is usually overlooked at the time of operation. If the pedicle is small, and the abdominal wall relaxed, changes in the centre of gravity of the tumor are readily produced by changes in the position of the patient; when she lies upon her left side it tends to rotate from right to left, since the infundibulo-pelvic ligament (which is its principal attachment) extends from the posterior wall of the pelvis anteriorly from right to left. The reverse is the case when she lies on her right side. This torsion is probably only temporary. After the neoplasm occupies the abdominal cavity the pressure of the intestines upon its posterior surface during peristalsis tends to increase the existing torsion; this pressure on the right side is exerted most upon the left side of the tumor and *vice versâ*. This theory was supported by a case of double ovariotomy of the writer's, in which the pedicle of the left tumor was twisted 180° to the right, and that of the right to the left.

THE TREATMENT OF UTERINE FIBROIDS ACCORDING TO APOSTOLI'S METHOD.

Two recent communications by well-known and successful abdominal surgeons are of considerable interest from the different conclusions at which the writers arrive.

KEITH (reprint from *British Medical Journal*) reports further progress in the electrical treatment of fibro-myomata. During the last three years and a half he has operated only upon fibro-cystic tumors, and believes that with care there ought never to be any doubt regarding the selection of proper cases. The best results are obtained in the case of small bleeding tumors of recent origin, which require shorter treatment than the old, large ones. He summarizes as follows: "This treatment *almost always* relieves pain. It *almost always* brings about diminution of the tumor—sometimes rapidly. It *almost always* stops hemorrhage—sometimes rapidly. The results are *almost always* permanent, and the growth of the tumor, if it be not lessened, is stopped. The general health is immensely improved. By '*almost always*,' I mean nineteen cases out of every twenty."

HOMANS (*Boston Medical and Surgical Journal*, 1891) records the results of his experience with the electrical treatment of uterine fibroids since December, 1887, including thirty-four cases, the subsequent histories of which were carefully traced. Of these the principal results noted were relief of pain and hemorrhage, and improvement in the general health. In ten cases the tumor continued to grow, in sixteen no change was noted, and in only two was there a marked diminution in its size; in the latter the menopause appeared soon after the cessation of the treatment. In general, he regards the treatment as merely symptomatic and rather unsatisfactory. It is not entirely devoid of danger, and is not capable of successful application by the general practitioner. " It may be inferred," he adds, after citing fourteen successful laparo-hysterectomies out of fifteen cases, "that I have found nothing sufficiently curative in electrolysis to make me lay down my knife and never take it up."

_____

INTESTINAL OBSTRUCTION AFTER OVARIOTOMY.

ANDERSON and HANDFIELD JONES (*Lancet*, 1890) report a case in which obstruction occurred seventeen days after operation. The abdomen was reopened three days later and a strong adhesion was found, attaching a coil of small intestine to the anterior abdominal wall. It was separated, the collapsed coil dilated, and the obstruction was overcome. The patient continued for a short time to have fecal vomiting, but eventually recovered. The writers distinguish two forms of obstruction following abdominal section, the first being almost immediate, the second developing after convalescence. In the first the symptoms are masked by those of peritonitis, and a secondary operation is usually fatal; in the second the diagnosis is easier and an operation promises relief. A second case is reported in which the obstruction was relieved twenty-five days after the primary operation.

COLLAS (Thèse de Paris, 1891) has collected twenty-three cases, eighteen of which followed ovariotomy. In eight cases a secondary operation was performed, four being successful. In fifteen the actual condition was only revealed at the autopsy. The symptoms of obstruction usually developed within ten days after operation, but in one instance six years elapsed. Peritonitic adhesions were the usual factors. The symptoms appeared suddenly and were not relieved by palliative treatment. The writer's deduction is that laparotomy offers the only positive means of relief.

_____

THE TREATMENT OF OSTEOMALACIA BY CASTRATION.

HOFMEIER (*Centralblatt für Gynäkologie*, No. 12, 1891) reports the case of a virgin, aged thirty years, who had osteomalacia of three years' standing, the disease being progressive at the time of operation, as shown by the presence of severe pains in the pelvic bones, inability to walk, and marked pelvic deformity. Menstruation regular and painless. Four weeks after removal of the ovaries the patient could walk without assistance, and the pains were much less severe. She received cod-liver oil and peptonate of iron; six weeks later she felt quite well, had no pain, and could walk a long distance. The pelvic organs were normal. The ovaries were atrophied, as in a woman after the menopause, and presented a similar appearance microscopically, only a few ovisacs being seen. The case was interesting, not only because the patient was a virgin (hence pregnancy could not be regarded as an etiological factor), and there was no disturbance of menstruation, or evidence of pelvic congestion.

As regards the effects of castration under such circumstances the writer admits, with Fehling, that it is impossible to give a satisfactory explanation. It may be due to some reflex action upon the vasomotor nerves supplying the nutrient vessels of the pelvic bones, the disease itself being regarded as a tropho-neurosis of the bones directly dependent upon ovarian activity. This theory receives additional support from a similar case reported by Truzzi. Fehling has collected twenty other cases of castration for osteomalacia, in none of which was there a failure on the part of the operator to secure at least a temporary benefit.

PARALYSIS FOLLOWING SUBCUTANEOUS INJECTIONS OF ETHER.

EBERHART (*Centralblatt für Gynäkologie*, No. 12, 1891) reports the following interesting case, which is of considerable interest to laparotomists, since ether is frequently used hypodermatically as a cardiac stimulant in cases of collapse during abdominal section.

In the course of an operation upon the cervix and perineum Eberhart's patient suddenly collapsed, whereupon two injections of ether were given, one on the anterior, and the other on the posterior aspect of the right forearm. The following day the patient had extensor paralysis of the middle, ring, and little fingers of the right hand, which disappeared in six weeks under faradization. It was inferred that a branch of the radial had been affected. Similar cases have been reported by Heymann, Mendel, and Remák; the latter attributes the paralysis to the direct irritation of the peripheral nerve by the ether. [We have long held the opinion that ether, although one of the most rapidly-acting cardiac stimulants, is too irritating for hypodermic use, even in emergencies in which it is invariably so employed. Even if paralysis does not result, persistent localized pain, paræsthesia, dermatitis, and abscesses are not infrequent results. We have found that deep injections of camphorated oil (one part to four), as recommended by the writer, were equally efficacious, and much less irritating.—ED.].

CYSTOPEXY.

TUFFIER (*Centralblatt für Gynäkologie*, No. 15, 1891) reported at the Société de Chirurgie several cases of cystocele treated by cystopexy, the technique of the operation being as follows: The bladder was first dilated with five ounces of boric acid solution, an incision two and one-half inches long was made in the hypogastrium, and a couple of catgut sutures were passed through the edges of the wound and through the superficial muscular layer of the anterior wall of the bladder. The abdominal incision was closed in the usual manner, and the patient was catheterized during the first week. In another case the bladder was suspended by four silk sutures, which included the serosa only, and were not passed through the skin.

Tuffier had operated thrice successfully by the extra-peritoneal method (as in epicystotomy), in one instance performing hysterorrhaphy, cystopexy, and anterior colporrhaphy upon the same patient. [This operation impresses us as being rather heroic treatment for a minor ailment. In the discussion of the paper Verneuil, Pozzi, and Richelot took the same ground. The same procedure was suggested and carried out by Dr. Henry Byford, of Chicago, at least two years ago.—ED.].

THE RELATION OF HEART LESIONS TO PELVIC DISEASE.

NEVIUS (*Centralblatt für Gynäkologie*, No. 15, 1891) calls attention to the frequent coincidence of cardiac and pelvic disease, mitral stenosis being most frequently observed. Since the pelvic symptoms usually absorb most attention, the cardiac complication is often overlooked. Among 419 women who were examined, 110 (26 per cent.) had mitral disease; of these, 55 per cent. had erosions of the cervix, 43 per cent. prolapse of the ovaries, 38 per cent. displacements of the uterus, and 43 per cent. menorrhagia or metrorrhagia. [We are forced to believe that the writer exaggerates the frequenoy of heart lesions in women with pelvic troubles, and would offer in support of this criticism the fact that in institutions like the New York State Woman's Hospital, in which the condition of the heart is carefully noted before operations, no such proportion has been observed. If this fact were well established, the number of gynecological operations, both in private and hospital practice, would be diminished at least one half.—ED.].

VESICAL PAIN AS A SYMPTOM OF PYONEPHROSIS.

·GUYON (*Centralblatt für Gynäkologie*, No. 15, 1891) reports two cases bearing upon this question. In one the extreme tenderness of the bladder in making pressure over the fundus, and in introducing a sound, the amount of vesical tenesmus, and the purulent character of the urine, seemed to justify the inference that the condition was primarily cystitis. Cystotomy was performed, and the pain was promptly relieved. The kidneys, which had previously been so large that they could be palpated, and were quite sensitive to pressure, rapidly diminished in size.

In the second case, in which the presence of enlarged kidneys, fever, and pyuria pointed to an existing pyonephrosis, cystotomy was followed by a disappearance of the symptoms, although the kidneys still remained large. The writer's deduction is that, as renal affections may be secondary to vesical inflammation, so the former may be relieved by treating the latter. [The writer's conclusions would be more valuable if his premises were more trustworthy. It is not clear that he possessed sufficient evidence upon which to base a reliable diagnosis of pyonephrosis. It would seem as if the disease in both instances was situated *below* the kidneys. Under similar conditions we recently made an explorative lumbar incision, and punctured the supposed pyonephrotic kidney, but found no pus. Subsequent observations showed that the symptoms were due to metritis. The recommendation to make an artificial vesico-vaginal fistula is none the less a good one in a doubtful case. —ED.].

EXTIRPATIO UTERI SACRALIS.

Under this term CZERNY (*Centralblatt für Gynäkologie*, No. 16, 1891) describes the operation of removing the uterus after resecting the sacrum, as practised by him in three cases. His technique is as follows: The patient being on the left side, an incision is made along either side of the sacrum. The coccyx, fifth sacral vertebra, and a portion of the fourth, are removed, osteoplastic resection not being recommended, since it retards the healing process. The peritoneum is divided, the coccyx is drawn downward, and the broad ligaments are ligated. The bladder is dissected off from above. The peritoneal wound is finally closed with catgut. The operation consumes at least two hours, and the healing process is slow; its advantages are not great, and it is only to be preferred in complicated cases—stenosis of the vagina, disease of the parametric tissues, etc.

MÜLLER (*Correspondenzblatt für Schweiz. Aerzte*, Bd. xxi., 1891) has performed the operation with success in three instances. The disadvantages of the operation are the necessary external incision and the preliminary separation of the rectum, and slow convalescence due to the size of the wound. It is sufficient to make an incision from the lower end of the sacrum to a point half an inch from the anus; it is only necessary to remove the coccyx, which will leave a much smaller wound. The advantages of the method are the perfect view of the field of operation, even in complicated cases, the possibility of controlling hemorrhage, and of avoiding injury to the uterus; finally, the peritoneal cavity is more easily and exactly closed. It is particularly applicable to cases of advanced carcinoma.

UNIQUE CASE OF FOREIGN BODY IN THE VAGINA.

SZIGETHY (*Orvosi Hetilap*, No. 52, 1890) reports the case of a woman, aged seventy-five years, who, thirty years before, in order to support a prolapsed uterus, introduced into the vagina a ball of string previously dipped in wax. This entirely relieved her, and was worn without discomfort, so that she forgot its existence, when it was forced out of place by a violent effort. When extracted, with some difficulty, it measured seven inches in circumference, and was covered with mucus, but otherwise unchanged.

PÆDIATRICS.

UNDER THE CHARGE OF

JOHN M. KEATING, M.D.,
OF PHILADELPHIA ;

A. F. CURRIER, M.D.,   AND   W. A. EDWARDS, M D.,
OF NEW YORK,   OF SAN DIEGO, CAL.

ASTHMA OF CHILDREN.

R. BLACHE (*L'Union Médicale*, 1890, No. 133) defines asthma as a bulbous disease, in which attacks are produced by impressive irritations of the vagus or peripheral nerves, particularly the trigeminus; the reflex action manifests itself by successive or simultaneous spasms of all the intrinsic inspiratory muscles, intercostals, scalenæ, trapezii, etc., and by a tetaniform contraction of the diaphragm.

Blache thus classifies the disease into three forms: Pneumo-bulbous asthma, essential or nervous asthma, emphysematous or alveolar asthma, catarrhal or bronchitic asthma.

Nervous asthma governs all asthmatical pathology of children. A class of asthma in infantile pathology which holds a place whose importance in-

creases every day as the pathogeny of the affections are better known, is the
class of reflex asthmas in general; these are the cases in which the bulbous
irritation does not leave the broncho-pulmonary filaments of the pneumogastric. The bulb is then impressed by an excitement springing from all
the peripheric branches of the vagus, but again from the other nerves—as
the trigeminus and the cutaneous nerves—so that nasal asthma, pharyngeal
asthma, amygdaline, gastric asthma, and cutaneous asthma belong to the
category of dyspnœas. Nasal asthma has only been known a few years;
Voltolini, in 1874, published the first facts relating to mucous polypi determining the approach of transient dyspnœa. Mucous polypi are rare in
children; but, on the contrary, adenoid tumors are very frequent and a usual
cause of nasal asthma. Hypertrophic rhinitis is also a frequent cause; this
may be a primary disease or follow successive attacks of acute coryza, or
infectious fevers, as measles and typhoid fever; it may be secondary to
another nasal lesion, malformation of the nose, deviating thickness of the
partition, foreign bodies, affections of the naso-pharyngeal canal, catarrh,
and adenoid growth. More than this, this rhinitis is at times connected
with diseases which attack the stomach (Bouchard, Ruault), the intestines
(Secchi, Buck), genital apparatus (J. Mackenzie, Joul).

With such a child, predisposed to bulbous irritability, either by diathesis
or heredity, and to nasal erectibility following the preceding lesions, an
attack of asthma may be brought on by congestion following cold, by the
action of vegetable or animal powders, by the influence of odorous matters,
by the contact of a probe on the pituitary gland, by an untimely nasal irrigation, and by remote causes, stomachic, intestinal, or genital excitations.

The treatment recommended for the attack is fumigation by belladonna
cigarettes, henbane, or the leaves of datura, stramonium, nitre paper, inhalations of oxygen, or ioduret of ethyl, but in many cases the hypodermic exhi-
bition of morphine will be required to produce even momentary relief. In a
general way, opium ought to be very prudently used with children; belladonna is much safer and can be used longer. Bretonneau and Guersant mix
one centigramme of the extract to one centigramme of the powder of belladonna, giving this each day and continuing for some time. The tincture of
lobelia inflata may be given in a dose gradually raised from 20 to 100 drops.
Moncorvo remarks that the endurance of children for the treatment permits
him to raise the dose 10 and 12 grammes in twenty-four hours. Blache has
obtained excellent results from tincture of grindelia robusta, which he gives
to children in doses of from 15 to 60 drops. Inhalations of vapor of pyridine,
advised by M. Sée, have helped Blache to lessen the force of the attack. According to Laborde and Daudrie, this substance lessens excito-motor force,
dilates peripheral vessels, and has a paralyzing action on the vaso-constrictor
nerves; hence, it increases the fulness of respiration, at the same time the
respiratory movements regulate themselves and diminish in frequency. The
curative treatment of asthma limits itself to the almost exclusive use of
iodine, particularly the iodide of potassium. The anti-dyspnœic effects of
this agent on the brain, and particularly on the bulb, are certain; Binz states
that it paralyzes the nervous functions and produces narcotism; in every case
it moderates the exciting power of the vital centre and regulates the distribution of the nervous influx.

Asthmatics presenting hyperæmia of the nasal mucous membrane are more easily affected with iodism. In cutaneous asthmas iodine may also be contra-indicated as aggravating the skin condition. At times the emaciation and loss of strength make it necessary to interrupt the treatment. Pyridine by aspiration, tincture of grindelia, arsenic, and aérotherapy by compressed air are, then, the only means which remain at the disposition of the practitioner. The iodine treatment is applicable to non-diathetic asthma; it is contra-indicated when the disease has a telluric or hereditary origin—for example, in the arthritic or gouty—a medication favoring incomplete nutrition or modifying the morbid secretions will be indicated. Asthmatics tainted with paludalism will require quinine in combination with iodide of potassium.

Blache agrees with Simon that the value of certain health resorts cannot be overestimated; the former gives preference to the waters of Mont-Doré, stating that their sedative and decongestive properties have produced good results, particularly in the pneumo-bulbous form; in herpetic asthma children as well as adolescents will find the sulphurous medication good. Bigorre, Saint-Honoré, and Alevard may be recommended.

———

REMOVAL OF A STONE WEIGHING 365 GRAINS BY VAGINAL CYSTOTOMY, FROM THE BLADDER OF A CHILD SIX YEARS OF AGE; URETER IN-JURED; OPERATIONS FOR CLOSING THE BLADDER DIFFICULT, BUT ULTIMATELY SUCCESSFUL.

In the *Pittsburgh Medical Review*, 1891, REAMY, of Cincinnati, records a remarkable case, in which, after the removal of a stone weighing 365 grains, *per vaginam*, it was necessary to perform four operations to close the resulting vesico-vaginal fistula, which was half an inch in length. The stone would have been removed by the supra-pubic operation if the operator had realized its size. The urethra was dilated to the size of the little finger; no paralysis followed.

The smallness of the vagina, together with the fact that the child was quite fat, made the operation for closure most difficult; and at the fourth operation the parts were much altered, considerable sloughing had occurred, and incrustation with urine salts; the edges of the wound were everted, ragged, and spongy.

The left ureter was seen to be discharging urine from the wall of the fistula. With much difficulty the ureter was dissected up, the mucous membrane of the bladder cut away sufficiently to uncover it; the free end of the ureter, liberated by the dissection referred to, was not cut off, but turned into the bladder. Seven No. 30 silver wire sutures were introduced into the fistula and allowed to remain two weeks; upon removal union was perfect. Though Parvin, Campbell, and others have turned an exposed ureter into the bladder, this is probably the first case in which this manipulation has been successful in a subject so young.

———

TWO CASES OF EPILEPTIFORM CONVULSIONS IN EARLY INFANCY.

BISSEL (*Journal Nervous and Mental Disease*, 1891) has observed two cases in very early infancy: the first a boy born of healthy parents, and the second a boy born of neurasthenic parents, whose mõther suffered from nervous prostration and comatose conditions; during the labor her conduct was that of a person suffering from acute mania.

Case I. presented the first symptoms when he was a week old. The convulsions, three in number, were slight and lasted two or three minutes ; but they increased in frequency from day to day, so that by the fourteenth day they were 70 in twenty-four hours; on the fifteenth day, 75; on the sixteenth, 79; on the seventeenth, 80; on the eighteenth day the intervals began to lengthen, and there were only 50 on that day, and on the next day but 8 light convulsions occurred; during the next five days they grew continuously less and less and eventually disappeared.

Total number of recorded convulsions, 366. During the entire period the patient took nourishment well, his appearance remained good, and his weight increased nearly two pounds. Medically he received a mixture of subnitrate of bismuth and deodorized tincture of opium, to control a few thin, copious passages from the bowels. To control convulsions, 2 grains of bromide of sodium, increased to 10 grains in twenty-four hours, were given.

Case II. weighed eight and one-half pounds at birth ; the greatest circumference of his head was 41 cm.

On the twenty-first day he had four well-marked convulsions; the spasms commenced at first in the hands and feet, with congestion of right hand and face; as the spasm passed the part became pale and the spasms would attack those parts that were reddening; during attacks the respirations were much impeded, there being twenty- and thirty-second pauses in the act; occasionally there would be a minute when the child did not breathe. The total number of convulsions for four days reached the remarkable total of 183. The fontanelles were tense, and measurements showed that the greatest diameter had increased from 41 cm. to 44 cm.; the fontanelles continued moderately tense and the bones widely separated for two days after the convulsions ceased.

The child received oleum ricini and small doses of bromide of sodium, as indicated.

Eighteen months later the boy was fat and well.

Note to Contributors.—All contributions intended for insertion in the Original Department of this Journal are only received *with the distinct understanding that they are contributed exclusively to this Journal.*

Contributions from the Continent of Europe and written in the French, German or Italian language, if on examination they are found desirable for this Journal, will be translated at its expense.

Liberal compensation is made for articles used. A limited number of extra copies in pamphlet form, if desired, will be furnished to authors in lieu of compensation, *provided the request for them be written on the manuscript.*

All communications should be addressed to

Dr. EDWARD P. DAVIS,
250 South 21st Street, Philadelphia.

THE

AMERICAN JOURNAL

OF THE MEDICAL SCIENCES.

AUGUST, 1891.

ADENOMA UTERI.[1]

By Henry C. Coe, M.D.,

GYNECOLOGIST TO THE NEW YORK CANCER HOSPITAL, NEW YORK.

In a former paper on " Malignant Disease of the Corporeal Endome-trium" (*N. Y. Medical Record*, April 5, 1890) I referred at some length to "malignant adenoma," which I then regarded as an extremely rare condition. Subsequent study and clinical observation have convinced me that it is probably less infrequent than I formerly supposed, although it often escapes recognition in what may be designated as the pre-malignant stage of the disease. So much confusion exists in the nomenclature of diseased conditions of the endometrium that I am sure that you will pardon me for selecting such an apparently technical theme if I succeed in placing the subject in a clearer light. I have chosen the general title " Adenoma Uteri" in order to call attention to the errors that have crept into the writings of some of the most careful pelvic pathologists through their including under this head a number of different conditions, ranging from simple hyperplasia of the endometrium to adeno-carcinoma. For example, Fürst[2] described three varieties of adenoma, viz.: *adenoma uteri simplex*, or simple glandular hyperplasia; *adenoma uteri suspectum*, or destructive glandular hyperplasia; and *adeno-carcinoma*, or typical glandular proliferation with epithelial infiltration and general destruction of the tissues. As the latest authority on gynecology (Pozzi) properly remarks, the application

---

[1] Read by title before the Obstetrical Section of the Amer. Med. Assoc., May 6, 1891.
[2] Zeitschr. für Geburtsh. u. Gyn., 1887, Bd. xiv. Heft 2, p. 364.

of the term "benignant adenoma" to simple glandular hyperplasia has been made by those who look at the subject almost entirely from an anatomical standpoint, and arbitrarily group together conditions which present similar histological appearances, without due regard for their clinical differences. The importance of this will be evident later when we discuss the question of the possible relation between endometritis fungosa and cancer of the corpus uteri. Still more confusion has been caused by the numerous references in the literature to "polypoid adenoma" (Muckel), "channelled polypus (de Sinéty), etc., terms which are applied to simple mucous polypi or even to endometritis polyposa· Winckel, usually so lucid, is by no means clear on this subject, but seems to favor Kloh's bewildering pathological division. Even such a forcible writer as John Williams might lead the incautious reader astray by causing him to infer that such polypi tend to become cancerous;[1] though he specifies the cervical variety, other writers are not so careful. It is by no means certain that the specimen described by him was a true case of cancerous degeneration ; and if it was, the development of epithelioma in the mucosa covering the surface of a so-called "glandular polypus" is a very different process from the transition of a true adenoma to carcinoma. Of course I refer always to intra-uterine, not to cervical, growths.

In the case of a mucous membrane which is so peculiarly the seat of localized and diffuse hypertrophies and pseudo-neoplasms as that which lines the uterine cavity, one must invariably apply the crucial test before deciding the question of the benignancy or malignancy of a certain growth. Is it confined to the mucosa in which it originated, or does it invade the deeper tissues? This it is often impossible to determine from an examination of curettings. Great injustice is done to pathologists in this respect. They are expected to decide positively regarding the character of an intra-uterine growth, when they receive only a few superficial fragments. Sometimes a lock of the patient's hair would be about as useful. No reliable microscopist would hazard a positive opinion in a doubtful case, unless he receives portions of the growth with the subjacent tissue; these can only be obtained by the use of the sharp curette. Reference will be made to this subject again under the head of diagnosis.

Briefly, then, I may state that I do not admit the existence of a distinct variety of intra-uterine neoplasm to which can be applied the term "benignant" as distinguished from "malignant" adenoma. I recognize only one variety—the adenoma malignum of Schröder, or diffuse papillary adenoma of Winckel, which I wish to show is anatomically the incipient stage of adeno-carcinoma ; that as regards their clinical symp-

---

[1] "Cancer of the Uterus." Harveian Lectures for 1886 ; London, 1888, p. 75.

toms they are practically identical, but that there is an important difference between the two as regards prognosis.

HISTORICAL.—Matthews Duncan is credited by Williams with having been the first to describe adenoma of the body of the uterus.[1] From his graphic description of the clinical symptoms, as well as from Slavjansky's careful report on the microscopical examination of the specimen removed, this would seem to have been rather a case of true adenocarcinoma—the final, rather than the initial, stage of the disease. Duncan himself, with his characteristic acumen, concludes: "I can entertain very little doubt that, whether the disease is as yet truly malignant or not, it will before many months are passed, show the terrible characters of undoubted cancer." We read that recurrence took place almost immediately, the patient dying five months after he first saw her. In the light of our present knowledge few would have hesitated to perform a radical operation, instead of the palliative one which simply hastened the fatal issue.

The next contribution to our knowledge of this class of neoplasms was made by Breisky and Eppinger,[2] who report and figure a most instructive case, in which the former thoroughly curetted a uterus for recurring hemorrhage, removing a number of cauliflower masses, which presented the typical structure of adenoma. The hemorrhage reappeared, and four months later a second curetting yielded a fresh quantity of material, which was softer and more friable than that which had been removed on the previous occasion, and on microscopical examination indicated clearly the transition of the adenoma to adeno-carcinoma, the cross-sections of glands showing their lamina choked with epithelioid cells that presented a marked contrast to the cylindrical epithelium with which the tubes were lined. There was also an invasion of the deeper tissues by the neoplasm, which had not been noted before.

Klebs in discussing this paper credits Ackermann with reporting the first case of adenoma uteri, but it appears that the growth was confined to the portio vaginalis.

Schröder[3] showed that he clearly recognized the condition, though he leaned toward the theory that there existed transitional forms between endometritis fungosa and what he denominated "malignant adenoma;" the latter, he noted, frequently developed into true glandular carcinoma. J. Veit[4] soon after described and figured a case which showed the transition from adenoma to carcinoma.

Winckel describes and figures a museum specimen of diffuse papillary

[1] Edinburgh Med. Journ., vol. xix. p. 92.
[2] Prager med. Wochenschrift, Bd. ii., 1877, p. 78.
[3] Krankheiten der weiblichen Geschlechtsorgane, 1879, p. 261.
[4] Zeitschr. f. Geburtsh. u. Gyn., vol. i., 1877, p. 189.

adenoma, without clinical history, and the writer of the monograph on Non-malignant Tumors of the Uterus in the *American System of Gynecology* reproduces the figure, but in the context fails to recognize clearly that it is a true neoplasm, not a mere hyperplasia of the endometrium.

Mann[1] should be credited with having recognized this condition, as he examined and described a post-mortem specimen.

Bartolet[2] had a similar case in which the diagnosis of papillary adenoma was made during life from an examination of curettings.

Thomas'[3] supposed cases are open to serious doubt. The very fact that one patient recovered after the curette had been used fourteen (!) times in five years, and that the other was curetted at frequent intervals during seven years. would at once exclude them from the present category. Moreover, only the curettings were submitted to microscopical examination.

Of Goodell's[4] three cases of "villous degeneration of the endometrium," the second was probably ordinary endometritis fungosa ; the first and third, from their clinical history, probably illustrated the transition from adenoma to adeno-carcinoma, as in my third case. Unfortunately, in neither of the instances was an opportunity afforded of examining the growth *in situ*.

Ruge and Veit[5] were the first to make a careful study of adenoma, and Ruge presented a communication on this subject to the German Gynecological Society in 1888. Fürst alludes to it incidentally in the paper already quoted. My own more recent observations were reported in my paper of last year, to which reference has been made. I there mentioned two specimens which I had examined (Dr. Wylie's and Dr. Bache Emmet's), to which are now added two of my own. Dr. Freeborn, Pathologist to the Cancer Hospital, tells me that he has seen a fifth. In all of these the entire uterus was removed.

The most recent communication on this subject is by E. W. Cushing[6] who clearly describes and figures the condition in question, recognizing its malignant character, as shown by its recurrence and eventual transition to the true carcinoma.

Beyond these I know of only five authentic specimens of papillary adenoma, described by any of the writers before mentioned, excluding all cases in which the diagnosis was founded upon the clinical history and the microscopical examination of scrapings alone. There may be

---

[1] Amer. Journ. of Obstetrics, January, 1878. p. 113.

[2] Philada. Med. Times, April, 1878, p. 354.

[3] Diseases of Women, 5th ed., 1880, p. 570.

[4] Lessons in Gynecology, 3d ed., 1887, p. 317.

[5] Zeitschr. für Geburtsh. u. Gyn., Bd. vi., 1881, p. 302.

[6] Annals of Gynecology and Pædiatry, May, 1891. p. 458.

others, but if so, they have been reported in such an imperfect way as to render them unreliable from a scientific standpoint.

In presenting these three uteri, removed by myself during the past year at the New York Cancer Hospital, I would call attention to the fact that they form a sort of ascending series. Case I. may be regarded as a typical specimen of circumscribed malignant adenoma, Case II. a beautiful example of the diffuse form of the same neoplasm, and Case III. illustrates the final stage of the disease—transition to adeno-carcinoma. As the histories have already been published, I shall present them merely in abstract for the sake of comparison.

Case I.—The patient was a single woman, fifty years of age, who had reached the climacteric seven years before. She had had slight atypical hemorrhages for five years before I saw her, and had been curetted twice during the previous year with only temporary benefit. The scrapings had not been examined microscopically. Diagnosis, probable sarcoma. She entered my service at the Cancer Hospital in December, 1889, being then in good general health.

She had severe paroxysmal pain in the pelvis, which recurred every day at regular intervals, but had no vaginal discharge whatever.

Tissue removed by the curette was examined microscopically but without positive results. I could only decide that the condition was neither endometritis fungosa nor round-celled sarcoma, and hence was led to believe that I had to do with cancer of the corporeal endometrium, although the long duration of the symptoms and the remarkably good condition of the patient were against this theory.

The uterus was extirpated *per vaginam* with considerable difficulty, though not large, because of the contracted vagina and outlet. Forcipressure was used. The patient made a good recovery and is now in perfect health, with no signs of recurrence. The anatomical condition is circumscribed papillary adenoma, neither does the microscope reveal any trace of transition to carcinoma. Yet the growth had begun to infiltrate the muscular layer, and the clinical symptoms, though of long standing, pointed unquestionably to its inherent malignancy. There is no doubt that a delay of a few months, with one or two more palliative operations, would have resulted fatally.

Case II.—Widow, aged fifty-three years. One child and three miscarriages. Menopause reached three years ago, soon after which she began to have an irregular sanguineous discharge from the vagina with occasional hemorrhages. She said that she had a "polypus" removed six months before, after which the flow ceased for a time, but soon returned. No pain whatever until a few weeks before her admission to the Cancer Hospital in November, 1890. Was in robust health. Examination showed the uterus to be moderately enlarged, freely movable, and insensitive to pressure; the endometrium bled easily. Fragments of tissue removed with the curette were too superficial to allow of a positive diagnosis, except that the growth was probably malignant. Total extirpation of the uterus *per vaginam*, with forcipressure. Normal convalescence, and patient discharged cured at the end of five weeks.

The specimen is a beautiful example of diffuse adenoma of the corpus uteri, which has just begun to infiltrate the deeper layer, but exhibits no histological evidence of cancerous change. The prognosis for a permanent cure, as in the former case, is excellent, although too short a time has elapsed since the operation to make the case valuable from a statistical standpoint.

CASE III.—Widow, aged sixty-three years. On entering the hospital she stated that she had passed the climacteric many years before, and had always enjoyed good health until seven months before, when she began to have a slight "show" at rare intervals, and her health commenced to decline without apparent cause. She had had no pain except severe backache for a few weeks. Slight inodorous watery discharge from the vagina. The os was dilated with tents, and the uterine cavity was thoroughly explored with the finger, revealing a diffuse cauliflower growth of the endometrium, portions of which were removed with the sharp curette, and examined microscopically. Diagnosis, adeno-carcinoma. Vaginal hysterectomy, with forcipressure. Discharged cured at the end of six weeks. Ten months later the patient had recurrence in the lumbar glands.

The specimen is clearly carcinoma of a particularly malignant form, that has deeply infiltrated the muscular tissue and has begun to ulcerate, rendering the prognosis much more unfavorable than in the two preceding cases. The after-history has confirmed the opinion which was then expressed, although at the time of the operation there was no evidence that the glands or perimetric tissues were involved.

ANATOMY.—It is unnecessary to dwell upon the histological appearances of such a familiar growth as adenoma. I have already stated that *endometritis glandularis hyperplastica* is not adenoma at all, which is readily demonstrated anatomically by the fact that in the former the mucosa is generally hypertrophied, there is enlargement, but not marked proliferation of pre-existing glands, and the process is absolutely confined to the mucous layer ; moreover the proliferation is always typical. That cancer may develop directly from such a condition is a question as yet *sub judice;* it may be affirmed by purely clinical observers, but when such careful students as Ruge and Veit declare that they have never yet met with an example of this transition, we must be content to regard it as not proven. On the other hand the development of carcinoma from true adenoma is unquestioned, as shown in Breisky's classical case; the malignancy of the neoplasm, even before the atypical proliferation of the glandular epithelium, so as to form solid columns, and the formation of outlying epithelial cell-clusters, is shown by its invasion of the submucous muscular layer and the disappearance of the interglandular fibrous tissue, in consequence of which adjacent glands are crowded together, forming glomeruli which Schröder has compared to a mass of earth-worms.

SYMPTOMATOLOGY.—I have no intention of claiming a distinct set of symptoms for the neoplasm under discussion, though Winckel has done so. On the other hand I would not affirm with Ruge that they are never distinguishable from those of cancer. I believe that malignant adenoma is a distinct pathological condition which, although it inevitably tends to pass into carcinoma, is not in its initial stage carcinoma, and would call attention to the fact which is clearly shown by the histories narrated, that there are some essential points of difference. Thus, it is evident that cancer of the body of the uterus would not exist for from three to five years without the occurrence of such retrograde changes as would either destroy life from exhaustion, or would seriously affect the patient's health. After continuing for so long a time there would certainly be more severe pain, more profuse hemorrhages, a foul discharge, septic infection, and involvement of the glands and perimetric tissues. Witness the contrast to Cases I. and II. presented by Case III. Furthermore, the negative evidence presented by the examination of curettings is of considerable value, since it is always easier to determine with the microscope the probable absence of malignant disease, than its presence.

DIAGNOSIS.—From a surgical standpoint I am not a stickler for the refinements of anatomical diagnosis in these cases. In proof of this I need only call attention to the fact that I performed total extirpation of the uterus in Cases I. and II., although by no means certain that I should find malignant disease, and was much relieved to find that my suspicions were justified. Such symptoms as those which I have mentioned, in a woman who has passed the climacteric, added to the fact that they rapidly recurred after thorough curetting, do not warrant further resort to palliative treatment. With the results of modern aseptic surgery before us, we are not justified in waiting until the diagnosis has been established beyond the shadow of a doubt, and the patient's health has been seriously undermined, before we decide upon radical measures.

PROGNOSIS.—As the history of the few *authentic* cases of adenoma uteri has shown, the course of the disease is usually slow and insidious, but, though less malignant than round-celled sarcoma and medullary carcinoma of the endometrium, its fatal termination is none the less certain. Sooner or later cancer is bound to develop with all its attendant evils, with which we are so familiar. The continued good health of the patient, her freedom from pain, local tenderness and a foul discharge should not deceive us. The end, though delayed, is inevitable.

TREATMENT.—Although maintaining a somewhat conservative attitude with regard to the question of total extirpation for cancer of the cervix, when it comes to cases of real or suspected malignant disease of the corpus uteri I would adopt the most radical measures. Fürst is right when he says that palliative treatment of the latter does more harm than good ; it simply aggravates the trouble. I believe

that every time that adenoma uteri is attacked with the curette it simply returns in a more malignant form ; the use of the galvano-cautery
may be less objectionable, but it is a blind procedure. " We have
scotched the snake, not killed it."

There is no class of cases in which vaginal hysterectomy offers such
good prospects of a permanent cure, as in those which form the subject
of this paper. The operation is exceptionally easy, as the uterus is
small and is perfectly movable, there is no involvement of the glands or
parametria, the patient's general condition is good, and above all, the
disease is *entirely* eradicated. It ought certainly to afford a surgeon more
genuine satisfaction to remove a uterus which is the seat of pure adenoma
that has not yet entered the cancerous stage, than to extirpate the entire
organ for commencing epithelioma of the portio vaginalis, when the
diseased tissue might have been excised by high amputation.

To conclude, the following deductions seem to be justifiable :

Benignant adenoma of the corpus uteri is a misnomer. Neither
glandular hypertrophy of the endometrium nor so-called adenoid polypus is a genuine adenoma. The only true adenoma of the corpus uteri is
essentially malignant both anatomically and clinically—anatomically
because it infiltrates the deeper tissues, and clinically because it recurs
after removal and eventually assumes a more malignant character.

Malignant adenoma is not at the outset identical with adeno-carcinoma, but may be regarded as the initial stage of the latter, having
many of the same symptoms. Rapid recurrence after removal by the
curette of an intra-uterine growth which does not appear to be distinctly
malignant histologically, and has existed for a considerable length of
time, should suggest the probability that it is adenoma, provided that the
patient, although at the age when cancer of the corpus uteri is most
common, does not have the foul discharge and cachexia attending
advanced malignant disease.

A positive diagnosis is possible only after digital explorations of the
uterine cavity and the removal with the sharp curette for microscopical
examination of a bit of the suspected growth, with the subjacent muscular tissue.

As soon as the diagnosis of a malignant growth is reasonably certain
total extirpation of the uterus should be performed without delay.
Palliative measures simply favor the more rapid transition to carcinoma, when the prognosis as regards a permanent cure becomes much
more doubtful.

A CONTRIBUTION TO THE STUDY OF PRE-COLUMBIAN SYPHILIS IN AMERICA.

By JAMES NEVINS HYDE, A.M., M.D.,

PROFESSOR OF DERMATOLOGY AND VENEREAL DISEASES, BUSH MEDICAL COLLEGE, CHICAGO.

THE question whether syphilis prevailed upon the American continent previous to the close of the fifteenth century has a larger measure than the interest of the antiquarian. It is one not without significance for the present, and proposes a problem to modern pathology.

The historical facts upon which it has been sought to rest both the affirmative and negative answers to the question are so well known that the briefest summary of them must suffice for the present purpose.

The ancient literatures of China, India, Greece, and Italy contain unmistakable proofs of the fact that at an early period of the world's history, certain genital lesions were recognized as resulting from sexual contamination. Many of the systemic results of syphilis, not merely in these writings but in those of the Middle Ages, are more or less graphically described. These descriptions are, however, for the most part fragmentary and disconnected; and the conditions they represent are often assigned to other and various disorders; rarely, if ever, are they identified as the results of a previous infection of some particular part of the body. Between, however, the years 1492 and 1494 an epidemic of syphilis spread over France, Spain, Italy, Switzerland, the countries bordering on the Rhine, and other parts of Europe, which eventually became as formidable in its effects as it was general of diffusion. Its prevalence was greatly aided by the campaigns of Charles VIII. of France, who, in his expedition to Naples, led an army of between eight and ten thousand men into the plains of Italy. He crossed into Piedmont on the 8th of December, 1494. His army was officered by young men of aristocratic connections, leading the loosest lives. The rank and file, following the example of their dissolute commanders, were successively quartered in most of the larger Italian cities, and, in the license of unrestraint, did not hesitate to pillage Rome. As a consequence, syphilis was offered to the study of physicians on a broader scale than ever before. Its phenomena were now carefully noted and its earliest and later symptoms recognized as phases of the evolution of a single specific disorder. Fracastor wrote his poem; Isla, his treatise; Sydenham, his letters. The affection soon passed from beneath the uncertain shadows of the mysterious into the calm scrutiny of science.

On the 4th of January, 1493, the Admiral Christobal Colon, better known to us as Columbus, sailed with his company from the West Indies in the Pinta and Nina. They reached the shores of Europe by the following March. Ruy Diaz de Isla, a physician of Andalusia, stated that he had treated some of this company for syphilis, the symptoms of which had first appeared on shipboard before the landing. On the 14th of June of the next year Nicholas Scyllatius reported syphilis as prevalent in epidemic form. The great captain, Gonzales Fernandez de Cordova, soon after left Spain, and in a second Italian campaign against the arms of Louis XII., brought his Spanish troops in contact with the French. Oviedo not only stated that the disease was introduced into Europe from the West Indies by the fleets of Columbus, but added that he was personally acquainted with some of the navigators who had acquired the disease from this source; and gives the name of one of these sufferers, personally known to himself as also to their majesties of Castile. He is also authority for the statement that Cordova, when he was sent to Italy, had in his army persons who were known to be infected.

Six years after Columbus sailed from Hispaniola the devout Las Casas writes of his Indian converts that they freely admitted the prevalence of the disease amongst themselves long before the advent of the Christians; and that the latter were far greater sufferers from the pestilence than the natives themselves. Sir Hans Sloane, who visited the West Indies in 1687, Robertson, the historian, and others whose names are as well known, have, after careful research, expressed their belief in the American origin of the malady. In our own country, Professor Joseph Jones, of New Orleans, may be cited as a classical writer on this theme. His explorations in Kentucky, Tennessee, and elsewhere have led him to conclude that syphilis existed in this hemisphere at a remote period of the past; but even if prevalent in the crowded West Indian Islands at the time of their first visitation by Europeans, did not for that reason necessarily exist upon the Northern and Southern continents. He cites, on the contrary, John D. Hunter, who, after a long captivity among the Indians, declared that they suffered from the disease, but that they had contracted it after communication with the white race.

Two interesting papers have also been contributed to this subject by Dr. Gustavus Brühl, of Cincinnati, Ohio, which embody the fruits of considerable historic research. They contain several interesting arguments having an etymological basis in favor of the existence of pre-Columbian syphilis in the Western Hemisphere. The writings of Sahagun, Torquemada, Roman, Mendieta, Pane and others show as to New Spain—first, that the bodies of those affected with syphilis were interred, as distinguished from those dead of other disorders, which were cremated; second, that the infected were not deemed fit for religious sacrifices; third, that they were represented at the festivals; and fourth, that the disease was counted a punishment sent from the gods for the non-performance of religious rites and other offences. The author also shows that the Mexicans not only recognized the connection between the earliest and later manifestations of the disorder, but distinguished between several types of the former, understanding also its remedial treatment far better than the Spaniards, even seeking thermal resorts for the purpose of securing relief. He quotes from seventeen Indian dialects, each of which has a primitive and native term for designating the disease, none of the terms thus employed suggesting their confrontation with a new malady, although soon after contact with the whites they were compelled to apply new names for many novel objects with which they were to become familiar. These new names either bear witness to the impression on their ears made by the speech of the Castilians, or describe some prominent.feature of the object to be newly named, a rule distinctly observed by them in the case of diseases known to have been imported from Europe to America, as for example, measles and smallpox. The singular confusion existing in the Mexican language of the sixteenth century, of the terms employed to indicate ideas of power, divinity, and the special disease here under discussion, possesses an interest in view of the fact that this is recognized in the dialects of Quechua and Aymerás three hundred years before Pizarro conquered the capital of the Incas.

But to the inhabitants of the Northern part of the Western Hemisphere, the chief interest which to-day attaches to this question rests upon the discovery of bones which have been disinterred in different parts of the country, many of them of great age, presumed to be prehistoric, some of which exhibit traces of disease thought to be syphilis. Such are those exhumed by Professor Jones, who claims that some of those taken by him from the Indian cemeteries are the "oldest syphilitic bones in existence." Others have been disinterred in California, Colorado, and elsewhere within the boundaries of the United States. Only one who has had the singular opportunity of examining all these specimens can speak with authority upon the conclusions which their study justifies. In the pages which follow reference is had only to those either examined by myself or to those represented by portraits in my collection. The following list of photographs may be regarded as fairly representative of these collections:

No. 1. Two incomplete human tibiæ from a mound in Alamada County, California, furnished me by the kindness of Dr. Billings, from the collection in the Surgeon-General's Office of the War Department, U. S. A.

No. 2. A group of tibiæ and fibulæ from a burial mound near St. Francis River, Arkansas, furnished me by the kindness of Professor F. W. Putnam, of the Peabody Museum of American Archæology and Ethnology in Cambridge, Mass. Figs. 2 and 3.

No. 3. A skull with other diseased and healthy bones, all from the same skeleton, from a burial mound in Colorado, furnished me from same collection. Figs. 4 and 5.

No. 4. Two tibiæ, selected from other bones of a skeleton in my own collection sent to me by Dr. J. W. Brown, Mr. Thomas M. Trippe, and Mr. Mentzel, exhumed from a prehistoric burial site on the Animas River, Colo-

FIG. 1. FIG. 2.

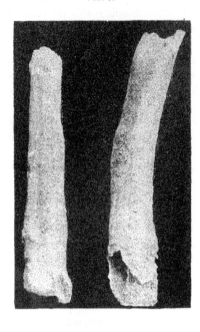 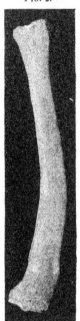

FIG 3 FIG. 4.

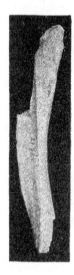 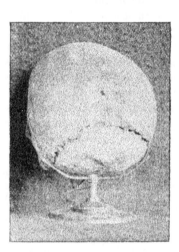

rado, about forty-five miles distant from Durango. In the process of exhumation of this skeleton the skull was found so far disintegrated that on exposure
it at once crumbled to fragments. Fig. 6.

Comparing the general features of the bones shown in these photographs with those elsewhere collected, figured, and described, as probably the seat of syphilitic lesions, I believe that they may be regarded as fairly representative of the entire group. For the purpose of readier comparison, I have also studied photographs of

No. 5. A left tibia, showing hyperostosis of the entire shaft, with some shallow depressions where it is supposed suppuration had occurred. The upper half shows abundant exostosis over all its surfaces, the joint being involved. Weight of bone thirty ounces. From a negro whose entire skeleton was involved in syphilitic changes. (Surgeon-General's Office.)

FIG. 5.   FIG. 6.

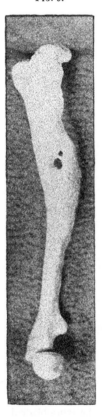 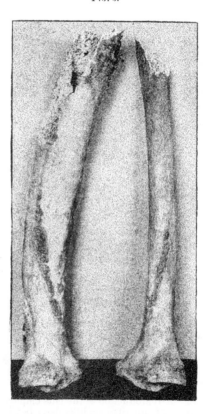

No. 6. Calvarium; the outer table showing numerous erosions, some large and deep, others small and superficial, which corresponded in the recent state with small pinkish gummata of the pericranium; a few perforations; many exostoses. The inner table shows many erosions and closely set osteophytes. From a colored man aged forty-two years. (Surgeon-General's Office.)

No. 7. Right tibia, showing marked nodular irregularity, resulting from gummatous tumors. The left tibia less strikingly affected with similar lesions. From a Saladoan. (Surgeon-General's Office.)

No. 8.   Lower ends of femora with patellæ, tibiæ, and fibulæ, showing results of inflammation, probably syphilitic; surface of bones, especially of front of tibiæ, very irregular, with marked depressions and new growth of bone; general osteoporosis.   Osteomyelitis; ossifying periostitis.   Removed from a mulatto woman aged forty-one years. (Surgeon-General's Office.)

No. 9.   Left tibia, the upper third of which presents subperiosteal necrosis and deeper fistulous passages; the middle third of the bone shows the same condition to a less extent; and in addition, especially on its posterior surface, an abundance of spongy osteophytes.   From a white man, age unknown; disease supposed to be result of exposure; leg amputated above knee; patient recovered. (Surgeon-General's Office.)

No. 10.   Right tibia; tibia osteoporotic throughout and ankylosed to astragalus.   From a white man aged forty-five years; had his right foot hurt while jumping, when fourteen years of age; hurt again in 1866 by being

FIG. 7.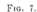

FIG. 8.

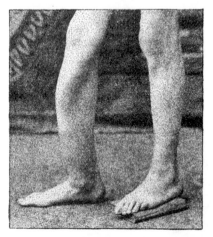

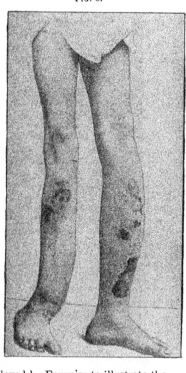

struck by a falling bar of iron.   Inflammation ensued; amputation in lower third of thigh.   Patient recovered. (Surgeon-General's Office.)

No. 11.   The lower extremities of a clinical patient, lately applying for relief at the clinic in Chicago, affected with inherited syphilis in the right tibia, exhibiting marked deformity, produced by enlargement and antero-posterior curve. Fig. 7.

No. 12.   A reproduction of the cuts employed by Fournier to illustrate the bone disease of inherited syphilis described by him as the sabre-blade deformity. (*Lame-de-sabre.*)   Fig. 8.

Viewing as a whole the group of exhumed bones whose photographs have been studied, it is clear that the morbid changes they represent are due to forms of inflammation described by Professor Jones as "periostitis, osteitis, endosteitis, caries, sclerosis, and exostosis."   "They are," using again the descriptive terms he employs, "thoroughly diseased,

enlarged, and thickened, with the medullary canal more or less completely obliterated by the effect of inflammatory action, with the surfaces
eroded in many places." Again: " In many the medullary canals are
equally involved with the periosteum." Some of these changes are
bilateral, involving—if not equally, to some extent—bones of like name
on the two sides of the body. In other cases several different bones of
one skeleton are diseased.

The most conspicuous of the features common to the greater number,
are the diffuseness, uniformity, and lack of sharp definition of the lesions,
represented chiefly by hypertrophy rather than atrophy. The first question then at issue does not concern the existence of these tangible metamorphoses. It is reduced to the inquiry, Are these metamorphoses due
wholly or in part to syphilis?

The distorted femur of the skeleton obtained from Colorado seems
to have been the seat of an abscess. I have suggested to Professor
Putnam that it may have resulted from traumatism by one of the triangular flints employed by the Indians as arrow-heads, wounding bone,
periosteum, or adjacent tissues. I am under the impression that he is
disposed to entertain the same view. In a sacrum and dorsal vertebra
to be found in a collection of bones taken from a prehistoric cemetery
in Madisonville, Ohio, the implements named are seen to have penetrated
the osseous substance to the extent of about half an inch.

As to the other modifications of shape and tissue exhibited in this
group of bones, there is a conspicuous absence of certain features which
are to be expected in bone syphilis, and which are seen, however imperfectly, in the group of photographs of bones known to be syphilitic.
Here are not the single or multiple, conical, roundish, or flattened,
smooth, hard, pea- to nut-sized and even larger nodules which may be
found in both the laminated and eburnated conditions. Here are not
the circumscribed swellings, well or ill-defined, found at the distal extremities of syphilitic bones, as, for example, near the wrist when involving
the radius and ulna. Here are not the atrophic areas whose definition
is scarcely less remarkable than that of the tumefaction which preceded.
Here is no suggestion of a poorly united fracture, no hint of a super-
added "splint," no trace of a circumscribed or even diffuse gummatous
involvement, leaving after degeneration, circinate, single, or multiple
relics of the process. We search in vain for bone-cicatrices; for smooth
or rough mamelonations of the surface, for localized sclerosis. We discover no centric rarefaction of the osseous tissue with a peripheral over-
growth. In the Madisonville collection, however, there are two tibiæ
suggesting the gummatous changes in the bones of the syphilitic subject,
illustrated in the photographs (already shown) of the skull with numerous erosions, and of the bones of the negro subjects. Professor Jones
describes also "rounded ulcerations with glazed surfaces," "tuberculated

ulcerations," "marked eburnifications," and "reticulated ulcerations," in which an ulcer penetrated a network of periosteal deposit with an annular border.

If syphilis actually prevailed among the aborigines of the Northern part of the Western Continent, it is natural to conclude that with only that measure of therapeutic relief which they could command, inherited syphilis must have been proportionately prevalent. It is well known, too, that in the last-named form of the disease bone symptoms are much more frequently encountered than in the acquired form. Yet I have been thus far wholly unable to secure a photograph or a description of any bone in America that can be fully identified as part of a prehistoric skeleton with the lesions of inherited syphilis unmistakably apparent. There is no bone illustrating these conditions, whether historic or pre-historic, in the collection of the Surgeon-General's Office. Professor Putnam informs me that he has many tibiæ of children exhibiting the curves to be seen in the condition described by Fournier as the "sabre-blade" deformity, and well illustrated in the photograph of a clinical patient lately shown before the class in Rush Medical College, Chicago. But in these curves the special changes described by Fournier, Taylor, Augagneur, Parrot, Ollier, Poncet, and others, often recognized in a general clinical experience, are not declared. There are no traces of the chronic or subacute, often symmetrical and multiple, simple or gumma-tous, osteo-periostites, and osteo-myelites, starting at the epiphyso-dia-physeal junction, and producing the smooth or irregularly undulating annular tumors embracing the bone. Even the "massive distortions" described and figured by Fournier in his classical work on *Late Inherited Syphilis* differ to some extent from those here represented, though suggesting a resemblance in the general contour of the deformed bones.

In order to investigate this matter more fully, I selected for patho-logical examination the tibiæ of the parts of a skeleton sent me from Colorado, not merely because they fully illustrate the general changes described by most authors as characteristic of prehistoric bones claimed to be syphilitic, but also because it is seriously claimed by the scientific men of special training who superintend the exhumation, that they antedate by a long period of time the relics of the Mound-builders and Cave-dwellers. The mode of their sepulture was different from that prevalent among the races indicated by these names, as also from that which has survived to our own day among the Zuñis.

Upon these bones, submitted to Dr. T. M. Prudden, of the laboratory of the College of Physicians and Surgeons of New York, I receive the following report:

"The bones were two apparently adult tibiæ, both lower ends of which were absent, being apparently crumbled off. Both of the bones pre-sented marked abnormalities which may be best described on the separate bones. The lesions of the left tibia are more extensive than those of the right.

"The *left tibia*. The shaft of the bone is bowed considerably forward at its middle and lower portions. The shaft, which is nearly cylindrical, is everywhere greatly increased in thickness, measuring from 4 to 4.5 centimetres in diameter in all parts except at the lower end, where it is slightly smaller. The whole bone is very light in weight.

" About the articular end, at the knee-joint, the bone presents erosions, irregular losses of substance and numerous larger and smaller bony out-growths—the latter being most marked about the front of the joint and especially about the seat of attachment of the ligamentum patellæ. The fibular articular surface is completely destroyed. The entire surface of the shaft is roughened and porous and beset here and there, especially along the lines of tendinous attachment, with larger and smaller rows and masses of the delicate bony outgrowths called osteophytes. These osteophytes are especially prominent along the lateral and posterior aspects of the shaft. Branching grooves in the surface of the bone and delicate projecting bony plates and spiculæ and ridges contribute to the roughness of the shaft.

"Transverse sections of the shaft of this bone at its middle third show that the bone, which from the outside appears to be largely hypertrophied, is a mere fragile cylindrical shell, the peripheral compact bone being almost everywhere thin and uneven, and the bulk of the shaft consisting almost wholly of irregular cancellous or spongy tissue.

" The more delicate central trabeculæ of the cancellous tissue, which apparently nearly or completely filled the narrow cavity have, except in a few places, largely disintegrated and fallen out with the lapse of time.

" Along many parts of the bone the cancellous tissue pierces the shell of compact bone—which though very thin in general encloses the shaft— and becomes continuous with the osteophytic outgrowths on the surface.

" The *right tibia* is smaller but heavier than the left. The shaft is in general irregularly ovoidal, its antero-posterior diameter in the upper and middle third being about 4 centimetres, its transverse diameter about 2.3 centimetres.

" The shaft presents, especially about its upper end, superficial erosions and osteophytic outgrowths similar to, but less extensive than those of its mate. The whole surface of the shaft is rough and porous.

" Transverse section between the upper and middle third shows an irregular inclosing shell of compact bone, from 1 to 5 millimetres in thickness. This superficial compact bone is in places riddled with larger and smaller very irregular Haversian canals; in places is quite dense and solid externally. On the posterior aspect of the bone along the oblique

line, the compact substance is pierced by the cancellous tissue, which
becomes continuous with the projecting osteophytes.

"Along the middle of the shaft, where it is most perfectly preserved,
the cancellous tissue completely fills the narrow cavity.

"The *microscopical examination* of the trabeculæ of the cancellous tissue
in both bones shows the usual appearances of such tissue, but the irregularity and apparent aimlessness of their grouping and arrangement indicate their formation under the influence of a chronic inflammatory process. Microscopical examination of the osteophytes shows the irregular
grouping and relative positions of the bone cells and bone lamellæ, which
is usually associated with such inflammatory structures. The microscopical examination of the more compact bone tissue from various
places in the shafts of both bones shows the utmost irregularity in the
arrangement, size, and direction of the Haversian canals and their surrounding lamellæ.

"The porous surfaces of the shafts show the eroded depressions, the
irregular entrances for bloodvessels, and in places the closely grouped

Fig. 9.

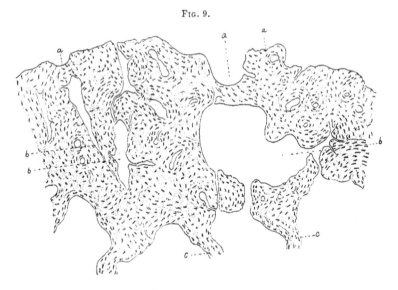

Howship's lacunæ which indicate the formation and absorption of the
superficial layers of bone under the influence of chronic periostitis. The
appearance of a considerably magnified transverse section of the more
compact bone of the right tibia, near its surface, is shown in Fig. 9.

"The articular surfaces of the knee-joint do not seem to have been the
seat of chronic inflammatory changes. But, judging from the large
osteophytic outgrowths about the upper end of the left tibia, it seems not
unlikely that this joint was stiff."

" Although there is no doubt that a certain amount of alteration in the external appearance of these bones has been produced by weathering or disintegration, yet the examination of their surfaces, even with a low magnifying power, shows most conclusively that they have been remarkably well preserved. The delicate sharp-edged openings through which the new-formed bloodvessels from the inflamed periosteum entered the bone ; the sharp-cut grooves along the surfaces in which the superficial bloodvessels lay as the new-formed bone spiculæ and lamellæ were built up about them, as well as the still finely preserved delicate projecting osteophytic masses, all show that to the vital processes of disease and not to disintegration or weathering are these various superficial changes due.

" If, then, we sum up the various departures from the normal which these bones present, in the form of an *anatomical diagnosis*, we find that they prove the existence of *chronic rarefying and formative osteitis, with osteomyelitis and chronic formative periostitis.*

" REMARKS ON MORPHOLOGICAL CHARACTERS AND CAUSATION.—It is evident that these are the bones of an adult who for a long time had been the victim of an extensive chronic bone disease in both legs, with a probable involvement of the left knee. This disease was so extensive and prolonged that it had led to the nearly complete making over of the shafts of both tibiæ.

" Under the influence of the inflammatory process the old bone was bit by bit absorbed, new bone being in greater or less degree formed near by to take its place. The new-formed bone, however, as is usually the case in chronic formative osteitis, has been only here and there developed in the proper amounts, situations, and relationships, so that it furnishes but a poor makeshift for and imitation of the original structure. Thus, while the right tibia, although the seat of profound disease, has fairly maintained its shape and functions, the left, although about twice as large as it should be, is a mere shell-covered spongy cylinder, which, yielding to the weight of the individual, has been bowed strongly forward.

" It seems probable that the disease was in progress at the time of the individual's death, because the evidences of repair are only such as are apt to go hand-in-hand with the destructive process in the chronic bone disease of this kind, as we know it to-day.

" Morphologically, the character and extent of the lesion in these bones is perfectly evident. When, however, we come to consider the probable cause of these extensive changes, the difficulties in arriving at a definite conclusion are very great. Whether the alterations are due to a specific cause—that is, to syphilitic infection, or to some other agency, it is, I think, not possible to say with even a measurable degree of positiveness. There is no evidence whatsoever in these bones that there has been either

caries or necrosis. There has been, so far as the bones show, simply
such a general rarefying and formative osteitis with formative periostitis
as to have produced the condition often described as spongy hyperostosis.
There is no evidence whatsoever, so far as I can see, of the presence at
any time of the more common and typical circumscribed nodular or
gummatous lesions, which are alone characteristic of syphilis of the
bones. There are none of those circumscribed local losses of substance,
associated with more or less localized sclerosis, which speak for the
former presence of gummata. On the other hand, there is, as is well
known, a more diffuse and general inflammation of the bone and periosteum which not infrequently occurs in the tibia, and which is believed
to be due to syphilitic infection. But even in this form of syphilitic
bone lesion, the sclerotic rather than the rarefying character in the inflammation, as is the case here, is, I think, apt to prevail.

" That the individual was not the victim of any phase of hereditary
syphilis which induced developmental malformations of these bones, is
evident from the sufficiently well formed upper articular extremities.

"Still, again, a simple non-specific general rarefying and formative
osteitis with formative periostitis leading to just such bone changes as
are present here, and with a predilection for the tibia is of no very
uncommon occurrence.

" On the whole, then, while I am disposed to think that there is nothing
in the morphological condition of these bones which would forbid the
assumption that the lesion might have been induced by the atypical form
of syphilitic inflammation, they present, nevertheless, no morphological
evidence to justify such a belief."

In the limits of this paper the effort has been made to restrict the
discussion to the main point at issue. What other diseases may be
represented in these morbid changes, in no way related to syphilis, is a
question for the general surgeon, the pathologist, and the practitioner.
Whether the septic forms of myelitis and periostitis with their consequent involvement of the bone tissue proper, may here be recognized as
due to the influence of the staphylococcus pyogenes albus and aureus ;
whether tuberculosis, or the exceedingly rare inflammations of bone due
to rheumatism, may be here assigned some place ; or, what is in this connection of more consequence, whether a special disease of the bones, not
syphilitic in character, prevailed among the aborigines, as it is said to
prevail to-day among the native tribes of some regions of this country,
there is not here space to inquire.

Admitting that among the bones exhumed in the Northern part of the
American continent, and found in the various collections of this country,
there are some which actually exhibit unmistakable lesions of syphilis,
the last problem prescribed for solution is: Are any of these bones not
merely syphilitic but unquestionably prehistoric? Are they parts of

the skeletons of North American Indians or of the whites mingled with the latter in the confusion resulting from race admixture in war, captivity, and many common enterprises? Are they, in point of fact, the bones of individuals dead before the first of the Spaniards set foot on the soil of San Salvador—or, in other words, of those dead before the year 1496? When we turn to the archæologists for a response, we are at once impressed with the fact that the romance once attaching to the prehistoric races of America has been dissipated by the researches of science. The conjecture that a people once dwelt on this soil of some pretension to civilization, building temples and cities comparable to those found in what we call the older world, has been removed by a more rigid study of the relics of the dust. The artificial mounds and stone dwellings, numbering thousands, some of very small and some of imposing size, and scattered throughout the country, were once thought to be the work of an ancient race of people commonly called the " Mound-builders" and the " Cliff dwellers," who were cited as a people showing evidence of an ancient civilization of no mean order and no common condition of culture. The bones which have been found in many of these mounds and in other places of sepulture, with the so-called works of art which these tombs contain, have been regarded as the remains of these primitive peoples.

These views have within a decade been shown to have a broader basis in the imagination than in tangible fact. From about the middle part of the Pleistocene period to the epoch of the first advent of the whites to the American coast, the history of man in America is seen to be the history of his slow and feeble evolution from a lower to a higher advancement in the Stone age. The best product of this process of evolution was reached by the North American Indian when he first looked seaward upon the sails of the Spanish fleet. There had been nothing superior to him before; and it is a question whether anything better has been since produced by this process of evolution from his race. He built no cities; he carved no vases; his work in metals was of the crudest sort. He and his fathers, his inferiors in culture, builded these mounds for sepulture and other purposes, sometimes as the foundation for communal dwellings. In some portions of the southwestern parts of the country where there is little vegetation and the plains are arid, he and his fathers excavated lodgings in the cliffs that hemmed in the canyons, or constructed them of the loose rocks that were easily separated from the walls of stone on either hand. But all the mounds are not prehistoric; and the same may be said of the excavated cliff dwellings. Even of the prehistoric mounds, some have been occupied in our own day, and some have been used for the interment of bones of individuals dead long after the admixture of the white and red races upon our soil. Of the glass beads, the tools and ornaments of copper, and other articles found in them suggestive of contemporaneous interment with the human bodies, many were manufactured by the whites and furnished to the Indians in the way of barter for peltries. It is also of importance to note that even within the mounds which are unquestionably of prehistoric structure and which undoubtedly at the first contained only the bones of a prehistoric race, there have been repeated intrusions, and these intrusive interments have resulted in depositing in such mounds, not merely bones of later generations surviving the Columbian advent, but, indeed, large bundles of such bones, some of them apparently collected from the most miscellaneous sources.

The wide door to confusion opened by the complete recognition of facts of this character cannot be ignored. It furnishes a possibility for errors which it would be difficult to number and impossible to overestimate.

In order to demonstrate in the case of bones obtained from any mound or burial-place of the cave-dwellers in North America, some of which exhibit evidences of syphilitic lesions of a suggestive or even unmistakable character, that the latter are proofs of a pre-Columbian prevalence of the disease, it is absolutely necessary to prove beyond question ; first, that such mound or burial-place was prehistoric in construction ; second, that such contained bones were interred at a prehistoric period ; third, and lastly, that after such burial there had been neither intrusive interment of bones nor other disturbance of mortuary relics after their first deposit.

From what precedes it is not difficult to conclude that positive proof of the prevalence of syphilis among the prehistoric races of America, based upon osseous changes, is scarcely yet at hand. With every passing year it may be remarked, the chances of securing such unequivocal demonstration are diminishing. As yet, we cannot say of any bone in our collections, that the demonstration both of its syphilitic character and prehistoric existence is without a flaw. We must, however, do full justice to the fact that an incredible amount of labor and of a praiseworthy American scholarship render it exceedingly probable to the mind of the unprejudiced that syphilis existed among the natives of the crowded West India Islands before the first visit of the whites. Even if some of the latter had been affected with a mild form of the malady, such as is described in the writings of the medical men of Europe before the fifteenth century, we can readily understand that the enormous culture-field offered by a race either virgin of that disorder or suffering from it in a mitigated form, might have been the effective origin of such a virulent epidemic as that which spread over Europe soon after the French invasion of Italy.

The appended titles are those of a few only of the works and papers that might be cited in this connection:

Brühl, Gustavus: "On the Pre-Columbian Existence of Syphilis in America," Cincinnati Lancet-Clinic, May 29, 1880.
—— "Pre-Columbian Syphilis in the Western Hemisphere," Cincinnati Lancet-Clinic, March 8, 1890.
Fournier, A.: "Syphilis Héréditaire Tardive," Paris, 1886.
Jones, Joseph: "Explorations of the Aboriginal Remains of Tennessee," Smithsonian Institution, Washington, 1876.
—— "Explorations and Researches concerning the Destruction of the Aboriginal Inhabitants of America," New Orleans Medical and Surgical Journal, June, 1878.
Lancereaux: "Traité de la Syphilis," Paris, 1873.
Langdon, F. W.: "The Madisonville Prehistoric Cemetery" [Author's edition], Journal of Cincinnati Society of Natural History, October, 1881.
Powell, J. W.: "Prehistoric Man in America," The Forum, New York, 1889.
Parrot: "Archiv de Physiolog.," 1871; Progrès Médical, 1880, and many subsequent papers to 1884.
Taylor, R. W.: "Syphilitic Lesions of the Osseous System in Infants and Young Children," New York, 1875.
Winsor, Justin: "Narrative and Critical History of America," Boston and New York, 1889.

NITROGEN MONOXIDE AND OXYGEN FOR ANÆSTHESIA IN MINOR SURGICAL OPERATIONS.

WITH A REPORT OF FIFTY CASES.[1]

BY WILLIAM WALDO VAN ARSDALE, M.D.,

ATTENDING SURGEON, EASTERN DISPENSARY, NEW YORK; LECTURER ON SURGERY, NEW YORK POLYCLINIC.

IN some physiological text-books we are told that mixtures of nitrous oxide and oxygen gas may be inhaled with impunity for any length of time, and when thus inhaled produce anæsthesia without unconsciousness. If this were true we would have in such mixtures the ideal anæsthetic that has for so long a time been the dream of many surgeons. A perfectly safe anæsthetic, respirable for hours by the patient, which would never fail to produce complete anæsthesia during any operation, and yet not render the patient unconscious, would be hailed as an advance in surgery.

In a recent paper read before the International Congress at Berlin, Horatio C. Wood spoke of such a "perfect anæsthetic," but added: "If such a drug exists (which has the power of paralyzing the sensory nerve-trunks without affecting other functions of the body) it yet awaits the coming of its discoverer."

[1] Read before the New York Surgical Society, with a demonstration on a patient of the method employed, Dec. 10, 1890.

Unfortunately, the above assertion in regard to the mixtures of nitrogen monoxide and oxygen requires considerable modification before it can be experimentally and clinically verified. If, however, there has been some advance toward finding the ideal anæsthetic referred to, this advance has been achieved by means of experiments conducted with such mixtures.

The use of pure nitrogen monoxide, so serviceable and efficient in dental practice as an anæsthetic, is not entirely so in surgery, even for minor operative procedures. It is true, for such operations as are of the very shortest possible duration, such as the incision into an abscess, it is a very valuable aid to their satisfactory performance, and one which we can ill afford to do without, whenever we have so great a number of such operations to perform that the question as to the amount of time spent on each one becomes an important one—as is the case in our public dispensaries.

But the short space of time during which complete anæsthesia, with loss of all reflexes, can be maintained by the administration of pure nitrogen monoxide interferes with the proper circumspect performance of the majority of operations generally classed together as minor operations (which we are called upon to perform in our clinics and dispensaries), especially when we make extensive use of the antiseptic method.

The opening and drainage, with incidental irrigation, of a palmar abscess, the cleansing and suture of an incised wound, the treatment of an abscess of the mammary gland, or of an acute suppurative lymphadenitis of the neck, cannot be satisfactorily conducted with the administration of pure nitrogen monoxide. I have myself used this anæsthetic in some 400 cases of the kind above described, and have always been oppressed by the sense of having to use undue haste in the performance of these small procedures.

But when such minor operations as the extirpation of ingrowing toenails, or the removal of cystic tumors of the scalp were to be performed, the administration of nitrogen monoxide in its pure form proved totally unsatisfactory and could not in any way compete with the use of cocaine.

Pure nitrogen monoxide, if given continuously, will produce complete anæsthesia with unconsciousness, on the average, in two minutes and eight seconds; and total cessation of respiration in about three minutes, on the average, which means death by asphyxia unless oxygen is speedily supplied. It is the deep cyanosis of the skin, and the dark-blue color of the blood flowing from the wound that induces the surgeon to abandon the anæsthetic before death ensues, and this, together with the fact that the heart continues to beat after respiration has ceased, constitutes the comparative safety of this anæsthetic—a safety which, however, exists only at the expense of the oftentimes unsatisfactory completion of the operation. The clonic spasms which occur before death are also liable to displace the mask and thus admit air into the lungs.

Although in many cases death may not occur so soon, in others it has occurred as early as after two minutes' inhalation of nitrogen monoxide. I recall only two cases where, before even the incision of an abscess could be accomplished, a state of asphyxia had obtained which was the cause, for some moments, of considerable anxiety on the part of the surgeon before the patients finally recovered. Both cases occurred in children, who generally take nitrogen monoxide very well.[1]

The physiological action of the nitrogen monoxide is now generally admitted to consist in shutting off oxygen from the blood. This action is not to be confounded with simple asphyxia after mechanical occlusion of the air-passages ; because in this latter case there is carbon dioxide present in the blood, which acts as a poison.

In asphyxia occurring after administration of pure nitrogen monoxide, there is simply a lack of oxygen in the tissues.

It is true, Ulbrich asserted that spectroscopic analysis of blood saturated with nitrogen monoxide showed no hæmoglobin to be present. But latterly Rothmann, by using more diluted solutions of such blood, established the presence of the hæmoglobin spectrum unimpaired, so that it must be conceded that there is no chemical action of the nitrogen monoxide upon the blood other than the simple shutting off of oxygen.

If, therefore, there is any interference with bodily functions in consequence of the inhalation of pure nitrogen monoxide, this may be due either to the specific action of the nitrogen monoxide (which is probably the cause of anæsthesia, as the experiments done with mixtures show), or it may be due to the absence of oxygen ; and this latter condition is probably the cause of the changes in the pulse and respiration, in the blood-pressure, and of the clonic spasms and tonic muscular contractions, observed after inhalation of nitrogen monoxide.

The action of the gas on the pulse and respiration has been described in a paper recently read before the National Academy of Medicine by Wood and Cerna, who found the pulse-rate decidedly slowed, while the arterial wave was enormously increased in size (due to stimulation of the inhibitory cardiac apparatus). The blood-pressure is extraordinarily raised, sometimes only momentarily and abruptly, and at various stages during the anæsthesia ; but present in the majority of cases.

The respiration very soon fails, and ceases entirely at a time when the heart is yet in full action.

When viewed as an anæsthetic to be admitted into general surgical

---

[1] From a verbal communication on the part of my colleague, Dr. Swinburne, I learn that he has observed four such cases, also occurring in children, in which considerable momentary apprehension was caused from an overdose of pure nitrogen monoxide, but in which perfect recovery followed.

practice it is evident that nitrogen monoxide in its pure state may never aspire to that position of usefulness occupied by ether and chloroform.

In the first place the danger attendant upon its administration for a longer period of time than three minutes, on the average, renders its use unsatisfactory.

Secondly, the action on the pulse at the commencement of the anæsthesia, and the increased blood-pressure, are serious drawbacks and a positive contra-indication to its use in a number of cases.

If anæsthesia, once induced with pure nitrogen monoxide, is to be maintained for any considerable length of time, this can be only achieved by admitting air in greater or smaller quantities into the lungs of the patient, by which means the occurrence of complete asphyxia may be repeatedly postponed.

This method has been in extensive use for some time. The administrator watches the skin of the patient, and when cyanosis becomes so deep that a further increase of the asphyxia appears alarming, sufficient air is admitted to postpone, for a time, the complete arrest of respiration. Or a certain quantity of air may be admitted, intentionally or unintentionally, along with the nitrogen monoxide from the first. It depends upon the skill of the administrator to keep the patient between the two evils of complete cessation of respiration and the awakening to consciousness with the return of the reflex motions and struggling.

With great skill and experience on the part of the operator, however, a prolonged narcosis can be maintained, presenting much the same effect as chloroform anæsthesia, and there are in the literature a number of such cases where anæsthesia was maintained for an hour and more.

But in all these cases cyanosis was continued and pronounced, and the blood that flowed from the wound was of very dark color.

When we consider that this cyanosis is actually due to the want of oxygen, and that we have to deal with a condition of incomplete asphyxia continued for a long period of time, it appears questionable whether its effects may not result from this practice. There is a state of asphyxia of the tissues, which leads to inflammatory changes with subsequent degeneration.

An Esmarch bandage applied to the limb of an animal will, by shutting off the oxygen supply of the blood, produce such great molecular changes in the muscles (disappearance of the nuclei and inflammatory conditions) that they can be seen and studied with the microscope, as Leser has shown. And this occurs after three hours' application of the bandage. It is, therefore, not out of place to question whether such tissue-asphyxia may not be induced quite as readily by prolonged narcosis by mixtures of nitrogen monoxide and air.

Another point may here be mentioned. When only a little air is admitted along with the nitrogen monoxide, as soon as this air has entered into the lungs carbon dioxide appears in the blood. So that these patients present the same conditions as do patients suffering from simple mechanical asphyxia. Now, we know when patients pass from asphyxia produced by carbon dioxide poisoning to complete suffocation. they do so without muscular spasms or convulsions. We see, therefore, that although the anæsthesia with mixtures of air and nitrogen monoxide may keep the patient more quiet as to muscular reaction, it does so at no small detriment to the system. Indeed, I much question whether the sugar found in the urine after prolonged anæsthesia with nitrogen monoxide is not the expression of such detriment to the system.

Still another disadvantage may be here considered, which often attaches to these narcoses maintained by the admittance of air with the nitrogen monoxide, and that is the subjective sense of strangulation on the part of the patient. This sense is not always pronounced, however, and does not usually interfere with the performance of the operation.

In view of all these disadvantages attaching to the administration of nitrogen monoxide, either in its pure state or when mixed with air, it is not strange that many attempts should have been made to obtain all the benefits of such an agreeable and safe anæsthetic as nitrogen monoxide has the reputation of being, without its drawbacks and disadvantages.

One of the most evident methods of avoiding the danger lying in the asphyxiated condition resulting from inhalation of the nitrogen monoxide is the admixture of pure oxygen with the gas. This method has been repeatedly tried and again abandoned, so that surgeons in general had lost all hope of practically introducing it into general use.

According to Von Bruns, Hermann was the first to mix the gases, taking seventy-eight parts of nitrogen monoxide and twenty-two parts of oxygen, thus imitating our own atmosphere in the quantity of oxygen. He found that this mixture produced anæsthesia without loss of consciousness. Subsequently Von Bruns tried this mixture for surgical purposes, but was unsuccessful.

The most distinguished effort in this direction was made by Paul Bert in 1878.

His method of reasoning was simple: Pure nitrous monoxide causes anæsthesia at atmospheric pressure, but also asphyxia. The latter can be obviated by the admixture of as much oxygen as is contained in our atmosphere—i. e., one volume of oxygen added to four volumes of the nitrogen monoxide. If, however, this admixture is made, the tension of the nitrogen monoxide in the mixture is not as great (by one-fifth) as it was before the admixture, and consequently no anæsthesia will be produced. In order to remedy this it is only necessary to increase the atmospheric pressure by just so much as the tension of the nitrogen monoxide gas is weakened by the addition of oxygen, namely, by one-

fifth atmosphere. If this be done the result of inhalation will be anæsthesia without asphyxia.

The practical problem presenting itself for solution was how to obtain
the atmospheric super-pressure. It was solved by Paul Bert by building a hermetically sealed glass cage with proper arrangements attached
for increasing the atmospheric pressure. Into this cage the patient and
the surgeons and assistants were all admitted, and here the gas was
administered.

The practical obstacles in the way of this method are the expense of
the apparatus, which alone amounted to 10,000 francs, and the difficulty
of its transportation.

With this arrangement, however, success was manifest. A large
number of operations were performed by L'Abbé and Péan, and the
following observations were made:

With an admixture of 20 per cent. in volume of pure oxygen to
the pure nitrogen monoxide, anæsthesia was almost instantly induced as
soon as the patient commenced inhaling it. It could be continued for
any desirable length of time. When inhalation was interrupted the
patient instantly recovered. After anæsthesia no headache, no nausea,
no digestive disturbance, was observed. No vomiting occurred. In
short, the compound appeared perfectly safe and innocuous.

We have here an ideal anæsthetic for surgical use, but the practical
difficulties in the way of its general introduction are insurmountable.

In the second year following, Raphael Blanchard published a monograph in which sixty operations of a major and minor character, some
of over one hour's duration, were reported, all done after the same
method of Paul Bert, and confirming his conclusions.

One year later, in 1881, Klikovitch, of St. Petersburg, began further
experiments with a mixture similar to that used by Paul Bert in obstetrical practice and during parturition. He came to the conclusion
that, for the purpose of rendering parturition painless, the inhalation of
the mixture without additional pressure was sufficient. The patients
retained their consciousness, although it was generally somewhat dulled.

The anæsthesia was not complete, however, the pain being merely
diminished in some cases and not entirely removed.

The conclusions of Klikovitch were: (*a*) that the mixture was entirely
free from danger for the mother and the child; (*b*) that pain was undoubtedly diminished; (*c*) that consciousness was not interfered with;
(*d*) that no vomiting or intestinal disturbance was induced; (*e*) that no
cumulative action of the gas mixture could be observed; (*f*) and that
the mixture could be administered even without the presence of a
physician; (*g*) but that the apparatus was not readily transportable and
that the procedure was too expensive.

These observations were corroborated by Tittel, of Dresden, and by

E. Cohn, of Berlin, and I may add that we have two further contributions to the literature regarding the use of the mixture during labor. The one by Swiecicki, who writes in favor of its use, and the other by Doederlein, who was not so favorably impressed by it. An attempted incision of an abscess of the mammary gland was a failure as far as the anæsthesia was concerned. Both used a compound consisting of 20 per cent. of oxygen and 80 per cent. of nitrogen monoxide, without atmospheric super-pressure.

The first successful major surgical operation with a less cumbersome apparatus than that of Paul Bert, appears to be one published in 1888 by Witzinger.

A mixture was administered composed of twelve volumetric parts of oxygen and eighty-eight of nitrogen monoxide and continued for eighteen minutes, during which time Von Mosetig-Moorhof performed a resection of the hip-joint. The operation had not been completed when the supply of the mixture gave out and chloroform had to be substituted. In another operative case, however, also of a major character, but occurring in dispensary practice, the compound failed entirely; while in two minor operative procedures the anæsthetic was administered with success.

In these cases the gas compound was not administered under pressure; but the percentage of oxygen was reduced from that employed by Paul Bert.

The clinical observations made during the operation of hip-joint resection were as follows: Narcosis was complete after one minute and two seconds. There was no preliminary stage of excitation. Respiration was calm; the pupils were dilated; there was total absence of muscular tonus. The conjunctival reflex was abolished. The action of the heart was regular and strong.

In the following year, 1889, Gersuny, of Vienna, published eight cases of surgical operations in which Hillischer administered a mixture of twelve parts of oxygen and eighty-eight parts of nitrogen monoxide. The gases were mixed immediately before inspiration by means of a specially arranged stopcock. In six of these cases the narcosis was maintained for from eight and a half to fourteen minutes. In two of them the duration was thirty-three and thirty-eight minutes respectively. The time necessary to induce anæsthesia varied between one and a half and ten minutes. In two cases asphyxia occurred, and the operation was interrupted. Two cases were complicated by vomiting. The pulse was full, between 120 and 140; the blood-pressure sank during narcosis. Respiration was 50, with marked cyanosis in two of the cases. No evil after-effects were noticed.

These few operations are the only surgical procedures I have been able to find recorded in the literature, where use was made of mixtures of oxygen and nitrogen monoxide.

The other cases refer either to experiments done upon animals, or else to the use of the mixture in dental practice. Both of these categories interest us here only in so far as our knowledge of the physiological action of the mixture has been increased by them.

The most prominent among the more recent experiments upon animals published are those done by Wood and Cerna.

They found that the blood-pressure was not raised when a mixture of nitrogen monoxide and oxygen, containing 10 per cent. of the latter, was administered; but that the pulse-rate was reduced, just as in the administration of pure nitrogen monoxide. They also found, however, that such a mixture failed to produce anæsthesia.[1]

As regards the length of time during which the anæsthetic may be administered, Martin, in 1888, narcotized a dog with a mixture of fifteen parts of oxygen and eighty-five parts of nitrogen monoxide, and kept the animal continually under its influence for seventy-two consecutive hours. The dog slept peacefully all the time.

When a similar mixture ($12\frac{1}{2}$ parts of oxygen and $87\frac{1}{2}$ parts of nitrogen monoxide) has been used on the human subject in dental practice for the purpose of painless extraction of teeth, it has been customary to mix the gases in a gasometer, and from these gasometers the mixtures generally escaped under slight pressure. A large number of such cases have been reported by Hewitt. In these cases, after a few inspirations, a slowing of the respiration was observed, but neither cyanosis nor stertorous breathing ever occurred. The pulse was full, strong, regular, between 80 and 90. These administrations were generally given for about two minutes; sensibility was sufficiently blunted to permit satisfactory work in extracting a tooth; muscular rigidity was sometimes present, and in some cases the anæsthetic failed completely.

In attempting to sum up the information given in all these data, and in the rest of the literature not quoted here pertaining to the mixtures, we are struck by the conflicting statements of different observers. The one statement, on which all appear agreed, is that the admixture of oxygen to the nitrogen monoxide does not cause an increase of the blood-pressure (Hillischer, 1866). The statements as to pulse and respiration vary. Asphyxia did not occur when the gases were previously mixed. But frequently the anæsthesia failed entirely, and often it was unsatisfactory; so that, with the exception of Paul Bert's cumbersome apparatus, surgical practice has as yet not profited much by these observations.

We may refer the lack of unity in the clinical observations made—to

[1] I learn from personal communication that Dr. B. F. Curtis, of this city, has lately performed similar experiments; but they have not yet been published, to my knowledge.

the variations in the methods and apparatus employed by the various administrators.

I now turn to my own experience with the mixtures of oxygen and nitrogen monoxide.

My attention was first called to these mixtures by my colleague, Dr. Moskovich, an expert in nitrous oxide anæsthesia and lecturer in the New York College of Dentistry, who told me, in June, 1889, of the experiments being made at that time in Russia.

I am indebted to the courtesy of Dr. Moskovich for administering the mixtures in all of the cases here reported, with the exception of but two.

The cases thus observed now number over fifty.

At first my efforts were directed toward verifying the facts first published by the physicians in Russia—Klikovitsch and others. Accordingly, I procured from a firm in this city a cylinder containing a mixture of twenty parts of oxygen and eighty parts of nitrogen monoxide, this being the mixture used by Paul Bert and others. The apparatus used was the same as employed for the administration of pure nitrous oxide gas; the S. S. White Inhaler No. 2 being used in connection with a seven-gallon rubber-bag reservoir. The first inhalation was taken by Dr. Moskovich himself, for a short time only, about two and a half minutes in all. After one minute he had lost sensation and consciousness; but there was no muscular relaxation. There was no trace of cyanosis, and subjectively no sensation of suffocation was experienced.

The next case was a successful one as far as the satisfactory completion of the operation was concerned: the incision and drainage of an axillary abscess, to which the patient, a young German girl, submitted without apparently feeling the least pain, although she retained consciousness all the time.

But the following three cases showed that the administration of this mixture produced excitation and incomplete anæsthesia, so that what still remained of the mixture was diluted with pure nitrogen monoxide in order to reduce the quantity of oxygen present to about half its original proportion, or to 10 per cent. With this mixture two successful operations were performed; the extraction of a foreign body in the hand of a woman twenty-four years of age, and the curetting of ulcerating tuberculous lymphatic glands of the neck in a man twenty-nine years of age. In both of these cases the patient was fully under the influence of the anæsthetic in from one to two minutes, and awoke at once at the removal of the inhaler. The anæsthetic was inhaled for four minutes without the least sign of cyanosis or asphyxia.

It was therefore believed that a mixture containing less of the oxygen would do better service; and a mixture containing 15 per cent. in volume of oxygen was prepared for me by the S. S. White Dental Co., of this city.[1]

This new mixture was administered twelve times. Dr. Moskovich kindly volunteered to inhale it, which he did for over five minutes consecutively. He took large inspirations and breathed naturally the entire time; the pulse was regular and full, not increased in frequency. There was no cyanosis or asphyxia. He remained conscious, however, or almost completely so, all the time. His subjective sensations were hammering and ringing in the ears; he could hear a loud voice, however, and feel a slight touch. The sensation of pain was greatly diminished but not entirely removed; anæsthesia was incomplete. A slight excitation was manifest to the by-standers; he followed our movements with his eyes, which were bright.

The cases treated with this mixture are the following:

CASE I.—J. K., female, aged nineteen years; abscess of the palm. Duration of anæsthesia six and a half minutes. Anæsthesia not complete; reflex movements of the hand noticed during the incision. The patient subsequently stated that she had not felt much pain.

CASE II.—B. W., female, aged seventeen years; abscess of the hand. Was partly unconscious; did not move the hand during the incisions. She subsequently said she had felt pain.

CASE III.—B. K., female, aged eighteen years; abscess of the hand. Was unconscious in three-quarters of a minute. One incision, which was not felt, and not remembered. On awakening after two minutes a hysterical excitation was manifested, which soon passed over.

CASE IV.—M. N., male, aged forty years; stricture of urethra. Patient of extreme neurasthenic condition, highly excited and nervous at taking gas. The excitement increased under influence of the mixture. After two minutes, mixture abandoned and pure nitrogen monoxide substituted. It was found impossible to bring the patient under its influence. Wild movements of the limbs, maniacal excitation, cries. Operation postponed to future date.

CASE V.—N. M., male, aged fifteen years; complete luxation of fore-arm backward. The mixture administered for examination and replacement. In one and a half minutes, unconsciousness; no muscular rigidity or spasm, no reflex movements. Immediate revival on removal of inhaler. No remembrance of pain. On questioning, answered that he did not know where he had been. No after-effects.

This patient subsequently took the mixture twice more, and each time with similar excellent results. Massage and passive motion produced no sense of pain.

CASE VI.—R. K., female, aged five years; large alveolar abscess. Took mixture for three minutes. Anæsthesia complete, but patient appeared not entirely unconscious. Incision. Immediate recovery.

CASE VII.—F. S., female, aged eight years; abscesses of the hand

[1] I take pleasure in acknowledging my indebtedness to the courtesy of this firm in supplying these mixtures, since by this means I was enabled to rely upon the accuracy of measurement and the good quality of the ingredients in each case.

and of the leg. Was given the mixture for six minutes. Consciousness and sensation had ceased after one minute; but slight reflex movements were noticed on incision through the skin.

CASE VIII.—L. E., male, aged three years; mastoid abscess. Unconscious after half a minute. Operation completed after three minutes.
No sensation, but muscular rigidity of the extremities continued the
entire time. Immediate recovery.

CASE IX.—H. W., male, aged twenty years; ingrowing toe-nail;
extirpation of nail. Anæsthesia complete. On recovery, nausea and
vomiting.

CASE X.—M. St., male, aged fifteen years; abscess of the jaw. The
patient was apparently not fully under the influence of the anæsthetic when the incision of the abscess was commenced. Reflex movements and muscular spasm. Time of narcosis two minutes and two
seconds. On recovery the patient stated he had not felt anything at all.

CASE XI.—A. S., male, aged twenty years; abscess at the back of the
neck. Administration for two minutes only; anæsthesia complete, but
muscular spasm and rigidity were present.

On reviewing these cases it became evident that this mixture is not
satisfactory for surgical work, when administered in this manner. Only
two cases of the eleven were satisfactory; in the others the muscular
rigidity and spasm and the incomplete loss of consciousness interfered
with the operation.

I therefore next procured a quantity of gas mixture from the same
firm containing ninety parts by volume of nitrogen monoxide and ten
parts of oxygen. With this mixture all further narcoses were conducted, and as far as the objectionable feature of the pure nitrogen
monoxide anæsthesia—the asphyxia—is concerned, it was always
avoided by the use of this mixture. No case presented any symptoms
of cyanosis, the patient retaining the normal color of his skin throughout.

One of the first cases in which this new mixture was used was very
successful.

CASE XII.—An adult man, suffering from an abscess of the neck,
took the mixture and immediately fell into a peaceful sleep. Deep,
normal respiratory movements continued and no excitement or muscular
rigidity was manifested. The operation was completed in three minutes.
The patient rapidly awoke on removal of the mask and had no consciousness of what had been done.

In the further cases treated with this mixture, however, the patients
behaved very much as with the foregoing mixtures containing fifteen
parts of oxygen to the hundred.

A state of semi-consciousness, combined with more or less muscular
rigidity, manifested itself and interfered with the uninterrupted performance of the operative procedures.

It was made out, however, at this time that the chief impediment to

the complete anæsthetization was the failure on the part of the patient
to take deep inspirations.   In the case of one or two patients (who
had no beards) who took deep inspirations, the anæsthesia was much
improved.   But the natural excitability of many of the patients about
to undergo a surgical operation is apt to prevent normal and deep respiration.[1]

As all these methods of administering mixtures of oxygen and
nitrous monoxide gas had failed to give satisfaction, it occurred to me
that by using pressure to force the gas mixture into the lungs of the
patient, the amount inhaled might be increased and at the same time
the tension of the nitrogen monoxide gas might be made greater.

This method is an entirely different one from that used by Paul Bert,
who placed the patient in an entire atmosphere of greater tension, but
did not influence the respiration in any way.

If, however, gas is administered under pressure, the mode of respiration is entirely changed.   It approximates more closely to the artificial
respiration which we have occasion to observe in our physiological
laboratories; but with this difference, that the pressure in our case is
constant, while there it is intermittent ; moreover, it is not great enough
to interfere with the natural expiration.

The practical question presenting itself was the construction of a
proper apparatus, which should be readily portable and should permit
of an exercise of pressure upon the gas reservoir that could be varied
as desired.

The difficulties attending the hermetical connection between the
mouth and nose of the patient and the reservoir bag were met by using
the S. S. White Gas-inhaler No. 2, which in adults can be held in place
so firmly by the administrator of the mixture that no air has access
alongside of the mask.

In two categories of cases, however, this adaptation of the inhaler is
interfered with.   First, in children, for the reason that the mask is too
large and admits air below the chin.   If it were considered necessary
to give the mixture to children under pressure, special inhalers of
smaller size would have to be used.   But in the case of children I have

---

[1] In one case the attempt was made to use morphine subcutaneously in order to
counteract the nervousness evidenced by the patient.   But this endeavor proved a complete failure.   The patient, a man, twenty years of age, was to have a toe-nail extirpated.   He was of a highly nervous organization and excitable temperament.   It was
found impossible to get him under the influence of the mixture, and, therefore, pure
nitrogen monoxide was substituted.   But this had no more effect upon the patient than
the mixture.   There was unconsciousness, but apparently no anæsthesia, no insensibility.   At each attempt to use the knife the patient would remonstrate, and move the
lower extremities.   The operation was finally completed, but on recovery the patient
vomited, and appeared prostrated for some time.   He said he had suffered much pain,
but did not know where he was.

found that the mixture works quite sufficiently well without additional pressure, so that I have not as yet had such an inhaler constructed. Secondly, in cases where the patient has a large beard, it is difficult to prevent the entrance of air alongside of the inhaler. For this reason the majority of cases, where the mixture was used for anæsthetizing such patients, were failures.

The amount of pressure necessary to induce anæsthesia is a question of some practical interest. According to Paul Bert's theory the tension with which the mixture is administered should bear the same proportion to the atmospheric pressure as the mixture bears to the nitrogen monoxide in the mixture. Thus, if we use a 10 per cent. mixture of oxygen and nitrogen monoxide, it will be sufficient to increase the pressure with which it is administered one-tenth of an atmosphere.[1]

In practice I have not as yet had opportunity to use so great a pressure—partly owing to the delicate construction of the reservoir bag used and partly owing to the arrangement of the mica valve in the inhaler used. The great majority of administrations of the mixture were given with the use of two simple boards of white wood, about two feet square and hinged together. Between these the rubber bag containing the mixture was placed, so that the gas was forced out into the inhaler at a pressure of about three-fourths of an inch of water on an average, this corresponding to a pressure upon the bag of three pounds, and when the gas was nearly consumed the bag was again filled from the cylinder *a tergo*.

Sometimes this pressure was employed from the commencement of the anæsthesia; but more generally the pressure was not added until the patient had inhaled the mixture for a minute or less and was considered under its influence. Then the weight of the upper board was brought to bear upon the bag.

The evident objection to this method of employing pressure is the following. When the two hinged boards approach each other the pressure upon the gas in the bag is increased, and when the bag is full and the boards become more separated in consequence, the pressure is diminished. The tension with which the gas escapes into the inhaler is consequently not equable. I have, therefore, of late contrived another simple arrangement of the two boards, by which they should remain always parallel to each other and thus render the pressure more equable.

---

[1] To state the problem more correctly, and since the volume of a gas is inversely proportional to the pressure, we may adduce the following proportion:

$$9 \text{ vol.} : 10 \text{ vol.} :: 1 \text{ atm.} : 1.111 \text{ atm.}$$

The total pressure on the mixture should then be 1.111 atmospheres; of this 1 atmosphere will be due to the nitrogen monoxide and 0.111 atm. to the oxygen. Expressed in millimetres of quicksilver, the pressure of the nitrogen monoxide would be 760, and that of the oxygen 84.3.

The upper board is provided with four stout iron wire rods, about two feet long, and attached near the corners of the board' after the manner of the legs of a table. These rods are unscrewed from their place for transportation. The rods pass through large holes in the corners of the lower board. The reservoir bag being placed between the two boards is thus exposed to a constant pressure amounting to five pounds and a half in the apparatus.

It will be seen that the administration of the mixture under pressure is a task requiring some skill and attention. In the first place, the mask requires to be held so firmly over the nose and mouth of the patient, that no air may enter alongside of the inflated rubber mounting. Secondly, the administrator should keep the reservoir-bag filled with the mixture during the entire time of the operation, so as not to cause any fluctuation of the tension under which the mixture is administered. At the same time he must watch the respiratory movements of the patient (as indicated by the valve in the inhaler), and the color of the patient's skin.

The first case in which the gas mixture was administered under pressure (in December, 1889), was a brilliant success.

CASE XIII.—The patient, a robust man of twenty years, suffering from a deep abscess of the finger, was given the mixture (containing 10 per cent. of oxygen), at first without pressure for three minutes. During this time he breathed naturally but retained consciousness, and could feel the prick of a pin as painful. Then moderate pressure was applied to the reservoir-bag (about two and a half pounds), and he immediately appeared to fall asleep. After one further minute there was complete atony, insensibility, absence of muscular spasm and rigidity, and absence of reflex movements. He recovered very rapidly after removal of the inhaler, and said he had felt nothing at the time of the operation.

Twenty-five further narcoses were conducted with the use of pressure-boards, and with the same mixture of ten parts of oxygen and ninety parts of nitrogen monoxide.

Many of these may be classed as brilliant successes, while others proved failures from one cause or another; and my attention was directed toward finding out, if possible, what occasioned the failures, so that they might be avoided.

I give the cases, as briefly as possible, commencing with the more successful ones.

CASE XIV.—R. S., female, aged thirty years; abscess of hand. Mixture given for fifteen seconds without pressure; then for three minutes with pressure. Patient completely anæsthetic and unconscious. Incision of abscess. Recovered rapidly.

CASE XV.—B. E., aged twenty years; two abscesses of the finger. Mixture given first for two seconds, then with pressure added for six minutes. Complete insensibility. Incision of abscesses.

Case XVI.—M. M., male, aged twenty years; abscess of hand. Mixture first given without pressure for twenty seconds, then with pressure. Complete anæsthesia and unconsciousness.

Case XVII.—M. S., male, aged seven years; foreign body under skin. Mixture given for twenty seconds without, then for one minute with pressure. Extraction, of the body. Unconsciousness and anæsthesia complete.

Case XVIII.—N. S., male, aged thirty years; foreign body under nail. Mixture first given for fifteen seconds, then with pressure. Extraction of body. Anæsthesia and unconsciousness complete.

Case XIX.—M. C., female, aged twenty-five years; suppurative mastitis. Mixture administered without pressure for twenty seconds, then with pressure. Unconsciousness and anæsthesia well marked, but slight muscular rigidity in the extremities. Four incisions into the gland. On recovery from the anæsthetic the patient had a laughing spell, and was greatly delighted at the fact of the operation being completed.

Case XX.—The same patient was subsequently treated for other abscesses of the mammary gland, three incisions being made at this time. The anæsthetic was administered in the same way with the same good effect; but on recovery the patient wept and felt pain.

Case XXI.—L. S., female, aged nineteen years, in the eighth month of gestation; abscess of the hand. Mixture administered for one minute without, then for five minutes with pressure. Two incisions were made. Unconsciousness and anæsthesia well marked; but a little muscular rigidity was noticed.

Case XXII.—A. B., female, aged (?); suppurative lymphadenitis of neck. Mixture given for thirty seconds without pressure, then for ten minutes with pressure. Incision of abscesses.

Case XXIII.—M. G., male, aged eleven years; foreign body in gluteal region. Mixture given with pressure. Extraction of two large splinters of wood.

In both of these latter cases some slight cyanosis was observed, the supply of gas in the cylinder being nearly exhausted.

Case XXIV.—M. N., female, aged twenty years; tubercular lymphadenitis of neck. Mixture given first without, then with pressure. The patient lapsed into a peaceful sleep; unconsciousness and anæsthesia perfect; no reflex movements or muscular rigidity. Incision.

Case XXV.—L. H., male, aged sixteen years; incised wound of wrist. Mixture administered with pressure from the first. Anæsthesia induced in one-quarter of a minute; kept up for three minutes. Complete unconsciousness and insensibility to pain. Anæsthesia resembling a perfectly calm sleep. No cyanosis; no muscular rigidity. Disinfection and suture of the wound. Quick recovery on removal of inhaler.

There were two or three other cases, not recorded in my notes, which may be mentioned here, where the mixture was exhibited in cases operated upon by my colleague, Dr. Schapringer.

Case XXVI.—This one was an operation for the occlusion of a lachrymal fistula in a girl aged about six years. The anæsthesia proved perfectly satisfactory, the excision of the fistulous tract and the placing of the sutures being done with perfect ease during the unconsciousness and anæsthesia of the patient.

CASE XXVII.—Another operation was the extraction of a foreign body from the external auditory meatus in an adult man, the anæsthetic being administered in the sitting posture, and giving perfect satisfaction. The patient neither moved nor manifested signs of insensibility during the operation ; although on questioning afterward he stated he had felt everything.

There were also some four further cases, of which, however, the notes have been lost.

Besides these successful cases of anæsthesia by this method of administering the mixture under pressure, there are several cases in which the results were less satisfactory.

CASE XXVIII.—L. G., female, aged six years; deep abscess of the neck, probably tubercular in character. Mixture administered without pressure for twenty seconds, then with pressure for four or five minutes in all. Incision and evacuation of abscess. The patient manifested a little excitement, breathed rapidly, and showed some cyanosis. (This was the residue of gas in the cylinder.)

CASE XXIX.—Adult female ; ingrowing toe-nail. Mixture administered for five minutes, during which time the operation for extirpation of the nail proceeded satisfactorily, when clonic movements of the extremities and manifestations of excitation set in. The operation was successfully concluded, and although consciousness was absent, the movements suggested the sensation of pain.

CASE XXX.—A. W., male, aged eighteen years; severe contusion of the elbow. Mixture administered at first for fifteen seconds without, then for three minutes with pressure, for the purpose of using massage and passive motion. No pain was experienced, but slight tonic spasm was manifest in the muscles of the arm during the anæsthesia.

CASE XXXI.—V. P., female, aged twenty-two years, of very excitable disposition ; suppurative axillary lymphadenitis. The mixture administered for two minutes and forty seconds under pressure before operation ; then for three minutes and twenty seconds, or for six minutes in all. Incision and drainage of the abscess. Loss of consciousness complete ; no cyanosis; but muscular rigidity present all the time. On awakening the patient lapsed into a hysterical condition, screamed, and was much excited. Vomiting also occurred.

CASE XXXII.—L. J., female, aged twenty-four years ; was present during the foregoing operation, and much excited and frightened in consequence ; suppurating mastitis. Mixture administered with pressure for five minutes and ten seconds in all. Remained partly conscious ; muscular rigidity marked. Substitution of pure nitrogen monoxide ; but patient could not be brought entirely under its influence.

There are, furthermore, some cases in which the action of the mixture under pressure were entirely unsatisfactory.

CASE XXXIII.—Male, aged thirty years; fistula-in-ano. Mixture given first without, then with pressure ; but the patient could not be got under its influence. Pure nitrogen monoxide was then substituted, but with no better result, and asphyxia occurring with convulsions, the operation was abandoned.

Case XXXIV.—B. S., male, aged thirty-one years; abscess of the hand. Mixture given under pressure. Incision of abscess. On removal of the inhaler a brief period of excitation of a maniacal character ensued, during which the patient uttered loud cries, walked across the room, and seated himself in a chair. On questioning, he afterward stated he had felt much pain. This patient was of a highly nervous temperament, but very muscular and robust.

Case XXXV.—Adult man, with large growth of beard; fistula-in-ano. Mixture given under pressure but failed in its effect. Pure nitrogen monoxide substituted; but even with this the patient could not be anæsthetized. Great muscular spasm supervened and the operation, consisting in actual cauterization of the fissure and removal of hæmor-rhoidal cicatricial excrescences, could be completed only with difficulty.

Case XXXVI.—In still another case, that of an Italian, aged eighteen years, the mixture as well as the nitrogen monoxide failed to have the desired anæsthetic effect, but no mention is made in my notes as to the cause of the failure.

In reviewing all these cases where the mixture of oxygen and nitrogen monoxide was given under pressure, we must first consider those cases in which the anæsthetic failed to act satisfactorily.

These cases may be arranged in four groups or categories.

The first group comprises those patients who manifest extreme nervousness and excitability of temperament before they are given the mixture. There appears to be some element in the mental condition of these patients which counteracts the sedative influence of the mixture.

We know that certain medicines act differently upon persons of different temperament and idiosyncrasies; and that pain is largely dependent for its subjective appreciation on the attention. So, in order that a mixture of oxygen and nitrogen monoxide should induce perfect anæsthesia, the patient should be at his ease and not in an excited or frightened state of mind.

In the case of a woman, who had taken the mixture with good anæsthetic effect a day or two before, the administration of the same mixture utterly failed, because she had been frightened by the screams of another woman while under an anæsthetic during an operation preceding hers.

Closely allied to this first group of patients is a second, comprising those patients that look forward to an operation about the genital organs or the rectum. I know not why it is that this class of patients should be more difficult to anæsthetize than others. I have often observed, however, that such patients take ether and chloroform far worse than patients expecting operations on other parts of their bodies; and I believe the fact that operations upon the rectum or the genital organs are more dreaded than those on other parts will explain the matter.

A third group comprises those patients who have a heavy growth of beard. This interferes with the close fitting of the inhaler to the face, and consequently air is admitted into the lungs along with the mixture. The patient cannot, therefore, be considered to breathe the mixture as it is prepared, and the desired effect is lost.

Perhaps it may be possible, by moistening the beard with water or in some other manner, to exclude atmospheric air in these cases.

A last group is represented by a number of persons, upon whom the mixture as well as the pure nitrogen monoxide has no sedative effect at all, or at any time, quite independently of their momentary mental condition. Every practitioner or dentist who has had occasion to use nitrogen monoxide in a large number of cases, has met with patients who cannot be brought under the influence of the gas at all. Generally they become more and more excited as the gas is inhaled by them, and acute maniacal attacks are sometimes observed, during which they utter howls and shrieks and make violent muscular exertions—oftentimes of an aggressive nature, and increased by restraint. Such conditions are comparatively rare, occurring in my own experience in about two per cent. of the cases, and always pass over rapidly without any detriment.

I ascribe the cause of failure in this group to habit. For I believe this condition stands in some relation to chronic alcoholism ; and judging by the difficulty we experience in bringing patients used to drinking large quantities of alcohol under the influence of chloroform and ether, I suspect a similar cause in these cases.

We therefore find the field for the administration of mixtures of nitrogen monoxide and oxygen considerably narrowed down, and are obliged to rule out, as unsuitable, quite an appreciable percentage of all the cases we may be called upon to treat.

In the majority of cases, however, in young, healthy individuals and in females, the anæsthetic mixture when administered under pressure was found to work well and to be much superior to the pure nitrogen monoxide for surgical purposes. It induces a state resembling a quiet deep sleep, in which the respiration is slow and regular, the pulse regular and full and not much, if ever, increased in frequency. The blood-pressure is not increased ; and insensibility to pain and unconsciousness go hand-in-hand.

It was my fortune to meet with a class of patients, as far as the foregoing observations are concerned, who were not sufficiently intelligent to observe their own feelings with any accuracy, or to inspire the confidence of others in their statements. It is one of the characteristic features of the nitrogen monoxide that while it induces unconsciousness to the surroundings it does not interfere with the activity of the memory and imagination.

The mixtures cause the patients under their influence to sleep, but also to dream, and more or less vividly—and some, on awakening are apt to mistake their dreams for reality. Under these conditions it is difficult to know whether, when a patient says he felt an incision, he actually has remembrance of pain felt at the time, or whether the pain still present in the wound on the rapid awakening of the patient is not mistaken for the pain of the operation. For this reason I think it advisable to continue the anæsthetic for some time after the operation is completed, especially when nerve-trunks have been severed.

This rapid recovery after administration of the mixture under pressure is not so marked as when no pressure is used; the longer time the pressure has been used, the more time is required for recovery. In any case, however, according to my own experience, the interval of time between the removal of the inhaler and the recovery of the patient is too brief to admit of the satisfactory use of the mixture, even with pressure, for the extraction of teeth. The pure nitrogen monoxide allows the dentist more time to work in, during the slower recovery of his patient out of his asphyxiated condition.

Some writers are fearful lest by keeping the mixture of oxygen and nitrogen monoxide under pressure in the steel cylinders, a higher oxidation of the nitrogen should occur, and nitrogen dioxide or other poisonous compounds be produced. As far as my experience reaches, I have seen no occasion for any apprehension, although I have given this question special clinical attention.

The contents of the cylinders procured from the company mentioned above appeared to act equally well whether they had been freshly prepared or kept on hand or stored for some time.

Some variation was observed, however, between the action of the first of the mixture escaping from the cylinder and that of the last. On opening the cylinder for the first time, the gas mixture contains more oxygen than the rest of the gas.

The first bagful is therefore not used at all, while the last two or three bagfuls of a cylinder act much the same as pure nitrogen monoxide, and should be given without pressure. The appearance of cyanosis in a patient under the influence of the mixture is a sign that the supply is giving out.

The large cylinder, holding three hundred and twenty and more gallons of gas, proved more satisfactory than the small ones, holding but forty; although they are less convenient for transportation.

In conclusion, I may say, then, that we have in the ten per cent. mixture of oxygen and nitrogen monoxide, an anæsthetic which may be administered with perfect safety and for a sufficiently long time to permit of the circumspect performance of most minor operations, but one which may be characterized as a weak anæsthetic. For although it will plunge the average adult into a state resembling peaceful slumber, in which anæsthesia and unconsciousness are well marked, it cannot gain the victory over states of great nervous excitement or dread, or certain habits and idiosyncrasies.

The anæsthetic action of the mixture is attained by administering it under pressure; and its usefulness is properly limited to the sphere of minor surgery in such cases where other anæsthetics are contraindicated or not desired, or where the saving of time is of great importance.

LITERATURE QUOTED.

Martin: Sur l'anesthésie prolongée et continué par le mélange de protoxyde d'azote et d'oxygène sous pression (methode Paul Bert). Académie de Sciences. L'Union Médicale, 3 sér. 45, 1888.

Witzinger: Ueber die Anwendung der Stickstoffoxydul-Sauerstoffnarcose bei grösseren chirurgischen Eingriffen. Vorläufige Mittheilung. Wien. med. Presse, 1888, 29, 47.

Swiecicki: Zur Stickoxydul-Sauerstoffanæsthesie in der Geburtshülfe. Centralbl. f. Gynäkologie, 1888, 12, 689.

Hillischer: Ueber die Verwendung des Stickstoffoxydul-Sauerstoffgemenges zu Narcosen. Deutsch. Monatsschr. f. Zahnheilk., Sept. 1887.

Ulbrich: Ueber die Lustgassauerstoffnarcose, mit Beziehung auf Hillischer's Veröffentlichung. Prager med. Wochenschr. 1887, 12, 27.

Hillischer: Zur Dr. Ulbrich's Aufsatz " Ueber die Lustgassauerstoffnarcose. Prag. med. Wochenschr., 1887, 12, 60.

Döderlein: Ueber Stickoxydul-Sauerstoffanæsthesie, Archiv für Gynæcol. 1886, 27, 85.

Klikowitsch: Ueber das Stickstoffoxydul als Anæstheticum bis Geburten. Arch. f. Gynæcol. 1881, 18, 81.

Tittel: Sitzungsbericht der Gynæcol. Gesellschaft zu Dresden, 5 Oct. 1882; Centralbl. f. Gynæcol., 1883, 7, 163.

Cohn: Ueber Anæsthesirung Kreissender, Deutsch. med. Wochenschr. 1886, 12, 268.

Zweifel: Bericht der med. Ges. zu Leipzig, 24 April, 1888. Schmidt's Jahrbücher, vol. 218, 275.

Hamecher: Schmezlose Zahnoperationen mit Chloroform oder Nitro-oxygen-gas. Deutsche Monatsschrift f. Zahnheilk., Leipzig, 1886, 4, 240.

Hillischer: Ueber die allgemeine Vewendbarkeit der Lustgas-sauerstoffnarkosen in der Chirurgie, und den respiratorischen Gaswechsel bei Lustgas und Lustgas-sauerstoff. Vortrag, gehalten in der 59. Versammlung deutsch. Naturforscher und Aerzte zu Berlin am 21. Sept. 1886. Wien, 1886. W. Frick.

Döderlein: Ueber Stickoxydul-sauerstoffanæsthesie, Tagebl. d. Versamml. deutsch. Naturforscher u. Aerzte, Strassb. 1885, 58, 111.

Brush: Nitrous Oxide as an Anæsthetic. Brooklyn, N. Y. 1890, iv. 289.

Debate on Anæsthetics: Journal of the Brit. Dental Assoc. Sept. 1889. Lond., Edinb., N. Y. 1889–90, 35, 544.

Hewitt: On the anæsthesia produced by the administration of mixtures of nitrous oxide and oxygen. Lancet, 1889, 1, 832.

Gersuny: Ueber einige Versuche mit Schlafgas, Wien. klin. Wochnschr. 1889, 2, 633.

Howland: Some new experiments in producing anæsthesia with nitrous oxide and air and nitrous oxide and oxygen in condensed air-chambers, illustrated by experiments on an animal. Proc. Amer. Assoc. Adv. Sci. 1888. Salem, 1889, 36, 280.

Rothmann: Zur Frage des Verhaltens des Stickoxyduls zum Blut. Vierteljahres. f. Zahnheilk. 1888. Heft 3.

Bert: Comptes rendus, 1879, t. 87, No. 20.

Blanchard: Thèse. Paris, 1880.

THE ETIOLOGY OF EMPYEMA IN CHILDREN:

AN EXPERIMENTAL AND CLINICAL STUDY.

By Henry Koplik, M.D.,

ATTENDING PHYSICIAN FOR DISEASES OF WOMEN AND CHILDREN TO THE EASTERN DISPENSARY,
NEW YORK.

(Concluded from p 50.)

EXPERIMENTS UPON ANIMALS.

Rabbits, diplococcus pneumoniæ.

1. Medium-sized, white rabbit, injected in pleural cavity, with a pure culture in bouillon of the diplococcus pneumoniæ; died in eighteen hours.

Autopsy.—Rigor mortis marked; chest on both sides showed pleurisy of a sero-fibrinous character; fibrin of a greenish-yellow tint; serum more abundant in left chest. Pericardium: pericarditis, with slight amount of fibrin. Peritoneum: a slightly increased serum; no fibrin; no evidence of inflammation. Blood gave upon culture and stain diplococcus pneumoniæ (pure). Pleuritic fluid, diplococcus pneumoniæ pure culture.

2. Black rabbit (small). Inoculated March 17th; killed by medulla while dying, March 21st. Injected pure culture diplococcus pneumoniæ in chest.

Autopsy.—Sero-fibrinous pleurisy, double sero-fibrinous pericarditis. Peritonitis, sero-fibrinous exudate. Spleen large and swollen. Blood and pericardial fluid pure culture diplococcus pneumoniæ.

3. Small white rabbit; injected about ten minims bouillon culture in chest of diplococcus, March 18th.

Autopsy, March 22.—Beginning rigor mortis. Slight pleuritis; very little serum and fibrin in pleuritic cavity. Sero-fibrinous exudate in peritoneal cavity (peritonitis). Spleen not very large. Blood gave pure culture diplococcus in agar and bouillon, no growth in gelatin, and found also by stain. Lung juice crude cover-glass gave exquisite capsule diplococci.

4. Rabbit, medium sized, injected with pure bouillon culture diplococcus pneumoniæ; died instantly; failure of injection.

5. Rabbit, medium sized; injected in chest same as 4; died on the fourth day.

Autopsy.—Pleuritis double sero-fibrinous; very severe. Pericarditis sero-fibrinous, pericarditis marked. Spleen large and soft. No peritonitis; no meningitis. Specimens of blood, pleuritic and pericardial fluid inoculated on agar, gelatin, bouillon, etc.; reaction by stain and culture of diplococcus pneumoniæ.

6. Rabbit, medium size, injected in chest with pure culture of diplococcus pneumoniæ; died in six days.

Autopsy.—Double sero-fibrinous pleurisy. Pericarditis sero-fibrinous. Peritonitis sero-fibrinous. Spleen large. Cultures made from blood and pericardial fluid; diplococcus pneumoniæ.

7. Rabbit, medium size, injected subcutaneously with pure culture of diplococcus pneumoniæ; no result.

8. Rabbit, black and white spotted, medium size; injected in chest with five minims of empyema pus in which diplococci pneumoniæ existed; animal died in thirty-six hours.

Autopsy.—Forty-eight hours after injection. Rigor mortis marked. Pleurisy slight; some fibrin in the left side at point where needle entered the lung. Peritonitis very marked with sero-fibrinous exudate; brownish serum in bottom peritoneal cavity. Cultures from peritoneum and pleura, pure culture diplococcus pneumoniæ.

9. Small, active rabbit, injected with pure culture diplococcus pneumoniæ obtained from animal 8.

Autopsy made before rigor mortis. Pleurisy marked; sero-fibrinous exudate on both sides. Pericarditis with adhesions; sero-fibrinous exudate. Spleen large. Peritonitis marked; sero-fibrinous exudate. Pure cultures of diplococcus pneumoniæ obtained from pleura, pericardium and blood.

10. Rabbit, medium-sized animal, injected with peritoneal fluid of animal 9 ; died in two days.

Autopsy.—Four hours post-mortem. Pleurisy left sero-fibrinous. Pericarditis slight. Peritonitis marked. Spleen enlarged. Cultures show diplococcus pneumoniæ.

11. Rabbit, large white doe, injected with twenty minims of peritoneal fluid of rabbit 10, in each lung ten minims; killed by medulla on seventh day in dying condition.

Autopsy.—Marked sero-fibrinous pleurisy on both sides and also pericarditis. Spleen large.

12. Rabbit, small-sized, lively animal; injected with peritoneal fluid of rabbit 8; first two days considerable dyspnœa, but recovered and was apparently well. Killed after a week; the only thing found were a few delicate adhesions between the coils of intestine; some clear fluid in bottom of peritoneal cavity.

13. Rabbit, medium-sized; pure culture injection; killed after fifth day.

Autopsy showed marked sero-fibrinous pleurisy; marked sero-fibrinous pericarditis, also advanced peritonitis, with sero-fibrinous exudate. Large spleen. Pure culture of diplococci obtained from blood, pleuritic and pericardial fluid.

14. Rabbit; died with a paralysis of posterior extremities; exhaustion; remains of an old pleurisy found; adhesions of the costal and pulmonary pleuræ. This animal was injected in the pleura with pure culture streptococcus pyogenes.

15. Rabbit; injected with pure culture streptococcus pyogenes in pleural cavity from Case XI.; died after two days.

Autopsy.—Kidneys larger than normal and congested, but the spleen was enormous in size. Cultures of blood gave streptococci.

16. Rabbit; subcutaneous injection streptococcus pyogenes (pure); death after three days.

Autopsy.—Jaundice, universal, of all tissues. Lungs contained small abscess in lower right lobe. Heart, normal. Liver, very small abscesses, studded throughout. Kidneys, cloudy swelling. Spleen much enlarged. Urine, bile pigment.

17. Rabbit; injected with pure culture streptococcus pyogenes, with no result; lived for months.

In addition to the above experiments, there were some injections into guinea-pigs of the diplococcus pneumoniæ; these resulted negatively, except one animal which had been injected with pleuritic fluid from a rabbit that had died in its turn from an injection of diplococcus. In this there were typical pleurisy, pericarditis, and peritonitis, with large spleen.

A few injections upon rats and mice subcutaneously resulted in case of diplococcus positively in one case. Injections into additional rabbits with pus obtained from a tubercular case gave nothing worthy of note.

Cases.

Case I.—Y. S., aged seven years, admitted into hospital. Mother has had phthisis; child has had measles, four years ago, since then a slight cough. Became sick suddenly two weeks ago; has been ill since with cough, pain in the side, chilly sensations, dyspnœa.

Physical signs (left side). Flatness from mid-scapula down. Bronchial voice and breathing (at middle scapula), below distant breathing. Signs of bronchitis on both sides; no signs of phthisis in front or on opposite side.

Operation eighth rib, resected in the post-axillary line; abscess was found to be higher up and encapsulated; adhesions had to be broken down in order to reach empyema. Examination of pus: crude cover and cultivation; streptococcus pyogenes. Cured.

Case II.—R. T., male, aged eight years; January 1st. Family history negative. He had scarlet fever four years ago; a year ago had a bronchitis; a month ago also bronchitis (?). Two weeks ago had fever, temperature 104° (physician). Complained of headache; next day had pain in the left side; dyspnœa; slight cough; no expectoration; temperature 103°. During the next week the temperature did not exceed 101.5°.

Admission to hospital, showed marked œdema of skin of left side, but on incision later (at operation) no infiltration of pus was seen; signs of fluid in left side.

January 2. Operation, resection as noted; there was no infiltration of the œdematous skin with pus. In spite of resection the lung would not expand.

January 3 to February 10. Temperature 100°, 101°, to 104°; pulse 110, 112, 138, to 152; respiration 32, 44, to 52. The boy did badly; there was a profuse discharge of pus, fetid in odor at each dressing, and lung did not expand. Several resections were performed upon this chest to favor retraction of chest toward lung and closure of the large cavity in the chest. There resulted much deformity, and at discharge from hospital there existed a discharging fistula.

Bacterioscopic results were limited to stainings of cover-glass specimens of pus and showed tubercle bacilli. Animal experiments negative.

Case III.—I. S., aged two years; male; February 18, 1890. Has had measles, a year ago; inflammation (?) of the lungs ten months ago; present illness began with fever six weeks ago; this fever after a few days was complicated by convulsions recurring at intervals. Cough was very marked and present during the entire illness; there was loss of flesh and strength, and increasing pallor.

Admission to hospital showed a weakly child, badly nourished, pale; temperature 100°; respirations 40; pulse 120. Physical signs of fluid in right side chest. Tenth rib exsected; about a pint of thick, green, tenacious pus evacuated.

Bacterioscopic result of examination, pus; diplococcus pneumoniæ (Fränkel and Weichselbaum).

May 11. Discharged cured.

CASE IV.—I. S., male, aged eleven months; has been sick for three weeks with fever, cough, dyspnœa, emaciation. Signs of fluid in right pleural cavity. Dulness to flatness. Loss of movement. Loss of fremitus. Loss of voice; pleuritic râles over whole side; syringeful yellow, thick pus removed.

Bacterioscopic examination. Staphylococcus pyogenes aureus. Result unknown.

CASE V.—P. M., male, aged two and a half years; March 3, 1890. Previous history negative. Present illness began a month ago with fever, cough, difficulty in breathing, and constitutional disturbances; fever continued marked during the first two weeks, then abated, but continued nevertheless; pallor, loss of flesh and strength, and generally becoming worse.

Admission to hospital. Anæmic, poorly nourished, anorexia, cough. prostration, and fever; temperature 101°; respirations 46; pulse 104, Signs of fluid in the left side and areas of consolidation (broncho-pneumonia) over the right side. Heart apex just inside the middle line.

March 4. Turbid flocculent serum removed from the chest. Cultures show diplococcus pneumoniæ. Aspiration, only four fluidounces (serous) removed in all, but patient continued to grow worse, temperature varying from 101° to 104°; respirations from 50 to 70; pulse 148 to 160.

16*th.* Needle in left side withdrew a creamy pus.

18*th.* Resection of rib, and about one ounce of pus evacuated, but patient grew worse; died March 27th from broncho-pneumonia on both sides.

Examination (bacterioscopic) of pus withdrawn March 16th, showed diplococcus pneumoniæ.

CASE VI.—I. K., male, aged three and a half years; March 13, 1890. Family and personal history not lucid. Present illness began nine weeks ago with fever and cough and difficulty in breathing; prostration, loss of appetite; patient complained of pain in the left side; loss of flesh and strength; there were night-sweats; patient has steadily lost ground.

Admission to hospital. Poorly nourished, anæmic, delicately built lad; no sign of rhachitis; temperature 101°; respirations 40; pulse 132 (dyspnœa). Physical signs showed fluid in left side. Heart apex pushed to the right, and sounds most intense behind lower end of sternum; no signs of phthisis at apices.

March 16. Operated resection of eighth rib; greenish odorless pus, with large masses of fibrin evacuated, as big as a child's hand.

28*th.* Discharged cured.

Bacterioscopic examination of pus, diplococcus pneumoniæ.

CASE VII.—M. B., aged two years; male; March 1, 1890. Family and personal history negative. The previous history is indefinite; the patient for some time has suffered from cough. Present illness dates a week back; contracted a severe cough, and dyspnœa became very marked; fever, night-sweats, loss of appetite.

On admission, patient is well nourished; suffers great dyspnœa, this symptom so marked as to give impression that œdema of the glottis was present, or obstruction in the larynx. Intubation attempted but failed, and tracheotomy performed. Temperature 100°. Examination of the chest revealed spots of broncho-pneumonia over both sides. March 5th to 15th, temperature 101° to 105°; respiration 40 to 76; pulse 140, with dyspnœa; increasing; attempts to remove tracheal tube resulted in renewed attacks of dyspnœa. March 15th, signs of fluid in left side of chest, and on March 16th, operated, and twelve ounces of pus, greenish, no bad odor, removed from left side. Eighth rib resected.

March 18. Discharged cured.

Bacterioscopic study and culture of pus revealed diplococcus pneumoniæ.

CASE VIII.—H. G., male, aged twelve years. Father, mother, and sisters and brothers in good health; previous history indefinite. It is not possible to obtain definite information as to the exact time of onset of present illness. He has for a few weeks past suffered from cough, fever, and night-sweats, pain in the right side upon coughing or taking deep inspiration; has been confined to his bed; no history of traumatism.

Admission to hospital. An anæmic but well-built lad, not at all emaciated. Physical examination revealed fluid, and needle withdrew pus in right side. Temperature 100°; respiration 40; pulse 140; resection of rib on right side and a pint of greenish fluid, not adhesive pus, removed; no fibrin clots were withdrawn; some adhesions between the costal and pulmonary pleuræ.

Bacterioscopic examination of pus revealed streptococcus pyogenes.

Result: Cure.

CASE IX.—Female, aged two and one-fourth years. April 10, 1890. Family history shows nothing. Present illness began three weeks ago with some eruption (?) upon the body; about a week later there appeared a cough, fever, distress in stomach and abdomen.

Admission to hospital. Anæmic child, with signs of rhachitis, cough, dyspnœa, and some cyanosis; temperature 101°; pulse 160; respirations 48. Physical signs of fluid in the right side, pus withdrawn, immediate operation, exsection; sixteen ounces of pus evacuated. April 12th to 22d, temperature varied from 99° to 103°; respirations 40 to 43; pulse 130 to 158; on April 22d, symptoms pointing to an invasion of the healthy lung by broncho-pneumonia appeared, and patient died with all the symptoms of pneumonia and exhaustion.

Bacterioscopic examination of pus revealed diplococcus pneumoniæ (Fränkel and Weichselbaum).

CASE X.—M. G., male, aged four years; April 18th. Family and previous history negative. Present illness began seven weeks ago with scarlet fever; three weeks later the patient developed general anasarca, this lasted until eight days ago; at the same time he had a severe cough, chills, and fever; constant sweating, lasting until the date of admission; loss of flesh and strength, also failure of appetite and frequent micturition.

Admission to hospital. Patient anæmic and emaciated, cough and dyspnœa. Temperature 99°; respirations 42, and pulse 140. Signs of fluid in the left side. Heart apex pushed to the right of the sternum.

Operation, exsection of rib; twenty-nine and a half ounces of pus of creamy character evacuated.

Bacterioscopic examination revealed diplococcus pneumoniæ.

Result: recovery.

CASE XI.—Male child, aged four months. May 9, 1890. Had been perfectly well until two weeks ago, at this time child was vaccinated; simultaneously with the vaccination, there appeared a burrowing abscess on the dorsum of the left foot which was deep and passed between the metatarsal bones. Eight days ago a febrile movement appeared and the patient was referred by me to a surgeon for treatment. There were at this time no lung symptoms. Three days ago the child developed cough and dyspnœa.

Status præsens: There is cough, dyspnœa, sighing respiration; pulse increased in rapidity; temperature 103°; abscess on foot still present; vaccine pustule still size of five cent piece and angry-looking. Examination of left side revealed chest full of fluid and needle withdrew pus, light yellow, thin, easily separating into two layers, clear and serous, upper and lower purulent.

May 10. Exsection of rib; six ounces of pus (milky) evacuated.

12th. Died; no autopsy.

Bacterioscopic examination of pus revealed streptococcus pyogenes.

CASE XII.—*May,* 1890. Male, aged twelve months; well developed; has been suffering from pertussis and just recovered; about two weeks before date was doing well, when suddenly there appeared a new cough with dyspnœa, and broncho-pneumonia of the right lung was diagnosticated. The cough and fever and dyspnœa still continued up to May 9th, when fluid was found in the right side. A needle introduced about this time withdrew a clear serum; temperature 103°; pulse 160, and rapid respiration. Transferred to the hospital, where child next day showed a measles eruption.

13th. Needle introduced into right side and pus was withdrawn; child was doing well, but on the morning of the above date, patient suddenly developed tympanites (peritonitis(?)) and died.

Bacterioscopic examination of pus of May 13th and serum of May 9th revealed diplococcus pneumoniæ.

CASE XIII.—Empyema; perforation; spontaneous recovery. Female, aged thirteen months. May 12, 1890. Previous history negative. Child was taken ill about three weeks ago with cough, fever, dyspnœa. The child had dyspnœa, and moaned when it breathed; there was a frequent cough and a temperature of 103½°; pulse 160. Examination of chest showed consolidation of the left upper lobe (dulness, bronchial voice, and breathing). Diagnosis: broncho-pneumonia. The patient seemed to improve up to a week ago, when the temperature and cough persisted, the dulness behind became more marked and spread toward the base of the lung; fremitus absent; voice and breathing bronchial. Needle introduced and pus withdrawn from left side, greenish-yellow, adhesive; heart not displaced; operation advised.

August 1. Child had escaped from observation, and having refused operation passed under care of others. It was brought to me, August 1st, for diarrhœal trouble; chest showed no signs of old trouble; lung had expanded; voice and breathing good, no friction sounds. There was a slight dulness only left over the affected side; fremitus good; no fever; child looks much improved. Mother says that after leaving my care the patient grew worse until she began to cough up large amounts of yellow matter (pus?). This continued some time at intervals; patient recovered; no cough.

Bacterioscopic examination of pus revealed diplococcus pneumoniæ.

CASE XIV.—*May* 13, 1890. L. H., aged eighteen months, male; previons history negative; father and mother well and in apparent good health. Nine days ago child developed a cough, fever and dyspnœa; the dyspnœa increased, fever continued, and there was restlessness at night. When brought to me the child was anæmic; had signs of rhachitis; there was much dyspnœa and moaning respiration, drowsiness, and partial stupor. Temperature 105°; pulse 165; respirations 56. Physical signs of fluid in right side below mid-scapula, needle introduced and a clear bloody serum obtained.

14*th*. Needle introduced, signs of fluid having increased, and withdrew milky pus.

15*th*. Exsection of rib, eight ounces of pus removed.

Bacterioscopic examination showed staphylococcus pyogenes aureus.

CASE XV.—D. H., male, aged five and a half years. Father and mother living, has had no special illness; present illness dates from October 6th, when there was fever and pain and dyspnœa; the pain was referred to the stomach; there was no distinct history of chill. When first seen, October 7th, patient was a well-developed child; no signs of past rhachitis; there was dyspnœa, a dry cough, fever; there was also some restlessness; complains of stomach pain. Temperature 103°; pulse 130; respirations increased. Signs in chest negative.

October 8. Temperature 104°; pulse 140; respirations rapid; pain in right side; rusty sputum. Diagnosis at this time: right lobar pneumonia lower lobe. At end of five days signs pointed to a resolution of an ordinary lobar pneumonia; temperature 102°.

19*th*. Signs of fluid in chest. The boy has not been doing well, and new signs appeared; loss of fremitus; flatness, bulging of right side; subcrepitant râles close to the ear, voice and breathing though coarse heard over whole chest; dyspnœa great; temperature 103½°; pulse 160; respirations rapid.

21*st*. Operation: simple opening in chest and tube inserted; about half a pint of pus evacuated; not fœtid; yellow color.

27*th*. Discharge fœtid and penetrating odor; the drainage bad and a resection was performed, November 5th. Final complete recovery.

Bacterioscopic examination of pus first taken from chest showed diplococcus pneumoniæ.

CLINICAL CLASSIFICATION.

The cases here recorded, from a clinical and bacteriological standpoint, divide themselves quite readily into groups.

GROUP I.—Here we can place those cases of empyema in which the bacterioscopic examination revealed the staphylococcus pyogenes aureus, or the streptococcus pyogenes. These microörganisms did not exist associated, but in so-called pure form and isolated in the exudate. The etiology of these cases is very difficult to make out, because this group does not include cases of empyema where an extraneous source of infection exists. Those cases of empyema in which the pleuritic exudate shows simply the presence of the staphylococcus or streptococcus alone, and where there is no history of traumatism with perforation of the skin, or where there is no suppurating focus of infection outside the pleural cavity, are most puzzling to explain because the bacterioscopic finding gives us no clue as to the origin of the disease. The staphylococcus and streptococci are microörganisms which exist in suppurating processes of the most diverse nature and situation in the body. I have four such cases to place under this heading. One female, aged seven years, and three male children, aged eighteen months, two years, and twelve years respectively. In none of these cases was there a history of traumatism of any kind. When they came under observation, they had been ill with symptoms of pulmonary trouble for periods varying from one to six weeks.

Assuming that an infection of the pleura is most apt to result from adjacent inflammatory processes, the most usual disease preceding or complicating such a pleurisy is pneumonia. Weichselbaum has demonstrated that in addition to the pneumococcus of Fränkel, there exists in the lungs of pneumonic patients the streptococcus pneumoniæ (or pyogenes) and the staphylococcus pyogenes aureus. Though we cannot as yet yield to these microörganisms the dignified position of being the direct cause of pneumonia, we find that they exist in the lung constantly as so-called mixed infections, as they do in diphtheria. Thu[1] has argued that microörganisms in pneumonic fibrinous pleuritis and pericarditis (pneumococci) first find their way through the lymph channels into the subpleural tissue and then into the pulmonary pleura, and finally gain the surface of the pulmonary and costal pleura ; from thence they may be carried into the mediastinal spaces and reach the tissue of the pericardium and even the muscular tissue overlying the costal pleura. It is true that the failure to find the pneumococcus in the exudate does not disprove the possibility that at some early stage of the empyema it might have been present ; however the tendency to-day is to consider the active predisposing causes exposure to cold and moisture. It is thought that though the above microörganisms may exist in the air passages, as has been proven in the nose and mouth of a healthy individual, they may remain inert until, cold and wet reducing the resistant vitality of the organism, they cause an empyema ; so a wound in the chest wall without perforation of the skin may exert a similar influence.

GROUP II.—The cases of empyema which fall under this group are the most interesting of all pleurisies. They are those which either complicate or follow a pneumonia. In the pleuritic exudate of such an empyema the diplococcus pneumoniæ (Fränkel and Weichselbaum) may be demonstrated as in all of my cases.

[1] Centralbl. f. bakteriol., 1889, Bd. v.

These were two female children, aged thirteen months and two and a quarter years respectively, and seven male children, aged twelve months, two years, two and a half years (two), three and a half years, four years, and five and a half years. They had been ill when they came under observation for periods ranging from one to nine weeks. In one case the patient had been under the observation, from the very beginning, of a skilful observer (Case XV.), and the diagnosis of lobar pneumonia followed by a pleurisy (empyema) was distinctly traced. As recorded elsewhere, the diplococcus pneumoniæ (Fränkel) could be easily recognized in the crude pus by spreading upon cover-glass; beautiful capsule appearances were also obtained. Pure cultures were isolated in every case and their virulence tested upon animals while the cultures were still recent. The experiments were in the direction of intra-pleural or pulmonary injections, so that appearances in the animal experiments resembled very much what is seen in the human subject. If such a pathogenic microörganism is found in a pleuritic exudate, it can be traced to only one probable source, the lung. It is scarcely necessary in any of these cases to prove clinically the existence of a pneumonia. If one will refer to the histories of the cases he will see that in some a pneumonia, either of the lobar or lobular type, must have been in active progress when the empyema was operated upon. At least the physical signs and symptoms indicated this condition of affairs in the lungs upon the opposite side to the empyema, if not in the lung corresponding to the empyema.

In one case, where the patient succumbed, the opposite lung was undoubtedly affected. In other cases, after operation, the temperature would not only persist, but persistent broncho-pneumonic processes were present; this was notably the history of Case III., who continued in the hospital for months, being finally discharged cured. In these cases, tuberculosis was excluded by all possible methods, both clinical and bacteriological. But in the majority of the cases in which the pneumococcus was found in the pus of the empyema, the evacuation of the pus marked the abatement of all symptoms and recovery of the patient, showing that the pneumonia, if it existed, had preceded the accumulation in the chest and had passed through its various stages. The pneumococcus has been found by Weichselbaum in lungs the seat of lobular pneumonia, as well as in those the seat of lobar process.

I have elsewhere described the macroscopic characters of the pleural exudates in the cases of empyema belonging to this group. But in two the pleuritic fluid when first withdrawn from the chest was serous in character, in one case even devoid of flocculi. In both of these cases, the exudate taken later with an exploring syringe was markedly purulent, and both cases were operated upon. In the serous fluids first obtained, as also in the purulent exudate, the diplococcus was found.

This shows distinctly that though an exudate may be serous at first, it may subsequently become markedly purulent, not on account of anything introduced into the chest on the occasion of the first puncture, but from the continued action of microörganisms already present (diplococcus pneumoniæ or streptococcus pyogenes, Fränkel). Again, pus from the chest has a tendency, without this cavity, to separate into strata, the upper one being serous and containing but few leucocytes; we may aspirate this stratum in a marked empyema, and thus can not draw any definite conclusion as to the nature of the exudate. If an exudate contain streptococci, even though serous, we can with certainty predict the advent of pus (Fränkel). We might make a similar assertion of fluids containing the diplococcus pneumoniæ. If a serous fluid withdrawn from the chest fails to reveal any microörganisms upon stain or culture, we can conclude that there is a probable tubercular element in the pleurisy (Fränkel). If such a serous exudate subsequently shows the presence of microörganisms (streptococci) and then becomes purulent, we can suspect contamination. With conscientious cleansing of a needle-syringe, we may fearlessly enter the pleural cavity without having in the least compromised the health of the patient. I am certain much misunderstanding has arisen on this subject through a misinterpretation of the real nature of some of these serous exudates. While some are devoid of microörganisms (tubercular), others are filled with pyogenic microbes, capable not only of producing suppuration, but maintaining it.

GROUP III.—This group, which includes empyema of tubercular nature, is most unsatisfactory in its various aspects. Fränkel, who spent much time and patience upon tubercular pleurisies in the adult, found cases in which examination of the exudate yielded a negative result. So common was this, that he concluded that a negative finding was much in favor of the tubercular character of the exudate. These exudates may be localized or involve the whole pleura. They may or may not be accompanied by lung areas of tuberculosis; in cases where the lung is involved, in the adult, the tubercle bacilli may be found in the sputum, but in children the examination of the sputum is not always practicable. If, as in children, the lung shows no positive involvement and the examination of the exudate is negative, diagnosis and prognosis are difficult. Ehrlich (*Charité Annales*, 1888) explains the absence of tubercle bacilli in two ways: 1. The fibrin formations in the exudate remove the bacilli by enclosing them. 2. Thickening of the pleura by adhesions causes a resistance to the transmigration of bacilli. In empyema, the bacilli are more numerous than in simple pleuritic exudates, because cells passing in myriads into the exudate are more apt to carry bacilli with them. Israel and Gerhart think that the bacilli rather become entrapped in the miliary growths of the pleura, and thus do not pass into the exudate.

I have but one case to place in this group, that of Case II., a boy of eight years, who had had several bronchitic attacks years before the advent of his empyema. The exudate had to be repeatedly examined in order to establish the presence of tubercle bacilli (stained by Ehrlich's method), but the experiments with animals were of a negative character. In this case the streptococcus pyogenes was also found in the exudate from the very first; this is similar to a case in the adult recorded by Fränkel. The formation of adhesions tying down the lung must have been exceedingly great, for operation found the lung unable to expand and repeated exsection of the rib had to be resorted to, in order to obtain partial closure of an immense suppurating cavity. The deformity resulting was most pronounced. I have made attempts in other children and this boy to obtain sputa for examination, but have not succeeded. I attributed my ill success in inoculation upon animals to the presence of contamination in the pus.

Thus, my group of tubercular empyema remains unsatisfactory, though diagnosticated with a certainty from the presence of tubercle bacilli in the exudate. The lungs upon examination yielded no evidences of involvement.

GROUP IV.—In this group we might class those cases of empyema in which some focus of suppuration situated in another part of the body may be with great probability pointed to as a source of infection. The infecting focus may be adjacent, as in the cases of Fränkel, where a retro-pharyngeal abscess or perforating peritonitis were the cause of the empyema, or the empyema may be one of the manifestations of a species of pyæmia (as in my own case). This was a male infant, aged four months, who was perfectly well up to within two weeks of its death. The infant was vaccinated and then developed a burrowing abscess of the foot, and after this the empyema appeared. No autopsy was allowed; it would have been interesting to see (though no pneumococcus was found in the exudate of the pleura) whether a pneumonia (pyæmic) was present with the empyema. The rapid death of the child speaks in favor of some virulent infection; an autopsy might have revealed several other hidden foci of suppuration.

The bacterioscopic finding and experiments in the above case are interesting. The streptococcus which was isolated and existed alone in the exudate was certainly very virulent. Two animals injected with a pure culture (15 and 16), both died. Both were injected at the same time with the same culture; the one in the pleural cavity, in this case, the animal died in two days; streptococci were found in the blood and organs, but there were no inflammatory exudates; the kidneys were swollen and the spleen was enormous in size. The second animal was injected subcutaneously, and the report of the autopsy shows metastatic abscesses all over the body with general jaundice and enlarged spleen

and cloudy kidneys. These results differ widely from those with streptococci obtained from cases of Group I. Here the animals survived and
autopsies after months showed no effects of infection, or as in rabbit 14,
only the effects of local processes limited in nature.

PUTRID EMPYEMA.

By this I desire to designate those cases of empyema in which there
was a putrid or fetid odor to the discharge, and in which this odor
persisted.

In both of my cases the exudate turned putrid after operation. In one
(XV.) the empyema followed a pneumonia, and in the fluid first withdrawn from the chest, the pneumococcus alone existed. In this case, on
account of the imperfection of drainage due to the first mode of operating,
there was retention of pus, the chest wound finally closed, and when reopened again for resection, the pus was very putrid.

The second case was that in which the pus showed the presence of
tubercle bacilli. There was no odor to the pus upon the first resection.
But there was not only lack of any expansion in the lung, leaving an
immense cavity in the chest, but the pus remained in this cavity. Here
the empyema became putrid, necessitating repeated washings of the chest
with creolin solution. In spite of this fact, the pus remained putrid.
Investigation succeeded in revealing the presence of a fluorescent green
bacillus, rather thick and short, which fluidified gelatin (much like that
found in water) and grew upon agar of Weichselbaum in a dark-green
layer with a rather mawkish odor to the growth. This is all that could
be found in addition to the tubercle bacillus and streptococcus previously
present. This shows that the most innocent exudate may turn putrid, as in
the case of pneumonic empyema, as well as the tubercular cases. It seems
rational to suppose that lack of expansion of the lung or retention of pus,
especially where the chest has been injected with so-called antiseptic solutions (in the above cases boric acid or creolin), are conditions peculiarly
favorable to the development of putrid exudates. I have seen air enter
daily freely into the chest cavity without causing the pus to become
putrid ; also the introduction of bacteria from the lips of the wound was
unavoidable, on account of the free moving of drainage-tubes and dressings and tampons over the mouth of the external wound. Yet drainage
being free, with full lung expansion, no putridity appeared. In the
future, the appearance of a putrid exudate in a chest in which primarily
the pus possessed no such characters, would make me think of retention
due either to insufficient drainage or want of proper expansion of the
lung.

PROGNOSIS.—We can safely say that the present status of our knowledge in these cases enables us to assure our patients with moderate
certainty as to the outcome of the illness of their children. Such

prognosis may be made at the bedside or within a very short period from the first examination of a case.   The simple means at the disposal of every clinician are adequate for the examination of crude specimens of pus, and delay of a day or two at the most is all that may be necessary for more deliberate investigation.   Nor do I think that we should take too much credit to ourselves for the recovery of a certain class of these cases which, under proper guidance, invariably get well. Thus, it would appear that the best prognosis is held out to those which belong to Groups I. and II.   More especially is this true of cases of meta-pneumonic empyema.   In one of these (XIII.), in which the purulent exudate filled the chest and was withdrawn from the same by exploring needle and contained pneumococci, the patient recovered ; having refused operation, the empyema perforated the lung and thus gained exit externally, pus being coughed up.   Subsequent examination of this case revealed nothing abnormal on the diseased side but slight dulness.   The lung had thoroughly expanded.   Fränkel records similar cases in the adult.   It would scarcely be well to expect too much from such *laissez faire* treatment, for a large percentage (Ziemssen's *Vorträge*) of cases which are allowed to perforate die.   The age of the patient and the presence or absence of any considerable pneumonia will weigh in each case.   Some authors are enthusiasts for the simple opening and drain in the chest ; others insist on the trial of repeated aspiration ; others contend that resection of the rib is the only safety of the patient and secures a rapid expansion of the lung.   The truth lies in the etiology of the cases of empyema.   In the meta-pneumonic exudates cases will do equally well by the various modes of treatment ; in other words, the pus evacuated by whatever means, there is an inherent tendency to absorption of what inflammatory product there is remaining and return to a normal status, as in the pneumonic lung.

The pneumonic exudates, if they hold out such brilliant prospect of recovery to the patient, are a striking contrast to the tubercular cases, where only a partial recovery is at best possible.   There are cases on record where, especially in children, an empyema (Ziemssen's *Vorträge*) of established tubercular nature has made an apparently good recovery, yet we must doubt its permanency.   We cannot rid ourselves of the idea that a large extent of surface like the pleura, once tubercular, must, if recovery takes place, be a latent danger to the patient.[1]   In other cases, the recovery results with fistulæ, retraction, and all the concomitants of permanently crippled respiratory apparatus.   The pyæmic cases are fatal as far as we know.[2]

---

[1] Klesch and Vaillard (Arch. de Physiol. et Path., 1886) have made autopsies upon pleurisies of a tubercular character which had apparently recovered, and were able to prove their tubercular nature at autopsy.

[2] I desire to express my sincere obligations to Dr. Barium Scharlau, of the Mount Sinai Hospital, for the clinical material which he so kindly placed at my disposal.

A REMARKABLE CASE OF SKIN DISEASE.

By J. Frank, M.D.,

ATTENDING SURGEON TO THE ST ELIZABETH AND COOK COUNTY HOSPITALS, CHICAGO, ILLINOIS.

Reported by W. C. Sandford, M.D.,

HOUSE PHYSICIAN TO THE ST. ELIZABETH HOSPITAL.

THE case which we are to consider is unique, not alone in the fact that the shedding of the cuticle and nails of the hands and feet was complete, but in its repetition for thirty-three consecutive years, on the same day of the month, and within a few hours of the same time of the day.

In a research in medical literature, in which we were kindly assisted by Dr. James S. Newburgh, we failed to find a parallel case; cases have been reported where the shedding was complete, but none which recurred at regular intervals.

The patient, John H. P., of Phillipsburg, Montana, called upon Dr. J. Frank, July 22, 1890, with a letter of introduction. Dr. Frank referred him to the St. Elizabeth Hospital, where he was admitted as a private patient on July 23, 1890. While here, the patient was seen by a number of prominent dermatologists of this city, and was studied with special interest by Drs. James Nevins Hyde, McArthur, J. S. Newburgh, and F. H. Montgomery.

The patient, a miner by occupation, has been exposed to all the hardships of camp life, but has borne them with ease, being well formed, and apparently in perfect health. Height 5 feet 9½ inches, weight 150 pounds, eyes dark, hair dark-brown, full set of natural teeth, special senses all normal, intelligence good, skin perfectly normal. No birthmarks were to be found.

His history, as given by himself, is briefly as follows: Father and mother both living; father sixty-eight years, mother sixty-one years. Maternal grandmother living, and in her ninety-seventh year. The patient is the second of a family of thirteen children, all of whom are living and in good health. Has never had any of the eruptive fevers, and has never required the attendance of a physician. Had two light attacks of gonorrhœa, and was salivated once by the breaking of a mercury retort, but took no treatment for either.

He was born December 29, 1857, during the Kansas and Missouri trouble. His mother was driven at night from her home in Franklin to the Meredenson River, four miles distant, where she was confined in the open woods, with no attendant but her mother. Mother and child were taken to shelter the following day. As there was nothing peculiar occurred during her pregnancy or confinement, the woman cannot account for the skin shedding of her child which took place later.

On the 24th of July following his birth he was suddenly taken ill—vomited, became hot and feverish, and in a few hours the entire surface of the body was scarlet-red. Symptoms increased for three or four hours, when they gradually subsided, and the patient was supposed to have recovered; but on the fourth or fifth day following the attack the entire cuticle was cast off, and a few days later the nails of his hands and feet were also shed.   This was repeated each year on the same date.   His mother took no notice of it at first, thinking it was one of the eruptive fevers.   When he was seven years old he was taken to a physician in Denver, who kept him under observation for a time, but gave no treatment.   He has never been attended by a physician except from curiosity.

The patient first remembers the shedding in 1865, when the cuticle and nails were cast off while at play.   These attacks have been repeated each year on the 24th of July, usually at 3 P.M., and never later than 9 P.M.

The paroxysm begins abruptly.   Patient has a feeling of lassitude and weakness of fifteen to twenty minutes duration, followed by muscular tremors, nausea and vomiting, a rapid rise of temperature, skin and mucous membrane of tongue and mouth become red and inflamed, and are hot and dry.   No perspiration appears after the paroxysm begins until the cuticle is cast off.

The acute symptoms begin to subside in from three to four hours, and are entirely gone by the end of twelve hours, with the exception of the redness of the skin which does not return to its normal color for thirty-six hours more.   The patient has been delirious three times during these attacks, once for nine days.

In his early life the cuticle began to be shed on the second or third day after symptoms appeared, and was complete by the fifth day ; but each succeeding year it takes a little longer, until now it is ten or twelve days before shedding is complete.   The cuticle can be detached in large sheets, and he has always been able to remove it from the hands and feet in one piece in the form of gloves and moccasins.

The nails are loosened and crowded off in about four weeks after the acute stage.

On the 24th of July, the day following his admission into the hospital, the above symptoms occurred with marked similarity.

By invitation from Dr. J. Frank, a number of physicians were present during the acute stage.   Among them were Drs. R. N. Hall, J. K. Bartholomew, H. M. Luken, L. A. Beard, Archibald Church, and W. F. Coleman.   At 2.45 P.M. the patient was seen by Dr. Luken and myself. He was apparently well, but assured us he would soon be sick.

3 P.M.   Was still walking in the hall.   Very nervous, and had a peculiar, anxious expression.

3.15 P.M.   Retired to his room.   Nervousness increasing; slight muscular tremors ; hands, wrists, and neck beginning to get red.

3.30 P.M.   His entire trunk, and arms down to the elbows, bright scarlet-red, resembling the appearance of a scarlet-fever patient, but cuticle is not elevated.

3.50 P.M.   Nausea; trembling over whole body; redness extended down to the great trochanters; mucous membrane of tongue and mouth also congested.

3.55 P.M.   Vomited two drachms of thick tenacious mucous, streaked with blood.   Was given a glass of warm water and a teaspoonful of syr. ipecac.

4.05 P.M.   Pulse 68 ; temperature 97° F.; slight flush over limbs, more noticeable over left.   He claimed to get an electric shock when the skin was touched. This was probably due to a hyperæsthetic condition or his skin.

4.10 P. M. Nausea, and attempt to vomit. The nausea subsides between paroxysms of vomiting, and patient converses intelligently. Right lower limb as red as trunk; left beginning to flush. Tongue and mucous membrane of mouth very red. Trembles greatly; cannot carry glass to lips. Given two glasses of warm water and a drachm of syr. ipecac.

4.15 P. M. Redness shows through the soles of his feet, giving them a yellowish-red appearance. Skin has a warm, greasy feeling. Perspires only under eyes and on forehead.

4.20 P. M. Left limb nearly as scarlet as trunk.

4.25 P. M. Vomited one pint of water and mucus.

4.30 P. M. Pulse 68; temperature 99.6° F.

4.50 P. M. All the body, excepting the forehead and beneath the eyes, scarlet-red, showing distinctly in the palms of the hands and soles of the feet.

5 P. M. Pulse 76; temperature 99.4° F. Vomited a small amount of mucus.

5.5 P. M. Nausea and acute pain. Given a glass of warm water. Trembled so he could scarcely carry glass to lips. Vomited immediately after taking water.

5.30 P. M. Pulse 76; temperature 99.3° F.

5.45 P. M. Vomited four drachms of thick gray mucus with extreme pain. Bowels moved; stool light-colored.

6 P. M. Pulse 76; temperature 99.3° F. Surface of body warm, but patient complains of being cold.

6.30 P. M. Pulse 88; temperature 101.2° F. Resting quietly. Took a light supper.

7.35 P. M. Pulse 92; temperature 101.4° F..

8.30 P. M. Pulse 92; temperature 102° F.

8.45 P. M. Given ten grains of antipyrine.

9.30 P. M. Pulse 88; temperature 103° F. Nausea and an attempt to vomit. Symptoms soon subsided. Patient rested quietly from 10 P. M. until 7 A. M. the following morning, sleeping most of the time.

10.30 P. M. Pulse 80; temperature 100° F.

11.30 P. M. Pulse 80; temperature 100° F.

25th, 12.30 A. M. Pulse 84; temperature 101.7° F. Given 10 grains of antipyrine.

2 A. M. Pulse 80; temperature 101.4° F.

5 A. M. Pulse 88; temperature 101.2° F.

7 A. M. Pulse 84; temperature 100.5° F. Still drowsy. Has a slight headache.

9 A. M. Pulse 80; temperature 99.8° F.

8 P. M. Pulse 84; temperature 101.5° F.

26th, 8 A. M. Pulse 84; temperature 99.5° F. Cuticle beginning to scale on scrotum.

8 P. M. Temperature normal. Skin has assumed its normal color. Redness faded in the same order as it appeared.

27th. The epidermis of the mucous membrane of the tongue and mouth came off. Tongue resembled a typhoid tongue after it has cleaned up.

28th. Perspires freely from forehead and under eyes. Cuticle over chest raised up in the form of blisters by the perspiration.

30th. Cuticle removed from trunk and arms to wrists.

August 1. Cuticle detached from lower limbs to ankles.

2d. Skin taken from right hand in the form of a glove.

3d. Left glove removed. Skin also loose on upper surface of feet ; soles still intact.

9th. Right moccasin removed.

11th. Left moccasin removed.

After the removal of the cuticle the skin was very soft and delicate, resembling that of a child.

Where the cuticle was thick, as on the palms of the hands and soles of the feet, the new skin was very sensitive, and to protect the feet he wore the moccasins for several days after they had been removed.

At the time of the dismissal of the patient from the hospital, August 15, 1890, it could plainly be seen that the nails would soon be cast off.

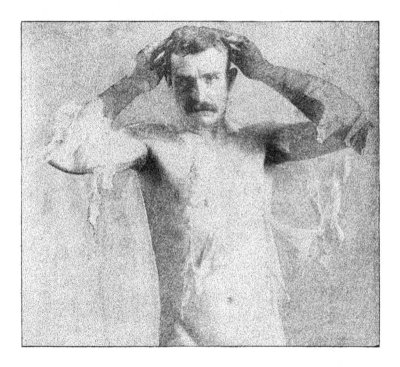

New ones were forming at their bases, and the old ones were loosening from the sides and underneath. A thin, blunt instrument could be passed beneath them to their bases without causing pain. Previous to leaving for his home a piece of integument was removed, under cocaine, from his arm, and a careful microscopical examination did not reveal anything abnormal.

Under date of August 29, 1890, Mr. J. P. writes the following: "I arrived at Black Pines the evening of August 22d, went to work that evening, and continued until the following evening. Am in perfect

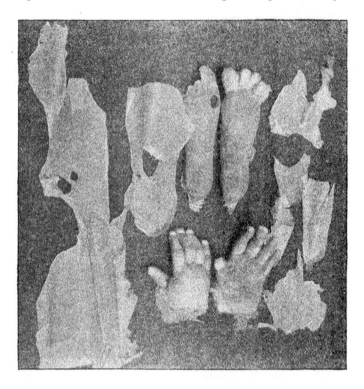

health. Enclosed find nails from little finger and second finger of right hand, detached August 26th. Will send the remaining nails in a few days."

September 19th I received another letter containing seven more nails. They were from the little finger and second and third fingers of left hand, detached September 2d; both thumb-nails removed September 5th; and the nails from the big toes, which were the last to come off, on September 8th.

The remaining nails became so broken while at work that they were useless as specimens.

ASEPTIC AND ANTISEPTIC GYNECOLOGICAL SURGERY, AS PRACTISED AT THE ROOSEVELT HOSPITAL.

BY GEORGE W. JARMAN, M.D.,

LATE HOUSE GYNECOLOGIST TO ROOSEVELT HOSPITAL; ASSISTANT SURGEON TO THE NEW YORK CANCER HOSPITAL; CLINICAL ASSISTANT IN GYNECOLOGY TO THE VANDERBILT CLINIC, NEW YORK.

RECOGNIZING the fact that many of the profession have either not had the benefit of a hospital training, or else received this training previous to the advent of antiseptic and aseptic procedures, I have concluded that an account of the entire details of operations in some hospital, from the reception until the discharge of the patient, might be of interest to those who have been compelled to "work out their own salvation." In December, 1888, the Roosevelt Hospital established a separate operating-room and reception-ward for gynecological cases, Professor George M. Tuttle having been appointed Attending Gynecologist, and it is from the experience gained in this department that I note the following details.

It has been the endeavor to perfect some plan of operation which would not only meet the requirements of the recent advancements in antiseptic surgery, but would also be practical in its application. Every surgeon must have been confronted with the dilemma of being compelled to depend on those who did not realize the importance of absolute surgical cleanliness, and from this fact it is evident that he must reduce the technique of his operations to a condition of practical utility.

A new operating-room which has been in use for several weeks greatly facilitates the work, which had previously been done in a room twelve by eighteen feet.

To simplify matters, I speak first of major operations and afterward of minor cases.

When a patient has been received into the hospital she is given a thorough bath, including the head; she is supplied with freshly-laundried hospital garments, and a complete history of her previous condition and present illness is taken and preserved for record. A physical examination is made and a description of any abnormal condition ascertained is added to the previous notes. Her urine is examined every morning and the result recorded. The operator is given a card upon the day of operation, showing the existence or non-existence of any abnormal characteristics. The nurse is required to enter daily upon the bedside-notes the temperature, pulse, respiration, and the amount of urine passed. Unless the case is one demanding immediate operative procedure, four to five days are spent in preparing her for the operation. Her diet consists of those articles which will leave the least amount of solid residue in the intestinal canal, such as soup, eggs, and a small amount of rare beef. Morning and evening she is given drachm-doses of compound licorice powder, until the evening previous to the operation, at which time all medication is discontinued. I specify the drug used since it has appeared to cause less flatus than others which have been tried.

In cases of doubt as regards the accuracy of the diagnosis the patient is examined while under the influence of an anæsthetic. The evening previous to the operation she has another thorough bath, the umbilicus receiving special attention. The pubes and the field of opera-tion above are carefully shaved. A folded towel moistened with a solu-tion of soft soap and water, equal parts, is placed over the abdomen, extending well down over the pubes, and is held in place by means of an abdominal binder. The next morning the patient is given an enema of soap-suds and a vaginal douche of 1 : 5000 bichloride solution. The towel is removed and the surface of the abdomen is washed with 95 per cent. alcohol and afterward with 1 : 1000 bichloride solution. A piece of damp bichloride gauze is now placed over the abdomen and is confined with a few turns of a roller bandage; this the patient wears to the operating-table. If the operation is to be performed in the after-noon, she is given a light breakfast and one hour before the operation one ounce of whiskey. Immediately before the etherization is begun she is catheterized, the urethral orifice having been previously sponged off with bichloride solution 1 : 5000.

The operating-table is an enamelled iron frame covered with two pieces of solid glass, which are inclined to its center, under which is a trough which empties into a basin below. The glass is covered with thick rubber pads.

Previous to the operation the nurses wash the operating-, instrument-, and dressing-tables with bichloride solution 1 : 1000. The instrument- and dressing-tables are covered with towels wet in the same solution. The instruments, with the exception of the knives, the needles, and all ligatures (except the cat-gut sutures) are wrapped in towels and boiled for one hour. The instruments and needles are transferred to glass trays containing a watery solution of hydronaphthol 1 : 1000. The liga-tures, including the silver wire, are kept under 95 per cent. alcohol. The catgut used in the hospital is bought in the raw state. After all foreign matter has been wiped off, it is placed in strong ether for four hours. This removes any oily material which may be present. It is transferred from the ether to bichloride solution 1 : 1000, and is allowed to remain for eight hours. It is again wiped off with a bichloride towel and is placed in absolute alcohol. It is kept *under* the alcohol and small quantities are removed from time to time and are placed in the 95 per cent. alcohol, ready for operations. No gut larger than No. 4 is used.

The sponges are also prepared in the hospital. While dry they are pounded lightly to remove the grit, after which they are placed in a solution of permanganate of potash, two ounces to the gallon, and are allowed to remain in this for two hours. They are next washed thoroughly in water and are transferred to a solution of hyposulphite of soda, three ounces to the gallon, to which has been added two ounces of hydrochloric acid, and are kneaded three or four times and at once washed in water until no odor remains. They are now stored in 3 per cent. carbolic solution.

The surgeon and his assistants, including the nurses, pay special attention to cleansing their hands and arms, using a stiff brush and soft-soap, being certain that the nails are thoroughly clean. After this the hands are washed in 95 per cent. alcohol and are then immersed in bichloride solution 1 : 1000. All then put on rubber aprons and cover these with linen gowns which reach to the feet. Great care is taken that the hands do not come in contact with anything which has not been rendered aseptic. Should it become necessary in arranging the patient on the table to touch parts which are not aseptic, the hands are at once washed in bichloride solution.

The patient being placed upon the table, with her feet on the foot-rest, rubber cloths covered with towels wet with bichloride solution 1 : 1000 are laid over her, above and below the field of operation. The bandage is then cut and the gauze is removed. The abdominal surface is sponged off with 95 per cent. alcohol, followed with bichloride solution 1 : 1000, no scrubbing-brush being used. Bichloride towels are fastened on either side of the field of operation, thus excluding all other portions of the patient's body. The operator and his assistants have near them two basins, the first containing bichloride solution 1 : 1000 and the other distilled water. From time to time during the operation the hands are dipped in the first and then in the second basin. The sponges are all counted previous to the operation and the number is noted on a blackboard, and before the wound is closed the nurse is required to account for all sponges used. A reserve set of sponges is always in readiness, so that if pus is encountered fresh sponges may be used after the irrigation.

Irrigation is resorted to under two conditions—if much oozing exists from the separation of adhesions, or if any septic (or possibly septic) matter has escaped into the peritoneal cavity. Distilled water only is used for this purpose, at a temperature of 112° F. A glass irrigator, holding three quarts, to which is attached by means of rubber tubing a glass nozzle fourteen inches long, with a smooth end, slightly curved, is the apparatus used. The tubing and the nozzle are always boiled with the instruments.

During the operation instruments not in use are kept under the hydro-naphthol solution.

Heavy, softly twisted Chinese silk is used for ligating the pedicle. The stump is always seared with a Paquelin cautery and is dusted with iodoform before being dropped back.

Drainage is resorted to if irrigation has been performed. Straight glass tubes, fenestrated throughout the lower third, and long enough to reach the bottom of the cul-de-sac, are employed.

If adhesions have been numerous and oozing persists after the irrigation, iodoform gauze is packed over the raw surfaces and is allowed to protrude from the lower angle of the wound. The wound is closed with No. 24 or 26 silver wire, depending upon the thickness of the abdominal walls. The suture is passed through all the layers, the fascia having been previously drawn forward by the assistant. A provisional wire suture is inserted at the site of the tube if drainage is employed. Interrupted silkworm-gut sutures unite the edges of the skin. This is the constant method in closing the wound, the different layers of the abdominal walls never being united separately.

The wound having been closed is thickly powdered with iodoform and is covered with iodoform gauze. Damp bichloride gauze is placed over this and is in its turn covered with borated cotton. (This borated cotton is prepared in the hospital and is made by boiling absorbent cotton in a saturated solution of boric acid.) The dressings are held in place by three pieces of four-inch rubber plaster, which pass entirely around the body of the patient. A many-tailed abdominal binder, made of muslin, confines the dressings.

If pus has been encountered during an operation, the instruments are scrubbed with soap and water and are boiled for one hour, after which they are wiped dry. Otherwise, they are simply scrubbed in the usual manner.

The drainage-tube has been a source of annoyance and danger to many, and I give in full the method pursued in emptying it:

The tube is filled with strips of iodoform gauze when the operation is completed. Within two hours the tube is emptied. The patient being on her back, the bed-covering is turned down to the lower part of the binder and a light blanket is spread over her chest. These are covered with rubber sheets, over which have been placed damp bichloride towels. The surgeon removes his coat, puts on a clean apron, and disinfects his hands and arms as if he were entering the operating-room. The lower two or three tails of the binder are removed and the dressings are cut down to the tube, exposing the strip of iodoform gauze. Before the strip is removed a piece of bichloride gauze is placed around the opening of the tube. As the strip is removed the gauze is placed over the opening and is kept there until a fresh strip is ready to be introduced. Several strips are inserted and withdrawn until they cease to return from the bottom of the tube stained. A long probe, with a fork on one end, is a simple and efficient means of carrying the strip to the bottom of the tube. The iodoform strips are kept in small glass jars, and no one is allowed to touch them whose hands are not perfectly clean.

These dressings are renewed, according to the amount of fluid present, at intervals of from two to four hours. As soon as a second or third strip used at any one dressing returns dry the tube is removed and the provisional wire is twisted. Should the gauze be used to pack any raw surfaces within the peritoneal cavity, it is removed as soon as the tube becomes dry, the latter being left for several hours after, in order that any fresh fluid which accumulates after the withdrawal of the gauze may be drained away.

Nothing is given the patient by mouth during the first twelve hours following the operation except small quantities of hot water to relieve the thirst. If she is suffering much pain, three or four minims of Magendie's solution of morphine are administered hypodermically. When the patient ceases to experience any nausea from the ether, small quantities of milk and lime-water are allowed, which amount is gradually increased according to circumstances. Nourishment is never given except at intervals of two hours.

An attempt is made to move the bowels as soon as any untoward symptoms, such as a rapid pulse, undue rise of temperature, vomiting or abdominal distention develop. Otherwise the bowels are moved on the third day. A one-grain calomel triturate, given every hour for three or four doses, is the medication usually resorted to, it having been found that the stomach shows a greater tolerance of this than other drugs that have been tried. In fact, it has appeared that the calomel in many instances has checked vomiting. An enema is administered eight or ten hours after the first grain of calomel has been given. Little or no medication is used after the operation, unless urgent symptoms arise which demand it. Nothing but fluid nourishment is given during the first week.

The sutures are removed on the eighth day, and the same antiseptic precautions are used as when the operation was performed. The patient is covered above and below the binder with damp bichloride towels spread over rubber sheets. The hands and arms of those who are to touch the wound or dressings are carefully disinfected and the instruments are boiled. The dressings are removed and the wound is sponged off with bichloride solution. After the sutures have been removed, the wound is again powdered with iodoform and a similar but lighter dressing than the primary one is adjusted. Great stress is laid upon the dressing being an occlusive one, and a mural or stitch-hole abscess is of rare occurrence in the ward. The second dressing is not removed for one week, after which all dressings are discarded and the patient is required to wear an abdominal binder.

In ordinary cases the patient sits up on the fourteenth day, and is allowed to leave the hospital on the twenty-first. But one patient during the past two years is known to have had a ventral hernia following laparotomy, and in this the fascia evidently was not carefully brought together at the upper angle of the wound. It is believed that this unusual freedom from herniæ is due to the care exercised in drawing the fascia well forward before the needle has penetrated the tissues.

A diagrammatic temperature and pulse chart is kept during the entire convalescence. A system of bedside notes indicating the exact condition of the patient, the number and character of the movements, and the amount of urine, is also kept. A specimen of the urine is tested, chemically and microscopically, every morning for one week following the operation, and longer should it contain any abnormal element.

The same care in regard to absolute cleanliness is carried out with minor operations. The preparation of the operating-room, the disinfection of the patient and arms and hands of the operators, is the same as in major cases In lacerations of the perineum through the sphincter the patient is subjected to treatment previous to the operation for at least five days. The bowels are freely opened and only fluid diet is allowed. The vagina is douched daily with 1 to 5000 bichloride solution. The perineum and adjacent parts are shaved and a damp bichloride pad is placed over the field of operation. After the operation the patient is catheterized every eight hours. The catheters used are made of glass, and are frequently boiled and kept in a bichloride solution. The nurse is required to carefully disinfect the urethral orifice before the catheter is introduced, and to place the tip of the finger over the end of the catheter before it is withdrawn, thus preventing any urine from escaping from the eye of the instrument. One or two small doses of opium are given after the operation to relieve the pain and to quiet any peristaltic action of the intestines. The wound is powdered frequently with iodoform, and a dry iodoform pad is kept over the parts by means of a T-bandage, and kept as dry as possible. The bowels are moved on the fourth day. On the evening of the third day one drachm of sulphate of magnesia is given at intervals of an hour until three doses have been administered. The next morning, if the bowels have not moved, one-half ounce each of castor oil and glycerin is given. The nurse is instructed to give the patient an oil enema as soon as any desire to have a movement is expressed. The enema is always given, both in these and other cases, through a soft rubber stomach tube, to which has been attached a funnel, by means of rubber tubing. The fluid to be administered is poured into the funnel and is allowed to appear at the eye before the tube is introduced. From this time forward the patient's bowels are kept open. The stitches are removed on the ninth or tenth day. During the past two years no failure of union of the sphincter has occurred.

Many cases of incomplete abortion are treated in this hospital and no labor is spared to render the patient and the operation as aseptic as possible. When such patients are received, if active hemorrhage is not taking place, they are given a thorough bath. The pubic and perineal regions are shaved. The condition of the heart is determined and a specimen of the urine is tested. Should these examinations justify it, the patient is anæsthetized. A thorough vaginal douche of 1 to 5000 bichloride solution is given. The surgeon, having rendered his hands and arms thoroughly aseptic, and wearing his operating-gown, proceeds to determine the condition of the os. Should he be unable to introduce his finger well into the cavity of the uterus, the os is forcibly dilated with a steel dilator.

When the product of conception is adherent, as much as possible is removed with the finger. A dull curette is used to free the cavity of any small fragments which may have escaped the finger, but the *finger* is always employed to determine the condition of the endometrium. The uterine cavity being empty, is irrigated through a double-current catheter with 1 to 10,000 bichloride solution at a temperature of 112° F. This usually causes firm contraction and a cessation of hemorrhage. In those cases in which the pregnancy is advanced beyond the fourth month and in which, by reason of lack of tone of the uterine tissue contraction fails to take place, strips of iodoform gauze are packed firmly into the cavity. It is the custom to operate upon all cases of incomplete abortion as soon as they enter the hospital.

No matter how slight the operation may be, the same scrupulous care is taken that everything coming in contact with the wound shall be absolutely clean. To secure this end, it will be seen that antiseptic and aseptic principles are combined—antisepsis previous to the operation, antisepsis in conjunction with asepsis during the operation, and asepsis after the operation.

REVIEWS.

A TREATISE ON THE DISEASES OF THE NERVOUS SYSTEM. By WILLIAM
A. HAMMOND, M.D., Surgeon-General U. S. Army (Retired List), etc.,
with the Collaboration of GRAEME M. HAMMOND, M.D., Professor of
Diseases of the Mind and Nervous System in the New York Post-Graduate
Medical School and Hospital. Ninth Edition, with corrections and addi-
tions. New York, 1891.

DR. HAMMOND'S book holds a unique place in American medical
literature. It was the first systematic treatise on diseases of the nervous
system to appear on this side of the Atlantic. In fact, it was the first
treatise of importance on its subject in the English language, for, if we
except a few works which scarcely rose above the dignity of monographs,
and the antiquated work of Abercrombie, the English themselves had
produced no special treatise at the time (1871), when Dr. Hammond's
first edition appeared. Certainly, if we except the somewhat fragmentary
writings of Prichard and Marshall Hall, they had produced none to
compare in value and completeness with the older work of Romberg,
and the almost contemporary treatises of Rosenthal and Hammond.
Their general medical text-books doubtless contained much excellent
and some original writing on nervous diseases. The contributions to
Reynold's *System* for instance were of enduring value, but they were the
works of numerous hands, and were inaccessible to many in that encyclopædia. Long before this time Sir Charles Bell had stimulated to an
unusual degree the study of nervous diseases, but his own writings were
largely anatomical and physiological, with a decided surgical bias. He
himself said: "I fear it will be a long time before combined efforts will
enable a medical author to arrange and accurately describe the diseases
of the nervous system." It is noteworthy that an American author was
the first to fully realize in the English language this brilliant scheme.

Dr. Hammond's book has enjoyed an unprecedented popularity with
the profession, not only because it was the first to take the field, but also
because of the striking personality of the author and the force, not to
say dogmatism, with which he expresses his opinions. This ninth edition
is an evidence of this popularity. It is also an evidence of the confidence which a successful author comes to feel in the continued indulgence and applause of his readers ; because the book in some of its parts
is not presented in the thoroughly revised and amended shape which
both its past record and the exigencies of the present time demand. This
is the more to be remarked because the author has had the collaboration
of his son, whose experience and ability amply fit him for, as his natural
pride must incite him to, the congenial and profitable task of revision.
Dr. Hammond's treatise no longer enjoys the field alone. It has many,

and some very formidable, rivals, and is bound to be measured by a standard which has changed much since 1871.

We have compared this with the fifth edition of 1881—the only one at hand—and find it practically almost the same. The former contains just two pages more than the latter, and most of these pages are identical, and printed apparently from the same stereotyped plates. It is thus seen that the book is rather a reprint than a new edition. How far haste of publication is responsible for this we do not know, but it is unjust to the merits, the reputation, and the claims of Dr. Hammond's treatise. Neurology is certainly a progressive science, and has made some notable advances during the last decade. The traumatic neuroses, we venture to say, are no longer in any other modern work treated of as anæmia of the posterior columns and of the antero-lateral columns of the spinal cord, according as they are respectively irritative and paralytic. This whole subject, which was elaborated by Dr. Hammond in his earlier editions with much plausibility and wealth of quotation from older writers, appears now in this edition rather antiquated. The author's position is certainly untenable. Again, cerebral localization, with its practical application in diagnosis and surgical treatment, has made great progress in ten years. The clinical work alone, done on this basis, has held the attention of the profession during that time as scarcely any other subject has done. It seems to us that the author has not done entire justice to this subject in his book. So, too, of multiple neuritis. Both the novelty and importance of the disease merit more than the cursory mention it receives in Dr. Hammond's book.

The relation of the infectious processes to various diseases of the nervous system is not ignored by Dr. Hammond. Tetanus is ascribed in this edition to the bacillus of Bonome. The researches of Pasteur in hydrophobia, however, are not credited with any definite results, and are dismissed with a very brief notice, while the description of the disease is long and diffuse, as in the former edition, and in itself presents nothing new. We have looked in vain for any adequate account of post-diphtheritic paralysis, and the various interesting nerve-lesions following other infectious diseases, as well as the acute delirious states occurring then, which could well be described in such a comprehensive treatise. These paralyses are briefly referred to, and classified under the head of anæmia of the antero-lateral columns of the cord—a pathology which is unreasonable, and, as the author himself says, has never been proved.

The chapter on syringomyelia has been added to this edition. The author inclines to the opinion that the majority of cases develop in subjects whose spinal cords were previously normal. Bruhl, however, has shown in his recent monograph that the congenital origin of these cases is most probable, and suggests the name *gliomatosis* for the proliferation of gliomatous tissue about the central canal in badly developed cords, to which class of cases he would confine the term. We have searched carefully but have found no description of Friedreich's disease of porencephalus or of the cerebral palsies of children.

Dr. Hammond's treatise will continue to meet with favor in the profession—to which its author therefore, owes the tribute of a careful revision of its successive editions. We believe that some of its pathology could have been profitably rewritten in this ninth edition, and that the many long quotations and detailed descriptions of the author's own cases, together with the merely theoretical and dogmatic statements in the book, could have been much curtailed, or even entirely replaced, by more careful descriptions of the morbid anatomy, symptoms, and natural history of some of the more recently studied diseases. Some space also could have been gained thus for detailed anatomical studies of the central nervous system, in which the book is rather lacking.

We have indicated what appear to us to be a few lingering defects in a book whose reputation is already thoroughly established. Its merits have long spoken for themselves. In succeeding editions, which we hope to see, the younger Hammond will no doubt see to it that the work is kept well abreast of the times, and that it continues to sustain the reputation of its author.   J. H. L.

SURGERY: A PRACTICAL TREATISE, WITH SPECIAL REFERENCE TO TREAT-
MENT. By C. W. MANSELL MOULLIN, M.A., M.D. Oxon.; Fellow of the
Royal College of Surgeons; Surgeon and Lecturer on Physiology to the
London Hospital; formerly Radcliffe Travelling Fellow and Fellow of
Pembroke College, Oxford, England : assisted by various writers on special
subjects.   Five hundred illustrations.   Pp. 1180.   Philadelphia: P.
Blakiston, Son & Co., 1891.

THE aim to make this valuable treatise practical by giving special attention to questions of treatment has been admirably carried out. Many a reader will consult the work with a feeling of satisfaction that his wants have been understood, and that they have been intelligently met. He will not look in vain for details, without proper attention to which he well knows that the highest success is impossible. As is quite proper at the present day, in a treatise on general surgery, little space is given to such departments as diseases of the eye, ear, larynx, skin, etc., and these subjects are treated by those specially fitted to do so.

The germ theory, in its application to surgery, receives the fullest acceptance. Septic fever and sapræmia (from absorption of ptomaines) are described as due to non-infective organisms, while true septicæmia is due to an infective germ. It is practically impossible to separate them clinically. Ulcers are classed with abscesses, as due to infective organisms. A burn, for instance, does not leave an ulcer, provided no other irritant is allowed to appear. Traumatic fevers should be clearly separated from those which are due to septic decomposition. Two forms are described : one, neurotic, as from emotion or peripheral nerve irritation; the other, caused by absorption from the wound of products probably related to the coagulation process.

Rabies is a specific disease for which " the only treatment of any service at all is the inoculation plan, discovered and perfected by Pasteur, and by which he has succeeded in reducing the mortality to 1.47 per cent. on the whole number (2164); and to a very much lower figure still, if only the later cases and those which applied for treatment soon after the injury are reckoned."

The use of antiseptic solutions is discussed in a very sensible way from the standpoint of practice, rather than of theory.

In the controlling of hemorrhage from deep-seated wounds, as those of the vertebral artery, packing from the bottom with iodoform gauze is advised, instead of attempting ligation. Punctured wounds of the deep plantar and palmar arches are to be treated by pressure. In the treatment of spina bifida, the author thinks that excision of the sac should very rarely be undertaken, and says that the only treatment which has met with any success is that of injection.

The work is especially rich in material which concerns the injuries and the diseases of bones and joints, to which is devoted one of the most admirably prepared and valuable portions of the book. An excellent chapter is that devoted to the treatment of fractures. The details of manipulation are so described, and such attention is paid to minor points, that anyone can follow out intelligently the advice given. The skilful use of a splint may be much more important than the shape or variety used. The writer is very fond of the plaster-of-Paris dressing; sometimes used from the first, with proper selection of cases, and immediate cutting, or in almost all cases after the first few days. Details given as to proper application are most practical. In the treatment of compound fractures the general attitude is toward a wise conservatism, determined by the light of modern methods. Compound fractures entering the knee-joint, as well as those of the thigh, still usually call for amputation, in spite of antisepsis, when they are due to direct violence. The limb can usually be saved, however, when the injury has been indirect.

After fracture of the spine, operation is opposed when indirect violence has caused the injury. The argument for this is hardly proven— that "the injury to the nerve structures is either so slight that an operation of such a nature is not justifiable, or so severe that it could do no good." In fracture by direct violence, on the other hand, "the operation should certainly be performed at once," if compression is suspected, without destruction of the cord. Especially is this advised in injuries of the cauda. He quotes the statistics of Thorburn—sixty-one trephinings for injury, only one a complete success; in seven only a *bona fide* improvement, and in six of these the improvement was in the cauda.

The operation for radical cure of hernia after herniotomy is looked upon with favor, Macewen's method being especially approved.

In acute intussusception, if enemata fail, laparotomy is advised within the first twenty-four hours, just as herniotomy is done if taxis fails.

In acute obstruction of the bowels laparotomy is to be done as soon as the diagnosis is definite, other treatment being worse than useless. As an important feature of the operation the author refers to the strong advice of Greig Smith to empty the overdistended bowel of gas by an incision or the use of a large trocar. This enormous distention will alone continue the obstruction by causing acute flexures.

No fewer than 200 of the 500 illustrations have been prepared expressly for this book. They are for the most part excellent in that they show clearly what is intended to be shown, which is of greater importance than size or display of workmanship.

The author's name is spelled with one "l" on the cover and with two on the title-page. G. E. S.

ELEMENTS OF PRACTICAL MEDICINE. By ALFRED H. CARTER, M.D.
Lond.; Member of the Royal College of Physicians, London; Physician
to the Queen's Hospital, Birmingham; Emeritus Professor of Physiology,
Queen's College, Birmingham, etc. Sixth edition, 8vo, pp. xvi., 496.
London: H. K. Lewis, 1891.

By brevity and condensation Dr. Carter has skilfully gotten a vast
deal of material into a relatively small compass, and this, too, without
more than the inevitable sacrifice of accuracy or completeness. The
present edition contains, in addition to the sections on general diseases, diseases of the respiratory, circulatory, alimentary, urinary and
nervous systems, chapters on general pathology and diseases of the skin.
At the conclusion of the work is a therapeutic index.

A number of minor defects and omissions do not materially impair
the value of the book. The organisms of Laveran receive no recognition in the discussion of malarial fevers; nor is reference made to the
pernicious types of malarial infection, hemorrhagic malarial fever, the
cerebral, pulmonary and gastric forms. The great value of morphine
and pilocarpine, given subcutaneously, in aborting the paroxysms of
these grave malarial fevers is also not mentioned. The subcutaneous
injection of pilocarpine also acts with almost specific certainty in erysipelas. It is rather doubtful if so-called gonorrhœal rheumatism will
yield to treatment useful in acute articular rheumatism. In the treatment of syphilis, mercury may be applied not only by inunction, fumigation, and internal administration, but also by subcutaneous injection.

That a section should be devoted to the general subject of carcinoma finds warrant in the statement that "it yet remains to be settled
whether, on the one hand, the newgrowth is but the local expression
of a constitutional taint; or, on the other, whether it is primarily a
local disorder, and only affects the general system secondarily." In
the symptomatology of diseases of the stomach a description is given
of "pain," which the probable omission of a word makes the text
say "is altogether absent." The smooth, white kidney and the granular, contracted kidney are given as the representatives of chronic
Bright's disease, and a common treatment is prescribed for both. We
are accustomed to believe that while iron is useful in the one case,
it is hurtful in the other. The lardaceous kidney is recognized as a
distinct form, but nothing is said of the occurrence of waxy casts in the
urine. It is true that we have no medicinal treatment for chyluria,
but the disease can be cured by removal to a climate in which the filaria
cannot live. The subject of dengue may have been omitted because the
disease occurs only in tropical countries, but the same limitation does
not apply to tetanus, which is as much deserving of a place in a work on
practical medicine as is hydrophobia. Notwithstanding the foregoing
criticisms, the book bears the stamp of a careful observer, an accurate
recorder and a versatile writer, and can be confidently commended to
the student as an "introduction to the study of systematic medicine."

                                                        A. A. E.

A GUIDE TO THE CLINICAL EXAMINATION OF THE URINE. By FARRINGTON H. WHIPPLE, A.B. Harv. 8vo, pp. x., 206. Boston: Damrell & Upham, 1891.

THE "aim in writing this little book" is stated as having been " to condense the essential features of larger and more diffuse books, and to present the subject in a more readily accessible and practical form," and in this aim the author has creditably succeeded.

At a time in the past not beyond the range of memory, examination of the urine was made only in obscure cases, and when the symptoms suggested the existence of derangement in the genito-urinary tract, and especially of the kidney. Now, however, such examination is almost universal in hospital practice, and quite general in private practice ; so that the investigation of a given case is not considered complete without a knowledge of the condition of the urinary secretion ; while the obstetrician who neglects to repeatedly examine the urine of a pregnant woman is held guilty of culpable neglect. With this advance in clinical study, manuals on the subject have multiplied, and thorough works on the practice of medicine devote considerable space to its discussion.

It should be borne in mind that the presence or absence of albumin in the urine is not always conclusive as to the existence or non-existence of disease of the kidney. Casts may be found when it had not been possible to detect the presence of albumin ; and examination of urine from an unequivocal case of nephritis will, from time to time, fail to detect the presence of either albumin or casts.

We do not believe that a clinical distinction between hyperæmia and inflammation of the kidney can be maintained. The presence of albumin and casts in the urine must be accepted as evidences of inflammation, from which, of course, recovery may take place, without leaving clinical traces of previous disease.

The subject of acetone is not at all referred to. A. A. E.

'CYCLING AND HEALTH—LA SANTÉ PAR LE TRICYCLE. By OSCAR JENNINGS, M.D. Paris, M.R.C.S. Eng. Translated from the French, third edition, Paris, 1889. By J. CROSSE JOHNSTON. Pp. 244. London : Iliffe & Son.

MADEIRA AND THE CANARY ISLANDS. A PRACTICAL AND COMPLETE GUIDE, FOR THE USE OF INVALIDS AND TOURISTS. With nine maps. By A. SAMLER BROWN. Second edition. Pp. 130. London : Sampson Low, Marston, Searle & Rivington, Limited, 1890.

STRATHPEFFER SPA : ITS CLIMATE AND WATERS. WITH OBSERVATIONS HISTORICAL, MEDICAL, AND GENERAL, DESCRIPTIVE OF THE VICINITY. By FORTESCUE FOX M.D. Lond., Fellow of the Medical Society of London. Pp. 165. London : H. K. Lewis, 1889.

'Cycling and Health contains, in epitome, the opinions concerning the 'cycle, " both of those invalids who have recovered their health by its use, and of those medical men who have turned their attention to the subject." The latter include such eminent Englishmen as Drs. B. W. Richardson and Lionel Beale. The author is evidently an enthusiastic 'cycler, who regards 'cycling as a first-rate remedy for a large number of ailments, some of which are varix, rheumatism, gout, obesity, constipation, diabetes mellitus, and various functional nervous disorders. The subject is presented so attractively that one can scarcely resist the desire to become a 'cycler, and thus enjoy some of the many benefits accruing from such invigorating exercise. The healthfulness of 'cycling and its superiority over indoor gymnastics is due to the open-air life the 'cycler leads, with sufficient exercise to properly employ the body and mind. It is superior to walking, since it is less monotonous and fatiguing, and is generally to be preferred to horseback exercise, because of its being far less expensive and troublesome. The book is well worth a perusal by those who have patients with rebellious ailments arising from too sedentary living.

The appearance of a second edition of *Madeira and the Canary Islands* in a surprisingly short time after the issue of the first may be accepted as a sufficient guarantee of its excellence, and that it fills the niche justifying its publication. It is intended, not alone as a *vade mecum* for travellers, but as a guide-book to physicians and laymen who desire complete condensed information concerning these islands as a health resort.

Strathpeffer Spa: Its Climate and Waters, its author informs us, is prepared for medical men and laymen interested in Strathpeffer and the Spa. It is, we should judge, an important contribution to the better knowledge of this health resort, and as such we commend it those who have in mind a visit to Strathpeffer.   D. D. S.

PROGRESS

OF

MEDICAL SCIENCE.

THERAPEUTICS.

UNDER THE CHARGE OF

FRANCIS H. WILLIAMS, M.D.,

ASSISTANT PROFESSOR OF THERAPEUTICS IN HARVARD UNIVERSITY.

ARSENIC AS A DRUG.

IN a lecture on this subject DR. JONATHAN HUTCHINSON points out some of the conditions under which this remedy is of especial service. It appears to possess specific power in persisting pemphigus. As a rule, no fresh bullæ are produced after the administration of the arsenic has been commenced, and the patient quickly regains health, with perfect soundness of skin.

In the treatment of common psoriasis, although the effect of arsenic is quite as definite and certain as in pemphigus, it is not nearly so immediately curative. Sometimes its effects are first manifested by the patches taking on a congested condition, and becoming very irritable. In a large majority of cases it will in the end, if well pushed, cause the eruption almost wholly to disappear. It seldom or never brings about a complete cure, and of late years we have been so much accustomed to reinforce it by efficient local measures that it is not always easy to estimate the proportion of our indebtedness to it.

As a tonic arsenic should be used only in small doses. In elderly persons, unless the disease imperatively demands it, it should not be prescribed. With the young, arsenic appears usually to agree well, and even very young children, although they but seldom need it, will bear full doses without ill effects. Amongst the facts which have been thoroughly established as regards the possible effects of arsenic it may be claimed that it is an undoubted cause of peripheral neuritis. Its influence in inducing herpes zoster, when given for the cure of other skin diseases, affords the most common example of this. It has been observed by those studying cases of poisoning by arsenic, and is especially noted by Christison, that local and unsymmetrical forms of paralysis not very infrequently result. During its medicinal use patients not infrequently complain of local numbness, more especially of portions of the skin of the lower extremities.   Numbness and tingling of the soles of the feet are by no means infrequent symptoms.

It is a very important question, especially in reference to chronic skin diseases requiring its use during long periods, whether arsenic is prejudicial or otherwise to the general health.   If given in small doses, with the exception of the risk that it may cause shingles, its effects are usually inappreciable, and there is no danger of its cumulative influence.   If arsenic be given in full doses for long periods, although it may be doubted whether there is any reason for styling it a cumulative drug, its employment is not without danger. There are certain symptoms which ought to lead us to take alarm.   If the patient has numbness of any particular part of the skin, or if there be decided loss of flesh, then it ought to be suspended.   Irritation of the conjunctiva is, of course, a well-known symptom of disagreement, but it may not be observed as frequently as some of the others just mentioned, and to them may be added a liability to diarrhœa, and, in a certain number of cases, extreme irritability of the bladder.

Under regular medical supervision a patient cannot well receive injury to his general health from arsenic.   If, however, a patient who has received great relief from his skin affection has obtained a prescription which he uses on his own responsibility, and with perhaps considerable increase in the dose ordered, it is then possible that serious or even fatal results may ensue.

As regards the influence of arsenic on the skin in persons previously healthy: Now and then we have opportunities to observe its action upon the skin when it is prescribed for maladies quite apart from the skin itself.   Its effects upon the nutrition of the skin, if the doses are large, is to make it brown and muddy-looking; it is also dry and harsh on the trunk and limbs generally, although there may be perspiration on the palms and soles.   The discoloration may be attended with actual pigmentation, and may increase until it almost resembles the tint of Addison's disease.

In extreme cases not only is there dryness and discoloration, but scaly patches may form on the knuckles, elbows and knees, much resembling common psoriasis, but less well circumscribed.   A much commoner result than this is, however, disturbance of the nutrition of the skin, not over the body generally, but over the palms and soles only.   On these parts, in addition to dryness, corns may form, and in certain very rare cases these corns pass on into epithelial cancer.   A peculiarly dry condition of the palms and soles, with tendency to the formation of corns, is by no means an infrequent result of long-continued courses of arsenic, and should lead to its discontinuance.—
British Medical Journal, No. 1588, 1891.

- - -

OPIATES IN ACUTE PERITONITIS.

DR. STEPHEN SMITH directs attention again to the importance of large doses of opium in treating acute peritonitis.

Under Professor Alonzo Clark's direction he treated six cases in 1840. The patients were seen every hour, the pulse and respiration closely watched. The quantity of opium was to be determined by the effects produced, not at all by the amount administered.   The condition of the patient to be secured was that of semi-narcotism ; this was to be determined by the degree of stupor and the respiration ; the patient must require to be shaken to be aroused to consciousness; and the respiration might fall to twelve per minute, but not below that figure.

At the outset each patient received one grain of opium every hour for three doses. No effect being perceptible, the dose was increased to two grains every hour, and continued for three doses. Failing with this dosage, the opium was increased to three grains every hour. In four cases this amount of opium had the desired effect, and it was continued in that amount. In the remaining cases it had to be increased to four grains every hour. One of these remaining cases yielded to this amount, and the opiate was continued at that rate. The sixth case was much more obstinate, and the opium was steadily increased until the dose reached was twelve grains every hour. This amount simply secured a light but continuous sleep, from which she readily awoke on placing the hand upon her wrist to examine her pulse.

The first four cases continued to receive three grains of opium every hour for three or four days, when the pulse fell to its normal standard, the tympanites subsided, the tenderness of the abdomen disappeared, and the patients were evidently convalescent. The opium was discontinued. They rapidly recovered and remained well.

In the fifth case, on the fourth night the patient was given so much opium, four-grain doses, that she was too deeply narcotized; she was without pulse, pale, and with only four respirations per minute. Active measures were taken to recover the patient from her profound narcotism. After several hours of continuous effort she was regarded as securely restored. All symptoms of peritonitis now rapidly subsided; the pulse had fallen from 112 to 92 per minute, the tympanites and tenderness had disappeared, and she expressed herself as feeling well. Within twenty-four hours all evidences of peritonitis recurred, and the treatment was renewed, three grains of opium being given instead of four. Semi-narcotism was readily produced, and after a brief period the symptoms again subsided; the treatment was suspended, and she was perfectly cured.

The sixth case proved an anomaly in tolerance of opiates. During twelve days the treatment was persevered in, the pulse remaining at about 120, the respirations 34 to 36, the abdomen greatly distended and tender to the touch, lancinating pains, the features pinched, perspiration at intervals, etc. During these twelve days the patient took the equivalent of 1950 grains of opium, and she neither vomited during that time nor had an evacuation from her bowels. At no time was she so narcotized that she would not awaken when a hand was placed upon her wrist. She remained in the hospital as an assistant in the laundry for six months after her recovery, and during that time she was in excellent health.

Professor Clark thus describes the method of medication : The plan is to begin with a dose that is safe, say two or three grains of opium, or its equivalent of sulphate of morphine, and in two hours notice its effect. If any of the opium symptoms have appeared, repeat the dose, if not, increase by one grain, and so on at intervals of two hours till the degree of tolerance in the patient is ascertained. After that the case can be treated by a diminished occupation of the physician's time—two or three visits a day. The dose is to be increased if the opium symptoms diminish, or discontinued if narcotism is approaching. The duration of the treatment will be sometimes no more than two or three days; it may be a week, or even a fortnight; and in one case the symptoms persisted mildly for forty days and then yielded. In this case the medicine used was sulphate of morphine, and the enormous dose reached, by steady and gradual increase, was one grain and a quarter every forty minutes, in a boy ten years old.

Of the several signs of opiumism there is none more valuable than the frequency of the respiration; and while the physician aims to reduce it to twelve in a minute, there are chances that he will see it fall to something below that.

Professor Clark does not explain the curative action of opium in peritonitis, but Professor Fordyce Barker, who had a large and varied experience in puerperal peritonitis in Bellevue, considered opium the most important of all agents in arresting and controlling this disease. By it the peristaltic movements are retarded or arrested, and thus the inflamed tissues have absolute rest, pain is annulled, emotional excitement is allayed, the nervous system is tranquillized, sleep is secured, and thus the depression of the vital forces resulting from the shock of the attack is lessened.—*Medical Record*, vol. xxxix., No. 22, 1891.

————

CACTINA.

Cactina is the proximate principle of the plant Cereus grandiflora, which is indigenous in tropical America. It is unirritating, a 10 per cent. solution applied to the conjunctiva produces no noticeable effect.

It is thought to increase the heart's energy and increase the blood-pressure in this way and also through stimulation of the vasomotor centre. It is said to resemble strychnine in its action upon the motor centres of the cord.

Clinical observation suggests that its greatest value is manifest in functional disturbances of the heart, as simple dilatation and cardio-muscular atony, without organic lesions A special indication for its use is during the critical periods of adynamic fevers, as it combines the elements of a heart and spinal motor stimulant.

Unlike digitalis, cactina may be administered continuously without fear of exciting gastric disturbance, and the objectionable cumulative action of the former drug is entirely absent. It may be employed in all varieties of functional cardiac disease and circulatory disturbances, and in organic heart disease, except in cases of mitral stenosis, where digitalis is to be preferred on account of its power of prolonging the diastolic period. In aortic insufficiency the short diastole produced by cactina allows no time for regurgitation of blood into the ventricle, whereas digitalis, by prolonging the diastolic period, favors just what we should seek to prevent.—*New York Medical Journal*, vol. liii., No. 24.

————

HÆMORRHOIDS.

Iodide of potassium	₅ss.
Iodine	grs. viij.
Glycerin	₅j.

Small plugs ot cotton steeped in this solution are applied every three or four hours to the piles.

By this treatment the inflammation subsides, and the hæmorrhoids diminish rapidly in volume, and finally disappear.—*Medical Press*, June, 1891.

MEDICINE.

UNDER THE CHARGE OF

W. PASTEUR, M.D. Lond., M.R.C.P.,

ASSISTANT PHYSICIAN TO THE MIDDLESEX HOSPITAL; PHYSICIAN TO THE NORTHWESTERN HOSPITAL
FOR CHILDREN;

AND

SOLOMON SOLIS-COHEN, A.M., M.D.,

PROFESSOR OF CLINICAL MEDICINE AND APPLIED THERAPEUTICS IN THE PHILADELPHIA POLYCLINIC;
PHYSICIAN TO THE PHILADELPHIA HOSPITAL.

Sudden Death from Spontaneous Rupture of the Aorta.

Martin-Dürr (*Archives Générales de Médecine*, 1891) reports the case of a woman of eighty-seven, who, two hours after dinner, was suddenly seized with pain in the back, on the left, which apparently subsided under treatment, though a sense of oppression of the chest and slight dyspnœa continued without disturbance of the respiratory rhythm. The intelligence was preserved throughout. Suddenly, two and a half hours later, the pain returned, and death took place immediately by syncope. At the autopsy, between the cæcum and the right kidney was found a cyst as large as an orange, with delicate, translucent walls, containing clear, limpid fluid of lemon-yellow color and highly albuminous. The splenic artery was as large as a little finger, extremely tortuous, nodulated and atheromatous; the liver was small and fatty; the gall-bladder contained a small cubical calculus. On removing the liver no blood flowed from the inferior vena cava. The internal and external iliac arteries and the abdominal aorta were in a high degree atheromatous. The right lung was emphysematous, adherent at the apex, and completely filled the pleural cavity. The pericardium was displaced toward the median line, and the lung pushed forward and upward. The left pleural cavity was filled with an enormous quantity of sanguinolent fluid and considerable clotted blood. The left lung was free, compressed, but crepitant. The pericardium and its cavity were normal. The heart was not hypertrophied, but laden with fat. The walls of the left ventricle were pale and of moderate thickness. The cavity of the heart contained neither fluid blood nor clot. The mitral orifice was normal; on the aortic valves were some calcareous nodules. The aorta was enormously dilated and contained numerous atheromatous patches. At the junction of the horizontal and descending portions, a little beyond the origin of the left subclavian artery, was an extensive opening almost four inches long, transverse to the axis of the vessel, in a spiral course involving its entire circumference and occupying the interval between two large calcareous plates. The margins of the torn surface were scarcely separated, and the peri-aortic connective tissue was infiltrated with blood, but at no point was the tear incomplete. The hemorrhagic infiltration extensively involved also the mediastinal connective tissue. It formed an ecchymotic area at the level of the third, fourth, fifth, and sixth dorsal vertebræ, to the left of the spinal column. The orifice of communication between the aorta and the pleural cavity could not be found.

Dürr has succeeded in collecting from the literature twenty-eight other cases of rupture of the aorta, in addition to the twenty-eight reported by Broca, the eighty reported by Peacock, and the fourteen reported by Pilliet. An analysis of these cases leads him to arrange them in three groups : 1, those without the production of dissecting aneurisms, which are rare; 2, those with the production of dissecting aneurisms, which are relatively common ; and, 3, those with the production of true aneurismal sacs, which are exceedingly rare. Spontaneous ruptures of the aorta are more common in men than in women, and especially common at advanced age. In many cases no exciting cause has been apparent; in some it was slight, and in others, violent effort, anger, emotion, or a large meal acted as a cause of rupture. Death may occur suddenly; or slowly, at once; or slowly in two periods, separated by an interval. The first is uncommon; the second, the least common ; the third, the most common. The most usual seats of rupture, in the order of frequency of occurrence, are the origin of the aorta, its ascending portion, the beginning of the arch or the origin of the innominate, the horizontal portion, the termination of the arch and the beginning of the descending portion of the thoracic aorta, and, finally, the abdominal aorta. The rupture is generally transverse. The blood is usually discharged into an adjacent cavity—most commonly into that of the pericardium ; much more rarely, into the left pleural cavity; occasionally, into the trachea or into the œsophagus. Sometimes the blood finds its way only into the peri-aortic and mediastinal connective tissue or beneath the left pleura, forming a tumor in the thoracic wall between the left lung and the. pericardium. The most common anatomical cause of rupture is atheroma of the aorta, often associated with dilatation. In the majority of cases the left ventricle is hypertrophied. Valvular lesions may or may not coexist. The diagnosis is scarcely possible. There may be severe pain in the pre-sternal region and between the shoulders, with intense anxiety and distress, while respiration remains normal and percussion and auscultation disclose no abnormality in the pulmonary functions.

Sudden Death from Rupture of Varices of the Heart.

Journiac (*La Médecine Moderne*, 1891) reports the case of a man of fifty-five, coming under his observation with delusions of persecution associated with hallucinations, probably of alcoholic origin. These manifestations speedily disappeared, a condition of dementia remaining. Nothing of note transpired during a period of more than five years. At the end of this time the patient was suddenly seized with loss of consciousness of brief duration, three or four seizures occurring rapidly in succession. A number of months later another attack occurred, which soon terminated fatally. Upon post-mortem examination nothing abnormal was found in the brain. The cavity of the pericardium was distended by an immense clot. At the left border of the left ventricle, a little below the auriculo-ventricular septum, was an ovoid tumor of the size of a small nut, dark in color, with a small opening at its summit, containing a loose clot; but between the cavity of which and the ventricle or a vessel no opening could be found. Above and below were a number of tortuous varicose swellings, none of which communicated with the ventricle. The branch of the coronary artery behind the tumor was normal. The heart itself was in other respects in good condition.

OBSTRUCTION AND INSUFFICIENCY AT THE TRICUSPID, MITRAL, AND AORTIC ORIFICES.

Before the Boston Society for Medical Observation, SHATTUCK (*Boston Med. and Surg. Journal*, 1891) reported the case of a domestic of forty-three, with a history of scarlatina at eleven, of muscular rheumatism at twenty-eight, and òf alcoholism. Following the attack of rheumatism there were asthmatoid seizures. Later on there were bronchitis, dyspnœa, œdema and ascites, derangement of menstruation, icterus, and diarrhœa. The area of cardiac dulness was increased, especially to the right. Over the aortic, mitral, and tricuspid orifices double murmurs were heard. The aortic-systolic was transmitted in the course of the great vessels; the diastolic, downward, along the sternum. The presystolic murmurs heard over the mitral and tri-cuspid orifices differed in quality. The jugular veins were distended and pulsated. Subsequently the tricuspid-presystolic murmur could not be detected. The area of hepatic dulness, at first increased, became diminished. Systolic retraction became apparent in the region of the apex of the heart. At the autopsy the pericardial cavity was found obliterated by old adhesions. The heart was enlarged; the aortic valve was incompetent; the pulmonary held water. The aortic crescents and the mitral leaflets were thickened, shortened and adherent, and the respective orifices narrowed. The tricuspid leaflets were thickened and shortened, with delicate vegetations at their margins; the orifice was narrowed. Delicate translucent vegetations occu-pied the pulmonary crescents along the lines of apposition. Two of the seg-ments were adherent. The left ventricle was neither hypertrophied nor dilated; the left auricle was dilated. The right ventricle was hypertrophied; the right auricle dilated. The aorta and pulmonary artery were atheroma-tous and dilated.

MALFORMATION OF THE HEART AND GREAT VESSELS.

MACAIGNE (*Bulletins de la Soc. Anat. de Paris*, No. 1, 1891) reports the case of a girl of eighteen, in whom, when eighteen months old, a cardiac affection was recognized. She could not participate in the games of children of her age. On the slightest exertion or emotion she became oppressed and cyanotic. For several years there had been cough and occasional hæmoptysis. The face was pallid, livid, puffy; the lips, nostrils, and fingers were cyanotic; the skin was pallid, but not cold; the cellular tissue was relaxed; the extremities of the fingers were clubbed. Dyspnœa was marked; the pulse accelerated. The cardiac action was regular and energetic; the impulse below the nipple. On auscultation a coarse, low-pitched, rasping systolic murmur was heard, with greatest intensity at the left third chondro-sternal articulation and at the inner part of the left second intercostal space, in the latter situation seeming more superficial; the murmur was propagated toward the middle of the left clavicle; the second sound of the heart was normal. On palpation a purring tremor could be felt over the area in which the murmur was heard with greatest intensity, particularly at the inner part of the second left interspace. The pulmonary percussion resonance was impaired on the left, below the clavicle, and in the supra-spinous fossa. Subcrepitant and sibilant râles were heard at both apices. There was cough, without expectoration. Several hæmoptyses occurred, following one of which the patient died asphyxiated. At the autopsy the apices of the lungs were found stuffed with tubercles, some of which were caseous; in the left apex were a number of small cavities. The leaflets of the pulmonary valve, which was competent, were replaced by a membrane projecting into the artery like a cone, of which the length was about a third of an inch and the diameter of the free orifice about one-sixth of an inch. The trunk of the vessel, at its middle, was an inch and a half in circumference; its walls thin and soft. The pulmonary artery divided regularly, but there was no trace of a ductus arteriosus. The thickness of the wall of the left ventricle was normal; of the right ventricle and between the ventricles, greatly increased. The tricuspid valve was well developed. The chordæ tendineæ were thickened, the papillary muscles and columnæ carneæ hypertrophied. The right ventricle communicated directly with the aorta, the conus being narrowed and limited in front and behind by two large muscular fasciculi. The interventricular septum was defective at its upper part; the free border was concave. The aorta was situated à cheval above the septum. The aortic valve was competent. The aorta was dilated. The right auricle appeared to be thrice as large as the left. The interauricular septum was defective. The duct of Botal was represented by three minute openings. On the septum were numerous bands, giving rise to an areolar appearance. The ductus arteriosus was wanting, but by the side of the aorta was a small cul-de-sac. No other arterial anomaly was discovered.

CHANGES IN THE SPUTUM OF PATIENTS TREATED BY TUBERCULIN.

AMANN (Centralblatt für Bakteriologie und Parasitenk., 1891), of Davos, describes the changes which he has observed in the sputum and in the contained tubercle bacilli of patients with diseases of the lungs treated by injections of the Koch fluid. His statements are based upon examinations of the sputa of 288 patients, 198 of whom received injections. It was found that the quantity of the expectoration and the number of bacilli were, as a rule, increased after reaction had occurred. The appearance of the bacilli was changed. The rods appeared broken up into numerous small fragments. The bacilli stained poorly, apparently from a diminution of their specific resistance to decolorizing agents. In 40 per cent. of the cases injected, reaction was followed by a diminution in the quantity of elastic fibres in the sputum.

_____

ALTERATIONS IN THE BACILLI EXPECTORATED BY PATIENTS.

VIERLING (*Wiener klin. Wochenschrift,* 1891) admits that the bacilli in the sputum exhibit certain changes in form and in behavior toward the aniline stains after injections of the Koch fluid, but denies that these changes are evidences of an alteration in the chemical constitution of the body in general and of the medium in which the bacilli live in particular, and concludes that the changes must be due to purely local causes. He reports a case in a girl, thirteen years of age, which terminated fatally, and in which, during life, alterations in the shape of the bacilli in the sputum were found, while the bacilli in the diarrhœic stools remained unchanged. It would be important to know whether the changes observed were the results of degeneration or of growth.

_____

ANGINA PECTORIS.

R. DOUGLAS POWELL (*Practitioner,* April, 1891, No. 274) argues that angina pectoris is a disturbed innervation of the heart or vessels, associated with more or less intense cardiac distress and pain, and a general prostration of the forces, always producing anxiety and often amounting to a sense of impending death. Considerable stress is laid on habitual high arterial tension as a factor in causation. Angina is not necessarily associated with coronary or other disease of the heart or vessels, although it is true that in fatal cases disease or obstruction of the coronary arteries is the most frequent lesion found, after which in order of frequency come fatty degeneration, aortic dilatation, aortic regurgitation, and aneurism. The author classifies the varieties of the affection as follows:

1. In its purer forms we observe disturbed innervation of the systemic or pulmonary vessels, causing their spasmodic contraction and consequently a sudden extra demand on the propelling power of the heart, violent palpitations, or more or less cramp or paralysis ensuing according to the reserve power and integrity of that organ—angina pectoris vasomotoria.

2. In other cases we have essentially the same mechanism, but with extra demand made upon a *diseased* heart—angina pectoris gravior.

3. The trouble may commence at the heart through irritation or excitation of the cardiac nerves, or from sudden accession of anæmia of cardiac muscle from coronary disease—primary cardiac angina.

4. In certain conditions of blood (often gout), or under certain reflex excitations of the inhibitory nerves, always, however, with a degenerate feeble heart in the background. We may observe intermittence in its action prolonged to syncope—syncopal angina.

Treatment.—In group 1, nitrite of amyl, and still more nitro-glycerin, are of great value, and may require to be combined with nervine tonics or sedatives, iron, zinc, valerian, bromides, etc. In groups 2 and 3, carminative stimulants, or digitalis with nitro-glycerin, are recommended; and of all tonics arsenic, as a rule, is the best.

BACTERIUM COLI COMMUNE IN THE PUS FROM A DYSENTERIC ABSCESS
OF THE LIVER.

VEILLON and JAYLE (*Compt. rend. hebdom. des Séances de la Soc. Biol.*, 1891) report the case of a patient admitted June 11, 1890, to the Hôpital Lariboisière, with the symptoms of abscess of the liver, having had dysentery in 1881 at Tonkin. From the pus removed by aspiration no cultivable organism could be obtained. Microscopic examination, culture in agar and gelatin of the pus obtained a month later by incision, however, revealed the exclusive presence of the bacterium coli commune. The patient recovered. This observation seems to demonstrate that the bacterium coli commune may invade organs adjacent to the intestine, when these are the seat of disease, without possessing special pathogenetic properties, though perhaps tending to retard recovery.

———

A NEW TEST FOR ALBUMIN AND OTHER PROTEIDS.

JOHN A. MACWILLIAM (*Brit. Med. Journ.*, No. 1581) states that the reagent is a saturated watery solution of salicyl-sulphonic acid, a white crystalline substance readily soluble in water and alcohol. It precipitates all classes of proteids: 1, native albumins (egg-albumin and serum-albumin); 2, derived albumins (acid-albumin and alkali-albumin); 3, globulins (*e. g.*, serum globulin and myosin); 4, fibrin (whether held in solution by dilute alkalies or by neutral salts); 5, proteoses (albumoses, etc); 6, peptones.

With all these the reagent at once forms a dense, bulky, white precipitate. This precipitate is not redissolved on boiling, except in the case of an albumose or peptone. The precipitate is readily soluble in a dilute alkali, provided a sufficiency of the alkaline solution be added. It is not soluble in weak acids, nor in strong acids unless a large quantity of strong acid (such as nitric) is added.

The method of testing is as follows: Take a small amount of urine (for example, 20 minims), preferably in a very small test-tube, and add a drop or two of a *saturated* watery solution of the reagent. If the urine is strongly alkaline an extra drop or two of the acid should be added, and if no opalescence or precipitate occurs it is well to test the reaction with litmus, and make sure that the urine has been made strongly acid. On adding the reagent, shake the tube quickly, so as to mix its contents ; then examine at once. The occurrence of an opalescence or cloudiness immediately or within a very few seconds (say two or three) is a test for proteids, intermediate in delicacy between the cold nitric acid test, on the one hand, and the acetic acid and heat test (under favorable circumstances), on the other. The development of an opalescence some time after (for example, one-half to two minutes) is a more delicate test than even acetic acid and heat, and shows the presence of minute traces of proteid, which are probably insignificant from a clinical point of view, as a rule.

Next heat the tube to boiling-point. If the opalescence or precipitate is caused by the ordinary "albumin" commonly present in albuminous urine, it does not disappear on heating; but, on the other hand, becomes markedly flocculent. But if the precipitate or opalescence is due to the presence of albumoses or peptones, it clears up on heating (before the boiling-point is reached) and reappears when the tube cools.

The author is satisfied from careful experiments, that—1, the precipitate is really a proteid one; 2, that it is always obtained when proteid is present in the various abnormal conditions of urine which may have to be examined; 3, that the precipitate cannot be caused by any other non-proteid constituent of the urine. Cloudy phosphatic urine clears adding the reagent.

Urine containing excess of urates gives no precipitate, nor does proteid-free bilious urine. As regards the presence of a large quantity of mucin this is not likely to prove a source of error. Moreover, it is probably only in the case of alkaline urine, when there is at the same time a marked irritation of some part of the urinary passages, yielding a greatly increased mucous secretion, that the amount of mucin in the urine can be sufficient to come into question at all. But in such conditions of the urinary tract the detection of a trace of albumin is probably of no significance. Normal urine gives no reaction with salicyl-sulphonic acid.

SURGERY.

UNDER THE CHARGE OF

J. WILLIAM WHITE, M.D.,

PROFESSOR OF CLINICAL SURGERY IN THE UNIVERSITY OF PENNSYLVANIA; SURGEON TO THE UNIVERSITY AND GERMAN HOSPITALS;

ASSISTED BY

EDWARD MARTIN, M.D.,

CLINICAL PROFESSOR OF GENITO-URINARY SURGERY IN THE UNIVERSITY OF PENNSYLVANIA; SURGEON TO THE HOWARD HOSPITAL AND ASSISTANT SURGEON TO THE UNIVERSITY HOSPITAL.

RELAPSE OF HERNIA AFTER VARIOUS OPERATIONS FOR RADICAL CURE.

Since BULL has had a more extensive experience with the radical cure of hernia than any other surgeon of this country his utterances upon this subject bear great weight. During the past three years, aided by his assistant, DR. S. E. MILLIKEN (*New York Medical Journal*, vol. liii., No. 22), he has carefully examined the histories of patients applying to the Hospital for Ruptured and Crippled in the hope of furnishing some statistical evidence of the value of different methods of radical cure of hernia. The tabulation made of relapsed cases numbers 119. In 73 cases the method of operation was definitely ascertained.

The average age in all the methods was about the same—from thirty-eight to forty-four years—showing that the extremes of life generally have been avoided. The duration of treatment, practically wound healing, in Czerny's method, where the pillars of the external ring and the integuments are carefully sutured, is almost as great as in the open method. This is an argument in favor of allowing the wound to granulate. It is particularly noteworthy that relapses occurred as late as two years and six months, and three years and four months, and that, on an average, no method shows immunity from recurrence for a longer period than fifteen months. This warrants the statement that future evidence as to the value of different methods must cover an experience of more than three years, and patients who have been without a recurrence for a year have no reason to expect to remain so permanently.

In one table eight cases are given, presumably operated on for radical cure, since the herniæ were reducible, and the operations were performed in the last five years. Relapse ensued after an average period of twenty-four weeks.

The next table gives twenty cases of irreducible strangulated hernia subjected to operation within eight years, without any data as to method. A radical cure may or may not have been attempted. Relapse occurred, on an average, in eighteen months.

These cases certainly demonstrate that many methods are defective and likely to prove disappointing if observed for a sufficient length of time.

Since ten years have elapsed since the modern operations have been in vogue there should be patients who have been more than five years without relapse. Some such patients could naturally be expected to appear at hospitals; no such records are present.

In the hospital books are recorded 46 patients who have been subjected to radical operations, and who present no sign of relapse, and who have been furnished with trusses; of these, only 5 have been under observation for three years, 8 for less than two years, and 32 for less than one year.

In a series of 136 radical cure operations reported by the author a year ago, there were only 4 cases that had been over four years without recurrence.

Eighteen cases are tabulated which were operated on for irreducible strangulated hernia, and in which no attempt at radical cure was made. This latter fact was ascertained from the date of operation (prior to the introduction of modern methods), or was known from the statement of the operator. The patients averaged 45 years. The period at which the relapse occurred varied from one month to 23 years, and was on an average 5 years. It is noteworthy that of 15 of these cases all wore trusses from the time of operation.

The author is not prepared to offer any statistical data bearing on the question of trusses preventing relapse or prolonging a cure. He states in general that the largest and most voluminous protrusions were met with in patients who had worn no truss; and furthermore, he had never seen any evidence of damage to structure by the pressure of the truss. In his own practice he always has his patients fitted with a truss immediately after the wound has healed, and directs that the pressure shall be very slight—that is, shall merely support the parts. Much that has been said against trusses can be laid to the score of the operation, and the condition that the parts are left in by it rather than to the truss. If suppuration is prolonged in the wound, and it is compelled to heal by granulation, a cicatrix of less vitality and less elasticity than the normal skin and subcutaneous fat is left. This structure is not tolerant of pressure. A primary union which restores the parts as nearly as possible to their normal condition will not be unfavorably affected by the truss. On the other hand, in a wound with much cicatricial tissue there is a natural tendency to softening and yielding, and this tendency should be hastened by the pressure of the truss without and the viscera within.

In cases treated by the open method the orifice of the relapsed hernia is not unlike that of ventral herniæ—that is, an opening in the wall without any canal, so that the hernia protrudes directly forward. This condition makes greater difficulty in the adaptation of a truss, which is further enhanced by the thinness of the yielding cicatrix. Although at first the cicatrix of the open operation can be recognized by its depressed situation and firm, contractile, tense character, at a later period it begins to yield in places or all along its line, and ultimately presents the features just mentioned.

Although these patients are not cured, the majority are certainly improved. They find much satisfaction in the fact that the protrusions are not so large as before operation; they experience increased comfort and security in the wearing of a truss. The author states that the figures given do not afford any valuable evidence as to the comparative reliability of different methods, but only emphasize the lack of promise to effect a cure. He believes that it is still wise to continue to strive for better methods. He advises that the term cure should be dropped, and the value of given procedures should be estimated by the relative proportion of relapses. That plan will be judged best which shows the smallest number of relapses in the course of the longest period of observation; such period should be at least five years. He further believes that all procedures should be so devised as to insure prompt healing of the wound, and that the support of a truss should be insisted on from the time the patient leaves his bed.

THE SEAT OF PUNCTURE IN PARACENTESIS ABDOMINIS.

TRZEBICKY (*Archiv für klin. Chirur.*, Bd. xli., Heft 4), in performing paracentesis abdominis at the point of election—that is, midway between the umbilicus and the anterior superior spine of the ilium—wounded a large bloodvessel which gave such troublesome bleeding that the life of the patient was threatened. The hemorrhage was arrested by compression of the common iliac artery. Incited by this experience, and by several reports of fatal bleeding following puncture at this point, Trzebicky conducted an experimental research upon a large number of cadavers. As a result of this he announces the following conclusions:

In the majority of cases paracentesis performed at a point midway between the umbilicus and the anterior superior spinous process of the ilium is perfectly safe, since neither the epigastric artery nor any large branch of this vessel is liable to be wounded. The artery commonly crosses this line at the junction of the inner with the middle third.

In a certain proportion of cases, however, the epigastric artery or one of its branches lies directly beneath the point of election.

The course of the epigastric artery is seldom exactly similar in the two sides of the body.

Since the artery runs within the sheath of the rectus muscle, its course depends mainly upon the position of this muscle. In case the two recti are separated by abdominal distention, the artery is displaced so that it lies very near the point of election for puncture. The rectus muscle does not, however, bear a constant relation to the artery. At times, even though the muscle is displaced to the side, the artery lies near the middle line.

Variations in the origin of the epigastric artery seem to have no influence on the course of the former vessel.

The artery is usually accompanied by a single vein.

Paracentesis abdominis should be performed either in the linea alba or in the outer half of the line joining the umbilicus and anterior superior iliac spine. In case the linea alba is selected, it is not important to keep strictly in the middle line, since there is an arterial branch which may be wounded if the trocar is entered, even slightly, to one side.

Catgut Infection in the Dry Treatment of Wounds.

KLEMM (*Archiv für klin. Chirur.*, Bd. xli., Heft. 4), on adopting the dry treatment of wounds, employed catgut as the material for placing buried sutures, and was surprised to observe as a result that abscesses developed at the site of operation much more frequently than was the case when he employed silk alone as suture and ligature material. At first this was attributed to some carelessness in operative technique, but even after the minutest observance of every precaution suppuration still occurred. For the first few days after operation there was no fever, no local pain or tenderness. On the sixth day, when the silk sutures were removed (the wounds were not drained), there seemed to be healing without disturbance by microörganisms. On the eighth or tenth day there was an elevation of temperature and swelling and tenderness in the region of the wound. On tearing open the latter an abscess was found, which, without exception, was found in the deeper part of the incision, where the catgut had been placed. The catgut employed was prepared by repeated washings in five per cent. alcohol-sublimate solutions until the latter showed no turbidity. The catgut was then stored in absolute alcohol, from which it was not taken until it was needed for use.

To determine whether this method of preparation rendered the gut sterile, a great many culture experiments were carried out. They all showed that the catgut thus treated was germ-free. Klemm next implanted in the deep tissues of dogs catgut prepared as first described and portions of sterilized silk of corresponding sizes. Examination some days later showed septic inflammation about the catgut implantations, whilst the tissues about the silk were in a normal condition. Culture of the catgut showed countless colonies of microörganisms. In the silk there were either none or very few.

From these experiments it is evident that catgut can be surely sterilized, but that, even though itself germ-free, it greatly favors infection of wounds. This infection, of course, takes place during operation, since it is almost impossible to keep a wound absolutely germ-free. The few germs which thus gain access find a favorable medium in which to grow in the softening, non-resistant catgut.

Bottini's Method of Treating the Enlarged Prostate.

MORROTTI (*British Medical Journal*, 1891, No. 1586) describes Bottini's method of treating enlarged prostate by means of the galvano-cautery. This method is designed to remove or lessen the mechanical obstruction to the outflow of the urine. To accomplish this a special instrument has been devised. This consists of an incisor apparatus and a battery. The former is a catheter-shaped metal tube, the lumen of which is divided into four separate compartments; two of these are for the conducting of electric wires, the other two are channels for the passage of a stream of cold water, which runs to the distal extremity of the instrument, thus preventing it from becoming over-heated. The conducting wires end in a cautery knife, which, when heated to a dull red, is applied to the hypertrophied tissue. This knife can be screwed backward and forward, and can be completely shielded by the curved point of the instrument.

In performing the operation the patient's urethra should be habituated to the use of the instrument before cauterization is attempted. Anæsthesia is not always necessary. Water need not be injected into the bladder unless this viscus is quite empty. The patient is placed in the lithotrity position and the instrument is used in the usual way. When the point is in the bladder it is turned downward, and is then drawn forward so as to cause the beak to hitch against the prostate and bring the cautery into contact with the part upon which it is desired to act. By exposing the knife, connecting the current, and gently elevating the handle of the instrument, the point is made to burn its way slowly through the prostate. When the sound of burning is heard the point should be moved backward and forward until the projecting lobe is completely divided. The knife should be allowed to cool; should be returned to its sheath; the instrument should then be passed into the bladder, and should finally be withdrawn.

Bottini has operated in this manner in 57 cases, with 3 deaths. In 32 cases a perfect cure was effected, in 11 there was improvement, and in 12 the result was *nil*. If the hypertrophy is only moderate the obstructing lobe should be entirely destroyed. In advanced cases the surgeon should be content with tunnelling a passage. Both these procedures are contra-indicated if kidney disease is present.

RUPTURE OF THE URETHRA FROM DISTENTION.

BAZY (*La Semaine Méd.*, 11 Ann., No. 14) has conducted a number of experiments to determine which portion of the urethra is most prone to rupture when this canal is forcibly distended. In the great majority of cases the urethra gave way at its bulbous portion, though in a certain proportion of cases the tear involved both the bulbous and membranous urethra. In the latter case the resulting effusion was poured into the rectum. In the exceptional cases, when the membranous urethra alone was involved, the extravasation was, of course, found in the space of Retzius. The ruptures were always on the floor of the urethra, or on its lateral walls. From this it follows that in case of tight stricture. even though the lesion is located in the penile portion of the urethra, if rupture takes place this is commonly located at the bulb.

In this relation the author again calls attention to the fact that terminal bleeding, that is hemorrhage following urination does not necessarily originate from the bladder, or from the neck of the viscus. Slight rupture of the anterior urethra may readily occur from the impact of the urine; especially is this the case when there is contraction of some part of the passage. The blood being mingled with a large quantity of water is not noticed at first. As the volume of the stream of urine diminishes it becomes more distinctly colored, till finally pure blood drops from the meatus. This form of hemorrhage must be diagnosed from that which originates in the bladder, as the latter is often of serious diagnostic import. The urethral hemorrhage is attended with burning, but is not marked by the straining and sensation of something that is left in the bladder which marks inflammation or disease of the latter organ.

OTOLOGY

UNDER THE CHARGE OF

CHARLES H. BURNETT, M.D.,
AURAL SURGEON, PRESBYTERIAN HOSPITAL, ETC , PHILADELPHIA.

THE AFFECTIONS OF THE EAR IN TABES DORSALIS.

DR. LEOPOLD TREITEL, of Berlin, has made a careful examination of the ears in a number of tabetic cases, and his conclusions are as follows (*Archives of Otology*, vol. xix.): In five cases of tabes, where the hearing was affected, only two the author considers as probably due to an affection of the auditory nerve. Careful study leads him to the conclusion that not only the perceptive apparatus of the ear, but also the conducting apparatus is affected. In one case, at least, there was reason to believe that changes had occurred in the mucous membrane of the tympanic cavity, "which depend on a retrograde metamorphosis, and may also be called sclerosis."

The author concludes that particular trophic fibres of the fifth nerve must be diseased, which may be affected alone, or together with sensory fibres. In one case trophic changes in the tract of the fifth nerve and the glosso-pharyngeal nerve were observed—two nerves which send branches to the tympanic cavity. From numerous observations Treitel is inclined to believe that "sclerosis of the posterior columns of the cord not rarely causes trophic changes in the middle ear, which may lead to disturbances of hearing." Such changes might be found frequently, if looked for, at necropsies. A number of facts seem to indicate the development of sclerotic changes in the middle ear from a tabetic cause.

It is fair to suppose that the aural affection is due to the tabetic disease, "when the disturbance in hearing is first noticed after the undoubted beginning of the tabes, no aural disease having previously existed, provided that the otological examination corresponds to the clinical history." The author cannot confirm the statement of Gradenigo,[1] "that especially in cerebro-

---

[1] THE AMERICAN JOURNAL OF THE MEDICAL SCIENCES, Nov. 1890, and Archives of Ohrenh., vol. xxx., 1890.

spinal diseases with amblyopia or amaurosis, an (electric) excitability of the auditory nerve is found."

So-called paradoxical conditions of hearing in deafness from tabetic or central causes, "where a screaming voice is heard only very near the ear, and the sound of the words, without the detail of the articulation, is still perceived, and even the scratching of a pen, the striking together of two metal pieces, etc.," are not admitted to exist in deafness from central causes alone, as they are often found in deafness from other causes, as, for instance, in sclerosis. In two patients with marked lessening of pain- and touch-perception on one side, no difference was found in the sound-perceptions of the two sides. "Whether for the producion of this condition a lessening of all the ' sensibilities is required is very questionable."

Chataigner's[1] conclusions are thus quoted : "The disturbances on the part of the ear (in tabes) may be of varying intensity. They are caused by a hyperæmia of the labyrinth, which may depend on a direct irritation of the auditory nerves, which extends from the centre toward the periphery, or of other nerves which exercise a vasomotor influence on the vascular system of the ear." The deafness in the former case may be total, in the latter partial. The disturbances in hearing may be the first symptom of 'the tabes." This view as to vasomotor influences leading to trophic changes in the middle ear harmonizes with that of Treitel.

NOTEWORTHY CHANGES IN THE NASAL MUCOUS MEMBRANE IN A CASE OF LEUKÆMIA.

SUCHANNEK, of Zürich, has examined post-mortem the nasal mucous membrane in leukæmia. The mucosa of both the respiratory and of the olfactory portion showed color entirely different from the normal one. Usually the respiratory portion is pinkish, in the olfactory region yellowish intermixed with pink. The leukæmic membrane, however, had a moist, glistening appearance, and possessed throughout its inferior part, up to the middle turbinated bone, a light yellowish-brown ; the upper portion, including the olfactory fissure, the superior turbinated bone, the part below the ethmoidal plate, the corresponding portions of the septum, *a dark-brown color*. The mucous membrane was also decidedly thickened throughout its whole extent. Microscopic sections showed lymphomatous nodules in the turbinated bodies, on the septum, and especially in the nasal roof. Normal olfactory epithelium was found—accompanied, however, by a total destruction of the glandular apparatus.—*Archives of Otology*, vol. xix.

CHOLESTEATOMA, PERFORATION OF SHRAPNELL's MEMBRANE, AND OCCLUSION OF THE TUBES: AN ETIOLOGICAL STUDY.

BEZOLD, of Munich (*Archives of Otology*, vol. xix.), under the above title contributes one of the most instructive and interesting papers it has been our good fortune to read. It has long been a question how concentric epidermic masses originate in the attic, antrum, and mastoid region. Virchow has thought that cholesteatoma might originate at these points by " an epider-

[1] Thèse de Paris, 1890.

moidal transformation of the mucous membrane of the middle ear," but this idea is "annihilated by the very localization of these tumors," which, up to this time, he has never found actually within the tympanic cavity itself. Bezold maintains that epidermic cells gain access both to the atrium and the attic of the tympanum, and thence into the antrum and the mastoid cells, from the external auditory canal through perforations in the membrana tympani.

"The moment that the sharp distinction between the cutis and the mucous membrane has once been lost by destruction of the surface of the membrana at any spot, we see the cutis of the remaining intact region gain ⋅the ascendancy over the mucous membrane, and extend with much greater rapidity over the entire district." Thus, when the membrane is entirely broken down, an epidermic layer from the skin of the external auditory canal may extend even into the mastoid cells (Schwartze). It appears that a favorite port of entrance of epidermic cells into the attic is through perforations in the flaccid membrane, above the short process.

Bezold then considers the origin of attic suppurations and perforations in the flaccid membrane.

It has always been difficult to say how suppuration in the attic, with perforation in the membrana flaccida only, originates. It was once supposed to come about like suppuration of the atrium of the tympanum, viz., through the Eustachian tube. But this has always been far from certain. Bezold rejects this latter theory, as does Walb (*Archiv. f. Ohrenh.*, vol. xx. p. 185, etc.), and he believes, with Walb, that purulent infection of this attic space in the tympanic cavity enters from the *external meatus, partly in the form of an otitis externa, with ulceration at the margin of Shrapnell's membrane,* and partly through a persistent foramen Rivini. This theory is strengthened by the fact that we often find evidences of closure of the Eustachian tube in cases of chronic purulency of the attic with perforation of the flaccid membrane.

Treatment.—It is maintained by the author that occasionally spontaneous cures occur in these cases. The surgeon's task, it is claimed, is either to enlarge the orifice into the attic by removing the upper bony margin of the perforations in the meatus, or by extraction of the malleus and anvil, or, thirdly, by making a new opening into the antrum. Entire removal of the epidermic (neoplastic) lining of the drum cavity is impossible.

TOPOGRAPHY OF THE NORMAL HUMAN TYMPANUM.

At the suggestion of Professor Blake, of Harvard Medical School, Dr. WILLIAM S. BRYANT, of Boston, has examined a number of temporal bones with special reference to the reduplications of the mucous membrane lining the tympanic cavity. Not one of the tympana examined—over one hundred —was free from these folds, and in several instances they occupied the whole cavity of the tympanum above the ossicles.

These folds are arranged by Dr. Bryant in three groups: 1. Those of the mastoid antrum, in which there is usually a central longitudinal band, with radiating lines and trabeculæ. 2. Those attached to the malleus and incus radiating from the three long axes of the bones. 3. Those of the stapes and round window, and the neighboring tympanic wall. "The mucous folds about the stapes join the crura together or connect the stapes with the walls of the pelvis ovalis. The mucous folds which are attached to the ossicula perform essentially the function of the ligaments, binding them together, or to the walls of the tympanum; and for this reason they might be classified as ligaments."

The article is accompanied by fifteen colored engravings, showing very graphically the results of Dr. Bryant's great industry in the study of these important structures in the drum cavity.—*Archives of Otology*, vol. xix.

REDUPLICATIONS OF TYMPANIC MUCOUS MEMBRANE.

Under this title DR. CLARENCE J. BLAKE, of Boston, draws attention to a series of important pathological conditions in the middle ear, and the results of their formation, upon the hearing (*Archives of Otology*, vol. xix. p. 213). As an important factor in the persistence of chronic suppurative disease of the middle ear, and also in the effects which that and various other non-suppurative diseases have upon hearing, Dr. Blake considers certain folds, bands, or reduplications of mucous membrane in the upper and posterior part of the drum cavity. These impair the mobility of the chain of ossicles, and of its complement, the membrane of the round window. These folds are divided into, first, a horizontal set, which impair drainage from the attic, and a vertical set, which are disposed around the stapes and the round window. This second class is important, because they interfere with the mobility of these essential parts of the conducting apparatus of the ear. A third set is described as striæ or reduplications, chiefly the former, in the neighborhood of the mastoid antrum. The two first are considered of most clinical importance. They exist normally in about 70 per cent. of all human ears, and are not to be considered pathological in themselves. Aside from an obstruction to drainage from the attic, the first class of reduplications "may be considered as playing an important *rôle* in the etiology of those diseases of the tympanic attic the majority of which start with a suspension of vasomotor inhibition in that region."

When a suppuration has been established, the presence of the mucous folds of the first class—the horizontal ones—may become an interference to free movement on the part of the ossicles after the suppurative process has closed.

The thickening and adhesions of the folds of the second class, viz., those about the stapes and neighborhood of the round window, interfere with the motility of these important parts. In cases where the membrana tympani is largely perforated, with spontaneous evulsion of the incus, "the considerable impairment of hearing, due to the immobility of the stapes from the adhesions and thickening of their mucous folds, an immobilizing effect still further increased by the unrestricted action of the stapedius muscle, has been improved by the division, first of the tendon of the stapedius, and then of these folds."

Dr. Blake thinks that in any case of chronic *non-suppurative* disease of the middle ear the operation of excision of the membrana tympani and evulsion of the malleus and incus is not necessary until other means are tried, as the stapes can be freed in some cases "by a division of the incudo-stapedial

articulation and tenotomy of the stapedius through an opening in the posterior portion of the membrana tympani sufficiently large to permit ready
access to the stapes and round window."

Hemorrhage into the Labyrinth, in Consequence of Ordinary Anæmia.

The same observer records also a case of the above-named character (*Ibid.*).
This case was examined only during life. A young woman, twenty years old;
four years previously had suffered from anæmia, with hemorrhages into the
stomach, intestinal canal, and retina. At the same time the hearing, previously perfect, became affected without any known cause, and also there
ensued tinnitus aurium and vertigo. The anæmia gradually disappeared,
the eyesight was restored, and the hearing became better, but not perfect.
The vertigo and tinnitus aurium also ceased. Examination lately by Dr.
Habermann revealed nothing abnormal in the membrana tympani nor in the
naso-pharynx. It was concluded that at the time of the hemorrhages into
the stomach, intestinal canal, and retina, there also occurred a hemorrhage
into the labyrinth.

DERMATOLOGY.

UNDER THE CHARGE OF

LOUIS A. DUHRING, M.D.,
PROFESSOR OF DERMATOLOGY IN THE UNIVERSITY OF PENNSYLVANIA;

AND

HENRY W. STELWAGON, M.D.,
CLINICAL LECTURER ON DERMATOLOGY IN THE JEFFERSON AND WOMAN'S MEDICAL COLLEGES.

Treatment of Anthrax by Carbolic Acid.

Poteenko (*The Practitioner*, 1890), praises the treatment of this disease by
the parenchymatous injections of a ten per cent. solution of carbolic acid.
Four severe cases were successfully treated, three or four Pravaz syringefuls
of the solution being injected, once daily, into the swelling and surrounding
tissues. The parts were kept covered with a dressing soaked in a five per
cent. solution of the same remedy. A few days sufficed for the relief of the
fever and other symptoms of systemic infection.

Aristol and its Uses.

Egasse (*Bull. gén. de Thérap.*, 1890) thinks that its value in lupus has been
overestimated. Neisser claims that it is not antiseptic. Observers are generally agreed that as an application to wounds it may well replace iodoform.
It is especially useful in simple and varicose ulcers. In psoriasis its action

is said to be as certain as chrysarobin, than which it acts slower and produces no irritation, and not much staining of the skin or clothing. It may be employed as a ten per cent. flexible collodion or ointment.

TRAUMATIC HERPES ZOSTER.

JANIN (*Brit. Med. Journ.,* vol. ii. p. 527, 1890) reports a case of this disease in a healthy boy aged fourteen years, which originated in a painful prick of a thorn in the shoulder. The puncture healed, but the site remained painful, the pain gradually spreading over the whole side of the back and chest. Eight days after the accident an exceedingly painful attack of herpes zoster appeared, occupying the third, fourth, and fifth intercostal spaces, and extending from the vertebral column to the sternum.

THIOL IN SKIN DISEASES, ESPECIALLY DERMATITIS HERPETIFORMIS.

SCHWIMMER (*Wiener klin. Wochenschr.*, 18, 1890) recommends thiol in the treatment of erythema, dermatitis herpetiformis, herpes zoster, acne rosacea, acne, papular and moist eczema, and burns; used generally in an aqueous solution 1 to 3. It proved especially useful in a case of dermatitis herpetiformis which had resisted other remedies. In erythema multiforme the remedy in powder form seemed preferable. The liquid form was best adapted to papular eczema. It is said that there is no unpleasant odor.

TREATMENT OF URTICARIA BY IODIDE OF POTASSIUM.

STERN (*La Semaine Médicale*, 1890) has treated five cases successfully, four of them being more or less chronic and rebellious to all previous treatment. None of the patients were either syphilitic or asthmatic. In one case, of four months' duration, the itching disappeared on the second day of treatment, and the cure was completed after two and a half drachms of the remedy had been taken. In two cases (one acute, the other chronic) the itching was at first increased, but a successful result was obtained in each case after the administration of seventy-five grains of the drug.

DERMATITIS AS AN EXCRETIONARY SYMPTOM.

WALSH (*Medical Press and Circular*, 1890) considers this subject and endeavors to show that excretory irritation is a not uncommon factor in inflammations of the skin. The conclusions arrived at are that—(1) Dermatitis may be set up in a certain number of cases by the excretion of irritant products from the system. (2) The irritant may be chemical or due to microorganisms. (3) That many of the inflammations of the hypo- as well as of the epiblastic tissues are simply expressions of excretory irritation. (4) That the severity of the inflammation and its result is in proportion to the specific action of the irritant on excretory epithelium. (5) That excretory parallels may be drawn between drugs and specific disease poisons, both as regards their harmfulness to epithelium and their channels of elimination. (6) Excretion not only affords a key to a certain number of skin inflammations, but also accounts for the success of many well-established methods of treatment which aim at changing the channels of elimination.

———

SCARIFICATION IN KELOID AND HYPERTROPHIC CICATRIX.

VIDAL (*Annales de Derm. et de Syph.*, No. 3, 1890) states that not only the keloid, but also the cicatrices made by the scarifications for the cure of the keloid disappear. The treatment of large tumors lasts for several months, while for recent growths six or seven operations may suffice. The scarifications must be continued until the cicatrix is supple and thin, and until all signs of induration have disappeared, otherwise the growth will re-form. The scarifications should be made at a distance of two millimetres, be cross-hatched at a right angle or obliquely, square or lozenge-shaped, and should penetrate through the depth of the keloid and not extend more than two or three millimetres beyond the margin of the growth. Local anæsthesia, produced by the application of liquefied chloride of methyl, is employed, the part being painted until whitened by freezing. As soon as the natural color inclines to reappear, a second, or even a third application should be made. By these successive applications the anæsthesia penetrates more deeply, and the scarifications cause only a very moderate degree of pain. The loss of blood is not much, being controlled by absorbent cotton. On the first day this is steeped in a solution of boric acid, and the next day the growth is dressed with a piece of *emplastrum de vigo*, and renewed twice daily. The action of the mercurial has been found favorable by the author.

———

THE TREATMENT OF RODENT ULCER WITH RESORCIN PLASTER-MULL.

BOECK records briefly (*Monatshefte für praktische Dermatologie*, Bd. xii., No. 4) two cases of rodent ulcer treated successfully with the plaster-mull of resorcin (Unna's formula). In the one case, a man aged seventy-two years, the lesion consisted of an ulceration of one and a half inches in diameter, situated on the cheek; in the other case, a patient aged eighty-two years, the ulcer was seated upon the temporal region. The plaster was kept constantly applied, a fresh application being made daily. Favorable change was to be noted from day to day, the time required for a satisfactory result varying from two to several weeks.

———

PEDICULOSIS PUBIS.

In a clinical lecture (*L' Union Médicale*, February 26, 1891) on pediculosis pubis, FOURNIER very properly decries the treatment of this condition with blue ointment, inasmuch as this method is not only dirty and otherwise offensive, but it commonly gives rise to the so-called eczema mercuriale, and may also, through absorption, bring about moderate or severe ptyalism. Much preferable and equally efficacious are—an ointment of calomel, 1 to 20; baths of corrosive sublimate; a lotion consisting of 400 parts of water, 100 parts of alcohol, and 1 part of corrosive sublimate; and one consisting of 300 parts of vinegar and 1 part of corrosive sublimate, to be applied diluted with one or two parts of water. As to the removal of the ova, the same method is to be practised as in pediculosis capitis—that is, with washings of warm vinegar, slightly diluted, and subsequent combings.

LEPRA AT HANOI (TONQUIN).

BOINET (*Revue de Médecine, Medical Chronicle*, 1890) finds that the disease exists along the watercourses, and that mud is a probable carrier of infection to the naked feet of the poor, the earth being impregnated by the sputa, crusts, and discharges from the lepers. The soil of the cemetery of Hanoi was found to be highly charged with the bacilli, the mode of burial being extremely careless. Native physicians scarcely acknowledge heredity. In the eighty cases examined, absence of heredity was found in sixty-one. The chiefs of the villages, forty years resident, deny having seen any case directly transmitted; nor are they themselves afflicted. Healthy young girls marry lepers and fail to contract the disease. A case is given in which grandfather and grandmother are lepers, while the father and five children, who have constantly lived in the community, have escaped. The eighty cases establish the *possibility* of direct contagion in fifty-one. Children of lepers removed soon after birth to an unaffected district remain free from the disease, while their brothers and sisters living in the leper community contract it. Such children, returning in adult life to the community from which they sprang, presently develop symptoms. The theory of the infection by means of the mosquito is regarded as being by no means impossible. The bacillus can find entrance into the mosquito, and has been found in human blood.

DISEASES OF THE LARYNX AND CONTIGUOUS STRUCTURES.

UNDER THE CHARGE OF

J. SOLIS-COHEN, M.D.,
OF PHILADELPHIA.

CARCINOMA OF THE LARYNX.

The clinical history of a carcinoma of the larynx is well exemplified in the record of a case under the care of DR. MAX SCHAEFFER, of Bremen (*Deut. med. Woch.*, No. 28, 1890). A man, fifty years of age, several of whose immediate relatives had perished with carcinoma, had suffered with psoriasis for twenty-eight years, with laryngo-tracheal catarrh for twenty-five years, and with hoarseness and soreness in the left half of the larynx for ten years. At the end of these periods, June 3, 1885, he was still well nourished and in good general health. His larynx showed slight infiltration and paresis of the left vocal band, with infiltration of both ventricular bands and of the left aryepiglottic fold. His respiration was somewhat weaker on the left side than on the right.

Under topical treatment these conditions subsided almost entirely during the course of the year. In October, 1885, a corneous granulation was noted for a while in the anterior third of the left vocal band, but it soon disappeared. February 2, 1886, only infiltration of the left ventricular band and paresis of the left abductor muscle were to be noted. November 13th, the left vocal band was so much hidden as to appear only as a projection the thickness of a catgut ligature. Eight months later, July 13, 1887, the voice was completely hoarse. There was a smooth infiltration of the left ventricular band fully over-covering the vocal band. At this time the diagnosis of sarcoma was made. December 13th, the infiltration was greater, and covered the orifice of the ventricle as well as the vocal cord; the left ary-epiglottic fold was somewhat infiltrated and looked œdematous. A month or so later, June 29, 1888, the infiltration had extended forward and had crossed the anterior commissure of the glottis to the opposite side, and the left side of the epiglottis appeared somewhat thickened and turned toward the right. The movements of the left half of the larynx were somewhat more sluggish than those of the right side. The patient complained of a sense of tension in the entire throat, and of difficulty in deglutition. Unilateral exsection of the larynx was now advised but refused. In September the vocal band had become visible and was exulcerated anteriorly and posteriorly, and a uvula-like tumor had become developed at the base of the epiglottis toward the right side. In October there was some bloody expectoration; some fœtor from the mouth; glutition of food was off-and-on painful; and the tumor at the anterior commissure had enlarged. The left arytenoid region seemed somewhat excoriated through the pressure of the tumor. The pus seemed to escape from an abscess cavity beneath the left vocal cord. Pressure over the left thyroid cartilage elicited lancinating pains extending toward the ear.

On November 8th, after performing a preliminary tracheotomy, and occluding the trachea, Dr. Hahn, of Berlin, split the larynx and found the region of the ventricular and vocal band of the left side transformed into a whitish-gray tumor composed of a smaller portion anteriorly in the median line and coalescent with a larger mass in the centre of the left side. The growth was not eroded and appeared to be fully circumscribed. It was removed by incision into the surrounding healthy tissue one-half to one centimetre from its borders, and the lower portion of the thyroid cartilage was also excised after separation of the external soft tissues with a raspirator. The wound of incision and the cavity of the larynx were firmly tamponed with iodoformed gauze which was secured with sutures through the integuments.

The patient did well for about a year. Then recurrence took place, and fifteen months after the excision, the new growth presented much the appearance of the first one at the period of the operation, and was rather more extensive.

June 6, 1890, a low tracheotomy became necessary; and the patient at last report was wearing a large-sized canula with comfort, with great improvement in respiration and with improvement in speech, but deglutition was very little bettered, inasmuch as the growth had extended into the left glosso-epiglottic fold.

The chief point of interest in this case is the slow development of the carcinoma, which for a long time obscured the diagnosis.

———

FRACTURES OF THE LARYNX AND TRACHEA.

At the time the compiler prepared the article on this subject for the *International Encyclopædia of Surgery*, but two cases of recovery after fracture of the cricoid cartilage appeared to be on record; the cases of Treulich and of Masucci. Two additional instances have recently been recorded. One occurred under the observation of DR. ALFRED SOKOLOWSKI, of Warsaw, which is reported (*Berl. klin. Woch.*, 1890) with many interesting details, especially in reference to its laryngoscopic phases.

A country girl, twenty years of age, wearing an apron over her shoulder and tied in a knot around her throat, after the fashion of the country, got the apron caught in the driving-wheel of a hay-cutter. Pain in the laryngeal region and dyspnœa were immediate, and were soon followed by severe cough, which continued for several hours, and was attended with expectoration in which was a good deal of blood. On the following day Dr. Sokolowski and his colleague Bukowski found her with cyanotic and œdematous visage, severe dyspnœa with respiration interrupted by severe stridulous cough, hoarse voice, and speaking with difficulty in a barely recognizable whisper. Considerable purulent sputum was expectorated with the cough. The entire neck was greatly swollen, and subcutaneous crepitation was felt in every portion on palpation. A deep vertical depression was felt in the left thyroid cartilage, pressure upon which produced pain and decided sensations of crepitus. Laryngoscopic inspection revealed a moderately swollen and congested epiglottis, beneath which two thick reddened projections were seen corresponding to the upper borders of the thyroid cartilage and occluding the interior of the larynx. Tracheotomy was at once performed by Bukowski. A perforation into the interior of the larynx was found occupying the lower angle of the thyroid cartilage, and due to comminuted fracture of the thyroid cartilage and of the anterior portion of the cricoid cartilage. This opening needed but slight enlargement downward to permit a large canula to be readily inserted through it. Two small fragments of cartilage became detached during the operation. Although recovery ensued, the patient has been unable to dispense with the canula. On performing laryngo-fissure to determine the cause of stricture, it was found that the entire cricoid cartilage had disappeared, and that what appeared in the laryngoscopic image to be the posterior wall of the larynx was in reality the anterior wall of the lower portion of the pharynx.

DR. C. M. DESVERNINE-GALDOS, of Havana (*Rev. de Ciencias Médicas* and *Annales des Mal. de l'Or., du Lar.*, etc., 1880), reports a case of laryngotracheal fracture, survived for several years, in which the vocal bands became united almost their entire length, only a space of two centimetres being preserved anteriorly, and in which the ventricular bands vicariously acquired the function of phonatory bands. The accident was produced by a fall from a trapeze upon a stove, an angle of which was struck directly by the chin and the larynx successively. Some bloody sputa were immediately expectorated, but dyspnœa did not take place for a number of days. There was no emphysema and no dysphagia. The larynx was flattened and deviated to the left side. Pressure over the thyroid cartilage provoked pain on the right side. Laryngoscopy revealed hyperæmia of the epiglottis, arytenoepiglottic folds, and the entire superior portion of the larynx, with infiltration more marked on the right side, and infiltration of the vocal bands and the arytenoid region. Tracheotomy was performed. The deep fascia had barely been incised when air escaped, denoting the existence of a fracture. The trachea was found flattened, with lateral fracture of three or four of the upper rings. The moment the canula was introduced sudden emphysema of the neck and face ensued, which gradually extended to the arms and trunk, in consequence of the frequent expulsion of the canula, which was too short. A special canula was introduced the day following, and the emphysema disappeared completely the eighth day.

Dr. Desvernine saw the patient for the first time late in 1887, when he was suffering with advanced pulmonary tuberculosis. The canula had been dispensed with for three or four years, and he breathed through a permanent infundibular fistule barely five millimetres in its exterior diameter. He spoke with effort in a bass monotone extremely limited in modulation.

The entire peri-laryngeal and laryngeal regions were normal, except that the vocal bands were completely in adhesion save for a minute orifice at their thyroidal extremities. The free borders of the ventricular bands formed an ellipse, the borders of which became approximated in phonation by a movement of elevation upon an accentuated convex plane. This phonatory function of the vocal bands had been observed at intervals during the long period of seventeen years. Operative interference to separate the vocal bands was declined. The patient died in 1888.

The autopsy disclosed that there had been a fracture of the thyroid and cricoid cartilages and of the upper four rings of the trachea; the solution of continuity of the cartilages having been complete. This explained the inability of retaining the short canula at the tracheotomy, the incision of which, parallel to the line of fracture, had partially liberated a band of elastic tracheal tissue three millimetres in length, which acted as a lever to drive the canula outward.

The ventricular bands had undergone development to double their ordinary thickness, their muscular fibres, as well as those of the aryepiglottic folds, being the seat of a most accentuated hypernutrition. The cricoarytenoid articulations were solidly ankylosed. The muscular fibres concerned in abduction and adduction of the vocal bands, as well as those concerned in their transverse and longitudinal tension, were in an evident state of atrophic regression, without presenting any characteristics of neurogenetic atrophy.

SPASMODIC TIC OF THE SOFT PALATE.

At a recent meeting of the Société Médicale des Hôpitaux (*Le Mercredi Médical*, 1890) M. DIEULAFOY presented a subordinate officer, forty-two years of age, and in perfect health, who had for two years an extremely marked spasmodic tic of the soft palate almost isochronous with the beats of the pulse. The only complaint was that of a certain amount of constraint produced by the spasm.

OBSTETRICS.

UNDER THE CHARGE OF

EDWARD P. DAVIS, A.M., M.D.,

PROFESSOR OF OBSTETRICS AND DISEASES OF CHILDREN IN THE PHILADELPHIA POLYCLINIC;
CLINICAL LECTURER ON OBSTETRICS IN THE JEFFERSON MEDICAL COLLEGE ;
VISITING OBSTETRICIAN TO THE PHILADELPHIA HOSPITAL, ETC.

An Epidemic of Puerperal Fever.

This unusual occurrence in a well-conducted clinic forms the subject of an interesting narration by DÖDERLEIN, of Leipzig (*Archiv für Gynäkologie*, Band xl. Heft 1), whose contributions on the bacteriology of sepsis are familiar. Three cases of lymphatic infection by the staphylococcus pyogenes aureus and streptococcus pyogenes occurred, the focus of infection being suppuration beneath an ill-fitting glass eye in a patient's orbit. In some manner the midwife who examined her infected her genital tract and that of two others, one of whom died. By control experiments upon animals it was observed that the union of the two microörganisms produced an especially virulent infection. From the standpoint of treatment the intra-uterine douche is of value as soon as high fever announces the infection; if delayed, the microorganisms are beyond the reach of the antiseptic and the douche is harmful. It is given by Döderlein by inserting a Cusco's speculum, washing out the vagina with sterile water and inserting a glass douche-tube into the uterus, through which sterile water is allowed to run until it is seen that the flow is uninterrupted. A 2 per cent. creolin solution is then used to thoroughly douche the uterus. For the treatment of puerperal peritonitis, he advises absolute rest, ice to the abdomen, antipyretics, and opium. He believes that internal examination for diagnosis should be as infrequent as possible.

Rapidly Fatal Puerperal Infection.

As illustrating the rapidity of puerperal sepsis caused by infection with streptococci, FRITSCH (*Deutsche med. Wochenschrift*, No. 16, 1891) describes the case of a patient on whom total extirpation of the uterus was performed during an epidemic of puerperal sepsis in the wards of the hospital. Death followed the infection in thirty-seven hours, the post-mortem revealing disseminated sepsis, with swarms of streptococci.

The Comparative Results of Hospital and Private Obstetric Practice.

At the recent meeting of the German Gynecological Society DORHN (*Centralblatt für Gynäkologie*, No. 22, 1891) gave the results of the comparison of statistics of puerperal mortality in German hospital and private practice. Although more complicated labors occur in hospitals than in private practice, yet septic infection is less frequent and mortality from preventable causes is less; this is due not only to antisepsis but also to the fact that hospital labors are conducted with less interference and with a better understanding of the phenomena of labor.

GONORRHŒAL INFECTION IN THE MOUTHS OF THE NEWBORN.

DOHRN (*Ibid.*) has observed five cases where gonorrhœa in the mother has been conveyed to the infant's mouth. Ulceration and the deposit of membrane followed, in which gonococci were readily found.

PRACTICAL RESULTS OF THE EXAMINATION OF MOTHER'S MILK.

In the *Archiv für Kinderheilkunde*, Band xiii. Heft 1, 2, MONTI writes at length upon the practical results of the examination of the milk of the nursing woman. He has found that a specimen of mother's milk in which both specific gravity and percentage of fat are high (1030 to 1035 sp. gr. and 3 to 5 per cent.), and which shows little variation during lactation, is suitable to nourish a healthy infant. It should be observed that both these factors must be present, as excess or deficiency of fat may result from pathological processes; and on the other hand, increased specific gravity, with diminished fat contents, renders milk unfit for nourishment. Regarding the microscopic examination of the milk corpuscle, Monti observed such great and constant variations that he regards it of little moment as a means of diagnosis. Many of the factors commonly supposed to affect the quality of milk, such as age, number of pregnancies, and length of lactation, he found without influence. Menstruation rarely affects the milk of a robust woman; prolonged flooding and debilitating causes lessen the size of the milk corpuscles.

COMPLETE PROLAPSE OF THE PREGNANT UTERUS.

A case of complete prolapse of the pregnant uterus at six months is reported by BERNE (*Lyon Médical*, Nos. 14 and 15, 1891). The patient was pregnant for the fourth time, and had suffered for several weeks from the presence of the prolapsed uterus between her thighs. Difficult micturition and leucorrhœa had resulted. Replacement was easily effected and maintained by a tampon; pregnancy continued to a successful termination.

[We recently had occasion to note the remarkable tolerance exhibited by the pregnant uterus in a case of total prolapse at the fourth month in a working woman, who sought treatment at an out-patient clinic. Reduction was easily effected and a fairly good position maintained by a tampon, the mass of which was carded jute covered by cotton, the whole smeared with a lanolin-iodoform paste.—ED.]

SOXHLET'S EXPERIENCE WITH STERILIZED MILK, WITH IMPROVEMENTS IN HIS METHOD OF STERILIZING.

In the *Münchener medicinische Wochenschrift*, Nos. 19 and 20, 1891, SOXHLET, whose name is so closely allied with the sterilization of milk, gives his conclusions regarding its value, and suggests an improvement in the manner of sterilization. Milk is placed in bottles, the whole in a tightly covered pail containing water. Instead of corks, he closes each bottle by drawing over its mouth a piece of sheet rubber, which is brought over the edge and secured by a rubber band which passes around the neck. The elasticity of the rubber allows air and steam to escape from the milk, while as the milk cools atmospheric pressure forces the rubber inward, closing the bottle. Milk is sterilized at boiling-point of the water in the pail for forty-five minutes. His experience leads Soxhlet to consider sterilized milk of great value, but not successful in all cases. Different sorts of milk can be sterilized with different degrees of success. The best milk is that of the ordinary meadow-fed cow; dry feeding (hay and grain) is not so good. The objections to sterilized milk lie in chemical changes affecting the emulsification of its fats, thus interfering with its digestibility. Good milk, when sterilized and kept closed, will keep several months.

[In common with American observers, Soxhlet recognizes the danger of contamination of milk by stable filth and bacteria from hay. Sterilized milk is far from being a perfect food, the gist of infant-feeding lying in careful study of each case, scrupulous cleanliness and regularity, the endeavor being to form a healthful appetite and gratify it.—ED.]

An Unusual Complication of Version.

In the *British Medical Journal*, No. 1589, 1891, HELME describes an arm presentation in a primipara where the membranes had ruptured and uterine retraction had taken place. Version was unsuccessful until it was observed that the contraction-ring resisted the movements of the fœtal shoulder. The prolapsed arm was then pulled down and the whole fœtus was pushed up into the uterine cavity, when the version was readily accomplished. In an occipital presentation or an ordinary shoulder presentation, the fœtal body forms the segment of a circle which offers no point of lodgment at the contraction ring.

The Treatment of Suppuration during Puerperal Sepsis.

The surgical treatment of puerperal sepsis complicated by suppuration is illustrated by a case reported by MOORE, of Victoria (*Australian Medical Journal*, 1891, p. 179). The patient was suffering from severe septic infection with peritonitis, the left side of the abdomen being especially dull on percussion and prominent. On opening the abdomen six pints of foul pus was evacuated; the uterus was near the umbilicus, the right upper portion of the abdomen being shut off from the abscess by adhesions. An opening was made posteriorly in the lumbar region and a drainage-tube was passed, and also one in front, at the lower end of the abdominal wound. Irrigation with boric acid solution was used. The patient made a slow recovery complicated by temporary retention of pus, on one occasion terminated by purulent expectoration.

At the recent meeting of the German Gynecological Society FRITSCH advised the following method of treatment for recent pelvic exudates of puerperal origin. Using a speculum, the operator locates the exudate and with tenaculum forceps draws the uterus downward and to the opposite side. An incision is then made into the most protruding portion of the exudate, a stream of sterilized water being directed upon the incision so soon as pus

comes. The opening is enlarged by the finger, the abscess emptied and irrigated, and the edges of the sac are stitched to the wall of the vagina. If
needed, iodoform-gauze tampons are used. The best after-treatment is frequent irrigation; drainage-tubes should be avoided. If difficulty is experienced in determining the point of incision an exploring needle may be used.
—*Centralblatt für Gynäkologie*, No. 23, 1891.

The Pathology and Treatment of Eclampsia.

Koffer and Kundrat report (*Wiener klinische Wochenschrift*, No. 20,
1891) the case of a young, strong primipara delivered spontaneously who was
attacked by eclamptic seizures eighteen hours after delivery. Death occurred
twelve hours later in marked cyanosis. At the autopsy Kundrat found hemorrhagic hepatitis, eclampsia having been caused by ptomaine poisoning of
hepatic origin.

[A similar case was reported by Paultauf and Kundrat in 1888.—Ed.]

In 52,328 births, Löhlein (*Centralblatt für Gynäkologie*, No. 23, 1891)
found 325 cases of eclampsia; average mortality 20 per cent. In discussing
methods of treatment, Cæsarean section is indicated when dilatation is not
sufficiently advanced to permit delivery, when the child lives and is vigorous, while other treatment fails to subdue convulsions, icterus supervenes,
and respiration and heart action are threatened. Medically, he relies on
heavy doses of morphine.

The Influence of Pregnancy upon Respiratory Metabolism.

Oddi and Vicarelli (*Lo Sperimentale*, Fascicolo No. 2, 1891), from an
interesting series of carefully tabulated experiments, conclude that during
pregnancy there is an increased consumption of hydrocarbons, derived from
the waste of nitrogenous material resulting from fœtal nutrition and growth.
This is observed in the study of the respired air during pregnancy with comparison of weight.

Tumors of the Placenta.

Alin (*Nordiskt medicinskt Archiv*, Häft 1, 2, 1891) describes three placental tumors observed in the obstetrical clinic at Stockholm. The cases in
which the tumors occurred were in other respects normal pregnancies and
labors. Alin finds that such tumors have nothing to do with the uterus or
membranes. Most of them are fibro-myxomata, rich in vessels, resembling
angiomata. They exercise no influence in most cases upon pregnancy or
labor.

Ectopic Gestation.

An ovarian pregnancy is reported by Eberhart (*Centralblatt für Gynäkologie*, No. 24, 1891) in the person of a multipara three months pregnant,
with symptoms of suppuration in the abdomen. The uterus was slightly
enlarged, a tumor as large as a hen's egg upon the left of the uterus. When
the tube and ovary upon that side were removed by laparotomy the tube was
found occluded, and an ovarian abscess was present. The microscope revealed
decidual cells in the wall of the abscess.

GYNECOLOGY.

UNDER THE CHARGE OF

HENRY C. COE, M.D., M.R.C.S.,
OF NEW YORK.

THE TREATMENT OF PELVIC SUPPURATION BY VAGINAL HYSTERECTOMY.

POZZI (reprint from *Gazette hebd. de Médecine et de Chirurgie*, 1891) opposes Péan's radical procedure, as recently recommended by Segond, who thinks that vaginal hysterectomy is preferable to abdominal section in cases of disease of the adnexa. The arguments advanced in favor of the former are the lesser danger attending it, its greater efficacy, and the absence of any external cicatrix. Pozzi does not deny that cases of pelvic suppuration may be cured according to Péan's method, but he does not believe that adhesions can be broken up and foci of pus evacuated as well as when the abdomen is opened. While it must be admitted that removal of the adnexa sometimes fails to cause atrophy of the uterus, as shown by the persistence of hemorrhage, the latter symptom can usually be removed by the curette, without the necessity of total extirpation.

The greater mortality of vaginal hysterectomy as compared with abdominal section, is shown by the published statistics of the two operations. In the former operation there is no opportunity to correct errors in diagnosis by an explorative incision, hence it is not a procedure to be generally recommended.

[It seems incredible to the English reader that the learned author, whom we now recognize as the representative of French gynecological surgery, should be compelled to bring forward so many arguments against a method which reflects little credit upon the humanity of the profession. No man in this country, however great his reputation, could report a case of total extirpation of the uterus for pyosalpinx without evoking indignant protests. In spite of statistics, we can only regard this heroic treatment as a distinct retrogression on the part of our French *confrères*, more to be regretted because of its distinguished adherents.—ED.]

VENTRO-FIXATION OF THE UTERUS WITHOUT OPENING THE PERITONEAL CAVITY.

CRESPI (*Gaz. degli Ospitali*, 1890, Nos. 20 and 22) has operated four times successfully by the following method : The patient is placed in the lithotomy posture with the hips elevated. A median abdominal incision is made, exposing the peritoneum. The uterus is then anteverted on a sound and is held in contact with the anterior abdominal wall, while several sutures are passed through the edges of the wound and into the muscular substance of the fundus.

WILLIAMS (*American Journal of Obstetrics*, 1890, No. 7) reports seven cases in which he adopted Kelly's suggestion of anteverting the uterus and passing two sutures of silkworm-gut through the abdominal wall and into the fundus by means of a large curved needle. . The sutures were secured externally by means of a silver plate, and were left *in situ* for three weeks. The displacement soon recurred in every instance.

KRUG (*N. Y. Medical Record*, 1891, No. 1) describes an ingenious operation which he calls "transperitoneal hysterorrhaphy," and has performed successfully several times. The patient being in Trendelenburg's posture, a sound is passed into the uterus and a catheter into the bladder. A median incision, not over two inches in length, is made just above the symphysis and the peritoneum is exposed. A Peaslee needle with a cutting point is then introduced at the left border of the wound, and with its edge the serous covering over the fundus uteri is scraped so as to leave a raw surface. The needle is then withdrawn slightly, is passed into the muscular substance of the uterus beneath the raw surface, emerges at the right edge of the abdominal wall, is threaded with silkworm-gut and withdrawn. Two sutures are sufficient to at once close the wound and to firmly attach the uterus in a position of anteversion. The entire operation should not occupy ten minutes, and can be supplemented by a perineorrhaphy if desired. The sutures remain for from four to six weeks. The writer affirms that with the patient in Trendelenburg's posture the intestines gravitate toward the diaphragm, so that it is impossible for them to receive injury. The catheter in the bladder indicates accurately the position of that viscus.

THE MECHANICAL CAUSES OF TORSION OF THE PEDICLE IN OVARIAN CYSTS.

CARIO (*Centralblatt für Gynäkologie*, 1891, No. 18) believes that the torsion may begin in consequence of a sudden muscular effort, as in lifting a weight during deep inspiration. The intestines are forced downward behind the tumor, and if they impinge on one side of it more than on the other, a partial revolution of the cyst occurs toward the side on which is the least pressure. Usually the resistance of the pedicle causes it to untwist and resume its former position after the pressure is removed, but if it is turned beyond 180 degrees further, torsion readily occurs.

THE ETIOLOGY OF VESICO-VAGINAL FISTULA.

WINTERHALTER (*Centralblatt für Gynäkologie*, 1891, No. 18) has collected 226 cases of vesico-vaginal fistula following labor, an analysis of which yields the following facts: 18.1 per cent. occurred in spontaneous, 81.8 per cent. instrumental deliveries. In 68.1 per cent. the forceps were employed, showing that their use is not unattended by danger. In the majority of the cases the pelvis was contracted. The writer advises craniotomy in preference to the forceps in cases in which impaction of the head is accompanied with œdema of the anterior lip of the cervix and of the external genitals, since under these circumstances 88.7 per cent. of the children are born dead. In a few cases the fistulæ were caused by pessaries.

GONOCOCCI IN AN OVARIAN ABSCESS.

ZWEIFEL (*Centralblatt für Gynäkologie*, 1891, No. 20) calls attention to the frequent coexistence of ovarian abscess and gonorrhœal pyosalpinx, though the fact of a common origin has never been proved. He has recently demonstrated beyond doubt the presence of gonococci in the contents of a Graafian vesicle, situated in the centre of a suppurating ovary. This important fact shows that the cocci possess a greater migratory power than has been supposed, that they are not confined to mucous surfaces, but under certain unknown conditions may be carried through the blood- and lymph. vessels to distant parts. This agrees with Bumm's experience in finding the cocci in peri-urethral abscesses and in the knee-joint in cases of gonorrhœal rheumatism.

FORCIPRESSURE IN ABDOMINAL SURGERY.

KOCKS (*Sammlung klin. Vorträge*, 1891, No. 21) claims the following advantages for the forceps: 1. If proper instruments are used, there is no surer way of controlling hemorrhage from the broad ligaments than by forcipressure. 2. The operation is shortened, hence the patient has less shock and less danger of septic infection. 3. The technique is greatly simplified, which is always of advantage to the operator. 4. Parenchymatous oozing is eliminated, and with it the danger of subsequent septic infection through the bleeding surface. 5. Clamps are easily rendered aseptic, while perfect asepsis cannot so readily be assured with silk and animal ligatures. 6. As the forceps are removed at the end of twenty-four hours, the abdominal cavity then remains free from any foreign body, hence there is no danger of suppuration or persistent irritation from the presence of ligatures. 7. Thorough drainage is insured.

SALPINGO-OÖPHORECTOMY.

ZWEIFEL (*Archiv für Gynäkologie*, Bd. xxxix. Heft 3) reports 77 cases of salpingo-oöphorectomy with a single death, statistics as yet unsurpassed by any other operator. He notes several interesting clinical facts, viz. : The majority of the cases of pyosalpinx were clearly of gonorrhœal origin ; the accompanying localized peritonitis probably results from mixed infection rather than from pure specific poison. Many patients with pyosalpinx suffer from catarrh of the large intestine of a peculiarly obstinate character, which may be due to specific infection, although this has never been demonstrated bacteriologically. The different bacteria which may cause pyosalpinx are gonococci, streptococci, and tubercle bacilli. The occurrence of an evening rise of temperature in a well-marked case of pyosalpinx is an important diagnostic point in tuberculous salpingitis. Salpingostomy, or simple drainage of the tube without extirpation, should not be practised if pus is present.

As regards the ultimate effect of removal of the adnexa, the writer states that where the ovaries were entirely removed menstruation ceased ; when it persisted it was in cases in which, on account of adhesions, a portion of the stroma probably remained. The majority of the patients reported that there was no change in their sexual feelings ; a few complained that these were extinguished. The psychoses, so often described, were observed in only one instance.

CLOSURE OF CERVICO-VESICO-VAGINAL FISTULA FROM THE SIDE OF THE BLADDER.

BAUMM (*Archiv für Gynäkologie*, Bd. xxxix. Heft 3) reports an interesting case in which he followed Trendelenburg's suggestion to close complicated fistulæ by exposing and incising the bladder, as in epicystotomy, and suturing the edges of the fistula from within. The patient had had extensive sloughing after a tedious labor, as a result of which there was a large cervico-vesical fistula with extensive cicatrization involving the entire vaginal fornix, so that it was impossible to expect a successful result from a plastic operation. The patient was placed in Trendelenburg's posture. A median incision was made just above the symphysis, the pre-vesical space was exposed, and the bladder was opened by a transverse incision two inches and a half in extent, through which the interior of the viscus could be thoroughly inspected. The mouths of the ureters were surrounded by the cicatricial tissue at the edge of the fistula, but were located by passing a probe into them. The borders of the fistula were denuded, an assistant aiding by making pressure upon them *per vaginam*. Eight silk sutures (having a needle on each end) were passed down into the vagina, where they were drawn through by the left hand of the operator, and subsequently tied with the aid of a Simon's speculum. The upper wound in the bladder was closed with a double row of sutures, muscular and sero-serous, a T-shaped drainage-tube being inserted. After tamponing the pre-vesical space with iodoform gauze, the abdominal wound was closed. The patient had a tedious convalescence, and six weeks after the operation there remained a large fistula at the site of the abdominal wound which never closed. It was necessary to perform a slight secondary operation in order to completely close a small cervico-vesical fistula.

PUBLIC HEALTH.

UNDER THE CHARGE OF
EDWARD F. WILLOUGHBY, M.D.,
OF LONDON.

THE ACTION OF COMMON SALT ON PATHOGENIC ORGANISMS.

This question, which, apart from its more purely scientific aspect, has a very practical interest in its bearing on the extent to which the salting or "pickling" of pork and other provisions may be relied on for the destruction of the germs of disease, was taken up about a year ago by Dr. C. J. Freytag at the instance of Professor Förster. It is well known that salt serves to preserve meat—*i. e.*, to prevent its spontaneous putrefaction, by abstracting water from the tissues and coagulating the albumin, though solutions of 10 per cent. dissolve out a portion of the myosin, which, together with the potash, salt, and extractives, may be recovered from the brine. But the question to be decided was whether it would destroy the vitality of microbes, as it certainly does that of parasites higher in the scale of animal life—in fact, whether it could be looked on as a disinfectant as well as a preservative. The ancient Greeks, as Dr. Anagnostakis has reminded us, employed solutions of salt as lotions in the treatment of wounds, and A. Seibert has recommended it for the local treatment of diphtheria. But R. Koch and Baumgarten had been surprised at the little or comparatively no effect of several substances, of which salt was one, commonly supposed to exert a destructive action on low forms of life; and Mertens had been equally disappointed in his experiments on the cocci of pus. These casual researches had, however, been conducted without adequate precautions, and Dr. Freytag determined to carry out his investigation exhaustively, beginning with the pathogenic bacteria of diseases proper to domestic animals, but possibly communicable to man in the consumption of their flesh. He made use not only of pure cultures of the bacteria, but of the tissues of diseased animals—e. g., the tubercular nodules found in the bodies of cattle suffering from "Perlsucht." To imitate the conditions presented by the process of pickling, he used so much salt that a portion always remained undissolved; in gelatin cultures this had the effect of liquefying the medium, when the bacteria and the undissolved particles of salt sank to the bottom of the tube, but with those in agar the colonies were simply covered by the finely-powdered salt.

At regular intervals of time fresh sowings were made from the salted cultures, and animals, kept in clean and airy cages, were inoculated from each. He insists on the fact that for many years no case of natural tuberculosis had occurred among the guinea-pigs, and only a couple of cases, more than two years ago, among the rabbits kept in the laboratory for experimental purposes.

The results in each disease were as follows:

Anthrax. The spores, raised on sliced potatoes, were, as Koch had already shown, in no way affected by continuous exposure to the action of concentrated solution of salt for six months. Not so the vegetative forms, which were invariably killed after two hours' steeping of the organs containing them in a concentrated solution. Although even a saturated solution failed to kill the spores, the limits under which their germination and further development were possible were presented by solutions of 7 per cent. to 10 per cent. of salt in Löffler's bouillon.

Typhoid. Koch-Ebert's bacilli, obtained from the spleen of a man who had died from enteric fever, and grown on sliced potato and on Koch's gelatin, retained their vitality and power of development in fresh media after six months' exposure to a concentrated solution of salt.

Rothlauf, or "pig scarlatina." These bacilli, provided by Pasteur, remained unaffected after two months.

Cholera. Koch's comma-bacillus. The growth of these was luxuriant, liquefying the entire mass of the gelatin; and the salt, when added in excess, was deposited. Sowings made from these tubes after four, six, twelve, and twenty-four hours were all alike without result. Another series of experiments showed that eight hours' exposure to a saturated solution was invariably fatal to these bacilli, and that the highest concentration in which they could live was 7 per cent, but that 5 per cent. (not 2 per cent., as Uffelmann had asserted), was required to check their growth in any perceptible degree.

Erysipelas. No effect was produced on the cocci of this disease by an exposure to a saturated solution for two and a half months.

Staphylococci of pus resisted a like solution for five months.

Diphtheria. The Klebs-Löffler bacillus in pure cultures made from a virulent and fatal case were unaffected after three weeks in a saturated solution.

Tubercle. Portions of the organs of a guinea-pig that had died of tubercular peritonitis, and the sputa of the same animal, were, after two or three weeks' exposure to a concentrated solution, inoculated into the abdomen of a healthy guinea-pig, which died of tuberculosis a month later. But lest this one might have been infected by the diffusion in the air of the room of the dried sputa of the other, Dr. Freytag made a fresh series of experiments precluding such an accidental source of fallacy, and found that gelatin cultures of the bacillus were not injuriously affected by the action of concentrated solutions for three months.

Nodules of "Perlsucht," after eighteen days' immersion in brine, were used for the inoculation of rabbits with invariable success; in fact, three months' steeping, a far longer period than is ever employed in pickling meat for human food, in no way lessened the infective power of the bacilli.

Galtier's experiments, which gave a different result, were made with the expressed juices, not with the organs or tissues themselves.

In conclusion, Dr. Freytag observes that though it might be urged that, the bacilli of anthrax being killed and the toxines assumed to be dissolved out into the brine, such flesh, if free from spores, might be eaten with safety, it would be in practice impossible to ascertain or to guarantee the absence of the spores.

The question of tuberculosis is, however, of greater practical importance, on account of the frequency of the disease and the fact that much meat from animals suffering from it in different degrees finds its way into the market.

Since boiling alone suffices to kill the bacilli—*i. e.*, provided the interior of the meat be raised to that temperature—the previous pickling, as suggested by the authorities at Lyons, is superfluous, and, indeed, by inducing a false security, would be worse than useless.

These experiments possess a peculiar interest for a country where the pickling of meats constitutes an important industry.—FREYTAG, *Zeitschr. f. Hygiene*, 1890.

Note to Contributors.—All contributions intended for insertion in the Original Department of this Journal are only received *with the distinct understanding that they are contributed exclusively to this Journal.*

Contributions from the Continent of Europe and written in the French, German or Italian language, if on examination they are found desirable for this Journal, will be translated at its expense.

Liberal compensation is made for articles used. A limited number of extra copies in pamphlet form, if desired, will be furnished to authors in lieu of compensation, *provided the request for them be written on the manuscript.*

All communications should be addressed to

DR. EDWARD P. DAVIS,
250 South 21st Street, Philadelphia.

THE

AMERICAN JOURNAL

OF THE MEDICAL SCIENCES.

SEPTEMBER, 1891.

FIVE CASES OF CEREBRAL SURGERY. I. AND II. FOR EPI-
LEPSY FOLLOWING TRAUMA. III. FOR INSANITY FOL-
LOWING TRAUMA. IV. FOR CEREBRAL TUMOR.
V. FOR DEFECTIVE DEVELOPMENT.

BY W. W. KEEN, M.D.,

ONE OF THE SURGEONS TO THE ORTHOPÆDIC HOSPITAL AND INFIRMARY FOR NERVOUS DISEASES, AND
PROFESSOR OF THE PRINCIPLES OF SURGERY IN THE JEFFERSON MEDICAL COLLEGE, ETC.

IN this paper I report, with some observations, five cases of operations
involving the brain, which have been done in the last eighteen months.
These are all the cases operated on by myself in the Orthopædic Hospital, except that in addition to these, one case (microcephalus) has
already been reported[1] and a second (probable tumor) is not yet terminated, and hence I shall report it hereafter. For most of the careful
histories of these cases I am indebted to Dr. F. A. Packard.

I would suggest that in operations on the brain it is of great advantage
to have a stenographer present at the operation, and so many surgeons
now have their regular stenographers that this can often be done very
readily. This is of especial value during the stimulation of the brain
by the faradic battery, when the stenographer can instantly note and
describe the exact point on the brain which is stimulated and the precise
phenomena in face, neck, arm, leg, trunk, etc., that occur on such faradization. It is very difficult to write quickly enough all the details that
are observed at such a time, and they are either lost or become confused,
and, even if this does not follow, the operation will be seriously delayed.
The stenographer can take such dictation instantly, together with memo-

---

[1] THE AMERICAN JOURNAL OF THE MEDICAL SCIENCES, June, 1891.

randa of measurements, etc., and possibly make a sketch of the convolutions exposed, with an accuracy which is greatly to be desired. Especially is this true at present, when the functions of such parts of the brain
as are stimulated are as yet, in man at least, not so accurately determined
as is desirable. The most correct measurements possible and all the
observed phenomena are, therefore, of the greatest value, and should be
minutely described.

The first two cases were both of epilepsy following trauma.

CASE I. *Traumatic epilepsy; operation; implantation of decalcified bone;*
recovery with partial integrity of bone, and no subsequent attacks for eight
months.—C. J., colored, aged about thirty-nine years. Her history is
very indefinite, owing to her want of intelligence. She was sent to the
Infirmary on October 8, 1890, by Dr. Merritt, of Easton, Md. She is
married and has had eight children; four are dead—one with spasms,
one with diarrhœa, one with marasmus, one, cause unknown. Three of
the four living children are healthy. Family history otherwise negative and uncertain, except that one sister is weak-minded, and at times
has to be kept in confinement.

In childhood she was playing on a cellarway when a window-sill fell
from a high window and struck her on the left side of the head, and
she remained unconscious for some time. No operation was done at the
time of injury, although it was spoken of. Her first spasm occurred
not long after the injury. In the first eleven years that followed she
had but two attacks—six years after the injury and five years later.
Then they began to be more frequent, and this frequency has been
steadily increasing until now they are only a month or two apart, and
sometimes she has two in one day. The character of the convulsions
has always been precisely the same. They begin with flexing of the
fingers of the right hand on the palm, followed by forced and extreme
supination of the wrist. She then either lies down or falls down and
screams. She loses consciousness completely, and knows nothing till
she finds herself crying and the right arm moving in a spasmodic manner. She does not sleep after an attack, nor is there any paralysis of
motion or disturbance of speech. She always has a severe headache,
however, at the site of the former injury for a day or so. She does not
bite her tongue. Once or twice she has urinated during an attack; no
defecation.

Her general health was good until last winter, when she had influenza. Intelligence poor, but perhaps, excepting memory, no more so
than usual. Between the attacks she is free from headache unless the
site of the injury is struck. Hearing is good; smell and taste subjectively unimpaired. Has dyspepsia, sluggish bowels, no œdema, no cough.
Menstruation regular.

Dr. de Schweinitz reports on the eyes: "Perfectly normal, oval discs,
fundus of each eye healthy. Visual field for form normal. Color fields
not taken."

Status presens: A fairly well-nourished colored woman. Face symmetrical; no facial palsy. Answers questions quite well. Tongue protruded straight. Arms symmetrical; is right-handed. Measurements
of two arms practically identical. Dynamometer: R. 97.5; L. 118.

Knee-jerk on right side much exaggerated; on left, slightly so. Sole tap, R. marked, L. absent. Front tap, R. marked, L. obtained with difficulty. Achilles' tendon reflex marked on both sides. Plantar skin reflex absent on both sides. Gait natural. On standing with her eyes closed there is marked swaying, but she does not fall.

3.5 cm. (1⅜ inches) behind and 5 cm. (2 inches) above the external angular process, on the left side, is an abrupt bony elevation. Toward the median line, from and behind this, there is a marked depression of a roughly triangular shape, the apex pointing backward. The anterior border of this depression is much thickened and the superior border lies 4.5 cm. (1¾ inches) to the left of the middle line. The posterior extremity lies 1 cm. (⅜ inch) behind the left fissure of Rolando. The antero-posterior diameter of the depression is 5 cm. (2 inches), and its vertical measurement is 3.7 cm. (1.5 inches). The cranial index is 77.7 and the fissure of Rolando, therefore, runs at 70.3°.

On October 15th she had a convulsion, which is thus described: "She screamed several times for about thirty seconds, then fell to right side, and right hand became first convulsed, the fit involving first hands and face, and lastly the legs. Jerking of the head was most marked. The legs twitched slightly, then she crossed the left one over the right. There was no frothing. She seemed to be conscious and tried to speak, but could not utter more than one word. The duration of the fit was three minutes. She knew it was coming on, and grasped her right hand above the wrist. The pupils were equally dilated and responded to light just at the end of the attack."

Operation, October 29, 1890. The usual semilunar flap, with the convexity upward, was made, and the depression was exposed. The bleeding from the scalp was, as usual, controlled by hæmostatic forceps. The defect in the skull was found to be covered by a thin membrane, which allowed the pulsations of the brain to be plainly seen, and this membrane was slightly attached to the margin of the opening in the bone. The membrane was matted together with brain tissue and a little of the brain tissue was torn away in its careful removal. Two or three apparent cysts were opened in the removal of the membrane. During this part of the operation the face was drawn strongly to the left, the right eye being a trifle open. The muscles of the left side of the face moved at times, the angles of the mouth being drawn strongly upward, the grimace then slowly relaxing. The patient seemed not to be completely anæsthetized and was groaning. No movement of arm or leg on either side was detected.

At the posterior lower part in the opening of the skull the bone was apparently 1.5 cm. (⅝ inch) thick, thinning just in front of it to 3 mm. (⅛ inch) thick. It was found that a fragment of bone had been depressed and grown fast, and thus gave the impression of greatly thickened bone. The projecting fragment was removed by forceps.

The entire face continued to be drawn tightly upward during this manipulation, the mouth markedly so, while this was not so marked at the angle of the eye, nor was the brow markedly contracted. The brain at the bottom of the depression was of a dark-gray color, with a brownish tinge, evidently being disorganized brain tissue. The cerebral surface exposed was of concave shape, the depression at the deepest part measuring 1¼ cm. (½ inch). The edges of the opening in the skull were irregular as well as thickened, and were removed by the rongeur forceps till it measured 6.3 cm. (2.5 inches) antero-posteriörly by 3.8 cm. (1.5 inches). At the first bite of the rongeur forceps the face on the left side became markedly contracted, while on touching the dura the contraction became much more marked. The right eye was a little open at the same time. This sensitive point on the dura was 7.3 cm. (2⅞ inches) to the left of the middle line and the same distance back of the external angular process. When this point was faradized the left side of the face became contracted, the right thumb persistently twitched, and the respirations became longer. The same effects were produced by faradizing the bone in the neighborhood. On faradizing the brain cortex for a very brief time just below the upper margin in the middle of the opening there was marked adduction and abduction of the thumb followed by extension of the fingers of the right hand, with clonic convulsive movements (flexion and extension) of the whole right arm. These movements persisted for nearly a minute after the stoppage of the current, and resembled the epileptic attacks. The point touched on the brain was 5.8 cm. (2¼ inches) to the left of the middle line, and 7.3 cm. (2⅞ inches) from the external angular process.

With a knife a circular incision was then made in the brain substance, including the point which had been stimulated, without producing movement of any part. The diseased cortical matter and some underlying white matter were removed with a sharp spoon until apparently healthy white matter was exposed. No phenomena were observed during this removal, the left face even gradually relaxing during the manipulation. The pulse was now 78. At this time the right eye was directed upward and outward, the left in a parallel direction, but to a less extent. On pinching the scalp with the forceps the same drawing up of the face took place as was noted when the battery was applied on the dura.

The battery was now applied to the white matter lying beneath, which had been exposed by the removal of the gray matter, and as nearly as could be ascertained, exactly below the point which had produced the brachial monospasm. This caused flexion of the ring and little fingers with abduction of the hand and flexion of the elbow, the phenomena stopping immediately upon the removal of the electricity instead of continuing and developing into a typical attack, as they had done before. There was no movement of the right face during the electrical or other stimulation, but there was constant contraction of the left face.

After all bleeding had been controlled and a small rubber drainage-tube inserted, a piece of decalcified tibia from a bullock, perforated by several openings, was fitted accurately to the defect in the skull, with the exception of a notch for the exit of the drainage-tube. The decalcified bone-plate was stitched to the scalp with chromicized catgut, superficial horsehair drainage inserted, and the scalp sewed with interrupted chromicized catgut sutures. A gauze dressing with rubber dam was applied.

On the day following the operation flexion and extension of the right hand were entirely lost in both fingers and wrist. She could prevent the hand from falling in extension, but not in flexion; that is, the flexors were entirely paralyzed, the extensors only partly so. Flexion and extension at the elbow were slight but present. Movements of the shoulder also present, but paretic. Right leg unaffected. Left angle of the mouth elevated slightly. Movement present in all face muscles;

eyelids could be closed. In speaking, the left side of the mouth was drawn upward slightly more than the right.

On the second day there was no area of anæsthesia. If anything, a pin-prick caused more pain on the right than on the left hand. There was no difference in distinguishing the two points of an æsthesiometer, being on dorsum of hands 2.5 cm. (1 inch), dorsum of second joint of fingers 7 mm. (¼ inch), outer side of forearms 6.7 cm. (2⅝ inches), outer side of upper arms 5 cm. (2 inches).

On the fifth day the drainage-tube was removed, and on the seventh the horsehairs and the sutures were removed, the wound being entirely healed. On the eighth day she was out of bed. On the tenth pulsation was still evident over the old defect in the skull, the lower half of the flap feeling soft, the upper half being more firm. There was slight improvement in the movement of the right shoulder, but not in the elbow, wrist, or fingers. The stitches through the implanted bone were removed on the eighth day.

On the nineteenth day she moved the fingers for the first time, the index finger leading, with slight motion in the thumb and middle finger. There was slight extension at the wrist. She stated that while gaping a few days previous to this the fingers had become markedly flexed. On the twenty-third day she left the hospital and went home, moving the three radial fingers more freely, but the two ulnar ones not at all. Wrist barely movable, especially in flexion; elbow could be almost entirely flexed or extended, but slowly and with difficulty. The decalcified bone had become concave in its lower part over an area the size of the tip of the index finger, but it was apparently secure.

June 11, 1891 (eight months). There have been no attacks since the operation, and her general health and mental condition are far better than before. Dynamometer: R. 25, L. 50; but for practical purposes the right hand is far more useful than would be judged by this difference. Its movements are complete in range, but lack power, and she cannot yet cut her meat at table. It is, however, constantly bettering. The trephine opening is well closed with firm tissue, but in part at least it yields to firm pressure to such a degree as to make it doubtful whether this is bony or not. It, however, affords an excellent protection to the brain.

CASE II. *Epilepsy following a trauma; operation; implantation of sheep's bone; recovery, with subsequent necrosis of implanted bone, but only three attacks in nearly six months, each caused by the operations.*—G. H., aged twenty-three years, was sent to the Orthopædic Hospital November 13, 1890, by Dr. H. M. Schallenberger, of Rochester, Pa. His mother died of consumption, aged forty-two; his father of renal dropsy. One brother died of consumption, aged twenty-eight. Otherwise the family history is good. While teething he had an unknown number of convulsions, but no others prior to his accident. In 1874, at the age of seven years, he was kicked on the head by a horse, and remained unconscious for a few hours. Trephining was soon afterward begun, but his physician says that it was not completed, owing to shock. Three pieces of bone, however, were removed. At least one had penetrated the brain for an inch. His recovery was slow and he was delicate for a year or more. So far as he remembers, his first fit was in 1876, two years after the accident, and his attacks have always been of the same character throughout. The attacks eventually became more frequent, being about once a week. After fourteen years of age they became less frequent, only coming about once a month; this not being the result of medicine. For the last six years they have only occurred about once in three months, except that in March last, without any apparent reason, unless possibly due to his having sat over a hot fire, there were three attacks in two days. His last fit was about the middle of last September.

There is no exciting cause for them, unless possibly coming into a warm room with a close atmosphere, and once or twice excitement has caused them. He has only had one attack during the night. He has often been struck in the neighborhood of the scar, though not on it, without producing any fit. At the beginning of an attack he has a confused feeling in his head, not lasting long enough usually to give him time to sit down; once he had time to cry "Look out!" Twice he has run a short distance during the premonitory mental confusion. Loss of consciousness comes on quickly without any cry. He usually falls forward and frequently injures his face; he always bites his tongue. He does not know that any part of the body is first or chiefly affected. There is no urination or defecation during the attacks. After a sleep of about an hour, followed by a weak and drowsy feeling and slight headache for a couple of hours, he is able to work the rest of the day.

Status presens: General health is good, although he appears to be not well nourished. His skin is pale; appetite good; bowels regular. His memory, he thinks, is not so good as formerly. No pain anywhere. Eyesight is not very good, but no worse than it has always been. His hearing is good. Dr. de Schweinitz reports that he "has a high grade of astigmatism, probably mixed. Pupils and external ocular muscles normal; discs rather gray-red in color, with some contraction of right visual field. The contraction is concentric and of no localizing importance. Pupils equal and react well to light." There is no facial palsy. Tongue clean and protruded straight.

Dynamometer: R. 153, L. 123. He is right-handed. No increase of biceps, triceps, or wrist tendon reflexes on the left side; wrist tendon reflex on the right side increased; others normal. No increase of muscular irritability in arms. Knee-jerk greater than usual, but equal on both sides. Ankle-clonus absent on both sides. Achilles' tendon reflex equal on both sides. Æsthesiometer: On dorsum of hands, two points felt at one inch on both sides; on dorsum of feet, 1½ inches, on both feet.

His head is of a natural shape and symmetrical, excepting for the scar. In the right parietal region is a large stellate scar, approaching an anchor in shape, the arms of the anchor being below and forming a shallow crescent with the convexity downward. At the junction of the pole of the anchor and the anterior arm there is a depression of 3.9 cm. (1½ inches) in the long diameter (obliquely upward and forward) and 2 cm. (¾ inch) in short diameter (transversely). The depression is 1.4 cm. (½ inch) deep. The edges of the depressed area are well defined and rounded off, with no sharp points. There is no pulsation to be seen or felt. The floor of the depression is hard and resistant. There is slight tenderness on pressure over the scar.

The longest portion of the scar (obliquely) measures 5 cm. (2½ inches), the short arm 2.5 cm. (1 inch). The centre of the depressed area is 9.6 cm. (3¾ inches) from the middle line and the same distance back of the external angular process on the right side. The cranial index is 79. The anterior extremity of the depression just touches the line of the Rolandic fissure at a point 8.3 cm. (3¼ inches) from the median line.

Operation, November 21, 1890. A semicircular flap was reflected, exposing the defect in the skull. In loosening the flap from the margin of this defect considerable cerebro-spinal fluid escaped *per saltum* synchronously with the pulse. The loose tissues filling the opening seemed to be more or less cystic. At least two or three ounces of the fluid escaped. A small loose spicule of bone was engaged in the membrane or tissue filling the opening. This tissue was next dissected away. The edges of the opening were greatly thickened, so that the squamous portion of the temporal was almost a quarter of an inch thick. The diploë in the parietal border of the opening was so marked that the bite of the rongeur was perceptibly divided into two distinct stages, one for each table. The thickened bone around the opening was bitten away till the opening measured 5 cm. (2 inches) obliquely antero-posteriorly, and 2.8 cm. (1⅛ inches) in a transverse direction. No dura covered the brain at the site of the injury. The brain tissue was now exposed. A moderate amount had adhered to the tissue filling the opening and had been torn away with it. The remaining portion was normal as far as eye and touch could perceive, and none of it was removed. One small branch of the middle cerebral was ligated. The convolutions could not be recognized, as they were to a large extent fused together.

The right hemisphere failed to fill the cavity of the skull to such an extent that not only was the surface of the brain depressed opposite the opening, but a space existed between the right hemisphere and the dura at least one-third of an inch across, so that one could look under the edge of the bone two and a half inches, away up toward the falx.

At this point my assistant, Dr. W. J. Taylor, removed a piece of bone from the skull of a young sheep which had been brought to the hospital and killed at that moment. The piece selected about corresponded in curvature to the curvature of the patient's skull, and the edges of it were bitten away by the rongeur forceps so as to fit the opening accurately. From the time this piece was removed from the sheep's skull till it was inserted in the patient's it was kept in a bichloride solution, 1 to 2000, at 100° to 105° F., and most of the trimming of this bone was done while it was immersed in this warm solution. Dr. Taylor, of course, used the same antiseptic precautions in his operation on the sheep as I did on the patient.

Two points were bitten out of the piece antero-posteriorly to allow for the passage of horsehairs for drainage, and two openings were made, not only for drainage, but also to allow the passage of two sutures, by which it was sewed to the flap of the scalp, and which were tied externally.

Before the opening was closed the brain was faradized at the following points: First, 7.1 cm. (2¾ inches) to the right of the middle line; 2.5 cm. (1 inch) behind the bi-auricular line. Second, 7.6 cm. (3 inches) to the right of the middle line, and 3.8 cm. (1½ inches) posterior to the bi-auricular line. The current was more than strong enough to move my own muscles, but no phenomena were observed.

The wound was then closed and the usual dressings applied, the gauze being of the strength of 1 to 2000.

In view of the large cavity between the skull and the brain I directed that he should lie with the right side of his head down, so that the blood should not accumulate in this cavity, but escape readily.

December 13*th* (22d day). On the night of the operation he had a severe and prolonged attack for nearly three-quarters of an hour, and ten days later, when terrified by a patient in the ward, who threatened to attack him, he had another fit, but only a slight one. Since then he has had none.

The drainage-tube was removed at the end of forty-eight hours and the horsehairs at the end of five days. For a week after the operation I dressed the wound daily, for the reason that a large amount of bloody serum accumulated between the flap and the bone, as was easily determined by palpation. This separated the bone from the flap except at the two points of suture and the area immediately about them, and, of course, accumulated under the bone between it and the brain, and caused me great anxiety lest the bone, being separated from its blood-supply, should undergo necrosis. Each day I was able gently to press out the fluid and bring the flap down to the bone, and as soon as I did so I could readily determine that the sheep's bone was not fast to the rest of the skull. At the end of a week the serum gradually ceased to accumulate. At the end of two weeks the bone was still slightly loose. I have not examined it between December 6th and to-day, when I found it, as far as gentle manipulation could determine, absolutely firm. The wound itself healed without trouble.

17*th* (26th day). He goes home to-day. In examining him yesterday I thought I detected a slight crepitus between the piece of sheep's bone and the skull. The external wounds have healed and he looks sound and well. He has no pain and has had no further attacks.

January 15, 1891 (2 months). He writes that a few days ago a small reddish blister appeared on the old scar. There is a slight bloody discharge from it daily. There is no pain, swelling, nor soreness. His general health is good.

April 25 (5 months). On his return to the hospital a few days ago I found over the site of the former operation a small opening in the scalp, with bare white bone exposed. The edges of the skin were blue and undermined with a small amount of pus, which was exuding. Under ether the edges of this opening were cut away, and on making a slight crucial incision through them the edges of the dead bone were reached, and it was easily removed. The piece of sheep's bone, which had originally been 2 by 1⅛ inches, had nearly disappeared, and the small fragment that I removed was rather less than half an inch in diameter both ways. Its edges were worm-eaten and soft. Underneath it was a distinct membrane in almost all respects resembling the dura. It was not opened, but by touch showed that under it was apparently a fluid. The wound was then wiped out with pure carbolic acid and dressed with ordinary bichloride gauze.

May 16 (21 days after second operation). The night of the operation he had a severe attack, since which time he has had none. The wound has healed readily excepting a very small area, scarcely the size of a pea. He is to go home in two or three days. He tells me that he feels immensely better than he did when he had the constant irritation of the gradually disintegrating bone. I have advised him to change his occupation, in order to have less stooping and lifting, either of which causes him considerable annoyance.

REMARKS.—These two cases suggest several points of importance. First, that in injuries of the brain immediate surgical interference may prevent the deplorable consequences which may arise, of which these two cases are illustrations. Of course, these particular accidents occurred at a time when surgeons were not equal to such interference; but they point out what the proper method of treatment of such cases should be in future. After wide and careful shaving and disinfection of the entire wound, not only the soft parts, but also the bone should be properly trimmed; and to this I would add that the lacerated brain substance should be removed, for experience is accumulating to a large extent to show that the scar tissue resulting from laceration is a very fertile source of epilepsy and other troubles, far more so than the scar which results from a clean incision in the brain tissue. Of course, no needless incursion should be made into sound brain tisssue, but better some of this, I believe, than to leave lacerated cerebral tissue. Even if some sound tissue be removed and paralysis follow, this will be only temporary; for after such excisions I have invariably found that the function has been restored in time, and generally nearly to the normal.

Secondly, if the dura be extensively lacerated, the lacerated portion should also be removed for like reasons. I would suggest that its place should be supplied from the pericranium by taking a considerable piece from the under surface of the flap of the scalp and sewing it to the dura, thus closing the gap. In doing this the osteogenetic (under) surface should be turned uppermost, so that if any bone should form, it should not grow downward toward the brain, but upward to fill the gap in the bone. A few interrupted sutures at the margin will fix it well in place. It will serve another important purpose also, namely, by closing the gap in the dura by early adhesions it will prevent the tendency to a fungus of the brain, so marked in every case where there is any considerable gap in the dural membrane, especially if there has been incision or laceration of the brain tissue. Since this idea occurred to me I have only had one opportunity of testing it, in a case operated on over three months ago at the Jefferson College Hospital. The piece of pericranium was cut entirely loose, turned downside up, and sewed to the dura, filling up the gap left by the removal of some of the dura, and up to the present time it has perfectly retained its vitality.

Thirdly, the question of immediately closing the gap in the bone by decalcified bone-plate. I do not know of any case at present in which this has been done as a primary step to remedy the defect in the bone tissue at the time of the accident. It seems to me, however, a very reasonable proposal, with probably only one serious drawback. In order that such a bit of decalcified bone shall retain its vitality, it is very essential that the wound shall be absolutely aseptic, and, of course, in a wound produced by an accident this is difficult to insure. On the

other hand, if the wound cannot be made aseptic the insertion of the
bone will not increase the danger to the patient.   I think, therefore,
that the attempt to close the gap in the skull by means of such a procedure should at least be attempted.   If the bone survives it is a clear
gain.   In both of the cases just reported I made a secondary attempt
to close the opening, by different processes, in the two cases.   In the
first case I inserted decalcified bone after the manner Senn has advised,
and with a very happy result, both as to the survival of the bone and
the health of the patient.   The facility with which this can be done is
far superior to the transplantation of bone from an animal, for we can
always have such decalcified bone in an antiseptic solution in a jar,
ready for an emergency ; whereas an animal cannot be so readily secured.   Moreover, it requires fewer assistants, for there is but one
operation to be done instead of two—one on the patient and one on
the animal—with equally strenuous antiseptic precautions.   As a minor
point, also, it is far less expensive.

In the second case I filled the gap with a piece of bone from a sheep's
head.   Had the case run a typical course I think success would have
attended the effort, but it was a most unfavorable case for such a trial.
First, because the brain tissue did not fill the cavity of the cranium, and
there was a hollow underneath the transplanted bone.   This hollow was
necessarily filled up by blood-clot of considerable size.   Had the brain
tissue and the bone been in contact I think the chances of the survival
of the bone would have been better.   Moreover, the large accumulation
of serum which took place between the transplanted bone and the flap
separated the bone for the greater part of the time during an entire
week from the flap of the scalp, and thus both on the under and upper
surface the transplanted bone was cut off from its blood-supply, excepting at the slight points of contact where the sutures passed through the
piece of bone and the scalp.   That it should apparently have survived
for three months, and then, with disintegration of the bone, attended
with suppuration, should have produced no endocranial mischief, I
consider a very encouraging fact as to future attempts.   I have had no
opportunity to try the novel suggestion of Fränkel, which has been
carried out by Hinterstoisser and Fillerbaum, to fill such openings with
a celluloid plate.   They state that it has been done three times with success (*Wiener med. Presse,* Jahrg. xxxi. No. 42).   Nor have I yet tried
König's method of chiselling loose the outer table of the bone along with
the flap of scalp, leaving this attached by its base, and swinging it around
to close the defect, while the site of the displaced osseo-cutaneous flap is
covered by a skin-graft by Thiersch's method.

Fourthly, as to the results so far as the epilepsy is concerned, the
time is as yet too short to give any definite opinion as to permanent
results, but yet thus far the improvement has been very manifest.

Fifthly, can we determine by faradism whether the brain tissue, which to the eye and touch seems normal, is really diseased or not? This is a question I am somewhat disposed to answer in the affirmative, although as yet I do not feel at all sure of my ground. My reasons for this possible belief are as follows: When the current is applied to a normal centre in the motor area and the electrode immediately removed, we obtain merely a contraction of the muscles represented at the point of such faradization, the muscular contraction ceasing upon the removal of the electrode, and also being limited to the muscles represented in this area. In Case I. it will be observed that when the current was applied for a moment to the *diseased* tissue a *typical epileptic fit* was produced, following the march of those which had been observed prior to the operation, involving other muscles beside those represented at the immediate point of the cortex which was stimulated, and continuing for half a minute or a minute after the electrode was removed. This same phenomenon I have observed in other cases. It is, however, also true that in some cases of focal epilepsy in which presumably the cortex is diseased, when the area is stimulated no such fit is produced. Whether there be any significance and value in the production of such a fit, such as the above question suggests, I do not know. I submit it for further observation and judgment.

Case III. *Trephining for delusional insanity following trauma; temporary improvement.*—T. N., aged forty-four years, German; mining boss. Family history negative; no insanity. Syphilis denied. Has been a drinking man, but has enjoyed good health until twelve years ago, when he was thrown from a horse, striking on the top of his head. No immediate serious symptoms followed, but after a time he began occasionally to hear imaginary voices, particularly when excited after drinking. Seven years ago (five years after the prior accident) he was badly beaten by some laborers, one of the injuries being a severe scalp wound and injury to the right parietal bone, together with other cuts in the scalp. He was taken to the Drifton Hospital, and was perfectly rational, but after two or three days became delirious from erysipelas. After a month's time the wound was healed. While in the hospital he had some delusions as to hearing. These continued after he left the hospital, and in January, 1890, they became very marked, so that he would sometimes leave his work to meet an imaginary person. These delusions last July culminated in an attempt at suicide. An imaginary voice told him that he was about to be killed by someone who was pursuing him. Another voice said to him, " Don't let them kill you, but do it yourself." Accordingly he procured a revolver and shot himself between the third and fourth ribs near the nipple line of the right breast, with a 38-calibre ball. The ball was extracted at the angle of the scapula.

He was again admitted into the Drifton Hospital, suffering from traumatic pneumonia and delusions. The wound entirely healed, but his mental condition remained unchanged. He could often foretell an attack by a peculiar headache which preceded the delusions, together with insomnia and refusal to eat. Delusions of sight were also present.

The patient was admitted to the Orthopædic Hospital and Infirmary for Nervous Diseases October 2, 1890, under the care of Dr. Sinkler, who kindly asked me to see the case with him, and to whom and Dr. Packard I owe the history. His physical condition at that time was good, but he complained of constant headache, especially in the right parietal region at the cicatrix. He had an anxious expression and heard voices constantly. No delusions of persecution. He was quiet and docile, and for the most part sat alone in the corner of the ward. On shaving the head a stellate scar was discovered over the posterior and upper angle of the right parietal bone; a depression in the skull can be felt through the scar. There were several other small scars on both sides of the scalp, but none of any great apparent importance.

The patient is right-handed. Dynamometer: R. 80, L. 90. Left hand steady, but right shows a tremor on squeezing the dynamometer. Dr. de Schweinitz examined the eye-ground and found it perfectly normal. Knee-jerk slightly exaggerated on both sides; station good. There is no word-deafness, word-blindness, aphasia, or agraphia.

Professor Cattell, of the University of Pennsylvania, kindly examined the patient, and made the following report: " He did not show an abnormal condition as regards sensation, movement, speech, or intelligence, although these all seemed to be somewhat subnormal. No difference in sensation areas, discrimination of weights, or pressure causing pain, was found in the two hands. Dynamometer pressure was, however, weaker with the right hand than with the left, and was accompanied with more tremor. Equal pressure was felt, greater on the scar and on the left side of the scalp than in the median line and on the right side, and about half the pressure caused pain at the former points as at the latter."

After a consultation of the staff it was decided to do an exploratory trephining.

Operation, October 17, 1890. The scalp was adherent to the skull under the cicatrix, with a marked depression 1 cm. (⅜ inch) in length and 3 mm. (⅛ inch) in depth. A one-and-a-half-inch trephine was applied at this point. The skull was quite vascular. The disc of bone removed was rather thin, but the under surface appeared normal. The bone was thickest at a point corresponding to the scar and the dura mater was more firmly attached at this point than elsewhere. The dura appeared normal. The brain did not bulge when the dura was opened, but appeared somewhat flattened at a point corresponding to the thicker part of the button of bone. The pia was somewhat œdematous. Several white patches were observed in the course of the veins. There were no adhesions on the under side of the dura, and passing the finger under the dura revealed nothing abnormal. The dura was therefore closed with interrupted sutures and the flap of scalp sutured in place. The button of bone was not replaced. A small cicatrix over the right parietal bone, three inches above the ear, was also excised. The bone was normal underneath.

The patient made an uneventful recovery, and got up in two weeks after the operation. The pain in his head was very much less, and he did not hear voices, nor did he have any other delusions after the operation. Discharged November 16, 1890. He returned home, and on December 1 was reported in very good condition, being considered by his wife and employer much more rational than he had been. He was able to do some light work.

May 28, 1891. Mr. Miller, Superintendent of the Drifton Hospital, informs me that he did admirably for some weeks, but about the 1st of May he left home, intending, he said, to go to the old country. As he has not been heard of since, and took a revolver with him, it is to be feared that his mental condition was as bad as ever.

REMARKS.—This case seems to be a good example of at least temporary good results achieved in some obscure functional diseases of the brain by exploratory trephining. Very possibly the slight pressure on the brain by the thickened bone or the irritation in the bony cicatrix itself, as well as the cicatrix in the scalp, may have been the cause of his marked delusions, so marked as to lead him to an attempt at suicide. But the resulting good was of very short duration.

CASE IV.—E. C. P., aged fifty-six years, American. Father died young from inflammation of the bowels. Mother died at eighty from debility. Patient is married and has four healthy living children. He had the ordinary diseases of childhood. There is no history of exposure to the sun. He has been subject to gastric disturbances. With this exception he has been entirely well until the onset of his present trouble. Syphilis denied.

Twenty years ago he fainted while in a hot room and struck his head against a cuspidor, receiving a scalp wound, which healed promptly. From the age of fifteen until the age of forty-six he was a jeweller, but for the last ten years he has been doing clerical work.

In May, 1889, his present illness began with pain over the eyes, most pronounced over the right side, and uninfluenced by any known circumstances. At first it was intermittent and of moderate intensity. This headache was the only symptom until August, 1889, when he had a spell of nausea for a week, and was compelled to remain in bed for three weeks. The headache was much intensified by this attack. While in bed he had several attacks of· vomiting without retching. This was the first of a series of such attacks, after which all his symptoms were intensified and new ones were manifested. While in bed it was for a time noticed that he had difficulty in selecting words—for instance, asking for a plate when he wanted a drink, speaking of his pillows as ribbons, frequently interchanging yes and no. He seemed to know that the word used was wrong, and recognized the proper word when suggested to him, although it could not be ascertained whether he himself was able to say the word suggested. This aphasia was present for three or four weeks, but then passed away, and was not noticed again till after Christmas, 1889. On first getting out of bed he had considerable giddiness, but never fell. Change of posture markedly increased the giddiness and headache.

Early in August his memory and vision began to fail. He remarked that he could write short words, but not long ones, owing to the fact that if long he could not see both the beginning and end of the word. At the same time he noticed that he was unable to see people or objects approaching him from the right side. He was able to walk with closed eyes, but could not readily touch the tip of his nose with his right forefinger, his eyes being closed. On getting out of bed after his first attack it was noticed that his right arm and leg were slightly paretic.

This has persisted to a greater or less extent ever since. After the first attack his appetite became ravenous and for a week he rapidly gained strength. At the end of a week after this attack he vomited his breakfast immediately after eating it, and the frontal and occipital headache, which had remained severe from the onset of his first attack, was much intensified, and he was compelled to go to bed again on account of this. The vomiting only appeared on the first day, but the nausea and headache continued. After the recovery from this attack his condition remained about stationary until October 25, 1889, when he began to improve, and was able to walk alone in the street, though he lacked confidence in himself, owing to the disturbance of vision and a slight dragging of the right leg.

December 1, 1889, he had an attack of nausea and headache, lasting three days, and after a lapse of ten days he had another. During the last attack some jerking of the right arm was noticed when he used it, as in brushing his teeth, and slight aphasia reappeared. His bowels were quite constipated. There was no weakness of the sphincters until after his admission to the hospital, when he had nocturnal incontinence of urine. No shortness of breath or palpitation ; no œdema; no cough. Sleep has been profound, but no somnolence. No emaciation.

He was admitted to the Orthopædic Hospital January 3, 1890, under the care of Dr. S. Weir Mitchell, who kindly asked me to see the case with him, and to whom and Dr. Packard I owe the history.

Status presens, January 3, 1890 : A spare man, with gray hair, blue eyes, and sallow skin ; temporal arteries somewhat tortuous and the walls slightly leathery. No arcus senilis. There is no scar on the head ; no tenderness to mediate or immediate percussion. No difference of percussion noted except that due to the varying thickness of the bone. Tongue clean and protruded straight. Breath offensive (possibly due to taking KI ?). Examination of chest and abdomen negative. There is slight rigidity of the posterior cervical muscles. Dynamometer : R. 75, L. 62 on one occasion, but on another, and probably more accurately, R. 75 and L. 85.

On exertion there is coarse, rapid tremor of the hands and arms. The outstretching of the arms causes a bilateral equal rapid tremor. When at rest there is no tremor. The superficial abdominal reflexes normal. Knee-jerk exaggerated on left side and somewhat more on the right. Ankle clonus present on both sides, most marked on .the right. No patellar clonus. Muscle reflexes poorly developed. The wrist, biceps and triceps reflexes could not be elicited. With eyes closed he cannot touch the tip of his nose accurately with either forefinger. Intellect sluggish ; answers slowly and in an abstracted manner, seeming to brighten up at times by a great effort. No alteration of hearing, taste, or smell.

When shown a pencil he called it " a pad from a table of envelopes," and later he called a key a " pad," although he both saw and handled it. Afterward when shown it again, he named it aright, but when shown a hairbrush called it a " key." He was told its proper name and again shown the key. When asked now what he would use the key for he said that " he would brush with it." His wife (with her eye-glasses on) then came in front of him, and when he was again shown the brush he said that it was " what is usually known as eye-glasses." On another trial he called the key a " penknife," and when asked whether he would use it to open a door said "yes." When asked to name it, he called it a "key-knife." Evidently the last preceding idea was carried over to the next object seen.

The letters A B were printed plainly on a piece of paper. He could not name them at first, but was evidently not paying attention. On a second trial he named and pointed to B, but also called A "B." He was then shown B again, and called it "C." When a key was shown him he could not name it, nor could he do better when the letters K E Y were shown with it, or by themselves. A pair of scissors and a piece of paper were handed him, and he was able to cut the paper properly with the scissors.

Dr. de Schweinitz reports as follows on the eyes: "Double optic neuritis. Discs swollen + 5 D. Some fresh hemorrhage at the outer side of right disc. Right lateral hemianopsia. Wernicke's pupillary reaction absent. No paralysis of external eye muscles."

Diagnosis: Cerebral tumor in the parieto-occipital lobe, and most likely in the angular and supra-marginal gyri, with pressure on the cuneus.

On shaving his head four scars were found, the first 1.9 cm. (¾ inch) above the inion, beginning at the middle line and running obliquely upward and forward for 1.9 cm. (¾ inch). Another scar, corresponding to the first, was present on the other side. 12 5 cm. (5 inches) in front of the inion, 1.3 cm. (½ inch) to the left of the middle line, is a small scar 1.3 cm. (½ inch) in diameter. 3.8 cm. (1½ inches) above the left meatus is a crescentic scar, the mouth of the crescent measuring 5 cm. (2 inches). Four inches in front of the inion in the middle line is a distinct blunt boss.

Operation, February 4, 1890. The median line, fissure of Rolando and the parieto-occipital fissure on the left side were marked on the scalp. At a point 1.3 cm. (½ inch) behind the latter, with the centre-pin 3.2 cm. (1¼ inches) to the left of the middle line, a 1½ inch button of bone was removed. The skull was very thick, but the button of bone showed no abnormalities. On examining the exposed dura, there was an indistinct sensation of hardness and tenseness below it. At the lower border of the trephine opening there was a decided adhesion of the dura. There was moderate but perceptible bulging of the tense dura, but no pulsation was visible. The dura was then opened, and as the opening was made the brain substance bulged markedly through it.

Faradism was then applied at various parts of the exposed cortex, without perceptible effect. An incision was next made through the cortex, when the left arm was pronated strongly several times. The right pupil was more dilated than the left, and there was lateral oscillation. An incision was then made in the brain substance at the postero-inferior border of the trephine opening, and the brain explored gently with the finger. There was a sense of an elastic, smooth, hard body about 6.3 cm. (2½ inches) below the surface, probably at the anterior border of the cuneus. A sharp spoon was introduced and an attempt made to determine the size and character of the hard mass, which was distinctly felt. Some pieces of the tumor were removed, but it was decided that on account of its size and depth it could not be removed, especially as the patient's condition was not good. The dura was united and the wound closed. The right angle of the mouth drooped, and there was slight rhythmical tremor of the right levator anguli oris.

He gradually sank, and died fourteen hours after the operation was concluded.

Post-mortem examination, February 5, by Dr. W. J. Taylor. Spleen normal, except an area of infarction ; liver small and flabby, with fatty changes ; kidneys congested and lobulated, with accessory renal arteries ; a small cyst in the pyramid of the left kidney. Vermiform appendix six inches long lying on the surface of the ascending colon, with a complete mesentery. Other organs normal.

Head : The wound looks in good condition. The scalp comes off easily, and no marks of injury can be seen on the skull. The dura rather opaque, slightly adherent, and congested, the smaller vessels showing plainly. Surface of brain apparently normal ; no congestion and no œdema on either side. Sinus empty ; considerable effusion exists in the vertebral canal.

Brain : A large area of broken-down brain tissue was found at the site of operation—about 5 cm. (2 inches) in diameter. Beneath this is a hardened mass as large as a filbert, the centre exactly 5 cm. (2 inches) from the end of the occipital lobe and 2.5 cm. (1 inch) from the middle line. The part of the tumor removed at the operation is posterior to this and midway between the remaining hardened mass and the point of the occipital lobe. The cavity left by the operation appears to be 1.8 cm. ($\frac{3}{4}$ inch) in diameter, and at the base the hardened mass can be felt extending into the point of the cuneus, where it is in contact with the falx, 1.3 cm. ($\frac{1}{2}$ inch) from the extreme point of the cuneus and the same distance from the middle line, covering an area of at least 1.3 cm. ($\frac{1}{2}$ inch) in diameter. There is marked congestion of the smaller vessels on the surface of the convolutions at the extreme point of the cuneus. Beneath and between the outer convolution of the cuneus is a clot 5 cm. (2 inches) long. The angular gyrus was removed at the operation. The tumor has no limiting membrane, but invades the brain substance, white and gray alike. Base of skull shows nothing abnormal. Dr. Charles W. Burr kindly examined the tumor, and found it an infiltrating glioma.

REMARKS.—The diagnosis of the location of the tumor in this case was made by reason of his apraxia and sensory aphasia and the hemianopsia. The diagnosis was exactly confirmed, as will be seen by the operation and the post-mortem, with the exception that the tumor was not superficial, but much deeper than had been supposed. I think we ought to have been led to deem it deeper than we did, by reason of its relation to the cuneus, since a tumor involving both the cuneus and the angular gyrus ought to have been localized as deep rather than superficial ; but in view of this condition and the possibility that the tumor might be removable, I think the operation was entirely justifiable. When I reached the depth that I did before I found the tumor, it was very clear to me that its removal was impracticable, and the post-mortem certainly convinces one of this fact.

Brain tumor, however, is necessarily and *per se* a fatal disease. Hence, I do not think that the fatal issue of this operation ought to be put over against the unknown possibility of the removal of the tumor until it was explored. I shall not soon forget the regret I experienced a few years ago, when at the post-mortem examination a tumor that I had declined to operate on shelled itself out of the brain during the manipulations for the removal of the brain; and the subsequent microscopical examination showed that the walls of the cavity in which it lay were not involved in the disease, although it was a sarcoma. Operation, which I unfortunately declined to do, might possibly have saved his life.

I cannot, therefore, even in the light of the autopsy, regret that this operation was done, as it hastened death but little. In the necessary uncertainty attending the diagnosis of cerebral tumors at the present time, I regard an exploratory operation in suitable cases as not only advisable, but needful. If we find an irremovable tumor, as a rule the patient will not die, and may even be bettered, as has been shown in a number of operations; and if he dies, it is anticipating by a very little what would have been the result without operation. If we do not explore in any reasonable case, we may find ourselves at the autopsy in the unenviable position which I recollect so vividly myself.

CASE V. *Trephining for defective development; death from hemorrhage and shock twenty minutes after the completion of the operation.*—M. F., aged eighteen years, kindly referred to me by Dr. John Van Bibber, of Baltimore. She first entered the Jefferson College Hospital February 10, 1890. After a careful study of the case I advised decidedly against operation, and she returned to Baltimore; but in March, 1890, she again came to Philadelphia and entered the Infirmary for Nervous Diseases, on account of the urgent request of her parents that an operation should be done. Her physician and some of my colleagues approved of an exploratory operation on the left side of her head, and I finally consented to operate.

Her history, as taken by Dr. Packard at the Infirmary, is as follows: The family history is negative, excepting that one of her nine brothers and sisters died of convulsions after an illness of thirteen hours, characterized by fever and right hemiplegia three hours before death; and another died at twenty-two, probably from tubercular laryngitis. At her birth, which was not instrumental, there was considerable difficulty and delay in delivering the head and the establishment of respiration. She had jaundice for three months after birth. At eleven months of age, while teething, she had a general convulsion. Prior to this time it had been noticed that she used the left hand more than the right, but until this convulsion it was unknown that the right arm and leg were partially paralyzed, the fact being discovered by the physician who attended her. At two years of age she fell from a baby-carriage, striking on her head, but without apparent ill effects. She began to talk at one year, but advanced slowly in speech. She began to walk at two years of age, dragging the right foot. At three or four years, right facial palsy and wasting of the right side of the face were noticed. During dentition she had five or six general convulsions. At three years of age she had an attack of *petit mal;* at irregular periods after this she had a few other attacks, and from ten years on they have been growing more severe and more frequent, until in the last month she has had five

or six. There is apparently an abdominal aura, as she grasps the abdomen with both hands at the beginning of an attack, and immediately
afterward the convulsion becomes general. For the last six months
choreiform movements have been noticed in all four extremities.

Her intellect is rapidly becoming more and more defective and her
memory failing. There is considerable headache at the vertex. Bowels
regular; no vomiting; menstruation regular. Her head is of peculiar
shape, looking as if it had been rubbed between two boards moving in
opposite directions, and the left side being markedly smaller than the
right. From the meatus to the middle line on the left side is 1.5 cm.
(⅗ inch) smaller than the right, and the left semi-circumference is 1¼
cm. (½ inch) smaller than the right. The right arm and leg are markedly smaller than the left, with contractures of the flexors of the hands
and fingers. Knee-jerk normal on the left side; much exaggerated on
the right. Slight ankle clonus on the right side; none on the left. Front
tap and paradoxical muscular contraction unattainable on either side.
The chest is somewhat deformed, the right side being largest posteriorly
and the left largest anteriorly. Sensation not satisfactorily tested, owing
to her mental state, but evidently much blunted on the right side, both
as to touch and pain.

Professor Cattell kindly examined her on March 8, 1890, and reports:
" The arrest of mental development and the asymmetry of the two sides
of the body were so extreme that exact measurements were neither
necessary nor easy to make. Reaction-time and rate of movement
could not be determined, as she was unable to hold a telegraphic key
in the right hand.

" Dynamometer pressure: right, 2 kgs. (obtained with difficulty);
left, 20 kgs. Sensation areas: Distance at which points can be distinguished, right hand 12 cm., left 2.5 cm. (normal). Pressure causing
pain was, right hand 1.6 kgs., left hand 3 kgs., forehead 1.6, head 0.6.
Very hyperæsthetic, especially for the right hand and head. The time
required to see and name colors was 1.467 seconds; words 1.819 seconds
—much longer than normal, especially for words."

Operation, March 4, 1890. Ether. The fissure of Rolando on the left
side and the median line were located with the cyrtometer and marked
with an aniline pencil. An allowance of 1.8 cm. (¾ inch) to the left of
the middle line was made for the probable dislocation to the left of the
superior longitudinal sinus, on account of the left atrophy. A 1½-inch
button of bone was removed, its inner edge being 1.8 cm. (¾ inch) from
the median line. The skull was very thick; the dura bulged slightly.
There was no especial spot of hardness or softness to be felt through it.
The dura was then incised for two-thirds of the opening, the base of the
flap being from the middle line. At one point, when the dura was
opened a free hemorrhage took place, amounting probably to four or
six ounces, evidently from a large vein. This was controlled with
hæmostatic forceps. The brain substance was of an opaque, pearly-gray
color, œdematous, but with no evidence of softening or cyst. The convolutions were very hard, feeling like tense worms. Three punctures
were made in the œdematous pia, followed by an escape of serum and
the subsidence of the pia to the brain tissue. The opening was enlarged
downward about a quarter of an inch by the rongeur forceps, when it
was noticed that there was a deep furrow extending downward and
forward, of evidently atrophied brain. During these manipulations the

hæmostatic forceps seizing the vein sprung open, and another free hemorrhage took place. I almost instantly placed my finger upon it, and got the bleeding vessel again controlled by the hæmostatic forceps; but the amount of blood lost before it was controlled amounted to about five or six ounces more. The patient became suddenly blanched, markedly cold, and collapsed. Hot saline solution was quickly injected into the cellular tissues, hot bottles applied, the legs elevated and the head lowered, and a hypodermic of $\frac{1}{60}$ of a grain of atropia sulph. given.

While my assistants were carrying out these directions a few interrupted catgut sutures were inserted in the dura; the forceps seizing the vessel remaining *in situ*, the scalp was sutured at a few points and a sublimate gauze dressing applied. Transfusion of salt solution was done, but before it could produce any effect the patient died, twenty minutes after the operation was completed.

Dr. C. W. Burr kindly examined the brain, and reports as follows: "Weight, when fresh, twenty-nine ounces Troy. The pia strips off easily. The entire left hemisphere is smaller than the right, measuring 18.4 cm. (7¼ inches) from the extreme point of the frontal lobe over the parietal lobe to the extreme end of the occipital lobe, while the right measures 23.5 cm. (9¼ inches). The convolutions are smaller than normal and the fissures irregular. The fissure of Sylvius is replaced by a deep wide valley extending almost to the occipital lobe, as if all the convolutions bounding it had atrophied and its walls fallen apart and its floor inward. Where the Sylvian fissure should be, the pia is attached closely. The temporal lobe is much shrunken; the fissure of Rolando is very short; the ascending frontal and ascending parietal convolutions are small and their lower parts absent; the corresponding crus cerebri and anterior pyramid is smaller than on the right side; the left hemisphere is harder than the right, and the left side of the skull smaller than the right. In the right hemisphere, apart from irregularities in the courses of the fissures, there seems to be nothing abnormal."

REMARKS.—In reviewing this case I regret very much that I did not adhere to my first decision not to operate; but her parents were so anxious that something should be done, in view of her steady mental and physical failure, that I finally consented. It was clearly an error of judgment. Moreover, the operation was not properly planned, especially in one respect: I allowed three-fourths of an inch for the possible displacement of the superior longitudinal sinus, which was one-eighth of an inch more than the difference in the measurements. This I thought sufficient, and rightly; but when I opened the dura, instead of making the base of my flap *from* the middle line, I should have made it *toward* the middle line, so that in lifting it I could have seen any large vessels emptying into the parasinoidal spaces, and so have avoided opening one of these spaces, as at the post-mortem I found that I had done, and this precipitated the hemorrhage which caused her death. That her death was caused by the loss of a moderate amount of blood is a matter of some importance to note, and should make the surgeon especially careful not so much to check as to avoid hemorrhage in any similar cases of operation on the brain. The hemorrhage was checked very quickly, but evidently hemorrhage from the brain, and especially a brain that is defectively developed, is much more serious *pro tanto* than from other parts of the body.

REST AND FOOD IN THE TREATMENT OF ANÆMIA AND ANOREXIA NERVOSA.

By James F. Goodhart, M.D., F.R.C.P.,
PHYSICIAN TO GUY'S HOSPITAL.

THE present paper includes two distinct groups of cases; but inasmuch as they are often found together, and are both treated, so far as I am chiefly concerned, in the same manner, I have ventured to bracket them under one heading, although I must discuss each separately. And first of all, Anæmia.

This is a wide subject, and is a symptom of many diseases. I do not propose to deal with it when thus *symptomatic*, but only when it is a substantive affection. And, even thus, I shall not take it in its entirety, for there is anæmia on the near side of middle life which requires one method of treatment, and there is the anæmia which, on the whole, affects the declining half of life, which is styled *pernicious* and which requires a different handling. It is to the anæmia of young adults, and, almost without exception, of women—the disease that has received the name of chlorosis, but which is not always by any means chlorotic—of which I am going to write.

One may feel inclined to ask, "What is there in this subject that we do not already know?" To that I would reply: Probably, nothing; but it is a subject on which men who are entitled to an opinion differ considerably as to the right treatment, and therefore anyone who has convictions on the subject, one way or the other, is at liberty tò air them. Not so very long ago no less an authority than Sir Andrew Clark read a paper on this subject in which he contended that anæmia was the result of the constipation which is its common accompaniment, and he advocated purgatives rather than iron as *the* remedy, although he *did* combine a little iron with his aperient pill. That paper traversed one of my most cherished convictions. There are not many occasions in medicine on which, perhaps, one can say, "I *know*," unhampered by any serious qualification. But, having been interested in these cases for many years, and having tested what I say in scores of cases, I venture to say I *know* that iron given properly will cure many of them and that attention to the constipation alone will not. I do not deny that the constipation is an important element in many cases and that it may make the anæmia worse, but I am certain that it is not the primary factor; that the anæmia is *not* essentially a result of fecal absorption. But there are certainly some who think that iron will not cure all cases. Then I say, that is because one or two considerations are lost sight of, and, as regards iron, because it is not given properly.

Now, treading upon a man's pet corn is not a bad way of causing a little excitement; therefore, let me mention certain common ways of giving iron which, as regards this disease, are not what I call giving it properly. Giving a dose of dialyzed iron three times a day is one of these. Many people are very fond of this preparation of iron; and when it was first introduced dialyzed iron seemed to me to promise well, for it was a mild preparation which might be expected to be taken without upsetting the digestion. I tried it extensively, and came to the conclusion that it was of very little use when compared with other preparations. "It won't do any harm," as a celebrated physician once said of a remedy to a lady of my acquaintance. "Thank you," said she; "I did not suppose that it would, but that was not exactly my purpose in coming to you." To order dialyzed iron is, as far as I know, playing with the remedy and wasting time. The mist. ferri comp. of the British Pharmacopœia is an *old-fashioned*, but, as far as it goes, a good medicine; but here, again, to give an ounce of it three times a day does not satisfy the requirements of most cases, for it only contains the equivalent of 2½ grains of sulphate of iron in carbonate to the ounce, and, although the better for this, patients are not thoroughly renovated, even after a protracted course of the drug. The sulphate of iron, again, is a good remedy, and has the great advantage that it can readily be combined with an aperient in a pill. But, good as it is, it has the drawback that it is difficult to raise the dose to the amount that I contend these patients require, for it has a tendency to act as an emetic. However, it *can* be pushed, if care be taken to do this slowly and steadily, for, like sulphate of zinc, tolerance is easily established and a sufficient dose can then be given. Some, again, are fond of the perchloride of iron, and it, also, is a valuable hæmatonic; but with *it*, even more than with the sulphate, the stomach is not tolerant of large doses in these cases, and therefore I do not give it. Some preparation, therefore, is wanted that *can* be given in *large* doses without disturbing the stomach, and, to my mind, such preparations are chiefly *two :* the saccharated carbonate of iron and the ferrum redactum, or reduced iron. There are numbers of people who will tell you that they cannot take iron, but it is seldom, indeed, that they have any difficulty with either of these preparations. They may either of them be given in half-drachm doses or more three times a day, and they may be given in pill or powder or lozenge. The powder is the least troublesome, and there is seldom any difficulty in thus administering it, if the patient be forewarned that, although dirty to look at, it is not bad to the taste. There are many people who cannot take pills; those who cannot will nearly always take the powder, and those who cannot take powders will take any amount of pills—indeed, the more the merrier. Perhaps I may be allowed to add that the pills should be made up with glycerin of tragacanth and coated with some of the soluble coatings now in use, lest they should pass through the intestinal canal unappropriated and the remedy thus come unjustly to be looked upon as a defaulter.

But there is yet another point about the iron treatment that is often not sufficiently insisted upon, viz., the *duration* of the course. Hundreds of anæmic people apply for treatment, and we ask, Have they taken iron? Oh, yes, say they, they are always taking it, and it does them no good. But when we come to inquire, they have taken a bottle, or perhaps two, and then left off for awhile. The average specimen of humanity still looks for his cure in his first dose, or, at least, somewhere within the depth of a six-ounce bottle; but it is needful to say that anæmia is not to be cured in so ready a fashion, and half the battle lies in a fair start. In dealing with these cases I always ask them, Are you prepared to carry out the requisite treatment? They, of course, profess themselves ready to do anything; whereupon I make them promise to take their medicine continuously for six weeks. Half-drachm doses, then, of the saccharated carbonate of iron or of reduced iron, given regularly three times a day over a course of six weeks, I consider to be so successful that I never can find heart to waste time (as I believe it is, for the most part) on other means of treatment, whether it be by potassii permanganatis or what not. Nevertheless, iron is a remedy that is not always successful in private practice. I have seen many cases, now, where I have been obliged to acknowledge that the iron treatment has been carried out in all respects properly, and yet the patient has not recovered her color satisfactorily. And in thinking the matter over there seems to me to be a difference in this respect between hospital cases and those in private. I look over the former and cannot remember one that has failed, and the only difference that I could think of was this, that they are invariably put to bed as soon as they come into the hospital and that they are also fed with at any rate a reasonable quantity of nourishment. In the better-class patient it is too often considered necessary only to give so much physic, food and exercise being left to the individual discretion.

Happily, Nature has some pretty stiff automatic checks, and the breathlessness of the anæmic is one of them; were it not so, anæmia of this sort would be a far more fatal disease than it is. But how can these patients expect to get well when they are so bloodless that they have nothing inside them to do a day's work upon, and yet they attempt to do that work. And what is that day's work? Well, "there is nothing the matter with them," so they do, after a fashion, much as other people do—that is to say, they think or are told that fresh air is good for them, so they drag themselves out to shop and walk. It is quite common to find young ladies thus affected going to early services at church, visiting in parish work, and as to not going to a dance because of their ailment, it would never occur to them for a moment. But after all, their chief exercise and exhaustion comes, I am persuaded, from the quite unnecessary tread-mill exercise they perform for the hundred and one things that they want which are downstairs when they are up and upstairs when they are down. And what do they do this upon ? Generally no breakfast—a cup of tea they consider a sumptuous meal ; a finger of meat, perhaps, for lunch, and, perhaps, again for dinner at the urgent importunity of their relatives ; and if they are particularly well looked after these tiny meals are supplemented by an intervening sup or two of beef-tea, whose one grand virtue is that it has been stewed so long that you can "cut it with a knife."

To summarize, these cases, if at all far gone in the bloodless condition, require :

First, absolute rest in bed for ten days or a fortnight—three weeks is none too much for some cases—and they should not be allowed to take much exercise of any kind for the six weeks that their treatment lasts.

Secondly, they must be fed with good, wholesome food—four meals a day—beginning with milk and egg, which can be taken in the fluid state, and thus stowed away almost regardless of appetite. Good meat and vegetables can soon be added, and each meal should see some addition until a reasonable quantity is taken.

Thirdly comes the iron, as already detailed ; and,

Fourthly, any mild aperient that may be necessary.

It is not my purpose to advert to the dangers that attach to the anæmic state. Whether they are few or many, it cannot be that this disease is an unimportant one, although it is so common and so generally remediable that one might well think it so. Unfortunately, it is so very common that the public have no idea of its importance as a disease, and therefore it requires some courage to send a patient to bed for a fortnight and to prescribe a Lent where physic shall replace the accustomed fasting.

But, as I am dealing with the point of curability of these cases, I should like to say that I have several times seen it stated that in distinguishing between pernicious and this form of anæmia that the pernicious form tends to relapse ; the chlorotic form, not. This has not been my experience ; quite the contrary. These cases frequently relapse after a time, and it is necessary to tell them that it will be so, and that at the first indication ot pallor or breathlessness, or, it may be, amenorrhœa, they must return to their remedy for a short course of three weeks or so. It is a curious disease, and, I believe, has a large nervous element as a factor in its production; but this I feel sure of, that, by its obstinacy and its tendency to relapse, it betokens a rather important constitutional vice, and that it is not a mere intercurrent affection that is treated and done with.

And now to turn to the other disease—anorexia nervosa: It will be remembered that this name was given by the late Sir William Gull to a series of cases which he recorded in the Clinical Society's *Transactions*, vol. vii. p. 22. These cases were very severe, associated with extreme emaciation, and more or less mental depression likewise; but, except for this, there was no apparent disease. A few similar cases have been recorded since, but all of them have been of such extreme degree, and associated with an amount of wasting so excessive—as may be seen by the woodcuts of the cases that have been published with the records— that I think there is no doubt that they have been looked upon as examples of a rare disease rather than as extreme cases of a very common one. At any rate, this is the point that I want to insist upon, viz.: mild anorexia nervosa is one of the very commonest diseases with which we have to deal, although it is, perhaps, not known by the name with which I would christen it.

The sort of case I have in mind is as follows:

A lady (these cases are always in women and most commonly but by no means confined to the upper classes), aged forty-two, who had never been strong, had been subject to fainting-fits, and had for long had recourse to strong purgatives for obstinate constipation, came to me for attacks of complete collapse; these were said to be so bad by her medical man, who came with her, that he really feared she would one day die.

I went into her history, and found that she was an extremely small eater, having an *objection* to meat, and being unable to take milk and eggs—a rather large order to cut entirely out of a daily dietary. Her attacks of collapse were thus described: She becomes faint and sick, with intense pain about the stomach, thighs, and spine. Her original weight was one hundred and sixteen pounds; she now weighs eighty pounds. Yet her vivacity seemed at times unimpaired, and she expressed herself as quite well and able to do anything.

This was her daily diet:

Breakfast. A cup of tea, without milk or sugar; a finger or two of toast, with very little butter.

Lunch. A very small piece of fish, a little bit of potato, a little salad, with plenty of vinegar; a little claret.

Entremet (afternoon tea, she fitly called it). A cup of black tea, without sugar or milk.

Dinner. Same as lunch.

Was I wrong, upon the facts before me, in characterizing her abdominal and spinal pangs as an expressive, not to say indignant, remonstrance on the part of her abdominal nerve-centres at the cruelty and ignorance with which they were being treated?

She was going out to India in three weeks from the time that I saw her, passage taken, and all things arranged. I mention these little details to enforce a point, viz., that you must be firm with these people; they don't appreciate the gravity of their condition, for use is a second nature to them, and they have got so accustomed to their miserable state of existence that they come and tell you, as this poor creature did, that they feel quite well. Further, they do appreciate very keenly the very disagreeable nature of the remedies proposed. I told her that, go to India or not, she must have six weeks of the *pâté de foie gras* treatment, and if the departure was a fixed and unalterable term it must be continued on board ship. She was put under the care of Dr. Andrews, of Hampstead. He concurred in the diagnosis, had her removed to a small home hospital, and carried out a six-weeks' course of feeding and massage; and I heard afterward that she went out to India later, quite well, having gained more than fourteen pounds in weight, but she relapsed again after a while, as such cases seem liable to do.

I will only burden you with this one case; but remember that I could give you case after case of the same kind, and that is one of the points I wish to make—it is a very, very common ailment.

The next point is, How are these cases brought about? A matter, I think, of the simplest physiology imaginable. These patients are invariably of a neurotic temperament, and in evidence of this I may point to the fact that the disease is almost entirely confined to the female sex, while other well-marked evidence may usually be found in neuralgia, flushings, faintings, etc. The point of this is, as it seems to me, that neurotic people are very commonly people of slow digestion. This is as much so in men as in women, but men very seldom take on this peculiar type of disease; they, for some reason or other, become hypochondriacs and over-critical as regards their intakes and their outputs, and particularly irritating to the medical mind by the very unnecessary detail into which they launch as regards the quantity and color of their fecal evacuations. In this respect, and also in their greater resistance to treatment, men are far less satisfactory patients than women. The neurotic of slow digestion suffers much from flatulence and its consequent distention, and, no doubt, digestion is to them a rather distressful process. The next step is that these people think that they have got the disease "indigestion," and as a very natural result they consult a doctor, and that appears, in a large number of cases, to be the very worst thing that they could do. And why? Because they are thereby confirmed in their belief that they *have* got indigestion. They *thought* they had before—that was bad enough; now they have authority for their belief, and they are on the straight road to perdition.

Having got indigestion they must, of course, diet themselves; perhaps they are already dieted by authority, but, if not, they very readily take to dieting themselves; and first one thing is left off and then another, as, failing to get relief, they still think they are taxing their stomachs too much. Last of all, they begin the round of physicians great on stomachs and their treatment. This means that for the most part they are still more rigidly fed by rule, and, in addition, they try, one after the other, the various remedies that are supposed "to go for" the stomach—the pepsins, the papains, the soda, the bismuth, the calumba, the mineral acids—according as the individual whom for the day they are confiding in thinks they have, according to his special bent, acid dyspepsia, atonic dyspepsia, gouty dyspepsia, or any other form of the many that have been described.

I have no special antipathy to these various drugs—they are all very useful in their way and if rightly used, even for these very cases I am discussing; but I want to insist, with all the force that is in me, that to treat these people for stomach affections is to do them positive harm. They are never cured by such means, and if they are moneyed people, as they often are, they go from one man to another until the whole round of great names is exhausted, suffer many things of them, and, in the end, think doctors as a genus a pack of fools, for they are worse than they were at the beginning.

We sadly want a little more common sense and real knowledge applied to the subject of diet. Our present practice stands self-condemned when we have to admit that of all the patients who apply for advice, three different printed sheets do for the lot. Such a method is clearly only a matter of routine; the individuality of the patient is out of the account altogether, and there are few things in which the individuality asserts itself more, which I may illustrate by two so-called dyspeptics whom I have seen quite lately: One, after detailing her discomforts, said: "But I am very peculiar, you know; I can eat *nuts* and *radishes* and all that sort of things." The other, after going through a long string of simple things which she could not digest, said: "But there is one thing that I can always eat." Quite thankful to hear it, for it sounded like progress, I inquired what it was, and she said, "*Lobster !*" I wish I had time to enter more fully upon this subject of diet and the many reasonless and, I believe, unphysiological dicta by which we are bound. But I am rather wandering from my subject.

However, these anorexia nervosas leave off first one thing, because they think it disagrees, and then another, and another, and so on until they are existing upon a most attenuated diet, and the wonder is that they are alive at all.

The explanation I would offer of these cases is a more fundamental one, and I take it from a common physiological fact of which we all have more or less cognizance. We all know that if we have to undergo an enforced fast, that at first very hungry, the appetite after a while goes off and we care not whether we have a meal or not. We often find ourselves in similar circumstances, too, when we have been unusually hard-worked or overdone: "Too tired to eat," we exclaim. In either case the bodily vigor has run too low, the nervous energy requisite for a healthy digestion is not forthcoming; therefore, the appetite is wanting, and food, if forced into the stomach, is only too likely to disagree. It is just so with these cases: they may have a sufficient flow of nervous energy to keep up appearances, just as a raving lunatic may be enabled to put forth an amount of energy which would not have been deemed possible by his associates, and then collapse after it; but they are always tired, and by so doing there is nothing left to charge the abdominal viscera. Hence, the flatulence, the distention, the pain, the indigestion, the constipation, etc.—the stomach is too tired to do its work. But, instead of thus going to the root of the matter, its work is made easier for it, either by diminishing the amount of food introduced or by predigesting what is presented to it, or by both combined. But the stomach is only a bit of human nature, and like its master—or its servant, rather, in this case—if its work is habitually made easy for it and it has little to do, it very readily accommodates itself to its altered circumstances. It would be unkind, indeed, of us to quarrel with it for taking advantage of the proffered ease, when it is so very good-tempered and bears so very uncomplainingly all the many indiscretions to which it is subjected in the opposite direction; and it gets small and lazy—a physiological sloth only—from having nothing to do. And unless you can dispute my fact that these cases are made worse by the advice that they too usually receive, which I do not think to be possible, the explanation of it seems to be patent. Of course they are; for to lessen the work is to accentuate the bad habit into which the organ has been allowed to drift. Clearly, then, the proper treatment of such cases is to restore the nervous energy of these patients, and, having done that, to gradually tax the stomach more and more, until by gradual efforts it is able to remove mountains.

To do all this it is absolutely necessary to send the patient to bed for some little time. It is clearly not conducive to successful treatment to allow her to waste or fritter away the little energy she has by dragging about in the dilapidated state of tissues in which we find her. All the vitality she has is wanted to be concentrated on her blood-making supplies; all waste, therefore, is to be curtailed, all possible energy husbanded, by keeping her in bed. Next comes, I was going to say, food; but I think medicine comes next in natural order, and *that, not* bismuth or remedies directed to any local failure, but strychnine and iron, as helping to restore the vitality of the patient. Then shall come food—and food which, although carefully adapted to the enfeebled organ, shall nevertheless be gradually and methodically increased, both in quantity and variety, until the healthy standard is again reached. Very little attention must be paid to the patient's suggestions in this matter; their fastidiousness will speedily drive you crazy; and it is very seldom indeed, although they vow they can never digest milk, that, under the altered circumstances in which they now find themselves, it disagrees with them in any way. Milk is the thing to begin upon, and cream may almost immediately be added to it. It is true, they will say the same of cream as they do of milk: it is bilious, etc. You can retort that even babies can digest it, so certainly they can; and, indeed, for weak stomachs of all kinds there are few things better than cream. Pounded meat and vegetables come next, and so on, according to all the details that have been so well advocated by Weir Mitchell.

There yet remain one or two little points in the management of these cases, and the first is to make them understand that in the generally lengthened process of fasting to which they have subjected themselves the cavity of the stomach has probably *contracted,* and that our process of stomach-stretching is not one that can be carried out without some little discomfort—indeed, I have no doubt that it sometimes causes a good deal of pain to the patient, so far as an outsider is able to gauge the degree of pain from which a neuralgic individual is suffering. Further, they must understand that a certain amount of distention of the stomach after food will be their lot through life, more particularly when their general health is rather low or they have been overdone or worried in any way. We are all familiar with that fact. Large numbers of people go about who habitually feel some slight fulness after food for an hour or two, and which subsides after that time, as the stomach settles down to its work and disposes of some of it. But to those of us who are robust, or know that it means little, it gives no trouble; it is only those who dwell upon it that it depresses and makes miserable. The next point is, that from the fixed idea that these people have as regards the injurious effects of certain foods upon their very particular food-bags, it is absolutely necessary to put them under the charge of a properly trained nurse and often to take them away from home. This latter part of the Weir Mitchell treatment may possibly be unnecessary, for they are for the most part intelligent and wanting to get well if only they can be shown how health is to be accomplished; but a nurse is an absolute necessity.

Having got the case thus far on her road of recovery there will come up, probably, the individuality of the patient, and with it a rather nice point to determine, viz., how much food a particular patient requires. We vary so much in this respect; and I believe it is the women who have habitually small appetites who supply the large majority of the sufferers I talk of—people who never have any desire for food, and who, measuring their needs by this low standard, gradually eat less and less, until they collapse. The rule of the life of such a one must be to try and take, meal by meal, some slight increase on the previous one, until the power to eat is cultivated.

Massage is useful as a restorative to the peripheral circulation and to the muscles, but it is not absolutely necessary.

THE BACK IN RAILWAY SPINE.[1]

By F. X. Dercum, M.D.,

INSTRUCTOR IN NERVOUS DISEASES, UNIVERSITY OF PENNSYLVANIA.

So much has been written upon railway injuries that it is not without some hesitation that I write upon this subject. It has, however, seemed to me that the physical condition of the back has been insufficiently discussed. Certainly far more has been said pro and con upon injuries of the spinal contents, and far more still upon the subject of traumatic neuroses. It has been my fortune to examine a large number of railway and allied injuries, and it has appeared to me that the condition of the back was often poorly understood and often unappreciated, while important points were sometimes entirely overlooked. Further, conditions are occasionally observed which are difficult of explanation, and to these I especially desire to call your attention.

At the outset of our inquiry, we are met with the problem as to what extent pain, a subjective symptom, should be admitted as a factor. We all know that pain of various kinds is met with in railway cases. Now it has seemed to me that we should exclude from this discussion all pains the existence of which cannot be confirmed by any physical evidence, and which rest solely upon the unsupported statements of the patient. Under this head come the vague aches, "weak feelings," and paræsthesias which may be absolutely genuine, but for the demonstration of which there are no known means.

On the other hand, all pain, signs of which are evoked without previous warning or suggestion, should be rigidly admitted. Under this head come all pains signs of which are evoked during palpation, pressure, percussion, and motion, either voluntary or passive.

To begin, it is impossible to separate sharply the symptoms elicited by palpation from those elicited by pressure. Curiously enough too, the very first symptom that presents itself for our consideration, namely, abnormal sensitiveness of the surface, or hyperæsthesia, constitutes a borderland symptom between the subjective and objective groups, the exact significance and value of which it is impossible to fix, and for the present, at least, this symptom must be set aside.

[1] Read before the New York Neurological Society, May 5, 1891.

Very different, however, are the symptoms so frequently elicited by pressure. Here the patient distinctly reacts in a manner that numistakeably indicates pain. At the outset, however, we must distinguish between two groups of symptoms radically different in their meaning and which are elicited according to whether the pressure is superficial or deep. In the first group we have the well-known tender spots of so-called spinal anæmia or spinal irritation and which are now recognized as being related to purely functional conditions. As is well known, they are elicited by comparatively slight pressure and most frequently over the dorsal and cervical spine; and further, in the vast majority of cases the area of tenderness is small and distinctly limited. Whatever specnlation we may indulge in as to their nature, whether we regard them as expressive of some nutritive or functional change in deeper structures or relegate them to the great group of the inexplicables of hysteria, there can be no doubt that these painful areas are genuine. If, without telling the patient just what is being done or what drug is being used, an injection of cocaine be made into a painful spot, the latter, in the fraction of a minute or longer, disappears. At the same time, the painful spots above and below not so treated remain unchanged. Surely upon this and other grounds the inference is justified that we have an actual, a *bona fide*, condition to deal with.

Without pausing to assign this symptom its proper place in the syndrome of railway spine, let us pass at once to the consideration of the symptoms elicited by *deep* pressure. In a large number of cases pain is not complained of unless the pressure made is decided. Care should, of course, be exercised in examining with deep pressure not to cause pain in the superficial structures, especially the skin. This can readily be avoided by pressing with the thumb, and, further, not with the point of the thumb but with its palmar surface. One would, of course, not think of using a pointed instrument or the knuckles in making this test.

The pain elicited on deep pressure differs, I need hardly point out, altogether from that elicited by superficial pressure. In the first place it differs in character. It lacks the acute sensitiveness of the painful spot. The patient reacts later and less suddenly. It utterly fails to resemble hyperæsthesia, which the painful spot in some of its features approaches. Secondly, it is more diffused, and instead of being found directly over the spine it is more apt to be found, and for some little distance, on one or both sides. Lastly, it very frequently bears in its position a distinct relation to the history of the accident. This I can best illustrate by citing one or two cases.

Case I.—A healthy young woman of twenty-four, while standing in a railway station, was struck by the pole of a loaded baggage truck. The truck was being pushed very rapidly and the end of the pole struck her directly between the spinal column and the right shoulder-blade. Two years and three months later, when first examined by me, I still discovered a very painful area upon deep pressure in this region, though I did not until afterward learn that it corresponded to the site of the injury. Superficial painful spots were not present in this case, nor was the patient in the least degree hysterical.

Another instance is the following :

Case II.—A finely developed man of twenty-seven, a brakeman, was caught between the bumpers while coupling freight cars. His back and left side were badly squeezed, though no bones were broken. Upward of two years later he presented marked pain upon deep pressure in the lower lumbar and upper sacral region, especially toward the left, and in addition deep tenderness over and above the left ilium. Neither hyperæsthesia nor painful spots were present. Both of these patients, I should say, had suffered from shock and still presented some asthenic symptoms.

Without pausing to multiply instances of this symptom or to discuss its meaning, let us pass to the pain elicited by percussion. It is at once evident that pain elicited by percussion is without significance unless both superficial and deep pain upon pressure have been previously taken into account or excluded. Percussion is, of course, best performed with a rubber hammer such as the Madison-Taylor hammer used in studying the knee-jerk. The patient lying prone, extended and relaxed, a number of very rapid and not very hard blows should be made directly over the spine with the point of the hammer, the idea being to elicit pain not by the force of the blows but by the faint though decided jarring produced.

Aside from the fact that this method will frequently elicit pain in the bony structures when other methods either cannot be well applied or result negatively, it is not improbable that even pain having its origin in the spinal canal itself may be brought to light by this means. Two instances in my experience favor this view. One was a man in my care at the Philadelphia Hospital, who fell from a wall some ten feet high, striking upon the lower portion of the back, and who subsequently developed a concussion myelitis. In him pain, absent in this region to other tests, was elicited in the lower dorsal and upper lumbar region by the hammer used in the manner described. The other case was the patient exhibited at the last meeting of the American Neurological Association, held in Philadelphia, who had been cured of paraplegia by the resection of a number of spines and laminæ. In this man pain on percussion was one of the most definite and valuable symptoms present, and in the course of the operation marked inflammation of the dura with adhesions to the subjacent pia were revealed, while the fragments of bone removed appeared healthy. These cases are very suggestive, and it certainly is not improbable that this method of percussion—that is, the jarring produced by slight though very rapid blows—may be of decided value in cases otherwise obscure.

Having briefly touched upon the examination of patients by palpation, pressure and percussion, let us now turn our attention to the important tests by motion.

In regard to pain elicited by voluntary motion the objection may properly be urged that here an opportunity is presented to the malingerer. However, there are, as will be pointed out, so many other means of ascertaining the truth at our disposal that difficulty in arriving at definite conclusions will rarely be experienced. In the first place if there be pain on movement there is an instinctive tendency to prevent all movement. The back is held very stiffly and very frequently indeed the patient adopts peculiar and striking attitudes. (This is well illustrated in Figures 1, 2, 4 and 5.) Further, if the patient complain of pain on voluntary movement, passive movement of the trunk in directions and at times not expected by the patient will generally act as a safe corrective to statements made by him. In addition certain physical conditions of the muscles are apt to be present; namely, the muscles in the painful area and its immediate neighborhood are apt to be in a condition of spasm either continual or coming on at such times when movement either voluntary or passive is attempted. This feature when present is most valuable, as it cannot be simulated and as it does away absolutely with the suspicion of malingering. Finally, the muscles which are in a state of spasm are painful when touched and are also in a condition of heightened reflex irritability.

Much depends upon the manner in which the various tests for motion be applied, and it may not be out of place to consider them in detail. They are flexion forward, lateral flexion, torsion and transmitted shock.

Having first practised palpation and pressure and gleaned such information as can be obtained from these sources, we should closely observe the back as the patient stands before us, supposing of course that he be not paraplegic. He is now directed to bend forward. . The points to which our attention should be directed are, the manner in which the act is performed, the amount of motion in the back itself, the stage in the act at which the patient complains of pain, if any, and the area to which the pain is referred, and finally the occurrence of muscular spasm. If rigidity be a marked feature the patient will often merely throw the back forward as one piece, motion taking place only at the hip-joints. (This is well illustrated in Figure 5.) If urged to make a more decided effort, the patient will frequently bend the knees, stoop, adopt, in fact, any expedient that will save the back. In cases less marked the patient will upon urging begin bending the back, but very soon will check the movement, protesting that it gives him pain. Very frequently also decided spasm makes its appearance in the muscles at this time. The spasm, when present, is usually most marked, unless otherwise determined by some detail of the accident, in the lower dorsal and lumbar regions. In cases still less marked than the above forward flexion may be almost completed before pain is complained of or, what is very important, motion may only be restricted in one part of the back. Thus a patient may hold the neck and shoulders very rigidly but flex the lumbar spine quite well, or there may be little or no movement in the lumbar region while the upper part of the spine is flexed considerably.

Supposing now that this test has not yielded decided results or that the patient in his unwillingness to bend the back has opened himself to suspicion, forcible flexion may justifiably be resorted to. Of course the adoption of this procedure depends absolutely on the good sense and judgment of the investigator. We should remember that the pain excited by forcible flexion is often extreme.

We next practise lateral flexion. Here the same points are of course to be observed as in forward flexion. It occasionally happens that in cases where forward flexion has failed to elicit symptoms, the latter are brought to light when the trunk is bent to one or the other side. This generally corresponds to some peculiarity of the accident. For instance, in the case of the brakeman already mentioned who was squeezed between the bumpers of cars, my notes read as follow : " No pain upon forward flexion. Marked pain upon flexion to the right. Pain referred to left side and extending from ilium to lower ribs." It should be remembered that it was the left side especially which had been injured.

Should forward and lateral flexion have failed to elicit symptoms or should the latter have been doubtful, torsion may be practised. An assistant kneeling before the patient should firmly grasp the hips, while the operator, seizing the shoulders, should gently but firmly rotate the trunk. If there be deep-seated soreness the patient will soon give signs of suffering. This method of searching for pain is a powerful one and is rarely of itself required, as most pains are readily elicited by the flexion tests. It may be, however, that in a given case the muscles of the back have suffered less than the fibrous tissues and smaller joints of the spine itself, and in such instances this test may be a very valuable one. While flexion both forward and lateral reacts upon the spine it reacts more powerfully upon the muscles. Torsion, on the other hand, reacts more powerfully upon the spine itself.

We now come to the test by transmitted shock. This may be practised in various ways. The patient standing as erect as possible, the operator places both hands with fingers interlocked on the head and then by a sudden downward pull sends an impulse through the spine. The amount of force exerted must be gauged by the reaction of the patient. The spine may be so very sore that the reaction to even a slight impulse is excessive, and needless suffering may be caused. A gentle pull should first be made, and if no response is elicited from the patient a more forcible one may be given.

If it be desired to eliminate the cervical portion of the spine from the problem, the patient may be seated and the impulse be transmitted through the shoulders. On the whole, however, this method will be found less satisfactory than the preceding.

A third method is to direct the patient while standing to raise himself upon the toes and then to let himself fall back heavily upon the heels. This method is also less valuable than the first. A man with a very sore back can absolutely not be made to execute this test properly. At most it should be used as a confirmation of pain elicited by other means.

We have thus far considered, though briefly, the various tests for eliciting pain. Not only is it possible with due care to settle the question of the genuineness of the symptoms by any one of the methods detailed, but it is also evident that there must be a general correspondence in the results of all the methods. We should expect, for instance, that the area of pain upon deep pressure should correspond, other things equal, to the area of pain on motion, or that the region of pain elicited by percussion should correspond to the region of pain elicited by transmitted shock. Admitting then for the present the reality of the symptoms, and without pausing to discuss their probable lesions, let us turn our attention to a few typical instances of the railway back.

CASE III.—J. C. J., colored, aged twenty-nine years, married, and a coachman by occupation, was in good health up to May 3, 1889. On that date, shortly after midnight, while driving an omnibus containing twelve passengers across the tracks of a railroad the vehicle was struck by a fast freight train. The coach was instantly demolished, three passengers killed, and the others more or less injured. Our patient says that he lost consciousness at the moment of the collision. Eight or nine hundred yards from the scene of the accident he was taken off the engine, on the front part of which he had been jammed.

He remained unconscious for five days. Consciousness then gradually returned, but he was for a long time dazed and confused. He felt great pain "all over," but especially in the head. Pain was also marked in the back and in the right shoulder. He also expectorated considerable blood. Little by little he began to improve, but it was not until six weeks after the accident that he was able to leave his bed. The pain in the head and back, however, steadily persisted. He was weak and nervous and could not sleep well. He seemed to improve a little, however, until December, 1889, when he seemed to reach a standstill. Three months later he was examined by the writer and presented the following conditions: When stripped his peculiar attitude was at once noted. (See Fig. 1.) His head and neck were thrown slightly forward and to the left, while the right shoulder was held much lower than the

left. At the same time a huge scar extending transversely along the
base of the skull from the right mastoid process to the median line was
found. Here, as his physician stated, he had received at the time of the
accident a deep lacerated wound. On the right parietal eminence
another scar an inch and a half long was also found. It was also noted
that in talking he did not turn his head but held it fixedly in the position already described. On touching the back it was found that the
muscles, especially to the right of the spinal gutter, in the neck, and to

Fig. 1.

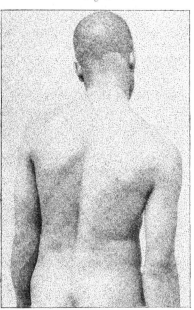

the left in the dorsal region, were swollen and hard. The spine was
exquisitely sensitive to superficial pressure, while deep-seated soreness
was made out over the muscles on both sides. Great pain was elicited
upon attempts at flexion, torsion, and upon transmitted shock. The
pain was especially referred to the cervical and the dorsal regions, being
worse in the former. All attempts at movement resulted in greatly increasing the muscular spasm. Spasm of the muscles could also be
excited by very slight handling. The right shoulder was somewhat
painful on motion. There was also marked diminution of the grip on
both sides, especially the right; the right hand registering 35, the left
62. In addition there was distinct awkwardness of movement of the
right arm and an excessive display of effort. Further sensation was
distinctly diminished on the right side as compared with the left and
the patient frequently made errors in locating the impression, generally
referring the point touched, if, say, on the middle phalanx of the finger,
to the proximal phalanx; or if on the proximal phalanx, to the meta-
carpus, and so on. Knee-jerks at first exaggerated, but soon exhausted.

No eye symptoms. Eye-grounds normal; no contraction of the visual field.

Patient complained greatly of headache and backache. Slept badly. Frequently had attacks of "terrors" at night during which he felt his heart beating very fast. Also complained much of dizziness, ringing in the ears, and said that he could not get his mind settled. Mentally he was much depressed.

Fig. 1 is based on a photograph taken in March, 1891, and it is seen that much of the original condition still persists. The attitude is still characteristic and muscular spasm and rigidity are still present, though in a lessened degree. The awkwardness of movement in the right arm has largely disappeared. Sensation on the right side is fully up to normal and errors of location are no longer made. There has also been some increase of general strength. Damages were awarded the patient about a year after the accident, but seemed to make no change in his condition other than to greatly improve his spirits.

The condition of the back was in this instance very typical. There was excessive rigidity, muscular spasm, great pain upon pressure and motion, and at the same time many of the general symptoms of persistent nervous shock so common in these cases. Especial attention should be directed to the fact that superficial tenderness was present in this case distinct from pain upon deep pressure.

The following constitutes another instance:

Case IV.—G. T., aged forty-six, single, and an upholsterer by trade; was in good health up to October 22, 1890. On that day he was sitting on the rail of the South Street bridge (Philadelphia). His hat blew off, and letting go his hold upon the rail to catch his hat, he lost his balance and fell a distance of thirty feet upon a mound of earth. He struck upon the back and head, became unconscious and remained so until he found himself in the University Hospital, to which he was removed on the same day. He was at first very much confused and suffered intensely from pains in the back and head, and his entire body seemed to tremble. On October 27th he was transferred to my ward at the Philadelphia Hospital. When first seen by me he walked into the the office of the nervous pavilions, walking without assistance. He seemed, however, weak and his steps were evidently shorter and slower than normal. He stripped to the waist without help. He complained of pain in the lower dorsal and lumbar regions, and here deep pressure revealed great soreness. Marked pain was also elicited in this region by flexion, torsion, and transmitted shock. Marked spasm of the muscles in this region was also noted on movement. In addition there was marked tremor of both arms and shoulders. He also complained of headache and seemed much depressed.

He was at once placed in bed on the rest cure. Milk in as large quantities as he could take was given, and for a time massage was attempted, but this had soon, owing to the painful condition of the back, to be abandoned. Instead of improving, however, his symptoms steadily increased in severity. His back became more and more painful. The muscles soon attained a condition of almost constant spasm, and as a consequence rigidity was very marked. The back also became sensitive to superficial pressure. Excessive sweating also set in. Tremor became more pronounced than ever. Four weeks after admission his symptoms had attained their height. The man was thoroughly and abjectly miserable. He was excessively depressed, cried easily, complained of headache, said that he could not sleep, dreamed sometimes that he was falling again from the bridge, had ringing of bells and hissing noises in his ears, trembled worse than ever, had difficulty in passing his water, frequently had sharp pains shooting through his back and head and even in his abdomen. In addition there was now decided loss of sensation in both feet and he was utterly unable to stand. His weakness was extreme. Sweating was excessive. Bowels constipated. Knee-jerks were much exaggerated.

He remained in this condition with but little change until the latter part of February.. He was now able, though at the expense of great suffering, to sit up long enough to permit his being photographed. (See Fig. 2.) Afterward he was immediately returned to bed. The photo-

Fig. 2.

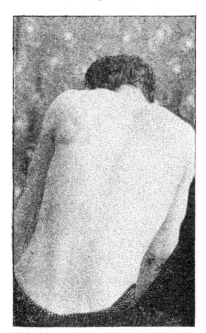

graph, though taken under the disadvantages of the diffused daylight of a hospital ward, shows, beside the peculiar attitude adopted by the patient, the spasm in the muscles. This spasm I should say had radiated to all the muscles of the back and even of the shoulder. An important symptom closely related to this spasm, and which should have been mentioned before, is the fact that the man spoke with great difficulty. His speech was short and jerky and seemed to give him pain in the back. It evidently caused him considerable effort and tired him

very much. Whether there was here a psychic element at play, or
whether the effort caused the spasm to radiate to the chest muscles and
perhaps also the diaphragm, it is impossible to say. The latter view,
however, seems to me to be the more probable.

The slight improvement in the patient's condition noted in February
has continued up to the present time. The patient, as a whole, is
stronger, sweating is less marked ; he is able to get out of bed and take
a few steps without assistance. The rigidity of the back, though still
present, is evidently diminished. Muscular spasm is, however, marked
in the lumbar region and the muscles still show excessive reflex excitability. Superficial spinal tenderness has largely disappeared, but pain
on deep pressure is still present. Knee-jerks still exaggerated. Sensation in feet and legs up to normal. Difficulty of emptying bladder;
though lessened, still persists. Mentally the patient has much improved
and when last seen was quite bright and cheerful.

The absence of litigation makes this case an exceedingly valuable
one. In a number of its features, too, it is unusually interesting and instructive. The fact that this patient steadily grew worse for almost five
weeks, and this, too, in the face of absolute rest and forced feeding, is
very remarkable. In spite of everything, his spasm, pain, rigidity and
asthenia steadily increased. It is somewhat difficult to frame an explanation, but the fact must be admitted. He is still in bed. Eye
symptoms, it should have been stated, were not present. There was no
contraction of the visual field.

CASE V.—A case somewhat similar is that of B. W., aged forty-two
years, married, and a carpenter and builder by trade, who presented
himself at the University Hospital, December 5, 1890. Last June,
while erecting a barn, he was struck by a large rafter in the middle of
the back, knocking him down and pinning him to the earth. He was
unconscious for a few minutes and later on was sick at his stomach.
Vomiting occurred repeatedly during the next four days, the vomit occasionally containing blood. During this time he was not confined to
the house, but continued outside directing his men at their work. He
said, however, that he felt giddy and was afraid to climb to a height. His
back, too, felt quite sore. About a week after the accident he began to
be troubled with headache, while the giddiness became more and more
marked. The soreness now spread all along his spine. His physician,
who accompanied him to the hospital, said that pressure upon the spine
now made him sick at the stomach and also caused his face to flush.
He was obliged to remain in-doors. He was unable to collect his
thoughts, could not concentrate his attention upon anything. Slept
badly, at night was restless and "delirious." He had also become very
weak.

Examination disclosed marked rigidity of the spinal column, excessive spasm and tremor of apparently all the muscles of the back,
great pain on pressure, especially at the site of the injury; pain on
movement in any direction; knee-jerks exaggerated on both sides;
ankle clonus present in both feet; paradoxical contraction of tibialis
anticus; excessive sweating and occasional flushing of the face. Mentally the man did not seem much depressed. He was bothered about

not being able to conduct his business, but otherwise seemed to take his condition quite philosophically.

This case is also interesting, because of the delay in the maximum onset of symptoms and also because of the bloody vomit. In accordance with our suggestion his physician placed him on the rest cure, and at last accounts he was considerably improved though still in bed. There was, of course, no element of litigation.

All three of these cases are interesting because of the entire absence of symptoms usually relegated to the domain of hysteria. In the following case, however, distinct hysterical symptoms are added.

CASE VI.—(See Fig. 3.)   H. M. G., aged twenty-three years, an employé in a rolling-mill; was in good health up to May 3, 1889. He was injured on that date in the same accident as J. C. J., the colored man

Fig. 3.

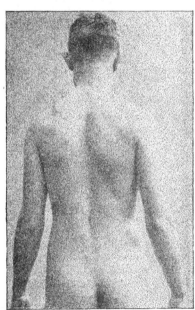

whose case has already been detailed. (See Case III.) He was sitting beside the colored man on the driver's box when the omnibus was struck by the engine. The last thing he remembers is the fact that they were crossing the railroad track. He then lost consciousness and some time later found himself lying on the platform of the adjacent station. Was confused but remembers that he asked to be taken home. That night he was very nervous and excited and continually imagined that "the train was coming on him." Had great pain in the head and back; could not move at all on account of it. For several days afterward he was "absent and bewildered." He could not pass his urine and had to be catheterized, while his bowels were obstinately constipated.   He was confined to the house, in bed and out, for a period of eight weeks. He was first examined on May 7, 1890, a year after the accident. He complained of constant pain in the head and back.   The spine was excessively rigid and very sensitive to superficial pressure.   General surface of the back hyperæsthetic.   Great soreness to deep pressure in small of back.   Pain in this region on flexion, torsion, and transmitted shock.   Slight lateral curvature to the right.   Decided spasm of the lumbar muscles on the left side.   Reflex excitability of the muscles of the back generally, very great.   Excessive knee-jerk and ankle clonus on both sides.   Cremaster and abdominal reflexes likewise excessive. Chin reflex also elicited.   Patient appears to be very weak.   Grip much below normal and very tremulous.   Both legs weak.   Patient limps badly with the left foot.   The instep is evidently very painful; the foot had been wrenched or badly bruised.   Sensation appears to be everywhere good, though patient occasionally makes errors of location.

He cannot work, cannot think clearly, cannot fasten his attention. Worries and feels badly.   Is very low-spirited.   Sleeps poorly, and dreams occasionally frightful dreams in which the horror of the accident recurs.   At those times his heart beats very fast.   Has at times ringing in the ears.   Pupils large and very mobile.   Visual field much contracted for both eyes.

I have had occasion to see this patient at intervals ever since, and repeatedly confirmed the above notes.   On a number of occasions he had convulsions, during which he appeared to be oblivious of his surroundings.   During the attack he would imagine that the accident was again occurring and he would cry out, " It is coming! it is coming! " evidently meaning the engine, and would be in a perfect paroxysm of fear. From descriptions that I obtained I judged the attacks to be distinctly hysterical.

The following case (Case VII., Figs. 4 and 5) presented mental symptoms probably hysterical in nature, associated with a *bona fide* railway back.

CASE VII.—G. H., aged forty-two, married, a carpenter by trade was in good health at the time of his accident, which occurred May 24, 1889.   He was seated in the rear end of a rear car of a train which was standing at a station.   He was leaning forward and turning to the left when another car, which was being added to the train, struck the car in which he was seated with great force.   His head and shoulders were violently jerked backward.   He instantly felt great pain in his back and cried out, " My God, my back!"   He supported his back with his hands, remained on the train a short while until his destination was reached and then tried to work.   However he was soon obliged to give up the attempt, for whenever he tried to use his saw or his plane the pain in his back became unbearable.   On the next day he made another ineffectual attempt to work.   He persevered for two hours and a half and was then forced to lie down for the balance of the day.   The next day was spent altogether in lying down, and from this time on he made ineffectual attempts at working, working fractions of some days and on others not at all until July, when he was obliged to desist altogether.

From September to December of the same year he again managed to work fractions of days, but always at the expense of great pain. Since that time he has been unable to work a stroke. He had grown decidedly worse. Was very weak and nervous, while his back was more painful than ever. He became very despondent and his appetite became very poor. He continued in this condition with but little or no change until February, 1891, when he had an attack of great mental excitement resembling mania, during which he manifested persecutory delusions and attempted suicide. The attack lasted from ten to twelve days, when depression again supervened. He became perfectly rational, but failed to remember any of the occurrences of the interim. Since this time he has had a number of convulsions which, from their description, were evidently hysterical in character.

Examined in March last he presented the following symptoms: His face is drawn and flat. Pupils excessively dilated. Eyebrows elevated and brow wrinkled, giving peculiar expression to face. Patient walks in

Fig. 4.

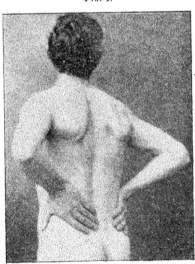

a peculiar manner, carrying his trunk very stiffly and supporting the small of the back with both hands. (See Fig. 4.) He rocks from side to side, throwing the right leg out and forward and slightly dragging the left.

The spine is exquisitely sensitive to superficial pressure, and deep pressure causes apparently intense pain. The muscles, especially in the lumbar region, appear to be very sore and in a condition of constant spasm. On handling them the spasm increases in severity and is evidently very painful. It is most marked on the right side. It is impossible to get the patient to flex the spine. He simply leans forward in the manner illustrated in Figure 5. Transmitted shock also elicits pain in the lumbar region. Knee-jerks plus on both sides, but readily exhausted. No anæsthesia. Bowels constipated; urine voided with much effort.

A remarkable and striking peculiarity of this patient is the difficulty he has in talking. His speech reminds one somewhat of the man who fell from the bridge, Case IV. It likewise is short and jerky and is evidently related, as in Case IV., to the spasm of the back muscles. If the man is in a condition of relative repose, the words can readily be understood and are merely uttered in a sharp, explosive manner. If, however, the spasm of the back muscles be increased by movement or by handling, the speech becomes so jerky as to be practically unintelligible, and indeed the patient is often compelled to desist from the

Fig 5.

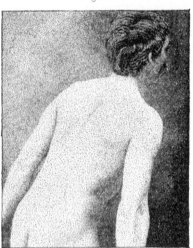

effort. It is exceedingly probable that this condition is owing to the fact that the spasm may radiate from one group of muscles to another and thus involve the chest and abdominal muscles. The involvement of the abdominal muscles is, by the way, quite evident at times. Further, when we reflect that the crura of the diaphragm arise from the very region of the spinal column which is proven by other tests to be the seat of the sprain, it becomes evident how readily the diaphragm might itself be affected with spasm, and this I believe, indeed, in the present instance, to be the case.

This patient, together with Case VI., resembles Cases III., IV. and V. very closely as regards the condition of the back and the associated symptoms of general asthenia. The fact, however, of the occurrence of the hysterical convulsions introduces another element to which full weight should be given. Regarding the physical condition of the back, however, let me repeat, there can be no doubt in either case.

I do not desire to tire by multiplying records and descriptions, but before entering into a discussion of the general questions involved, I will briefly present another case because of a condition not noted in the others, and because of the valuable lesson it teaches as regards the possible duration of the railway back.

CASE VIII.—F. W. S., male, aged twenty-seven years, married, a barber by trade; was injured February 23, 1887, during a collision between two street cars, the latter pursuing routes at right angles to one another. The collision was so violent that the car in which our patient was sitting was derailed and thrown over to the curbstone of the sidewalk, while his position was such that the full force of the blow was

FIG. 6.

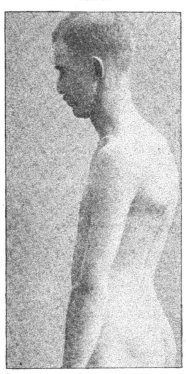

received by his back. He was thrown violently to the opposite side of the car while another passenger fell with and upon him. He was not rendered unconscious, but got up and walked to a neighboring store. He stood waiting for about three minutes and then boarded another car on which he rode about a mile. On leaving this car he became faint and weak and had to cling to surrounding objects for support. He was finally assisted to his home by a stranger and at once went to bed. Here he remained for six weeks. Backache, headache, disturbed sleep, and frequent micturition were symptoms from which he suffered.

He was first examined November 11th of the same year. Flexion, torsion, and transmitted shock, as well as pressure, elicited pain in the lumbar region. Marked muscular spasm was also noted on motion. In addition there was marked general weakness. The grip was weak and tremulous and there was also decided weakness of both legs, especially the right. Weakness, however, was not by any means confined to the extremities, but was also marked in the truncal muscles. (See Fig. 6.) The weakness of the back muscles was indeed so decided as to give rise to marked lordosis, and to this condition I desire particularly to call attention. Rigidity was not a marked feature at the time of the examination, and spasm was only excited by motion. When left to themselves the muscles everywhere became relaxed, resulting in the condition mentioned.

The associated symptoms in the case were similar to those already familiar, and need hardly be mentioned. There were present exaggerated knee-jerks and ankle clonus, while a chin reflex was also elicited which curiously enough involved in its response a contraction of the platysma myoides. No marked sensory symptoms. Mental condition that of depression. Sleep bad and frequently interrupted by the desire of voiding the urine. Frequent micturition a constant and distressing symptom. Urine free from sugar, but perhaps a little increased in amount. Sexual desire and power in abeyance.

Damages were awarded this man in November of 1887. In February, 1889, almost two years after the accident, I examined him again. There was no material change in his condition. There had been some gain in weight and there was much improvement in his mental condition, but pain in the back and muscular spasm were elicited as before. The reflexes were still exaggerated and ankle clonus was still present. The chin reflex, however, was less readily elicited than before. There had been some gain in general strength, but he was still unable to work more than two hours a day. Frequent micturition still present and necessitating his rising four or five times at night.

On May 29, 1890, he was again examined, as also in March, 1891, when the photograph was made (see Fig. 6), now fully four years after the accident. Little change has taken place in his condition. The pain in the back on flexion is somewhat lessened, though forced flexion provokes muscular spasm as of old. Pain can still be elicited by torsion and transmitted shock. The reflexes are still exaggerated, though less so than formerly. Micturition, however, is still as frequent as ever. General asthenia is still very marked, and, as he tells me, he still spends the greater portion of his time in lying down. Lordosis is perhaps a little less marked than formerly, though, as seen in the figure, still very evident.

The various symptoms presented by the six cases I have instanced can be conveniently grouped as follows: First, those due to the physical condition of the back; second, the symptoms of functional derangement and asthenia; third, psychic and hysterical symptoms. To the first group belong—first, pain on deep pressure; second, pain on motion and transmitted shock; third, muscular spasm and rigidity; fourth, muscular weakness.

Now the pain elicited by pressure, motion, or shock is evidently the result of a deep-seated injury either to the ligaments of the spinal column or to the muscles, probably to both. Practically it is impossible to differentiate between the two, nor is it important. We should remember, in thinking of the muscles, that they are normally in a state of tension, especially when the trunk is erect. Indeed, the physical condition presented is that of a bow with many strings. It is not difficult to understand how, under these circumstances, jars and blows should cause serious though perhaps minute strains of the muscles, especially in their tendinous insertions, and these, as we know, are excessively numerous. Further, it is not impossible that at times even the intervertebral cartilages and the joints formed by the articular processes may be the seat of sprain. I should certainly regard this probable in cases that reacted inordinately to transmitted shock and torsion.

To muscular spasm and rigidity are to be assigned the same value which is assigned to the muscular spasm observed in a sprained, a dislocated, or a broken limb. The muscular weakness, resulting occasionally in lordosis, is to be ascribed to the general weakness resulting from the shock and also to the direct effect of the trauma upon the muscles themselves.

To the group of symptoms of functional derangements and asthenia belong of course the various symptoms of general weakness, both mental and physical, tremor, sweating, inability to properly expel or to retain the urine, etc., but it is not our business to deal with them here.

To the group of psychic and hysterical symptoms we must of course relegate the hypochondria, the night terrors and the convulsions. These likewise it is not our business to discuss.

One important problem, however, still presents itself. Why is it that some of these cases do not attain their maximum severity for days and weeks after the accident? This was especially illustrated in Cases IV. and V. Both of these men suffered comparatively little at first, but after a time the symptoms were of the most pronounced character. I confess that this problem is somewhat difficult to answer. It has, however, seemed to me exceedingly probable that there was here a direct extension of inflammation from the original site of the trauma along the sheaths and tendons of the muscles. It is difficult to escape from this inference, inasmuch as there was a marked spread in the area of pain on deep pressure. Hand-in-hand with this there is beyond all doubt a radiation in the muscular spasm, a radiation too which may reach not only muscles immediately adjacent, but those even relatively remote, such as the muscles of the abdomen or the muscles of the shoulder.

Before closing I desire to touch on a point of great practical importance. We are almost invariably asked as to the probable duration of the symptoms and as to the prospect of entire recovery. Of course, an absolutely definite answer can never be given. It is a question of probability and of degree, and therefore one in which legitimate differences of opinion may obtain. However, taking the cases I have presented it is evident that chronicity must be admitted as established beyond cavil. Case IV., the man who fell from the bridge, has now been six months in bed and though somewhat improved is far from well. Case V. is now of ten months' duration and is still under treatment. Neither case involves litigation. Cases III. and VI. have each received damages, and yet two years after the accident, though slightly improved, each preserves the prominent features previously present. Case VII. is, I believe, still unsettled. However, it is improbable that anyone qualified to judge would fail to recognize the physical condition of the back. This, at the end of two years, is still very marked. Finally, Case VIII. still presents at the end of four years the more important points fully intact. Some improvement must be admitted with regard to all of them, and yet the photographs taken, all very recently, speak for themselves.

In regard to the disappearance of so-called "litigation symptoms," made so much of by Page and others, my observation has been that when a claim for damages has been settled, the mental condition improves very much. A man who, perhaps, is poor is suddenly raised to a condition of relative wealth. No wonder that hypochondria often disappears and is replaced by buoyancy and exaltation. It were strange indeed if it were otherwise. After a while, however, I have seen the old mental condition partly reëstablish itself while the physical condition had undergone no change save that which could be accounted for by the slow repair of time.

Lastly, the cases which I have presented were selected because of the marked and pronounced condition of the back. I do not, however, wish to create the impression that every case should present the back symptoms to an equal degree in order to be considered genuine. As a matter of fact, in a large number of instances of *bona fide* railway back the symptoms are far less evident than in the cases here detailed. To cite illustrations would add unnecessarily to the length of this paper. I will simply repeat that careful application of the various tests for eliciting pain and spasm cannot fail to evoke a reply if trauma be really present.

INOCULATIONS FOR YELLOW FEVER BY MEANS OF CONTAMINATED MOSQUITOES.

By Charles Finlay, M.D.,
OF HAVANA.

At the time when my former article was written[1] I observed that the figures there given were not considered by me, "from a statistical point

---

[1] "Yellow Fever: Its Transmission by Means of the Culex Mosquito." AMERICAN JOURNAL OF THE MEDICAL SCIENCES, October. 1886. p. 395.

of view, to afford any definite clew either in favor or against the prophylactic value of my inoculations." In fact, neither the number of
my experiments nor the length of time during which the parties inoculated had been under observation could at that time justify any scientific
deductions. Now, however, the case is different; I have on record a
series of sixty-seven persons, including all those whom, in collaboration
with Dr. Delgado, I have inoculated since 1881, by means of contaminated mosquitoes, in the manner explained in my previous article. All
were Europeans, with few exceptions natives of Spain, young adults
recently arrived in Cuba and presenting the usual conditions which
imply liability to contract yellow fever. Among the sixty-seven a considerable number, fifty-two, are considered as acclimated, either from
the fact that they have resided in the infected quarters of the city of
Havana (the old town) during periods varying between three and seven
years, or in consideration of their having experienced fevers which are
attributed to the yellow fever infection, though of a mild type in the
vast majority of the cases. Two parallel groups, one of thirty-three
inoculated persons and the other of thirty-two *not inoculated*, both offering to all intents and purposes such similarity (as to susceptibility and
exposure) as can seldom be obtained, afford a reliable foundation for a
fair and unbiassed comparison. I consider, therefore, that the time is
now come when some practical inferences may be drawn, and, as far
as they go, I am happy to say that they agree with my former expectations.

The statistical method of demonstration is, at best, a tedious and a
slow process, but it can boast of great triumphs, such as are recorded in
the instances of Jenner and Pasteur, who have had to rely exclusively
on its results in order to bring over to their views the balance of scientific opinion and public favor. They represent, moreover, two distinct
applications of that method. Jenner vaccinated indiscriminately a vast
number of subjects in order to verify subsequently the immunity enjoyed by the majority when exposed to the variolous infection. Pasteur,
on the other hand, adopted the system of carefully registering every
person inoculated by his method after being bitten by a rabid animal,
and afterward comparing the statistical results observed in them with
the average proportion of hydrophobic cases developed in the non-
inoculated after similar bites. I have chosen Pasteur's plan, believing
it to be the more reliable and more applicable to our case. It cannot
be denied, however, that, limited as we have been in our field of experiment, our numbers cannot compare with those of the glorious French
investigator, nor that we labor under a disadvantage in having to deal
with a disease which so far has not been proved to occur, under ordinary circumstances, in lower animals. Thus obliged to confine our
investigations to the human species, it could hardly be expected of us

that we should carry our scientific zeal to the point of seeking, through a bolder application of our inoculations, to determine a violent attack of the disease—thereby carrying conviction, no doubt, to the sceptical mind, but at the risk of having betrayed the confidence placed in us.

A somewhat specious objection was recently raised against our mosquito-inoculations, on the plea that the proboscis of the insect not being susceptible of sterilization many accidental germs might be inoculated together with or instead of those of yellow fever, supposing the latter to exist in the proboscis of the contaminated mosquito. To this hypothetical imputation I can oppose many facts. In none of our numerous inoculations has such an occurrence been observed, nor has it ever been proved that the acclimated inhabitants who are constantly being stung by those insects acquire thereby any specific infection. I have on several occasions introduced into sterilized tubes provided with agar jelly mosquitoes that had stung acclimated persons. In most of these experiments, after several days' confinement, the insect died for want of food, and yet not a single colony appeared upon the jelly; when any growth was developed it mostly consisted of fungi, the spores of which had probably been introduced accidentally while transferring the insect from one tube into another. From this curious result I infer that the insect has some means of rendering its outer surface aseptic, and probably does so through a very peculiar operation which I have often seen it perform. This consists in collecting with its hind or middle legs a secretion expelled from the posterior part of its body, and besmearing very persistently with it every part of its body—legs, wings, head, and proboscis. I also believe that we are justified in admitting that the liquid which the insect employs to lubricate its complicated sting, and which being poured into the wound occasions the painful sensation felt by its victim, must vary in its chemical composition in different species of gnats, thereby accounting for the difference in the sensations occasioned by their sting. It is quite possible, therefore, that the presence of that liquid may constitute in the sting of the culex mosquito an appropriate soil for the development of the yellow fever germ, whereas the same germ would remain sterile in the sting of other species of culex.

Another objection of a clinical character was made to our considering as cases of mild yellow fever the attacks of non-albuminuric fever observed in our inoculated subjects, either within the plausible limits of incubation or later on, with the result of rendering them immune against subsequent attacks of albuminuric yellow fever. To this objection an answer is given by the present statistics themselves, inasmuch as among fifty-six inoculated and non-inoculated subjects mentioned therein and who have resided during periods varying between three and seven consecutive years in the city of Havana, *one-half* have acquired their immunity exclusively through non-albuminuric attacks suffered during the first three years after their arrival here.   If the objection turned out to be well grounded, it would only prove that what we had considered as a partial immunity had been a complete one in ninety per cent. of our inoculated subjects.

I have distributed our sixty-seven inoculated subjects into six groups:

GROUP I. Fifteen—whose observation is yet incomplete, not having resided three years in Havana, nor experienced any form of yellow fever.

GROUP II. Twelve—who experienced, within a period of days varying between three and twenty-five, after the inoculation, an attack of fever with or without albuminuria.

GROUP III. Twelve—who did *not* experience any pathogenic effects within the twenty-five days following the inoculation, nor any other febrile attack subsequently, that could be referred to the yellow fever infection.

GROUP IV. Twenty-four—who did not experience pathogenic effects within the twenty-five days, but subsequently had fevers of a mild type, either non-albuminuric or with slight or transient albuminuria.

GROUP V. Three—who experienced no pathogenic effects after the inoculation, but were subsequently attacked with regular albuminuric yellow fever (severe in two cases), but recovered.

GROUP VI. One—who not having experienced pathogenic effects after the inoculation, was attacked some months later, and after exposure to an infection of unusual intensity, with fatal yellow fever.

After excluding the fifteen incomplete observations of Group I., fifty-two cases remain to be considered which may be conveniently arranged under three heads:

Mild acclimation (Groups II., III., IV.) .	48 cases	= 92.2 per cent.
Acclimation with regular yellow fever—			
cured	3 "	= 5.9 "
Fatal yellow fever	1 "	= 1.9 "
	52		

The next point was to obtain reliable data for comparison.   I was fortunate in receiving from two religious communities placed under my medical charge the authorization to practise my inoculations on such members as would be willing to submit to them.   These communities are those of the Jesuit and Carmelite Fathers, established in the city of Havana.   Their members are partially renewed almost every year by the arrival of new-comers from Spain to substitute others who have resided several years here.   Since 1883, every year except 1885 I have inoculated some of the new-comers, while others did not go through that ordeal.   During the period 1883–1890 the Jesuit Fathers have had thirty-six inoculated and seven not, and the Carmelites had thirteen inoculated and twenty-five not inoculated. Of the inoculated none have died of yellow fever, whereas five of the non-inoculated have died of it (one Jesuit and four Carmelites). After deducting from the inoculated thirteen cases still under observation, we have thirty-three inoculated and thirty-three not inoculated members of the same communities, having arrived in the same years as the former, leading the same life and exposed to the same chances of infection.

	Inoculated.	Not inoculated.
Mild acclimation (Groups II., III., IV.)	31 = 94 p. c.	21 = 65½ p. c.
Acclimation with regular yellow fever —cured	2 = 6 "	6 = 19 "
Died of yellow fever—none of the inoculated, but of the non-inoculated		5 = 15½ '
	33	32

The conclusions which the above statistical results, together with the comparative observations, appear to justify are as follows :

1. The inoculations with one or two recently contaminated mosquitoes, in the manner practised by ourselves, is free from danger, inasmuch as the numerous trials which have been made have produced at most (in about 18 per cent. of our cases) a mild attack followed by immunity.

2. We must attribute to the influence of the inoculations with contaminated mosquitoes : 1. The mild acclimation observed in 94 per cent. of our cases, whereas the same desirable result has only occurred, cœteris paribus, in 65½ per cent. of the non-inoculated ; 2. The reduction of cases of regular yellow fever to the proportion of 6 per cent. instead of 19 per cent. ; and 3. That of fatal yellow fever to less than 2 per cent. instead of 15½ per cent., one single death from yellow fever having occurred among the sixty-seven persons inoculated by us since 1881 until the present date.

3. The contaminated mosquitoes appear to lose either partially or completely their contamination after they have stung healthy subjects ; whereas the contamination appears to become intensified by successive stings of the same insect on yellow fever patients.

4. The inoculations performed during the colder season should not be considered to afford sufficient protection, but should be repeated on the approach of the hot season.

UREA AND SEROUS MEMBRANES.

BY C. S. BOND, M.S., M.D.,

RICHMOND, INDIANA.

IT has been known for years and has been a part of the clinical experience of all careful observers in this field, that in chronic Bright's disease, serous membranes in various parts of the body were attacked by inflammations and that these secondary conditions resulted often in the great distress or death of the individual. The pericardium became inflamed, serum accumulated and within a few hours the patient was dead. A sudden peritonitis would develop in an apparently convalescing person and the day of doom had come to the patient. An acute attack of pleurisy would set at rest another slowly tortured with the familiar dropsy, dyspnœa, and fluttering heart. Thus I might review the clinical history of many of these sufferers, and glance briefly at these inflammations in various and often remote parts of the body by way of illustration, but more than this mere mention I deem not necessary.

These inflammations at this time in the disease are doubtless due to a combination of causes, and are generally common factors with the lesion in the kidney. The waste-laden blood is carried to tissues which it has for a long period of time failed to supply with sufficient nourishment, and even the small morsel it now offers is so mixed with the offending excrementitious products that they are not able to assimilate it. The bloodvessels themselves have undergone àn atheromatous degeneration that, together with the contracted arteries, causes such increase of blood-pressure that the heart has enlarged and still fails in its irregular efforts to supply the necessary nourishment. No great wonder, then, that these highly vascular and therefore most imposed upon membranes should cry out with pain and even finally succumb.

It is well known from an extended observation both of the clinical features of this disease and of the many carefully recorded tests of the excretions from the kidneys, that the excreted urea which such organs eliminate in constantly diminished quantity is, when taken with the other symptoms, the most reliable guide in diagnosis, even though the patient be passing albumin and casts. It is also known that this same relation holds good in cases not passing albumin and casts, and that the severity of the clinical features of the disease can be determined often by a knowledge of this excrementitious product, after many recorded tests have been made, without the presence of the patient.

The purpose of this paper, therefore, is to recite cases which, to my mind, make clear that serous membranes are not only involved in inflammation during the pronounced evidences of Bright's disease, but that they are often involved seriously before the times of passing albumin and casts, and that these inflammations cannot be properly considered in a diagnostic way without a thorough knowledge of the amount of urea excreted daily for a long period of time for individual cases. Finally, these cases will show that these membranes are involved in the general disturbances which are now so indefinitely known to be associated with diseased kidneys, by the common knowledge of the clinical and excreted evidence.

PELVIC PERITONITIS.

CASE I.—In January, 1887, I was called to see a woman in great haste on account of some acute pain in the abdomen. She was about twenty-three years of age, well nourished, married; had had no children, or abortions; no history of gonorrhœa or syphilis. For some weeks past had had slight dyspnœa on exertion, with headache. She had no other history of disease and considered herself well to this date, with exceptions noted. Physical examination showed patient in recumbent position with legs flexed on abdomen, suffering from severe pain. Pressure upon the abdomen caused increase of pain. Slight distention of bowels with gas. Examination *per vaginam* of pelvic organs disclosed great tenderness in pelvic floor, with serous effusion, most marked in front and right side of uterus. Patient, after chilly sensations, had now a temperature of 103°; pulse firm and small, beating 120 times per minute. Had slight nausea and the characteristic face. Had been attacked without traumatic or other known cause a few hours before my visit, and was now anxious to be relieved from pain. One-third of a grain of morphia was administered hypodermically and pain was allayed for several hours, after which morphia was taken by mouth to modify pain. The day following my first visit pain still continued more or less intense, unless under the influence of the anodyne. Examination *per vaginam* now disclosed more serous infiltration and consequently a more firm pelvic floor. Within a few days the characteristic "deal board" hardness and fixation of uterus was established and pain began to subside slowly, with frequent exacerbations, and terminated in recovery by slow absorption, which extended over a period of several weeks. At the close of this period patient still complained of headache, slight nausea, dyspnœa on exertion and general weakness, although she had apparently recovered her former health. Examination of her urine at this time showed no albumin or casts, after repeated trials, but the quantity of urea excreted in twenty-four hours ranged from twelve to eighteen grammes within this interval, and patient again, after six months from first attack, and soon after these examinations, lapsed suddenly into her former condition of pain and serous effusion. It now occurred to me that there was an intimate relation between the diminished quantity of urea excreted and this inflammation, as other parts of the history were negative, and in addition to the hypodermic injection of morphia I gave a second hypodermic of pilocarpine, which caused free perspiration, and this was followed by an active saline cathartic, which was repeated within twenty-four hours, and the bowels were thoroughly emptied. After three days of this kind of treatment hostilities on the part of the peritoneum had ceased, and what promised to be a more serious attack than before, terminated thus abruptly. After this experience it was determined to try, as far as possible, to avert another attack by giving attention in the interval to the excretions. Nitro-glycerin, saline cathartics, and sudorifics were vigorously used until the normal standard of from twenty-five to thirty-five grammes of urea was excreted daily and the patient so far recovered her health as to claim to be entirely well. At this time she became pregnant, and during the whole of her pregnancy she protested herself well; although I repeatedly inquired concerning her health and warned her of her probable troubles at delivery, she did not feel that she had any distress that she could not easily attribute to her condition. At about the eighth month of gestation I was called to her confinement, and after three hours of fruitless efforts, while the os was yet but slightly dilated, she had the first convulsion and continued unconscious until the child was delivered, having three other convulsions in the interim. At this time the urine showed no albumin or casts, but only 9.6 grammes of urea within twenty-four hours were excreted. Patient recovered rapidly on saline cathartics and former remedies, and since that time, May, 1889, has had but one or two slight attacks of peritoneal pain, and is well, so far as appearance and urinary tests can discover, except having a mitral regurgitant murmur, developed at or near the time of confinement, with slight enlargement of the left side of the heart. As repeated examinations of the chest were made before that time, I know the date of its appearance, and it may be well to state that no history of rheumatism can be obtained.

CASE II.—Mrs. B., aged forty, married, had had five children, no abortions. Had no history of gonorrhœa or syphilis. Had had several attacks of what a physician had called "bad misplacement of the womb," accompanied with very severe pain, before my visit. Attacks extended over several months; she was hardly up until another seizure. Before this visit had not had an attack for a month or six weeks and was in a fair state of general health. Now she had excruciating pain in region of pelvis, with knees flexed against abdomen, with increased pulse and elevated temperature. Examination *per vaginam* revealed a very tender pelvic floor with slight serous effusion on right side of uterus, which advanced from day to day, producing general hardness. As all other causes for this condition were absent, I examined the urine, to find that patient passed only 7.2 grammes of urea in twenty-four hours. Albumin and casts were never found in her urine. In ordinary fever, following acute conditions in other parts of the body, and in cases of pelvic peritonitis from other causes, urea is increased in amount. After anodynes to relieve pain, pilocarpine, saline cathartics and diuretics were used vigorously and patient made a rapid recovery. A careful record of her examinations now shows an ebb in the urea excreted, and a renewal of her former attacks, which gradually grew lighter, until, when she removed from observation, she had not had an attack for almost a year, and was apparently well, excreting from twenty-three to thirty grammes of urea in twenty-four hours.

Two other well-marked cases have come under my observation as still further illustrating these conditions, and I no longer have any doubt of the relation of these factors. One of these cases has had repeated attacks and always at the ebb of urea excretion, promptly recovering under the treatment suggested, and thus can be prevented, for long intervals, from having even slight attacks. I do not want to be considered as saying that any considerable part of the whole number of cases of pelvic peritonitis is due to this cause, but I do mean to say that such cases are frequently enough met with, even in a limited private practice, to cause a very serious reflection on the part of the profession.

PERICARDITIS.

CASE III.—In August, 1889, I was called to a man, twenty-six years of age, who was found unconscious in a water closet the previous day; had been seen by other doctors and pronounced a case of morphia poisoning. Patient was of good habits, and had no history of syphilis, rheumatism, or indeed any disease, except a profuse diarrhœa for a day or two previous, for which morphia had been taken. Examination now showed patient to be profoundly unconscious, pupils slightly dilated, pulse 110, respiration 20, slight twitching of muscles in forearm, temperature 100°. Examination of urine showed no albumin or casts, but patient passed only 9.6 grammes of urea in twenty-four hours. Saline cathartics and diuretics soon caused patient to rally, and when otherwise apparently well he still complained of the usual dyspnœa, vertigo, nausea and insomnia at times, and a record of his excretions showed at such times a very small quantity of urea excreted. At no time did he pass albumin or casts, although very frequent examinations were made. Patient was a candymaker, and went to work at his trade, against advice, in a neighboring town in last November. In January of this year he returned to the office again, suffering from what he called a bad cold, which was really another explosion of disease. Records show at this time ten grammes of urea, dyspnœa, vertigo, vomiting, twitching of muscles over body, and within two days pericardium began to fill with fluid, heart beat muffled and 110 times per minute, temperature 101°, respiration 26, dizzy and soon became unconscious, and within the night died. Post-mortem showed chronic interstitial nephritis and pericarditis with extensive effusion.

CASE IV.—This was a man, sixty-five years of age, well nourished; no history of syphilis or rheumatism; had considered himself well until within a few weeks of this consultation. Had had within this time dyspnœa, exhaustion on slight exertion, dizziness, and nausea. Had, at this first visit, a temperature of 102°, pulse 100, which had been preceded by a slight chill. Had slight distress in chest, accompanied by dyspnœa. Examination of the chest revealed an inflamed pericardium with slight effusion. The effusion during the succeeding days became very pronounced and caused quite uncomfortable dyspnœa and interfered with the heart's action. Not wishing to grant the idiopathic origin of this disease in this case and not finding another alternative, I, remembering Case I., examined his urine, to find no albumin or casts but that he passed only eight or ten grammes of urea in twenty-four hours, and that this condition extended over several days, contrary to the rule in idiopathic cases, which pass large quantities of urea. Indeed this case had almost fallen into obscurity by simulating to belong to such a class. Two other attacks followed this one within the following year and were marked by small quantities of excreted urea. The first of these was lighter than the original, and the last was lightest of all. The treatment from the beginning was nitro-glycerin, diuretics, saline cathartics, and sudorifics. The vertigo, general weakness, nausea, and dyspnœa that at first distressed patient during the intervals, gradually subsided, as excretions improved, until patient now considers himself well, as he has not had an attack of pericarditis for almost two years and the other symptoms are almost entirely relieved.

Two other well-marked cases of this variety have come under my care with similar results.

ARTHRITIS.

The relation between serous and synovial membranes is so close that I relate two cases of extensive inflammatory conditions in these membranes, as I believe them to be connected with this subject:

Case V.—A man, twenty-one years of age; had no history of rheumatism in parents; had not had syphilis, gonorrhœa, or any serious illness until four years ago, when the present sickness began; had no bad habits—neither drank nor chewed; married, had healthy child. Had always been a farmer in easy circumstances. Four years ago had an attack of so-called rheumatism, vertigo, and general malaise. Joints of lower extremities at this time were swollen and tender; could not walk for several days, and suffered at times with them. Was treated for rheumatism in a neighboring town, and after several weeks recovered. At the same time dyspnœa and the other symptoms passed off and patient resumed his occupation, occasionally relapsing into the condition of dyspnœa and other similar symptoms. Two years ago he had a similar attack to that first mentioned and it ran an analogous course; apparently recovered, with exceptions of general weakness and dyspnœa on slight exertion. Last January I was consulted and made the following record: Joints of lower extremities slightly tender, but not much swollen, and no concretions on motion. Legs were slightly œdematous between articulations, and this had been much more marked, patient thought, during former attacks. Had marked dyspnœa, dizziness, and nausea. Had insomnia and malaise. Symptoms had been increasing in severity for the past ten days, and he feared one of his former severe attacks. The history caused me to examine the urine. I found neither albumin nor casts, but he was excreting only ten grammes of urea. Heart and other organs healthy, except slight roughness of mitral valves. The treatment before mentioned several times in this paper averted what promised to be a serious attack, and after a few weeks all distressing symptoms were gone and patient considered himself entirely well. All medication for rheumatism had not relieved any of these symptoms promptly, and some remained constantly. Patient went to Nebraska to follow his calling and consequently passed out of my charge. During the summer had another attack, and, from what I can learn from the family of his symptoms, must have died from chronic disease of kidneys, accompanied with many of former symptoms.

Another well-marked case of this kind of inflammation is now under observation—a woman, aged twenty, who has not walked for more than a year. Joints are tender and slightly swollen, but the intervening tissue is much more so. There are no concretions in the joints, no thickening of ends of bones. She has the accompanying symptoms of dyspnœa, nausea, vertigo, and a feeling of general weakness, with pale lips. Muscles are not atrophied; heart, lungs, and other organs healthy. Has no history of rheumatism, syphilis, or gonorrhœa. Parents healthy. Patient has been treated for past three years for these relapsing attacks, and is now an invalid. Examination of urine shows that patient passes but twelve to fourteen grammes of urea daily. No albumin or casts or other evidence of disease of kidneys, save those noted above.   Patient has been under observation but two or three weeks, and under saline cathartics, sudorifics, and diuretics, she is rapidly improving and gives promise of walking again soon, after having been confined to the house for over a year, and having been treated for rheumatism by six or seven doctors, with all the nostrums known to the profession, without avail.

ENDARTERITIS.

CASE VI.—In April, 1886, I was called to see a woman, sixty-five years of age, who for several months past had been "gradually growing worse," as she states.   Had now vertigo, blindness, nausea, and general weakness; could not walk about home without great exhaustion.   Had no history of either rheumatism or syphilis in herself or parents.   Did not drink alcoholic beverages.   Had to be in bed at times because of irritable heart and extreme dyspnœa causing much exhaustion.   Had intercostal pain and headache at times.   Passed at this time but 6.7 grammes of urea in twenty-four hours.   On diuretics and saline cathartics patient improved in a short time and was able to do some work and be out of doors.   Urea excreted in four months after first visit amounted at one time to twenty-four grammes in twenty-four hours, and patient was comfortably well.   In December, 1886, she had another explosion of former symptoms, which came on suddenly, and in addition to old symptoms had delusions and hallucinations.   Same treatment again seemed to improve patient, but one night she slipped from the house and drowned herself in the river which flowed near by.   Post-mortem showed extensive atheromatous degeneration of bloodvessels in head and many other regions of body.   Kidneys were slightly smaller than normal, but gave no more evidence of disease than other organs, and bloodvessels were not as much changed here as elsewhere.

CASE VII.—In September, 1886, I saw a woman, forty-six years of age, who had no history of rheumatism or syphilis; the mother of several healthy children ; had been for several months distressed by headache, vertigo, nausea, great dyspnœa upon slight exertion, intercostal neuralgia, and general weakness.   Examination of urine at this time showed no albumin or casts, but she passed only 4.1 grammes of urea in twenty-four hours.   Within two months she grew apparently better. Passed 19.2 grammes of urea, but passed trace of albumin with casts. Within the year following she developed marked insanity.   At this time the radial arteries were atheromatous.   The heart was slightly enlarged and with an irregular effort was doing the best service it could. Patient was sent away and died, therefore no post-mortem was made ; but I have no reason to doubt the diagnosis.

CASE VIII.—A man, fifty-nine years of age ; had always been healthy until about a year previous to my seeing him in July, 1886.   Had no history of rheumatism or syphilis.   Had healthy family of children. Drank no alcoholic beverages.   Had a continuous aching in lumbar and intercostal regions, together with occasional nausea, vomiting, dyspnœa, and vertigo, which had continued for several months with varying severity.   Had atheromatous condition of radial and temporal arteries. Passed from 12.7 to 15.2 grammes of urea in twenty-four hours for several weeks.   Appetite generally good.   After several months in this condition he had a sudden paralysis of left side, and after some months more without relief from symptoms he had another stroke, from which he finally died.   No post-mortem, but no question remains of the gen-

Three or four other cases with similar histories are upon my records of the past six or seven years, and I have no doubt of the pathological changes underlying these clinical pictures, nor have I grave doubts of the steps leading up to this final fatal conclusion.

CASE IX.—A clergyman, sixty-eight years of age; always an active man; never had any constitutional disease but this. Has always maintained the dignity of his profession, and is the father of several healthy children. About one year ago he began to be dizzy. Had slight dyspnœa on exertion. Has now irregular heart action. Sometimes it beats only forty times per minute for several days in succession, and quite irregularly even then. Has hardened radial arteries, slight vertigo, and insomnia. Passes only twelve to eighteen grains of urea in twenty-four hours. Passes no albumin or casts, and careful physical examination reveals to my mind no other diseased organs or tissues.

This man is still under my care. What can I tell him and his friends will finally befall him? Will he die of apoplexy, Bright's disease, endarteritis, or a combination of these, if no other disease intervene? He evidently is now at the point where all these roads meet, and it is still an open question on which one the fell destroyer will most rapidly make his approach, after he has been retarded as long as possible by the use of drugs. What shall I name this hydra-headed disease? Meigs styles it endarteritis. If in a short time he passes albumin and casts, in accordance with what Bright said many years ago, all practitioners now would unite in calling it Bright's disease. If he die from pericarditis, pleurisy, or peritonitis, without passing albumin or casts, they could not be called secondary to a primary Bright's disease; nor with this general evidence, together with the excreted evidences of ill-health, could we say that these diseases were idiopathic. We therefore need a new name that shall cover these symptoms of disease. We have abandoned dyspnœa, vertigo, and dropsy in our list of diseases, and have placed our outposts but a little further into the darkness which surrounds this whole subject, and now the facts that are brought to light from beyond these distant landmarks are demanding new names for the newly discovered conditions that shall take into account the full connotation of the term. During the time of Bright there were vaguely grouped several acute and chronic affections of the kidneys, which had in common one important characteristic—that the urine contained albumin. Almost every year since that time changes have been made in the classification to more nearly correspond to the pathological conditions, until it was discovered that patients could have otherwise this identical disease without passing albumin, and finally even albumin is beginning to be lost sight of in our rapid march toward the source of all these symptoms.

In endeavoring to find the first departure from health in the direction of these extensive after-changes in vessels, organs, and tissues, many theories have been advanced, and are of importance only so far as they can be incorporated into the clinical conditions of these patients.

George Johnson believes that chronic Bright's disease is a constitu-

tional malady, as shown by a morbid condition of the blood, which causes changes in the secreting cells of the kidney, and then finally to changes in bloodvessels in kidneys and other organs. DaCosta and Longstreth believe that there are lesions of the renal nerve plexuses and possibly in other ganglia that should lead finally to these extensive changes in the kidneys. Semmola believes it to be a morbid change in nutrition, and that the kidney changes are due to a constant excretion of albumin. Gull and Dutton believe these extensive changes to be due, as a primary factor, to a fibrosis of the arteries and capillaries. Meigs has made perhaps the most lasting guess by first basing it upon a most worthy study of numerous pathological specimens of arteries from the different classes of these patients, and he inclines to the belief that the initial step is an endarteritis of many or few of the bloodvessels, which in the beginning or after a longer or shorter time may, and probably will, involve the arteries of the kidneys. Thomas believes that some irritating substances in the blood, as alcohol, large quantities of phosphates, urates or uric acid, lead, and oxalates, have a tendency, after a long time, to produce the contracted kidney.

If, now, anyone who has made a careful study of this whole subject, with ample clinical advantages and without bias, should be called upon to decide from these views and many others which might have been named, I am inclined to the belief that no decision could be reached as to who was most nearly in accord with all the observed phenomena of these diseases. The want of a constant sign that would be unvarying in its relation to the clinical evidence on the one hand, and the pathological changes on the other, seems to me to be much more important. It is with this object in view that I have tried to show the intimate relation which seems to exist, under all these varying conditions of this many-sided disease, between the abnormally small amount of urea excreted and these serous inflammations which precede, accompany, and follow Bright's disease. If I should be led to express a purely fanciful notion of this relation, I should be compelled to say, for want of a more plausible explanation, that urea is in some way the cause of these inflammations, or, the cause of the suppression of this excrementitious product causes such inflammations. I am inclined to this view, as the same clinical evidence exists in the patient in a more mild form, but still pronounced, as is well known to exist in some of its forms in toxic conditions resulting from an undeniable uræmia, and because at the other extreme we find this clinical evidence in very close relation to the excreted evidence before any visible sign of inflammation has begun, and are enabled to follow these patients until the first serous invasion has taken place in an apparently healthy, well-nourished, young patient oftentimes, as shown by my tables published in THE AMERICAN JOURNAL OF THE MEDICAL SCIENCES, January, 1890.

REVIEWS.

A PRACTICAL TREATISE ON FRACTURES AND DISLOCATIONS. By FRANK
H. HAMILTON, M.D., LL.D., Surgeon to Bellevue Hospital, New York.
New (eighth) edition, revised and edited by STEPHEN SMITH, A.M., M.D.
8vo., pp. 832. Philadelphia: Lea Bros. & Co., 1891.

THE eighth edition of Dr. Hamilton's well-known treatise has been
improved in practical value by the judicious revising and editing of Dr.
Stephen Smith, of New York, and still retains its old position, which is
that of the most comprehensive and reliable work upon this subject in
the English language. With the possible exception of the section on
fractures contained in Agnew's *Surgery*, there is no other teaching on
the subject which combines accuracy of statement, fulness of detail, and
sound practical judgment as does this work.

In looking over it for evidence of the contributions of the present
editor the following seem worthy of mention :

Dr. Smith quotes, with approval, the opinion of Dr. William Hunt,
in reference to active and prompt laryngotomy or tracheotomy after
fractures of the cartilages of the larynx, and adds the suggestion of
Pick in relation to the employment of Trendelenburg's tampon-canula
to aid in maintaining the cartilages in position after they have been restored.

In reference to fractures of the vertebral arches he quotes the cases
of Macewen, Horsley, Gordon, and Dandridge, and adds : " Unsatisfactory as operations have thus far proved to be, there are exceptional
cases in which they will prove useful. Macewen has thus expressed
the opinion that is entertained by the most advanced· surgeons on this
subject : ' Traumatic lesions are, as a rule, so gross, and the destruction
so complete, that in such operative treatment can be of little service.
Still there are cases in which traumatism has produced localized pressure, primary or secondary, which can be relieved.' "

This can scarcely be regarded as entirely satisfactory in the face of
the rapidly accumulating statistics of operations upon fractured vertebræ, showing a slight but progressive increase in favorable results. It
is well, however, in a treatise intended for the guidance of the general
practitioner, to err on the side of caution and conservatism.

In relation to fracture of the bodies of the vertebræ the recent results of treatment by suspension and plaster-of-Paris jacket are briefly
discussed, and the experiences of Kónig, Wagner, Burrell, and others
are recorded.

The addition of the description of Bryant's ilio-femoral triangle is in
our opinion of distinct value. We have found it in our own experience
one of the most valuable methods of determining with the least possible disturbance of the patient the exact seat of a shortening known to
exist somewhere between the ilium and the condyles of the femur.

The interesting observation of Dr. Sutton, of London, in reference to the etiology of Pott's fracture, is quoted with apparent approval: " Dr. Sutton notices the comparative length of the external malleolus in man and adds: 'If this malleolus in man is compared with that of mammals, which so closely approach him in anatomical characters, it will be found to descend much lower.' He states that no one has ever described an example of Pott's fracture in a monkey, nor, indeed, in any mammal save man ; he concludes that Pott's fracture is peculiar to the human kind, and occurs as a distinct result of the extraordinary length of the fibula malleolus, in that it affords excessive leverage when the foot is suddenly and violently twisted laterally, the force applied to the distal end causing the fibula to snap at some point in its lower fourth."

In reference to the correction of deformity after badly set Pott's fractures, the methods of Erichsen (subcutaneous division of the fibula and forcible adduction) ; Le Dentu (refracture and the employment of an osteoclast) ; Fenger (removal of a piece from the tibia and re-fracture of the fibula) ; and Sabine (subcutaneous osteotomy of both bones) are detailed.

In 1888 we saw in the wards of Professor Lister, in London, an interesting case which, in a letter to *The Medical News*, we described as follows : " One of the most striking cases which I saw was an operation for the relief of the deformity caused by badly treated Pott's fracture. The fibula had been broken at the usual point, and there had also been a fracture through the base of the external malleolus; the foot was so greatly everted that the limb was absolutely useless to the patient ; this condition had persisted for more than a year. At the operation the soft parts were turned forward down to the bone by an incision following the posterior border of the fibula and of the external malleolus ; the fibula was divided at the point of fracture, the triangular space existing between the lower edge of the fibula and tibia, which was filled up with fibrous material of almost bony hardness, was cleared with the gouge, chisel and sharp spoon ; the soft parts over the internal malleolus were then turned forward by a similar incision, and the mass of new bone, which was easily recognized, and which filled up the gap between the two fragments of the malleolus, was chiselled away. After this the application of considerable force by means of pulleys brought the foot suddenly, but perfectly, into position. The subsequent course of the case was absolutely uncomplicated, and the patient, at the end of three weeks, already had considerable motion without pain in the ankle-joint."

We have recently done practically this same operation in a patient who had a similar deformity and with most excellent results.

In reference to dislocation of the acromial end of the clavicle upward Hamilton gives the usual unfavorable prognosis. The editor adds a description of the ingenious dressings employed by Dr. Powers, of New York, and Dr. Pilcher, of Brooklyn. We have had two cases, in both of which by the application of a dressing resembling these we have succeeded in getting an almost perfect result. In one of them, now more than eighteen months old, no difference between the shoulders is discoverable. In the diagnosis of this dislocation it may be useful to note that the vertical circumference of the shoulder is slightly increased, but to a less extent than in dislocations of the humerus ; that the distance from the acromial end of the clavicle to the external con-

dyle is increased, and that the distance from the same point to the supra-
sternal notch remains unaltered.

Unfortunately, like most other surgeons, we have had a much larger
number of cases in which permanent disability of moderate extent resulted. Dr. Smith gives the following excellent amplification of Hamilton's statement that in compound dislocation the treatment should
include "a judicious employment of antiseptic precautions and of
drainage." The rule of practice should be as follows: "1· Determine
the amount of injury which the structures about the joint have sustained. If the vessels and nerves are so far uninjured that the limb
can be saved, determine upon reduction or resection. 2. In either case
cut away tissues so bruised or torn that death is likely to ensue. Disinfect all the exposed surfaces with hot sublimate solutions (1 : 4000),
the water being injected forcibly with a bulb-syringe. The solution
should be of a temperature of not less than 130° to 140°, or so that the
hand can scarcely be retained in it. If of the proper temperature the
irrigated tissues will be changed to a dull-gray color. The greatest
care is necessary to force this solution into every part of the joint, and
among the tissues. 3. Reduction or resection should now be effected
with little strain upon the tissues. 4. Ample drainage should be provided, the drainage-tube or tubes extending to every recess. 5. The
wound should be closed by the union with suture of all divided tissues
which can be brought into easy apposition. 6. Antiseptic dressings,
enveloping the parts sufficiently, should be applied; and to maintain
rest a plaster-of-Paris dressing may be required, as at the knee or ankle.
These dressings should not be changed for three or four weeks, unless there is evidence of disturbance in the wound. The tubes should
be removed in four or five days by opening fenestra where they are
located."

All this seems very sound, the only criticism which suggests itself to
us being the direction to leave the dressings undisturbed for three or
four weeks, unless there is evidence of trouble in the wound. It is
certainly true that in the great majority of cases a safer routine
method would be to inspect carefully at an earlier date than this, with,
of course, all possible precautions as to unnecessary movement.

Many valuable additions have been made in almost each chapter of
the book, and we may repeat our hearty indorsement of it as a safe and
reliable guide to the general practitioner. J. W. W.

De La Malaria. Par Dr. Edouard Pepper, L.F.P., Algiers. Précédé
d'une Introduction par M. le Professeur Peter. Paris: G. Masson, 1891.
A Contribution to the Study of Malaria, as Observed in Algiers.
By Dr. Edward Pepper, L.F.P.

The author of this interesting volume is an American physician of
recognized attainments in France, who having won distinction in the
Franco-Prussian war, and being in impaired health, has made Algiers
his residence. He has profited by the opportunity there offered to study
malarial infection, and dedicates his treatise to his friend Professor Peter,
of Paris.

In his introduction, Professor Peter emphasizes the fact that the patient's peculiarities influence very greatly the course and symptoms of his disease. He regards the malarial germ as an accompaniment, but not as the cause, of the disorder, and supports this opinion by an extensive clinical observation.

Dr. Pepper precedes his account of malaria as seen in Algiers, and its treatment, by a description of the country from the standpoint of the medical scientist, and the narration of the circumstances which led to an epidemic of malarial infection which came under his observation. He states most explicitly the best hygiene for foreigners living in Algiers, and this portion of his book cannot fail to be of great interest and value to any who may visit the country.

In the prophylaxis of malarial infection he has found precautions as to diet, clothing, and bathing of importance; also the use of a few drops of an arsenical solution, taken with coffee or any agreeable beverage, when the patient is fatigued.

His description of the symptoms of severe malarial infection is excellent, and might well be incorporated in standard works on diagnosis.

In the treatment of malaria in infants, he has found hydrobromate of quinine of use in early infancy; the hypophosphite in older children, and the valerianate in girls approaching puberty. The author writes fully regarding his use of quinine in adults, discriminating between the different salts and indications for their use. He has not often exceeded sixty grains in twenty-four hours in ordinary cases; in pernicious malarial infection he has given fifteen grains of the acid hydrochlorate hypodermically, accompanied by forty-five grains of the sulphate by the stomach at the same time.

In what is styled "bilious remittent" malarial infection, he has had good results from rectal injections of carbolic acid, with hypodermics of quinine, giving from fifteen to thirty grains of carbolic acid in twenty-four hours. Arseniate of strychnia with quinine is of great value in the profound nervous depression which accompanies severe infection. The author's formula, which has been adopted by the marine service of several tropical countries, is as follows:

R.—Sodium arseniate   .   .   .   .   .   . gr. 3
    Strychnia sulphate   .   .   .   .   .   . gr. 1½
    Distilled boiled water   .   .   .   .   . fl℥ 10½

To be used without filtering.

In the hypodermic use of the acid hydrochlorate of quinine he has found the best formula fifteen grains of the salt to half an ounce of saturated camphor-water, freshly prepared. In briefly mentioning these points we merely indicate to our readers some of the many instructive details which Dr. Pepper incorporates in his interesting treatise. The clinical histories in full of sixty-four cases form the basis of his deductions regarding treatment, and illustrate his methods.

We are interested to know what definition of malaria an acute observer like the author, placed in such favorable conditions to study malarial infection, may formulate of this common but not clearly defined malady. He states (p. 280) : " Malaria is an infectious, feebly contagious malady, caused originally by telluric action, assisted by meteorologic influences affecting the electric status of the body and the nervous system; the infection gains access to the blood through the respiratory organs, less often through the digestive tract." The book is handsomely published, and will adorn and enrich the library of the physician or the traveller. E. P. D.

PRACTICAL TREATISE ON ELECTRICITY IN GYNECOLOGY. By EGBERT H. GRANDIN, M.D., Chairman of the Section on Obstetrics and Gynecology, New York Academy of Medicine; Obstetric Surgeon, New York Maternity Hospital; Obstetrician, New York Infant Asylum, etc., and JOSEPHUS H. GUNNING, M.D., Instructor in Electro-therapeutics, New York Post-Graduate School and Hospital; Gynecologist to Riverview Rest for Women; Electro-gynecologist, Northeastern Dispensary, etc. Illustrated. Pp. 171. New York: William Wood & Co., 1891.

THE appearance of a new monograph upon the application of electricity to diseases of women is a proof of the importance which this therapeutic agent has assumed in gynecological treatment. In reviewing in this journal the recent work upon the same subject, we took occasion to question the advisability of recommending the use of what may be called the refinements of electro-therapeusis by the general practitioner, and we are still of the opinion that even gynecologists who have not made a special study of the theory and practice of electrolysis, and are provided with all the expensive apparatus necessary for its proper application, ought to refer their patients to an expert who is prepared to make a rigid scientific test of the method. The statistics of tyros in this department are valueless from a scientific standpoint; they only serve to place the subject in a false light before the profession. It is fair neither to our patients nor to medical science for us to employ electricity simply for "effect." In no other branch of therapeutics is it so true that "a little knowledge is a dangerous thing." Of all the manuals on this subject which have appeared, we regard the present one as the safest and most conservative. "The agent is considered," we read in the preface, "not from the standpoint of a specific, but as a valuable adjuvant to routine therapeutic methods"—a claim to which no fair-minded man can take exception.

The first chapter, including nearly one-third of the book, is devoted to a discussion of theoretical questions and descriptions of apparatus, and is unusually well illustrated. The brief closing paragraph on contra-indications to the use of electricity might with propriety have been extended to several pages; it is extremely important for the general practitioner to learn clearly in exactly what class of cases electricity should *not* be used, though we doubt if any but an expert gynecologist is really competent to recognize this at the examining-table.

Chapter II., on "Routine Uses of Electricity," will undoubtedly prove of the more practical value to the ordinary reader than will the succeeding carefully elaborated chapter on "Electrolysis." We are glad to see that the authors regard dysmenorrhœa rather as a "symptom complex," than as a single symptom referable purely to a gross local lesion or abnormality. It is only by viewing the subject in this way that we can understand the undoubted analgesic effect of the continuous current. The point is made that the tension faradic current, with the bipolar intra-uterine electrode, is not to be used indiscriminately,

but only " where the flow is scanty and insufficient stimulus is a probable source of the dysmenorrhœa." Stress is laid upon the fact that
the galvanic current, when used in cases of chronic oöphoritis accompanied by severe local pain, simply relieves the neuralgia, but does not
exert any miraculous curative effect upon an ovary which is the seat of
actual organic disease. While affirming that the proper application of
electricity restores tone to the relaxed supports of a displaced uterus,
the authors do not share in the enthusiasm of some electro-therapeutics,
who claim that displacements can be cured by this agent alone. "A fact
to be emphasized is that the use of electricity does not, as has been
claimed, enable us to dispense with pessaries."

The section on the electrical treatment of diseases of the adnexa
ought not to give offence, even to the avowed opponents of conservatism,
since the authors simply plead for a fair trial of this agent before resort
to abdominal section. "To make one of these suffering women comfortable," they conclude, " if not to entirely cure her, by means of electricity, redounds more to the credit of the gynecologist than if he
sterilizes her and still does not cure her."

To those who desire a lucid statement of the theory and practice of
electrolysis for uterine fibroids we commend Chapter III. So much
that is obscure and confusing to the general reader has been written on
this subject that it is gratifying to have the entire matter satisfactorily
explained.

A monograph written by two individuals must necessarily be somewhat uneven. In the one before us, however, the dual element is seldom
noticed, each author adhering to his one line of work. The style is
clear, unpretentious and effective. The book is an honest book by
honest men, and, as we said before, can be relied upon as a safe guide
to the inexperienced, while the specialist will find in it not a few useful
hints. The illustrations are numerous, well-executed, and possess the
rare merit of freshness.   H. C. C.

Du Chimisme Stomacal (Digestion normale—Dyspepsie), par Georges
Hayem, Professeur de Thérapeutique à la Faculté de Médecine de Paris,
Membre de l'Académie de Médecine, Médecin de l'Hôpital Saint Antoine,
et J. Winter, Preparateur du Laboratoire de Thérapeutique à la Faculté
de Médecine de Paris. Pp. 274. Paris: G. Masson, 1891.

Chemistry of the Stomach (Normal Digestion—Dyspepsia). By
Georges Hayem, Professor of Therapeutics of the Faculty of Medicine
of Paris, Member of the Academy of Medicine, Physician to the Hospital
Saint Antoine, and J. Winter, Preparator of the Therapeutic Laboratory
of the Faculty of Medicine of Paris.

This little work embraces original researches in the chemistry of the
stomach, in two principal parts. The first comprises the consideration
of the normal, and the second of the abnormal chemical functions of the
stomach.

After an exhaustive general review of the various chemical theories
of the digestive process, in which great stress is laid by the authors on

the conclusions of Richet that the principal part of the hydrochloric acid is secreted and contained in the stomach as organic compounds of chlorine, they deal with a discussion of the methods of analysis of the gastric juice.   The principal point of interest of this centres on the quantitative determination of free hydrochloric acid of the stomach.   The method of Bidder and Schmidt they consider to be simply demonstrating that a certain amount of chlorine is present in the gastric juice otherwise than combined with mineral bases, also the quantitative results of Prout's researches as derived by his method of distillation, by which they claim the hydrochloric acid is by heat liberated from the organic bases it is combined with.   The clinical results of Ewald and Boas they think illusory, and of qualitative value only, as the organic chlorine compounds are by them neglected.   All the previous methods, qualitative and quantitative, they condemn as not taking into consideration the organic compounds of chlorine, which with them, as with Richet, appear to have become foregone conclusions, and a matter of the greatest importance in the chemical work of the stomach.

The authors describe at length and base their subsequent observations on the process of M. Winter, which we will describe here briefly, as it forms the principal point of the whole controversy on the subject. This method is intended to furnish: 1. The total chlorine; 2. The fixed chlorides (mineral compounds of Cl); 3. The difference between the two as hydrochloric acid, both free and in combination with organic matter; 4. The difference between the total of the two latter and the amount of HCl that can be dissipated by a temperature not exceeding 100° C., as the chlor-organic compounds.

The determination of the three values to be ascertained is by titration with the deci-normal solution of silver nitrate.   Three specimens of 5 c.c. each of the gastric juice are obtained.   To the first is added an excess of sodium carbonate, after which it is evaporated, and finally incinerated. The titration of this yields the total chlorine, to which they assign the letter T.   The second portion is evaporated over the water-bath to dryness, and then for one hour more; the residue is mixed with sodium carbonate, incinerated and also titrated.   This gives the fixed chlorides plus the non-volatile hydrochloric acid (organic chlorine compounds). This subtracted from the total chlorine (T) leaves the amount of free hydrochloric acid, termed H.   The third part is evaporated and incinerated without addition of sodium carbonate.   It gives on titration the fixed chlorides, designated as F.   The third result, subtracted from the second, leaves the amount of chlor-organic compounds, including also *ammonium chloride.*

The authors claim that if carefully done this process will always give accurate and reliable results, which in their cases, with normal secretions, have been remarkably constant.   It might seem that they had at last solved the Gordian knot, and presented alike an accurate and ready method for quantitative estimations of the HCl in gastric juice, as well as established the presence of HCl not volatile at 100° C., in excess of that fixed by mineral bases.   The constancy of their results would also tend to make the organic chlorine compounds a factor of importance, and thus they would bring us at once to a new epoch in our knowledge of gastric chemistry, could they present to us also the evidence of the existence of their organic chlorine compounds in the *fresh—i. e.*, not heated and evaporated—gastric secretion.   When they claim the results of Prout as erroneous, owing to the liberation by heat of HCl from loosely combined organic chlorides, the same fault must inversely attach itself to their method, in so far as they may be said to *produce* the organic chlorine compounds in their process of analysis. While this is not proven, it certainly cannot be, or is not, disproven by them, as their principal factor upon which they base their conclusions is at best hypothetical. That there are in the gastric secretions albuminoid matters is not to be disputed; that these change under the effect of heat at and below 100° C. is another fact; that under such conditions bases form which combine with the free HCl of the gastric juice is very probable, and that their deduction therefore of an existence of organic chlorine compounds in the *fresh* gastric juice is not established becomes apparent.

The experiments of Prout and so many others are in fact much more conclusive, and lean toward the assumption that in the fresh gastric juice HCl is present in its free state. It might be said that the constancy of their value C (chlor-organic compounds) may be claimed in support of their theory, but this might as readily be explained by a constancy of the albuminoid matter in the gastric juice and the bases produced by their process of evaporation.

The chapter on the normal evolution of the gastric digestion is quite ingenious and interesting, but it is, after all, only a defence of their theory of the preëxistence of organic chlorine compounds in the gastric juice. They value the digestive power of the gastric juice by the relative proportion of the organic chlorine compounds with the abnormal (not HCl) acids. Thus they arrive at a formula in which A is total acidity, H free hydrochloric acid, and C organic chlorine compounds; these yield the digestive utility of the gastric secretion, as $\dfrac{A-H}{C}$, to which they give the term, and according to its decrease or increase over the normal, which they found as 0.86, they classify pathological peptic acts as respectively hyperpepsia and hypopepsia. These, in turn, they subdivide in three degrees, of which the last of the latter is equivalent to apepsia. They also give a class of simple dyspepsia, in which the peptic disturbance does not arise from a marked variation of the chemical values.

A most disturbing element in their deductions appears in speaking of the factors to which the total acidity of the gastric juice is due; they declare on page 105: "After our experiences, the free hydrochloric acid, the organic acids, and the acid phosphates present together a value which represents in the normal state but a small part of the total acidity. *The greatest part of the total acidity comes from the hydrochloric acid compounds with albuminoids in solution;*" whereas, on page 241, in referring to cases where the total acidity is nothing, and the organic chlorine compounds are given respectively as 0.055 and 0.202, they say, "While the total acidity is nought, the chloro-organic products are *deprived entirely of the acid function.*" If a factor for gauging the peptic act is subject to such abnormal qualitative conditions, it can, in our opinion, scarcely be classed as the controlling element of digestion; besides, it may be presumed, that in part, if not altogether, as most probably in the last cases cited, these organic chlorine compounds are principally ammonium chloride derived from the free HCl secreted in the stomach, acting during the evaporating process (by which it becomes concentrated) on the nitrogenous compounds of the gastric juice.

This volume is, however, a most remarkable one, full of original thought, and the casuistic presented shows an almost unparalleled industry on the part of the authors. Their lines of research are so entirely original that the perusal of their work is of the greatest interest to those who give more earnest study to gastropathies.

To admit that the authors are right in their premises would upset all present doctrines regarding digestion and its perverted state, and at once start a gastro-pathology, which, in its complications, would lead to utter confusion. We admit the brilliant conception and the laborious elucidation of the leading idea, which it seems hard to supersede in some of the great minds of the French medical schools. Ever since the hydrochloric acid digestion of albuminoids was proven there have been periodical attempts to prove the supposed existence of the organic chlorine compounds. So far this has not been done, and Professor Hayem leaves this point as problematical as it was after the researches of Richet.

To students of gastro-pathology we can recommend this little work as most interesting reading, though we differ essentially with the hypothesis it attempts to prove.   L. W.

REPORT OF CARLOS F. MACDONALD, M.D., ON THE EXECUTION BY ELECTRICITY OF WILLIAM KEMMLER, *alias* JOHN HART. Presented to the Governor of New York, September 20, 1890. Pp. xx.

THE importance of its subject justifies a reference in these pages to this brief document. To those whose notions about the execution of criminals by means of electricity have been derived from the sensational romances of the daily press, this report will prove an excellent corrective.

The autopsy was held about three hours after death, but, with the exception of the local desiccation caused by too prolonged contact with the heated electrodes, nothing was discovered but the ordinary appearances produced by a fatal charge of electricity.

In spite of minor defects in the apparatus, and its mode of application, which were inevitable by reason of inexperience, it is the opinion of the distinguished reporter that—

"Compared with hanging, in which death is frequently produced by strangulation, with every indication of conscious suffering for an appreciable time on the part of the victim, execution by electricity is infinitely preferable, both as regards the suddenness with which death is effected, and the expedition with which all the immediate preliminary details may be arranged. . . . The execution of Kemmler, from the time he entered the room until the second contact was interrupted, occupied not more than eight minutes; whereas, executions by hanging usually require from fifteen to thirty minutes. In fact, it not infrequently happens that the heart continues to beat for that length of time after the fall of the fatal drop. Then, too, far more time is consumed in placing the prisoner on the gallows, pinioning his limbs, putting on the black cap, placing the noose about his neck, and carefully adjusting the knot under his left ear . . . than would be required for arranging the preliminary details of an electrical execution."

If anyone should still object to the alleged failure to annihilate existence at the first electrical contact, let him contrast the expedition with which the possible failure was corrected and converted into an unquestionable success, with the horrible delays that attend the replacement of a broken rope in execution by hanging. Contrasting the details of the present report with the records of execution by other methods, the electrical method has everything in its favor. Read, in the blood-stained annals of history, how in the agony of death, high-born noblemen and gentle women, breaking away from the block, have been chased around the scaffold by the executioner with his bloody axe, and have only been felled by a succession of blows upon the head, shoulders, and neck. Witness the frightful scenes of a military execution : bodies perforated with bullets, yet weltering in conscious pain until life is finally ended by the sergeant's merciful pistol-shot through the head. Nor does the expeditious work of the guillotine prevent horrible anguish on the part of the wretch who is hurried from his bed into the cold prison-yard at dawn of day, strapped to a plank, and shoved under the knife that severs his bleeding head from a struggling trunk. Rough and painful are the preliminaries of all these processes; whereas, in the case before us, the victim of the law was quietly and comfortably placed in a chair, with no terrifying apparatus in sight. One contact, and all possibilities of sensation and consciousness were instantaneously annihilated. He could not have known that he was dying. This, certainly, is a perfection of euthanasia that even anæsthetics and poisons cannot procure.

As a result of the experience acquired in this execution Dr. MacDonald recommends :

"1. The statute providing for the execution of criminals by electricity should be amended so as to provide for but one plant, to be located in the central part of the State, in a building especially constructed for the purpose. This building should contain the necessary electrical apparatus, an engine, execution-room, solitary cells, and quarters for the guards and other necessary officials, the apparatus to be in charge of and operated by a competent, accredited electrician.

"2. The engine and dynamo should be especially constructed for the purpose, and should be capable of generating an electro-motive force of at least 3000 volts, in order to insure the maximum voltage that would be necessary, and at the same time cause no injustice to any electrical lighting company, such as is likely to be the case so long as commercial dynamos are used in executing criminals.

"3. The volt-meter should be located in the execution-room, and a competent and responsible official should be detailed to take the readings of the meter before and at the instant the current is applied. The voltage should not be less than 1500 nor more than 2000, and should be a matter of official record. The prisoner's [electrical] resistance should also be taken immediately before bringing him into the execution-room.

"4. The statute should require an official report of each execution to be made to the Governor within ten days after the execution takes place." H. M. L.

PROGRESS

MEDICAL SCIENCE.

THERAPEUTICS.

UNDER THE CHARGE OF

FRANCIS H. WILLIAMS, M.D.,
ASSISTANT PROFESSOR OF THERAPEUTICS IN HARVARD UNIVERSITY.

TREATMENT OF EPILEPSY BY THE CONJOINED EMPLOYMENT OF BROMIDE OF POTASSIUM AND OF AN AGENT CAPABLE OF RENDERING THE NERVOUS CENTRES ANÆMIC.

Under this head POULET, of Plancha-les-Mines, in the last *Bulletin général de Thérapeutique,* writes of a combination of bromide of potassium with Calabar bean, which has given him success in the treatment of obstinate cases of epilepsy where the bromides alone had failed. A favorite formula of his is the following:

> Bromide of potassium . . . . . . 100 parts.
> Tincture of Calabar bean . . . . . 35 "
> Water . . . . 470 "

Dose: A tablespoonful, to be increased to a tablespoonful and a half, then two tablespoonfuls, daily.

A tablespoonful contains about fifty-seven grains of bromide, and about sixteen minims of the tincture. The medicine may be given in divided doses instead of in one full dose, half a teaspoonful being given at first twice, then three times, then four times a day.

Poulet reports five obstinate cases treated in this manner. These were cases where bromide alone failed to cure:

1. The fits were formerly six or eight a week (*grand mal*). After a year of the new treatment, no return of the epilepsy. In this patient the tincture of Calabar bean is occasionally replaced by eserine, in the dose of one-sixty-fourth of a grain to each fifteen grains of bromide; the result has been the same. No contraction of the pupil has been observed during the administration of the medicine.

2. A most obstinate case; had been epileptic for eight years, eight or ten fits a day. Failure of bromides, given alone, also of bromides and picrotoxine. Definitive cure under bromides associated with tincture of Calabar bean.

3. Also a case of chronic, inveterate epilepsy. Several months' treatment by the combination specified has given exemption from all convulsive accidents.

4. A case of grave epilepsy at the menopause. Frequent daily vertiginous attacks ending in convulsions and stupor. At first the disease was successfully combated by bromide of potassium associated with picrotoxine; this combination afterward failing, sulphate of atropine was substituted for picrotoxine (ninety grains of bromide of potassium and one-sixty-fourth of a grain of atropine daily). The latter treatment has been kept up for a year, with complete cessation of the vertigo.

5. A case of cardiac epilepsy. The *grand mal* attacks were followed by hemiplegia with stupor and hebetude (*état de mal*). A combination of bromide and digitalis caused disappearance of the epilepsy (120 grains of bromide associated with 30 minims of tincture of digitalis in divided doses daily).

Poulet terminates his article by the following conclusions:

The bromides remain the sheet-anchor in the treatment of epilepsy, and by the term *bromides* we have especial reference to the bromide of potassium, which alone is truly efficacious.

There are, however, a great many epileptics whose attacks are only mitigated or posponed, not completely suppressed, by bromide of potassium.

In such cases if we associate the bromide with some medicament which possesses properties identical with those of the bromide (that is, being capable of anæmiating and decongesting the nerve-centres and paralysing the system of voluntary muscles) we generally obtain results which are perfectly satisfactory in essential epilepsy, and even in partial or Jacksonian epilepsy, on condition that, in the latter, we begin by the specific treatment of the determining cause. The substances that have been most successful are Calabar bean, picrotoxine, and belladonna. In cardiac epilepsy digitalis must be added.

We may indifferently substitute sulphate of eserine for the preparations of Calabar bean, sulphate of atropine for those of belladonna, and digitaline for digitalis.

———

Some New Uses for Saline Preparations.

Dr. John Strahan points out some uses for saline preparations which would not be recalled to the minds of many practitioners.

Thus, in pleurisy it is known that salines produce an outpouring of fluid from vessels in the intestinal canal, as well as a greatly increased secretion from all the glands of the mucous membrane. Nothing better reduces abnormally high arterial tension, because, if the abdominal vessels are much filled, pressure must fall generally. Thus a saline purge will often relieve renal congestion, and thus act as the best diuretic. Even in the healthy a saline purge will often greatly increase the quantity of urine, although a great quantity of fluid has been discharged by the bowels. For such purposes salines should be given in only as much fluid as will dissolve them. Their affinity for water must then be met by exosmosis through the intestinal capillaries. In some cases of general anasarca, whether cardiac, renal, or merely anæmic, the effects of a few half-ounce doses of sulphate of magnesium is very striking and can only be approached by puncture of the swollen leg. Such treatment is often of advantage in acute, subacute, or even chronic pleurisy.

The salines will act just as freely and as promptly in the case of a patient under the influence of morphine or opium as if such drugs were not present, which is often an advantage, and which can hardly be said of any other purgative. An ounce of sulphate of magnesium will produce a full watery movement in two or three hours, and without the slightest griping or pain, in a man who is narcotized by opium.

Milk diet is a valuable accessory to this method of treatment; so also in general renal and cardiac dropsy and anasarca the salines act as efficient diuretics by removing stasis of the renal veins, and in ascites from portal obstruction salines are still more useful, as they act directly on the organ concerned. The œdema of the lungs and œdema of the brain, which so often imperil life in Bright's disease, are usually more quickly and decidedly benefited than by any other plan of treatment, while it is known that free purging in cases of dropsy or anasarca is not followed by weakness and exhaustion, as it would be in other cases, or even in health. As a rule, it is best to prescribe the sulphate of magnesium in mixture with dilute sulphuric acid and extract of licorice, which quite disguises the taste. If the sulphate is ordered, four- or even two-drachm doses every four hours will cause a profuse but painless diarrhœa which is perfectly within the control of the medical attendant.

Again, in uræmic cases, and irritable and inflamed states of the stomach and intestines, salines may be freely and painlessly employed when no other purgative would be dreamed of, except, perhaps, calomel. The circumstances which exclude salines, with all other purgatives, are inflammation and probable perforation of the vermiform appendix, perityphlitis, and peritonitis from perforation. Fecal impaction and simple typhlitis are, on the other hand, strikingly remedied by salines when other purgatives may cause enteritis or peritonitis, while croton oil, jalap, senna, etc., cause violent excitation of the muscular coat of the bowels, and thus often intense pain in the bowels of the healthy. If the irritability of the stomach be so great that constant vomiting prevents the administration of salines through the mouth, they may then be given by enema, and two ounces of sulphate of magnesium as a purgative enema will be thoroughly satisfactory with its quickness, thoroughness, and its perfect painlessness. A good formula is: Sulphate of magnesium two ounces, glycerin one ounce, water enough to make four ounces; this is unirritating, and is perfectly reliable. The glycerin in this formula is undoubtedly a useful adjuvant; but while glycerin produces solid stools, the salines in the formula lead to the excretion of large amounts of liquid, and consequently a fluid passage. In stricture of the intestine, as in cancer of the rectum, nothing can equal salines which cause fluid stools—generally painless ones; for salines liquefy the feces, so that they may pass through the narrow gut without pain or straining, thus avoiding danger of perforation or rupture.   This also applies to all diseases of the rectum attended by diffi-cult defecation, such as ulcers of the anus.

In lead colic, in acute dysentery, and in rectal and pelvic hemorrhage, especially if the latter condition is due to constipation, they may be used.—*Provincial Medical Journal*, vol. cx., 1891.

In Acute Bronchitis.

A simple expectorant mixture in acute bronchitis is:

 ℞.—Ammon. muriat.   .   .   .   .   .   ℥ss.
  Mist. glycyrrhiz. comp. .   .   .   .   ℥iv.—M.
 Sig.—Take a dessertspoonful every four hours.

The dose is smaller in the extremes of life, and in severe coughs it is given every three hours.

Tablets of the muriate of ammonium and the compound licorice mixture are very efficient.   When the secretions are with difficulty brought up, the use of senega is advised.

When the secretions are abundant and not easily coughed up, turpentine in emulsion is an excellent remedy, not so pleasant, perhaps, as terebene or terpine hydrate, but rarely failing to do good in properly selected cases.   The formula, with occasional modifications to suit particular cases, is:

 ℞.—Ol. terebinthin.   .   .   .   .   .   ℨij. to ℨiij.
  Mucil. acaciæ .   .   .   .   .   .   q. s.
  Aq. cinnamomi   .   .   .   .   .   ℥j.
  Aquæ   .   .   .   .   .   q. s. ad   ℥vj.—M.
 Sig.—A tablespoonful in a little water every four hours.

Ofttimes the cough is of such an irritating character that these ordinary expectorant mixtures avail little; then recourse must be made to a narcotic in some form.   Codeine, a very useful alkaloid of opium, has the advantage of not constipating as much as morphine.   A good combination is:

 ℞.—Codeinæ sulphat. .   .   .   .   .   grs. viij.
  Syr. prun. Virginian.   .   .   .   .   ℥ij.—M.
 Sig.—A teaspoonful in a little water three or four times a day and at bedtime if necessary.—*Therapeutic Gazette*, July, 1891.

Whooping-cough Treated by Atomization.

Dr. H. Ernest Schmid states that he now relies entirely upon atomiza-tion for the treatment of whooping-cough in all stages of the disease.   The spray which he uses is made up as follows:

 ℞.—Carbolic acid   .   .   .   .   .   .   grs. vj.
  Menthol, 4 per cent. solution   .   .   .   ℨiv.
  Cocaine, 3   "   "   .   .   .   .   ℨiij.
  Glycerin   .   .   .   .   .   .   ℨj.
  Cherry-laurel water   .   .   .   q. s. ad   ℥j.—M.

This solution should be thoroughly used, brutally if necessary, by an atomizer every three hours; force may be employed if necessary, and disregarding any apparent strangling upon the part of the little one during vigorous atomization, the nozzle of the instrument should be directed as far into the mouth of the patient as possible. During the struggling and sputtering and strangling some deep respirations will before long be made, and the object is accomplished. At first, in most cases, a violent paroxysm of coughing may result from the spraying, especially if much force has to be used with the child, but these soon cease and palpable effects are soon noticed by the parents. The point is to be able to impress the importance of perseverance. Dr. Schmid has seen whooping-cough arrested by this means after one thorough spraying, the cough continuing without the whoop for a while, and perfect recovery has followed in one or two weeks. From his success, he feels justified in claiming that the method promises to be more efficient than other means of treating the disease.—*Medical Record*, June 13, 1891.

TREATMENT OF CONSTIPATION IN CHILDREN BY ABDOMINAL MASSAGE.

KARNITZKY describes this method of treatment in both acute and chronic constipation in children from eight to twelve years of age. He concludes that abdominal massage may produce effects upon the alimentary tract, in connection with digestion, which are not inferior to those produced by purgatives. Habitual constipation may be easily cured by massage without the aid of purgatives, and the more readily the younger the child. The younger a child is the milder should the manipulations be and the shorter the séances, which should be from three to ten minutes, according to the age of the patient. Longer séances are inadvisable, and may even be harmful and aggravate the condition of the patient. Abdominal massage may be regarded as the best means of treating constipation in children. Purgatives should only be used in exceptional cases.—*Journal de Médecine*, 1891.

ALOIN.

PROFESSOR HANS MEYER, of Marburg, has examined chemically and physiologically the aloïn obtained from various kinds of aloes. From the Barbadoes and Curaçoa he obtained the same crystalline substance. Natal aloes yielded a somewhat different aloïn. In experiments on animals and on man the aloïn was given per os and also subcutaneously. The aloïn can be detected in the feces and urine by tests which are given at length and which are extremely delicate. Experiments showed that aloïn acted with certainty as a purgative, whether given by the mouth or subcutaneously. The dose in both cases is about the same, which is explained by the fact that aloïn, when given hypodermically, is excreted from the blood chiefly into the bowel, only a mere trace, or none, being found in the urine. In man, dogs, and cats, there is no albuminuria after subcutaneous injection, but in rabbits—in which animals aloes does not cause purgation—subcutaneous administration is always followed by inflammation of the kidneys, albuminuria, and death. Its purgative action is as slow when it is given hypodermically as it is per os. Natal aloïn by subcutaneous injection is always active. In man on an ordinary mixed diet it had but little effect, but in man fed exclusively upon an animal diet it was much more active. The reason probably is that in the latter case the putrefactive processes in the intestine are much more marked, and the aloïn is decomposed into a more active substance. All the experiments seem to point to the conclusion that aloïn itself is not an active purgative, but that it becomes gradually decomposed in the intestine into a more active body, and hence the slowness of its action.—*British Medical Journal,* 1891.

DIURETIN AS A MEANS OF REMOVING DROPSY.

DR. ROBERT H. BABCOCK has used diuretin with good results in three cases, and considers that in this remedy we have a useful drug. The alkaloids caffeine and theobromine are diuretics of great power, but the former has the drawback of primarily increasing arterial tension by its stimulation of the vasomotor centres. An objection to caffeine in large doses, say five to ten grains three or four times a day, lies in the nervousness and insomnia of which patients are apt to complain. Moreover, the system becomes speedily accustomed to its effect, necessitating the employment of increasing doses.

This remedy is readily soluble in warm water, and had better be administered thus or in pill form, since, if exposed to the air, as in powders, it undergoes a change. The daily dose is large—sixty to one hundred and twenty grains in twenty-four hours. It may be given in divided doses of fifteen grains each.

His conclusions are that diuretin is a diuretic of great power and promptitude, suitable to all forms of dropsy. Since it does not increase arterial tension, it is likely to succeed where digitalis, caffeine, and their congeners fail. In cases of cardiac dropsy with great feebleness of the pulse and erythema, it will strengthen and regulate, rather than depress, the heart's action.

It appears to cause no irritation of the stomach or kidneys, and requires to be given to the extent of from ninety to one hundred and twenty grains daily, and preferably in small doses frequently repeated.—*New York Medical Journal,* July 11, 1891.

TREATMENT OF CHYLURIA BY THYMOL.

TWO cases are reported, in which the filaria sanguinis was found, where complete cure followed the internal use of thymol. The first case was that of a man twenty years of age. The urine was white. Quinine and many other remedies were tried without any result; the urine remained milky and the patient's fever continued. Thymol was given every four hours in doses of five-sixths of a grain. Fifteen days later the dose was doubled. A month after this treatment the patient was cured and no more filariæ were found in the blood. The other patient was relieved under the same conditions after a month's treatment, taking the same dose three times a day.

These two cases suggest that the thymol destroys these organisms in the blood and in the tissues. The author has tried the effects of thymol upon other pathological organisms, such as the bacillus of tuberculosis and of leprosy, but without any result.—*Bulletin général de Thérapeutique,* 1891.

MEDICINE.

UNDER THE CHARGE OF

W. PASTEUR, M.D. LOND., M.R.C.P.,

ASSISTANT PHYSICIAN TO THE MIDDLESEX HOSPITAL; PHYSICIAN TO THE NORTHWESTERN HOSPITAL
FOR CHILDREN;

AND

SOLOMON SOLIS-COHEN, A.M., M.D.,

PROFESSOR OF CLINICAL MEDICINE AND APPLIED THERAPEUTICS IN THE PHILADELPHIA POLYCLINIC;
PHYSICIAN TO THE PHILADELPHIA HOSPITAL.

MALTA (REMITTENT) FEVER.

GADDING (*British Medical Journal*, 1891, No. 1585) gives an analysis of forty-two cases occurring on H. M. S. Agamemnon.

The writer describes three types: Enteric type, always severe and generally supplying the fatal cases. Remittent type, with high initial temperature, marked remissions and tendency to relapses. Hybrid type, supplying 60 per cent of the cases. The primary attack is often trivial and of short duration. Rheumatism of an obstinate character is a common sequela and relapses of a severe nature are common. These cases are variously described as " Malta fever," "sweating fever," "typho-malarial," and "undefined climatic fever."

Etiology: The disease commences almost invariably in the spring. A few cases followed exposure to a hot sun. In four cases trifling injuries, bruises, and sprains appeared to determine the attack. Exciting causes: Malarial poison plays an important part, but true ague is not often seen. The disease is no doubt largely filth-produced, and improved drainage and water supply have lessened the virulence of type. The poison concentrates its force on the lymphoid structures of the alimentary canal (tonsils and Peyer's patches), thus accounting for the resemblance to typhoid fever; but the disease must not for this reason be assumed to be typhoid.

Duration: One week to six or seven months. Only eight made perfect recoveries, and were from one to six weeks under treatment. No eruption was noted in any case.

Symptoms and complications: Acute orchitis was noted in seven cases. Rheumatism occurred in nearly all at some period of the attack, and was often a troublesome sequela. Pneumonia was observed in three cases, the signs rapidly clearing in two. One death occurred from secondary pneumonia.

Diagnosis: The majority of cases point strongly to a malarial origin. The chief points of difference from true "remittent" are: (1) absence of splenic and hepatic enlargement; (2) powerlessness of quinine to cure, and (3) character of the complications—rheumatism, orchitis, tonsillitis, etc. The disease really defies all treatment. The one efficient remedy is change of climate.

In the opinion of SURGEON DAVID BRUCE, M.S., founded on an experience of 400 cases in the Military Hospital at Valetta, Malta fever is in no sense a

malarious fever; it is a species of fever perfectly distinct from enteric or
malarious fever, having its own definite parasitic cause, and is as worthy of
specific recognition as diphtheria or tuberculosis. The writer states that in
every fatal case of true Malta fever a definite microörganism is demonstrable
which has not the slightest resemblance to the amœba-like parasite of malaria.
It can be cultivated with the greatest ease from the spleen and other organs,
and has never been found in the organs of cases of malarious fever or any
other disease. No description is given of the microörganism in question.

DOUBLE EMPYEMA.

HANDFORD, of Nottingham (*British Medical Journal*, 1891, No. 1585),
reports the case of a boy, aged seven and a half years, in whom double empyema followed on an illness of three weeks' duration. The left chest was
opened and three-quarters of an inch of rib removed. Dyspnœa was much
relieved by the evacuation of pus. Ten days later the right chest was emptied
in a similar way. Both tubes were left out at the end of nine weeks, and the
patient made an excellent recovery.

FIBROID PNEUMONIA.

AULD, of Glasgow (*Lancet*, 1891, Nos. 3537 and 3538), under this title
describes two cases of an affection of the lungs which "has only within recent
years begun to be recognized." The affection is in no way connected with
those variously known as chronic broncho-pneumonia, chronic pleurogenous
pneumonia, pneumo-koniosis, and phthisis pulmonalis.

Anatomically, though not clinically, the disease is identical with chronic
pneumonia succeeding acute pneumonia. It has also been termed "parenchymatous pneumonia," or "primary indurative pneumonia." Cases of this
disorder have been described by Ludwig Bühl, in 1872, and M. Heitler, in
1884, and also by Eppinger, Wagner, and Talma. English medical literature
contains a few isolated examples.

From the consideration of his two cases, together with the indications
afforded by those quoted above, the author concludes—(1) that there is a pneumonia, a lobar affection of the lungs, insidious in its origin and subacute or
chronic in its course, characterized essentially by induration of a creeping
fibrinous exudation and by interstitial changes, and accompanied by proliferation and fatty degeneration of the pulmonary epithelium, and also not
unusually of the bronchial epithelium; (2) that anatomically the disease is
in every respect identical with chronic pneumonia succeeding an acute
attack; and (3) that the morbid anatomy of the disease has in its earlier
stages such distinctive and unequivocal features as to give the affection an
assured position and to permanently exclude the possibility of confounding
it with any other chronic affection of the lungs. Insomuch as this disease—
whether preceded by an acute pneumonia, or being chronic from the first—
has as its leading feature the development of a nuclear fibrous tissue in, with,
and about a pneumonic exudation, it is most titly termed "fibroid pneumonia."

The subacute cases usually terminate fatally in about six weeks, after running a course not unlike that of acute phthisis. Tubercle, when present, is limited. In one of the author's cases there was no tubercle, and the bronchial pus contained the capsulated diplococcus pneumoniæ. In the other case there was apical cicatrix and adhesion, with included cretaceous matter and general fibrosis of other organs.

In the writer's opinion it is chiefly, if not exclusively, after an acute onset that fibroid pneumonia may assume the chronic type. The subacute cases are distinguished from chronic broncho-pneumonia by their comparatively short duration; but there are admittedly great difficulties in the way of making a clinical diagnosis of this disease, among which may be mentioned its rarity and the similitude in general of its physical signs and symptoms to those of phthisis.

Points of Affinity between Rheumatoid Arthritis, Locomotor Ataxia, and Exophthalmic Goitre.

Spender (*British Medical Journal*, 1891, No. 1587) mentions that nearly every case of rheumatoid arthritis in early or middle life shows marks of cerebral sympathy in one or more ways: pigmentation, sweating, tachycardia or high tension, neuralgia. Pigmentation is common, and of various hues. A bronze smear across the forehead, dark streaks beneath the lower eyelids, or staining of the cheeks or neck are met with: discolorations which closely resemble those occurring in exophthalmic goitre. Leucadermia is met with in both diseases. Discoloration of the skin is, however, rarer in arthritis than in exophthalmic goitre.

Tachycardia is a not uncommon feature of early cases of arthritis. In nine out of eighteen cases of undoubted rheumatoid arthritis the average pulse-rate was above 90. The heart's action was not accelerated by emotion or moderate exercise. There were no murmurs. Venous hum was frequent. Attention is drawn to the occasional coincidence of thyroid enlargement in rheumatoid arthritis, especially where there is a dark stain on the neck.

Tremor and muscular spasm are common to both diseases, though far less frequent in arthritis.

Functional disturbance of the pneumogastric nerve is an important bond between arthritis and locomotor ataxia. Gastric crises, cramps of the stomach and vomiting, a pseudo-asthma, or a transient dyspnœa and difficulty of swallowing may occur in the early stages of both diseases. But the closest analogy between them is in the nature and character of the pain. The author inclines to the view that rheumatoidal and Charcot's joint lesions are identical.

Bradycardia, or the Slow Heart.

Seymour Taylor (*British Medical Journal*, 1891, No. 1589) says: Bradycardia is defined as being that condition in which the heart-beats do not exceed forty per minute. A classification of causes is difficult, owing to the wide pathology and varied associations; hence he proposes to subdivide the cases into two headings: *A*. Occurring in health; *B*. Occurring in disease. (*A*.) As regards health. It frequently occurred in tall, muscular men, who were or had been athletic in their habits. In them it was not inconsistent with prolonged life and great mental vigor. It was important to note that in such examples the bradycardia was not attended with dyspnœa. It was not infrequently an accompaniment of old age, but an age which might be attended with no other sign of decay or degeneration. There was also a group of cases which, for want of a better term, might be called "functional." They were usually an accompaniment of indigestion, or some other disorder of stomach or other organ. They were temporary only, and were not attended with any signs of heart lesion. (*B.*) Cases the result of disease. Here the assertion that disease tended to quicken rather than to lessen the heart's action was admitted. Yet there were some disorders which produced an opposite effect. For example, it was occasionally seen in (1) disease of the heart-walls; (2) obstruction of coronary vessels; (3) as a sequel of certain fevers and blood diseases; (4) in relation with diseases of the respiratory beat and mechanism; (5) as a manifestation of grave neurotic changes—epilepsy, traumatism, etc.; (6) in abdominal injuries and operations; (7) as the result of certain drugs and poisons.

SENILE CHOREA; MANIA; RECOVERY.

FERRIER (*Lancet*, 1891, No. 3538) records the case of a woman, aged seventy years, who had an attack of left-sided chorea in 1890. The present attack affected the right side and began at Christmas-time with a severe bilious attack, and was accompanied by great irritability of temper and sleepnessness.

On admission to hospital there was typical chorea of the right side. The thoracic and abdominal viscera were healthy. The same night the patient became acutely maniacal and had to be isolated and put into a straight waist-coat. She was taken home after three weeks in practically the same condition. About nine weeks later the chorea began to subside, and the condition of cerebral excitement rapidly passed off. The treatment consisted mainly in the administration of bromide of potassium, arsenic, and quinine.

ON THE TREATMENT OF INTUSSUSCEPTION BY INJECTION OR INFLATION.

MORTIMER (*Lancet*, 1891, No. 3534), while fully admitting certain obvious advantages, draws attention to some of the dangers of this plan of treatment. Inflation does not appear to be safer than injection. An even pressure should be employed in all cases to lessen the chance of exciting peristalsis and rupture. With a view to ascertain the limits of safety of the mode of treatment, post-mortem experiments were made on infants. It was found that when the resultant pressure distending the colon rose to two and a half pounds to the square inch (irrigator raised five feet) there was apt to be cracking of the peritoneum. In some cases there was complete rupture of the bowel at a slightly higher pressure (irrigator at six feet). The writer criticises adversely the conclusions of Dr. W. E. Forest, of New York, in regard to the amount of pressure which it is safe to use.

An interesting case is quoted in which post-mortem experiment was made on a case in which invagination had occurred during life. The subject was an infant aged three months, who presented the usual signs of acute intussusception. Inflation was performed with a Higginson's syringe and the tumor gradually disappeared. The symptoms recurred after some hours and ended fatally. On examination the stomach and intestines were much distended; there was no peritonitis; the apex of the intussusception was below the splenic flexure. A tube was tied into the rectum and the irrigator raised to two feet. The intussusception was reduced in a few minutes with the exception of one inch ; the end of the ileum, the cæcum, and part of the vermiform appendix remaining tightly ensheathed by the colon. After fifteen minutes the irrigator was raised to three feet. A slight further reduction took place, but in four minutes the colon ruptured in three places just below the intussusception.

In another case, in a child aged eight months, about ten ounces of water were injected three times from an irrigator held at three feet, and on the two following days a pint of water was run in at a lower pressure. Post-mortem, three ruptures were found in the descending colon. The writer argues against inflation or injection as a prelude to laparotomy.

CEREBRAL SUPPURATION FOLLOWING INFLUENZA.

DR. J. S. BRISTOWE (*British Medical Journal*, 1891, No. 1592) reports two cases in which the patients were attacked two to three months before death with symptoms indistinguishable from those of influenza.

· In the first case, that of a carman, aged twenty-four years, cerebral symptoms came on early and continued with variations and ingravescence to the end. In the second, that of a school-girl, aged fourteen years, headache was an early symptom, but it was only latterly that the symptoms indicated the presence of grave cerebral disease.

The facts which lead the author to conclude that the cerebral abscesses in these cases were referable to influenza are: (1) Acute onset with symptoms indistinguishable from those of typical influenza; and (2) That none of the usual causes of abscess of the brain were or had been present.

In Case 1 the abscess—the size of a small Tangerine orange—was situated in the upper part of the left hemisphere. There was no disease of the ear nor any other condition tending to throw any light on the origin of the abscess. In Case 2 the abscess—which was about the same size—was situated in the right occipital lobe and adjoining part of the sphenoidal lobe. The ears and frontal sinuses were quite healthy.

In an addendum Dr. Bristowe mentions briefly three other cases in which influenza terminated fatally with symptoms of cerebral disease which may have been due to suppuration.

THE SIGNIFICANCE OF CHEYNE-STOKES RESPIRATION AS A SYMPTOM IN CARDIAC DISEASE.

DR. M. A. BOYD reports a case of cardiac hypertrophy and dilatation with systolic aortic bruit in which Cheyne-Stokes breathing occurred, presenting several features of interest.

The phases of the respiratory phenomena observed were as follows :

(1) An apnœal period characterized by deep sleep, lividity of face, quick pulse, feeble contractions of heart, perfect rest from all agitation, mental and bodily.

(2) An inspiratory period, with rousing of all the patient's faculties, extreme restlessness, slowing and strengthening of the pulse, apparently stronger contractions of the heart, less lividity of the face, and then a final deep inspiration.

(3) An expiratory period, with inspirations gradually getting shorter and expirations longer, pulse getting quicker and heart feebler in its contractions until expirations cease and the chest is empty, and restlessness gives place to sleep, which continues through the apnœa following.

The author lays stress on the variations in the pulse or cardiac rhythm during the different periods, and draws attention to the fact that though the respiratory effort during the ascending period is an inspiratory one, during the descending period of the effort it is chiefly expiratory. He is of opinion that the cardiac conditions necessary for the production of this form of breathing are not alone dilatation of the aorta, but also dilatation of the right ventriele with commencing degeneration or weakness of its walls; also hypertrophy of left ventricle with or without dilatation, but with degeneration of its muscle or enfeeblement from any cause, so that it is unable to empty its contents into a dilated and inelastic aorta.—*Dublin Journal of the Medical Sciences*, 1891, No. 235.

INFLUENZA EPIDEMIC OF 1889-90.

In the official Report just published, DR. PARSONS, who undertook the inquiry, tracks the general course of the epidemic from the northern hemisphere in a direction east and west, and it is explained that this took place mainly against the prevailing winds.

The theory of its relation to some Chinese inundations and of an aërially travelling miasm across the Asiatic and European continents is not borne out by the information procured; but, on the other hand, there is an abundance of evidence to show that it travelled mainly along the lines of human intercourse, attacking large towns and centres of population first, and that the disease travelled only just as fast as any humanly conveyed infection with a similar incubation period might have been expected to travel.

On the question of infection Dr. Buchanan, in his introduction to the report, writes : " Probably no evidence has ever been put on record in such abundance as that accumulated in Dr. Parsons' report, to show that, in its epidemic form, influenza is an eminently infectious complaint, communicable in the ordinary personal relations of individuals with one another. It appears to me that there can henceforth be no doubt about the fact."

Dr. Parsons does not appear to be impressed with the evidence in favor of the existence of any direct relation between influenza and the disease in horses known as " pink-eye."

Over-crowding and impure air must be regarded as having a powerful influence in developing the epidemic, whilst poverty and absence of warm clothing have largely conduced to the fatality of the disease.

The contagium of the disease does not appear to be of a very stable kind, and one characteristic of its instability lies in its uncertain and varying incubation period. Speaking generally, the evidence adduced points to a period of two to three days as the most common period of incubation, and to twenty-four hours on the one hand, and to some four days on the other, as fairly common extremes.

The poison may find admission into the system through the lungs, but Dr. Bezly Thorne, whose views are quoted at length in the report, is of opinion that the conjunctiva is the structure which the infecting material or microbe most generally, if not always, attacks.

THE PRACTICAL ELECTRO-THERAPEUTICS OF GRAVES'S DISEASE.

H. W. D. CARDEW, M.R.C.S. (*Lancet*, 1891, No. 3540), is of opinion that many cases in which drugs have proved valueless are amenable to electrical treatment.

For this purpose galvanism is superior to faradism. A very weak current (two to three milliampères) is sufficient. Each application should last six minutes and frequent applications (three times a day) should be made. The anode should be placed on the nape of the neck, the centre of its lower border corresponding to the seventh cervical spinous process, and be firmly held in that position during the application. The kathode should be moved up and down the side of the neck from the mastoid process along the course of the great nerves. The application is followed by a reduction in the frequency and force of the heart-beat, prolongation of the diastole being most marked. The slowing of the pulse-rate does not usually last for more than half an hour. The diminution in violence of beat lasts longer. As the case progresses and improves these effects become permanent.

THE TREATMENT OF TUBERCULOSIS BY MEANS OF SUBCUTANEOUS INJECTIONS OF EUCALYPTOL, GUAIACOL, AND IODOFORM.

PIGNOL (*Compt.-rend. hebdom. des Séances de la Soc. de Biol.*, 1891, No. 10) reports that for three years he has applied eucalyptol, alone or in combination with iodoform and creasote or guaiacol ; guaiacol and iodoform, without eucalyptol ; and creasol and guaiacol, subcutaneously, in the treatment of tuberculosis, with most satisfactory results. He uses as a menstruum sterilized liquid vaselin, olive oil, or oil of sweet almonds—preferably one of the latter two—containing twenty per cent. of the medicaments in varying proportions, of which at least from three to ten cubic centimetres are injected daily. The injections are made with antiseptic precautions into the retrotrochanteric fold. The best results were obtained from a combination of guaiacol and iodoform.

PICOT (*Bull. de l'Acad. de Méd.*, 1891, No. 9) has reported the results of treatment in twenty-five cases of pulmonary tuberculosis and eight of pleurisy by means of subcutaneous injections of iodoform and guaiacol, dissolved in sterilized olive oil and vaselin, each cubic centimetre of the solution containing one centigramme of iodoform and five of guaiacol. The injections, each of three cubic centimetres, were made into the supra-spinous fossa daily, and were unattended with unpleasant local results. As an evidence of the absorption of the medicaments, the presence of iodoform could be demonstrated in the urine, guaiacol not being eliminated by the kidneys. As a rule, the injections occasioned no general reaction, but in certain cases, especially in those with fever, profuse perspiration followed, succeeded in turn by a sense of comfort and a lowering of temperature. In exceptional instances abdominal pain and diarrhœa developed in the course of treatment, but subsided on suspending the injections. In three cases of advanced phthisis, in which death took place, the changes found in the lungs were indicative of a reparative tendency. The tubercles presented an appearance of beginning fatty degeneration; the cavities were clean and dry. In one case the ulcers in the intestine showed a disposition to cicatrization. Neither in the lungs nor elsewhere was there any evidence of a fresh eruption of tubercles as a result of the treatment. In the remaining cases of phthisis the cough diminished, the sputum became less, and the number of bacilli in the sputum smaller, the body weight increased, the night-sweats disappeared, the general condition improved, and the physical signs receded. In the cases of pleurisy the results were equally good. Effusion speedily disappeared, and recovery was rapid.

DIABETES AND VASCULAR SCLEROSIS OF THE PANCREAS.

LEMOINNE and LANNOIS (*Arch. de Méd. expérim. et d'Anat. pathol.*, 1891, No. 1) made a study of the pancreas in four cases of diabetes : three of these belonged clinically to the so-called pancreatic type; one was in a case of long standing. In the last, the liver and kidneys presented alterations similar to those found in the pancreas. In the other three the liver contained several limited areas of interlobular sclerosis not involving the hepatic lobules ; the kidneys presented no lesion; the pancreas, however, presented marked changes. In all, the lesions of the pancreas were topographically the same. Sections of pancreatic tissue, hardened in Müller's fluid and stained with hæmatoxylon or carmine, exhibited interacinous and intercellular sclerosis— a true interstitial pancreatitis—having for its point of departure the vascular system and notably the venous and lymphatic system of the gland, and giving rise to consecutive degeneration of the cellular elements. This differs from the conditions found after ligature of the duct of Wirsung, in that the dilatation of the duct is followed by its fibrous transformation, the vascular sclerosis appearing late and as an accessory phenomenon. In the cases in which the pancreatic duct has been ligated the absence of sugar in the urine has been expressly noted. These facts give support to the opinion of M. Lepine that the pancreas, like the liver, has a double function. The liver elaborates not only bile, but also glycogen ; the pancreas separates not only trypsin, amylopsin, and steapsin, but also a glycolytic ferment—the first three at the free extremity of the cell, the last at that pole of the cell in relation to the vascular supply.

HEMIATROPHY OF THE TONGUE OF PERIPHERAL ORIGIN.

Before the Canadian Medical Association, at Toronto, BIRKETT (*Montreal Medical Journal*, 1891, No. 9) reported a case of hemiatrophy of the tongue of peripheral origin. The patient, a bank clerk of twenty-three, nine years previously, following an attack of mumps, noticed a large and painful swelling behind the angle of the jaw on the right side. Subsequently there was some difficulty in speech, and the tongue, when protruded, deviated to the right. Five years later it was observed that pressure upon the swelling led to flushing and sweating on the right half of the face and to a sense of dryness of the throat. At the time the patient came under observation, when the mouth was opened, the tip of the tongue pointed to the left, but when the organ was protruded, the tip deviated to the right. The right half of the tongue was smaller than the left, and presented reactions of degeneration, but there was no fibrillary contraction, and the sense of taste was unimpaired. There was paresis of the right half of the soft palate, and the mucous membrane of the fauces, soft palate, and walls of the pharynx were insensible to titillation. Sensation, however, was unimpaired at the posterior extremities of the inferior and middle turbinated bones and on the lips and mucous membrane of the mouth. The right vocal band occupied the cadaveric position, scarcely moving in abduction and adduction. Movement of the right half of the epiglottis was defective. The pulse was ninety-six in the minute. The pupil was smaller and the palpebral fissure narrower on the right than on the left. Vision was myopic—on the right by 1 D.; on the left by 0.25 D. From a careful study of the case Birkett believes the lesion to be peripheral, the result of inflammatory changes in and about a cervical gland behind the angle of the jaw and involving the hypoglossal, the vagus, and the accessory nerves, the pharyngeal plexus, and the superior ganglion of the cervical sympathetic—all on the right side. The following deductions are made:

1. The hypoglossal is the motor and trophic nerve of the tongue; 2, the glosso-pharyngeal nerve is concerned in the function of taste; 3, branches of the pharyngeal plexus supply the mucous membrane of the naso- and buccal pharynx with sensory fibres; 4, the motor nerve of the levator palati and azygos uvulæ muscles is probably the accessorius; 5, the superior ganglion of the cervical sympathetic contains (a) dilator fibres to the iris of the same side; (b) vasomotor fibres; (c) sweat fibres; and (d) secretory fibres to the mucous glands of the pharynx.

Pulmonary Abscess.

In a paper read before the St. Louis Medical Society, Porter (*Journal of the Amer. Med. Association*, 1891, No. 10) expressed the view that pulmonary gangrene or abscess following embolism is not necessarily multiple; that gangrene may follow embolism of a pulmonary artery; and abscess, embolism of a bronchial artery. When the products of disorganization can be readily discharged, with the probability of cicatrization taking place, operation may be deferred; but when there are evidences of rapid breaking down, when fever, restlessness, and depression are marked, prompt and active measures are indicated. When the abscess is extensive and operation necessary, Porter prefers to excise a large piece of rib over the cavity and make a free opening in the pleural sac. A smaller incision may be made in the lung. Two cases of gangrene, successfully operated upon in the manner indicated, are reported.

MORVAN'S DISEASE.

CHURCH (*Journal of the Amer. Med. Association*, 1891, No. 10) reports a case of so-called Morvan's disease, with a brief review of what is known on the subject, the literature of which is scanty. The affection is characterized by a destructive process, progressively and symmetrically involving the digits, ulceration with exfoliation of bone taking place, and resulting in deformity, sometimes preceded by pain and attended with anæsthesia. In the only case of the disease in which an autopsy has been reported, an excess of connective tissue was found in the posterior horns, posterior columns, and gray matter of the cervical cord and in the peripheral nerves. Nothing is known as to its etiology. The disease is to be distinguished from scleroderma, anæsthetic lepra, symmetrical gangrene, and syringomyelia. The treatment is symptomatic.

CONGENITAL OCCLUSION OF THE ŒSOPHAGUS; COMMUNICATION BETWEEN THE TRACHEA AND ŒSOPHAGUS.

GRANDOU (*Bull. de la Soc. Anat. de Paris*, 1891, No. 3) reports the case of a newborn infant, which, applied to the breast several hours after birth, took the nipple without difficulty. Each time it nursed, however, the infant became congested and purple; it then abandoned the breast, and almost immediately vomited the milk it had taken. Efforts at feeding with a spoon and gavage were no more successful. Death took place on the sixth day. On examination the superior portion of the œsophagus was found to be normal; lower down was a dilatation an inch and a half in length, below which the œsophagus was replaced by a firm cord, two-thirds of an inch long and a quarter of an inch thick, adherent in front to the trachea. Beyond this the œsophagus resumed its calibre for a distance of a little more than two inches, at its termination emptying into the stomach. Opening the trachea from in front an orifice with bevelled edges, the plane of which looked upward and forward, was found on the posterior wall, a little more than an inch below the cricoid cartilage. This orifice communicated with the lower portion of the œsophagus and through it the mucous membrane of the trachea was continued.

PARTIAL NEPHRITIS.

CUFFER and GASTOU (*Revue de Médecine*, 1891) describe as partial nephritis a condition succeeding the acute or active manifestations of a renal lesion, in which a fixed and invariable amount of albumin is present in the urine, although the patient is in all other respects in perfect health. Five cases illustrative of the condition are cited. Pathological evidence is wanting, but an analogy is made with the lesions found in amyloid disease, in arteriosclerosis, and in plumbism, in which diseased and healthy structure alternate or the disease is less decided at one part than at another. The condition must be considered not as a disease, but as an infirmity, for which treatment is useless and may prove hurtful. It is important, however, for the patient to avoid those influences which are known to affect the kidneys injuriously.

The prognosis is not grave if appropriate precautions are taken. The conclusions formulated are that persistent albuminuria is a result of a past nephritis, in the chronic stage, and that the persistence of a fixed amount of albumin in the urine, incapable of diminution, is evidence of a partial nephritis.

SURGERY.

UNDER THE CHARGE OF

J. WILLIAM WHITE, M.D.,

PROFESSOR OF CLINICAL SURGERY IN THE UNIVERSITY OF PENNSYLVANIA; SURGEON TO THE UNIVERSITY AND GERMAN HOSPITALS;

ASSISTED BY

EDWARD MARTIN, M.D.,

CLINICAL PROFESSOR OF GENITO-URINARY SURGERY IN THE UNIVERSITY OF PENNSYLVANIA; SURGEON TO THE HOWARD HOSPITAL AND ASSISTANT SURGEON TO THE UNIVERSITY HOSPITAL.

STAB-WOUNDS OF THE SPINAL CORD.

DR. OTTO BODE (*Berliner klinische Wochenschrift*, Jahrg. xxviii., No. 22) gives an interesting account of the diagnosis, course, and proper treatment of stab-wounds of the spinal cord. He cites the case of a man who, in a street fight, received several wounds on the head; on the back of the neck there was one about five centimetres long, running obliquely down to the spinal column and exposing at its bottom the atlas and axis. At the moment of wounding the patient fell to the ground, lost consciousness for only a minute, but remained paralyzed on the right side below the point of wounding. When called upon the right lower extremity responded slowly and reluctantly, but for walking or standing was weak and useless. There were no areas of anæsthesia, nor any disturbance of the special senses. The bladder and rectum were normal; priapism not present. The muscles of respiration on the right side were decidedly implicated. The faradic excitability of the muscles remained normal. For three weeks this condition continued apparently unaltered. At the expiration of this time the patient began to gain more and more use of the paralyzed limbs, albeit at the same time the reflexes became greatly exaggerated, and at the least touch the muscles jerked. The patient was under observation for three months; the paralysis was practically gone, and even the reflexes had returned to normal, and in a year's time no evil effects of the wound remained, save at times a slight tremor in the muscles which had been paralyzed. The wound was treated solely by the antiseptic dressings.

From the anatomical relations of the vertebræ and their ligaments, Dr. Bode proceeds to show that in the cervical region when the neck is bent down, as it usually is when a man receives a wound there in a fight, the cord can be wounded at almost any point of its circumference, or, indeed, may be wholly severed, without injury to the vertebræ. From the motor

disturbances and the direction of the external wound in his case, he diag-
noses a partial severance of the anterior column and the anterior part of the
lateral column on the right side. Therefore, he maintains that it is not possible that the lateral columns in the cervical cord carry both sensory and
motor fibres, since in his case there were absolutely no disturbances of sensation.

Dr. Bode cites several cases of perfect healing of wounds of the spinal cord
involving not quite half its diameter, which were recognized during life to be
wounds of the cord, or were subsequently clearly demonstrated at the autopsy
by the cicatrices.

He goes on to explain that the appearance of symptoms which set in generally on the second to the third day after the wounding, and which might
easily be mistaken for traumatic myelitis, is due to what Schiefferdecker
describes ("Ueber Regeneration, Degeneration, und Architektur des Rücken-
marks," *Virchow's Archiv*, Bd. lxii.) as traumatic degeneration following
wounds of the spinal cord, and setting in on the second to the third day.
The degeneration begins as a disintegration of the elements of the nerves
into glossy flakes. This process extends from the cut surfaces about four to
six millimetres above and below. Hence, in the case of wounds in the
neighborhood of the fourth cervical vertebra, although the phrenic nerve be
not at first implicated, yet at the end of the second or third day that complication may arise.

The increase of the reflex excitability, Dr. Bode explains as due to what
Schiefferdecker describes as secondary degeneration, which manifests itself
about the fourteenth day, and which, by cutting off the influence of the
reflex inhibitory fibres running down the lateral columns in the cervical cord,
gives rise to an increase in the reflexes. Schiefferdecker describes a third
form of degeneration, which he calls cavity formation, and to this Dr. Bode
ascribes the fibrillary tremors in the limbs formerly paralyzed.

Retention of urine and feces is not uncommon following wounds in this
region. The organs either return to normal, or else incontinence sets in.
The height of the wound has no influence hereon. Priapism almost always
occurs where there is vasomotor disturbance. Elevations of temperature are
not found on the anæsthetic areas of the skin, if there be any, but only on
the areas where there is motor paralysis. This proves that the vascular nerve-
supply runs down the same paths as the motor fibres. Dr. Bode cites a very
interesting case where he found variations of temperature of the affected
part entirely independent of the temperature variations in the rest of the
body.

He maintains that it is impossible to locate with absolute certainty the
position of the wound on the cord from the symptoms, since some hemorrhage affecting the parts immediately adjoining is inevitable, and, furthermore, unless the assailant's knife be very sharp, it must make more or less of
a contusion on the cord before it cuts through the elastic pia mater.

To sum up, the most conclusive symptom is a sharply defined paralysis
below the point of wounding, coming on at the moment the wound is
received.

As to treatment, he says the external wound should be enlarged and left·
open. Above all, free drainage should be encouraged, even to the loss of

meningeal fluid, and the blood and secretions of the wound should be kept aseptic. Finally, the wound should be allowed to heal by granulations, or sewn up secondarily.

Intestinal Anastomosis by Means of Vegetable Plates.

After reviewing the well-known objections to all the mechanical arrangements designed to accomplish intestinal anastomoses, DARBON (*Medical Record*, vol. xxxix. No. 26) states that he has discovered what may be called an entirely serviceable emergency plate in one made from a raw potato. He has experimented on a large number of dogs, and so far as this work goes has evidently well proven not only the reliability of his plates, but the value of certain modifications he has made in the operation of intestinal anastomosis. A pair of the potato plates can be made by his method in ten minutes. The material can always be procured. It has no tendency to swell; it is rigid, and remains so longer than the majority of other materials devised for this purpose. For use upon the human gut the plate should be made about one-third of an inch in thickness, and should be cut so long that the opening is about twice the normal diameter of the gut to be operated upon. To prevent the threads from cutting through they should be very coarse, and the needle before passing through the plate should traverse a scrap of rubber drainage-tube or a minute bit of cloth, which, by its broad surface, prevents the large knot tied on the end of the thread from pulling through. Instead of first making the incisions into the gut, which subsequently serve as the artificial opening, the plate is inserted into the lumen of the bowel through its divided end and the needles are made to traverse the gut-wall at their proper positions. When the two plates are thus placed in the two extremities of the bowel, at least two inches from the cut extremity, the corresponding threads of the two plates are tied together, thus apposing the two peritoneal surfaces covering the plates. These surfaces previously should be well scraped with a knife, so that prompt adhesions may take place. After the plate-threads are tied, at least one line of sutures should be run around the plates, great care being taken not to pass the needle into the lumen of the bowel. The author prefers a basting-stitch, since it is easier to apply, employing three stitches to the inch. When these stitches are placed, into one open gut-end a strip of wood is passed; this is for the purpose of cutting against; the opening is then made through the apposed gut-walls enclosed by the rings. To do this a scalpel is inserted into the open end of the gut, and as long an anastomotic opening is made as the plates will allow. The strip of wood prevents cutting too deeply. After this incision is made, water should run freely into one end and out of the other. Under gentle hydrostatic pressure, closing the outlet end with the finger and thumb for a few moments, the line of suture should not leak if properly made. The free ends of the bowel are next scraped, inverted, and secured in this position by a double line of running sutures.

Finally, a stitch or two is taken between the blind ends and the gut against which each rests, first scraping the peritoneal surfaces which are apposed. This prevents the possibility of another loop forcing its way into this angle with the result of undue tension of the stitches at the plate-ends. The author states that he has without extreme haste done lateral anastomosis by this method, including tying off the mesentery and excising several inches of the gut, in half an hour, counting from the first incision into the belly-wall to the knotting of the last parietal suture. He claims as original: the material from which he makes his plates; his method of inserting the plates and making the anastomotic opening; his method of suturing; his method of denuding the peritoneum by means of the knife-blade, and his method of protecting the suture at the plate-ends by causing adhesion of the blind ends of the adjacent bowel. To those who have had much experience in laboratory work, the technique described would in some points commend itself.

Union of the Divided Ulnar Nerve by Plastic Operation.

Dittel (*Wiener klin. Wochenschr.*, Jahr. iv., No. 18) reports a successful plastic operation upon the ulnar nerve, although there was considerable loss in the continuity of this structure. The patient received a severe wound of the arm, which, together with extensive injury to the skin and muscles, destroyed about two and a half inches of the ulnar nerve. The peripheral end of this nerve could not be found. The wound was closed under antiseptic precautions. Examination on the following day showed that the sensibility of the skin supplied by the ulnar nerve was practically unimpaired, and that there was very slight difference in the muscular power of the right and left arm. This was evidently due to nervous anastomosis. Four weeks later an electrical examination showed that the muscles supplied by the ulnar nerve were completely paralyzed. By no form of current could contraction be induced. An operation for the restoration of the continuity of the nerve-trunk was at once undertaken, since it seemed desirable to accomplish this before marked degenerative changes could set in. By careful dissection the proximal and peripheral ends of the nerve were exposed. About three inches from the extremity of the peripheral nerve-end a thin-bladed scalpel was thrust directly through the centre of its trunk; by carrying the blade upward the trunk was split in two equal halves. The incision stopped short before reaching the extremity of the nerve. In a similar manner the proximal end was split. By transverse cuts half the nerve was freed and carried upward from the distal end, downward from the proximal end, until the extremities of the ends thus split off were brought in contact. Sutures were applied. To cover the large defect of the soft parts resulting from the original injury, a flap of skin was transplanted from the upper portion of the arm. Suppuration set in. The wound was dressed by the open method. Eight weeks after operation an electrical examination was made as to the condition of the muscles supplied by the ulnar nerve. The results were negative. Two weeks after this, however, the muscles reacted to electricity. At the time of reporting the case contractions could be excited, not only by application of the current to the muscles, but also by excitation of the nerve-trunk.

Brenner (*Ibid.*) also reports a successful neuroplastic operation ten years after injury to a nerve.

The patient exhibited a bluish discoloration and decided emaciation of the left index and middle fingers, the nails of which were thickened and turtle-backed. Both fingers were flexed at the metacarpo-phalangeal articulations; tendons and joints were found to be normal on manipulation. The palmar surface of both these fingers and the ulnar surface of the thumb were completely anæsthetic; the other portions of the skin of the hand were normal. Ten years before, the patient had received a stab-wound on the flexor surface of the wrist-joint. The scar of this wound lay directly over the course of the median nerve; beneath it there was a hard knot the size of a cherry; this often occasioned great pain. It was diagnosed as a neuroma, and excision was determined upon. On dissecting this tumor free, it was found attached to the extremity of the central portion of the median nerve. On dividing this connection, the cross-section of the nerve seemed perfectly healthy. It was then determined to find the distal end of the nerve and restore the continuity of this structure by a plastic operation. The two extremities of the nerves were split almost to their terminations. The halves of the split trunk were freed at the points most distant from the terminations of the nerve; the flaps thus formed, made long enough to completely bridge the gap existing between the nerve-ends, were turned down and up, respectively, and were sutured to each other and to the freshened extremity of the two nerve terminations. The wound was closed, and healed by primary intention. Two weeks after operation there was return of sensibility. A year later sensibility was completely normal, and the contracture of the fingers was no more observable. The trophic disturbances, however, did not disappear.

EROSIVE BALANO-POSTHITIS.

An erosive circinate form of balano-posthitis. quite different from the ordinary type of the disease so often observed complicating gonorrhœa, is described by BERDAL and BATAILLE (*La Médecine Moderne*, an. ii. No. 22). They find that there is a distinct inflammation of the epithelial covering of the foreskin and glans penis, characterized by the facts that it is inoculable and contagious; that it is not secondary to irritation, but is essentially primary and due to a microbe; that it has a definite course, starting in one or more erosions and extending centrifugally in circinate lesions; that these lesions are circumscribed by white, friable borders; that there is a very free purulent secretion in which spirilla can be found, and that this inflammation occasions lymphadenitis and polyadenitis. These are all characteristics sufficiently distinct from the salient features of ordinary balano-posthitis, which is neither inoculable nor contagious, is always secondary to mechanical or chemical irritation, has no definite course, begins not as an erosion, but as an area of acute hyperæmia, has little tendency to spread, and rarely produces extensive lesions.

Certain cases of herpes at times closely simulate the erosive circinate form of balano-posthitis; but in herpes the white, friable margin is wanting to the lesions, and, as Leloir has shown, on pressing an herpetic erosion between the fingers there is a free exudation of serum. This is not the case in circinate balano-posthitis. Mucous patches may so closely simulate the form of balano-posthitis described as to render a differential diagnosis impossible until sufficient time has elapsed to determine the nature of the disease from its clinical course.

There is also a certain rare form of chancre which produces lesions very like the circinate erosive balano-posthitis: this is the epithelial phagadenic chancre, manifesting itself in the form of an erosion which may extend over the greater part of the glans penis.

The treatment of erosive circinate balanitis consists in destroying the epithelial cells—the breeding-ground of the parasites which occasion the disease. This is best accomplished by nitrate of silver, bichloride of mercury, or strong solutions of carbolic acid. Other antiseptics are of little value.

DUPUYTREN'S CONTRACTION.

In a series of lectures delivered upon the contraction of the fingers and toes, ANDERSON (*The Lancet*, 1891, vol. ii. No. 2), after a careful study of the pathology and treatment of true and false Dupuytren's contraction, arrives at the following conclusions:

There are two forms of disease comprised under the name of "contraction of the palmar fascia," the one traumatic in origin, dependent upon changes in the integumental and fascial structures, and occurring at all ages; the other unassociated with obvious traumatism, tending to multiplicity of lesion, and almost confined to middle or advanced life.

The latter condition, true "Dupuytren's contraction," is not, strictly speaking, a contraction of the palmar fascia, but consists of a chronic inflammatory hyperplasia, commencing in the subcutaneous connective tissue and involving secondarily the palmar fasciæ and the deep fibres of the corium. The morbid bands are, for the most part, formed at the expense of the normal tissues.

This condition does not appear to be connected primarily with pressure or friction of the palm by tools or other objects employed in manual occupations, but is probably due to a specific infective agent which effects its entrance through epidermic lesions made by the finger-nails, or otherwise.

It is almost essentially a disease of advanced and middle age, more common in men than in women, occurring in all classes, tending to progress slowly through a long course of years, and to return after operation.

It is connected with a special diathesis, inherited or acquired, which cannot yet be expressed in any known terms; but neither gout, rheumatism, rheumatoid arthritis, nor any other of the ordinary constitutional ailments has been shown to have any causative relation to the disease.

It appears to be almost, if not quite, unknown in certain parts of the East, as in India and Japan.

THE MICROÖRGANISMS OF THE NORMAL URETHRA.

Since Lustgarten and Mannaberg stated that in the healthy urethra of man were constantly to be found microörganisms which in form, grouping, and color reaction closely resemble gonococci, much discredit has been thrown upon the reliability of this latter microbe as an indicator of the presence of true gonorrhœa in any given urethritis.

PETIT and WASSERMANN (*Annales des Maladies des Organes Genito-urinaires*, 1891, Tome ix. No. 6), in a series of carefully conducted researches, both microscopic and bacteriological, failed to find in any case the microörganisms characterized by Lustgarten as pseudo-gonococci. They found a number of bacilli, micrococci, and sarcinæ, which they believe are saprophytes—that is, are accidental hosts, and which vary in accordance with the nature of the soil in which they grow. In 1000 examinations they failed to find pseudo-gonococci. Frequently, however, they observed sarcinæ, which on super-ficial examination might well be taken for gonococci. These, however, are not decolorized by Gram's method; there are also certain sarcinæ which are readily decolorized by Gram's method, but they are so much larger than the gonococci that they cannot readily be confounded with the latter.

Steinschneider has long since shown that it is not alone upon one feature that the gonococcus is to be recognized, but upon the facts that these organisms are grouped around nuclei in the interior cells, are decolorized by Gram's method as formulated by Roux, and are recolorized by Bismarck brown or by Loeffler's blue.

In summing up the results of their experimental investigation, the authors state that the normal urethra is always inhabited by various organisms; that the same varieties are not found in different urethræ; that different varieties are found in the meatus and in deeper parts of the canal; that none of the varieties found in the healthy urethra are pathogenic, and that the greater number of microörganisms of the normal urethra decompose urea.

OPHTHALMOLOGY.

UNDER THE CHARGE OF

GEORGE A. BERRY, M.B., F.R.C.S. ED.,
OPHTHALMIC SURGEON, EDINBURGH ROYAL INFIRMARY,

AND

EDWARD JACKSON, M.D.,
PROFESSOR OF DISEASES OF THE EYE IN THE PHILADELPHIA POLYCLINIC; SURGEON TO WILLS EYE HOSPITAL, ETC.

AN EXPERIMENTAL STUDY OF THE INFLUENCE OF THE RETINAL AND CHOROIDAL CIRCULATION ON THE NUTRITION OF THE EYE, PARTICU-LARLY THAT OF THE RETINA, AND OF THE CONSEQUENCES OF SECTION OF THE OPTIC NERVE.

Under the above title DR. WAGENMANN contributes a long paper which occupies 120 pages of the last number of the *Archiv für Ophthalmologie*, xxxvi. H. 4. The investigation was undertaken at the instigation of Prof. Leber.

The experiments, which were made on rabbits, gave the following results:

1. Section of the optic nerve above the entrance of the central artery produced at first practically no alteration in the ophthalmoscopic image. Afterward a pallor of the disc became visible, and in the course of some weeks atrophy of the nerve bundles. After this lesion the circulation in the retina remains unchanged, but the retina shows a slight grayish veiling owing to

loss of transparency. The degeneration and disappearance of the nerve fibres can be followed anatomically. The degeneration spreads to the ganglion cells, but so slowly that well-preserved cells are to be found even after six months.

2. Section of the optic nerve with its vessels produces an immediate pallor of the papilla, a narrowing of the vessels, and disappearance of their blood-column. Generally, after the lapse of a week or two, there is an imperfect restitution of the circulation in the retina. This is effected by means of newly formed vessels springing from the choroidal ring, from the nerve-sheath, and from the episcleral ciliary vessels. The section of the retinal vessels is not followed by any opacity of the retina. The subsequent changes in the nerve are in no way distinguishable from those which take place after section of the trunk above the point of entrance of the central vessels.

3. Section of the long and short posterior ciliary arteries on the one side produces a rapid degeneration of all the corresponding layers of the retina. This shows itself at first ophthalmoscopically, and a few hours after the lesion, as a grayish retinal opacity. The nerve fibres above are relatively but little involved. Owing to the reëstablishment in a few days of the choroidal circu-lation a complete degeneration of the one side does not take place. Thus, on microscopic examination, the most varying degrees of degeneration are found in close proximity to each other. The outer layers suffer most severely. A subsequent migration of pigment takes place into the degenerated portion of the retina.

4. Section of the optic nerve and its vessels, and at the same time of the ciliary vessels of one side, leads to a rapid degeneration of the nerve-layer of the retina on that side, the same layer on the other side only atrophying slowly.

5. Section of the optic nerve and vessels and all of the ciliary vessels causes a rapid degeneration of the whole eye.

The author admits that one cannot unreservedly apply the inferences as to the sources of the nutrition of the retina to which these experiments on rab-bits must lead, to the case of man. He points out in particular that whilst the division of the retinal vessels alone did not cause any opacity of the rab-bit's retina, the sudden removal of the blood supply caused by embolism of the central artery in man is invariably accompanied by a marked opacity. There is this difference, however, that the veins are not blocked in the latter case, and although no case of fresh embolism has as yet formed the subject of microscopical examination, it is highly probable that the opacity met with is merely an œdema. In other respects, viz., in recovery of transparency by the retina and in the absence of any subsequent pigmentation, the condition of embolism in man is in accord with the experimental result on section of the vessels in the rabbit. Anatomically, too, it has been found that as the result of embolism the nerve-fibres and ganglion-cells slowly disappear.

––––

ON THE CORTICAL VISUAL CENTRE IN MONKEYS.

MAZZA has studied this question in the Physiological Laboratory at Genoa (*Annali di Ottalmologia*, xix. 6). He was struck by the fact that no previous experimenters had taken proper precautions to examine the field of vision.

After several attempts he succeeded in devising a plan which forced the animal to make use of direct fixation. This consisted in fixing a shell in the shape of an artificial eye, but perforated by a central aperture in the conjunctival sac in front of the eye. These shells were modelled from wax and caoutchouc. With such a shield, which had only a limited movement, in front of the eye, if the animal saw anything out of the direct line of vision one could feel sure that it did so with a peripheral portion of the retina. The experiments were made with a regular perimeter, the animal being fixed by means of a specially constructed apparatus. Removal of the cortex cerebri of the angular gyrus only produced a temporary concentric restriction of both fields of vision. Removal of the cortex of the occipital lobe produced a persistent hemianopia.

On the Validity of Weber's Law in the Case of the Light-sense.

DR. SCHIRMER, by modifying the details of the usual method of testing the light-sense, has been able to show that Weber's law holds good with reference to this as well as to other senses. The light-sense referred to is what is now generally called the light-difference perception, or L. D.—*i. e.*, the extent of the power of distinguishing luminous impressions of different intensities. The statement of Weber's law is that "appreciation of the difference of two similar excitations of different magnitudes is not dependent upon their actual but upon their proportional differences." Former experimenters, and notably Aubert and Helmholtz, have denied the validity of this law in the case of the light-sense. Schirmer points out that the discrepancies between the results of these experiments and Weber's law are due to their not having taken into consideration the necessity for allowing for the adaptation of the eye for different light intensities. His own experiments, after providing for adaptation and performed with an ingenious modification of Masson's disc, led to the following results:

1. Weber's law is valid for the light-sense within a range of illumination of from oné to one thousand standard candles at the distance of a metre from the illuminated surface. The eye must be allowed its full power of adaptation : so that the validity of the law is subject to the fulfilment of certain physiological conditions.

2. Physiological adaptation alone is capable of explaining why Weber's law should hold good, but Schirmer's experiments do not exclude the possibility of the participation of a certain psycho-physical process (such as Fechner assumed) in bringing about the result.

3. The adaptation of the normal eye does not all along keep pace with the diminution of daylight as dusk comes on.

An Experimental Study of the Nutrition of the Crystalline Lens and the Development of Cataract.

By examining the first stages in the development of artificial cataract in the lenses of living rabbits, by the method of magnification with a strong glass lens behind the ophthalmoscope mirror, MAGNUS (*Archiv f. Ophthalmologie*, xxxvi. 4) has been able to throw some light on the process by which the crystalline lens is nourished, and to make some valuable suggestions regarding the etiology of idiopathic cataract.

The artificial forms of cataract studied were those produced by the internal administration of naphthalin, sugar, and salt.

One dose of three to four grammes per kilometre of body weight given to not too young a rabbit is sufficient to give rise to changes in the lens after six hours. According as it was desired to produce a greater or less degree of opacity this was repeated more or less often. The lenticular changes made their appearance always before any visible changes occurred in the fundus. Although both lenses usually show the changes about the same time, they are occasionally to be found well marked in the one while the other remains perfectly normal. Two distinct phases are to be distinguished in these changes.

In the first there are to be seen a number of transparent bands, in the second well-marked and progressive opacities. They both begin at the equator of the lens, and apparently the very first traces are met with in two zones, the one lying immediately behind and the other immediately in front of the equator.

A characteristic feature of naphthalin cataract is that the opacities are capable of clearing up, and do so invariably if the naphthalin be stopped after only two doses have been given. Even a well-marked opacity of this nature occupying the whole extent of the superficial layers of the posterior cortex may entirely clear away. The clearing up always takes place in exactly the same manner, proceeding from the equator and posterior pole.

As the recovery of transparency can only well be supposed to be due to the return to its normal condition of the nutrient fluid of the lens, the nature of the clearing process affords, Magnus argues, important conclusions as to the places of entrance of these fluids into the lens. It is thus rendered very probable that the position of the posterior zone of opacity and the posterior pole are important in this respect.

Further experiments with salt and sugar led to precisely similar conclusions. Altogether, the experiments led to the following results with regard to the conditions of nutrient supply in the case of the normal lens:

1. The nutrition processes are effected more actively and more completely in the posterior section than in the anterior section of the lens.

2. A zone lying posterior to, and parallel with, the equator appears to be that through which the most extensive supply of nutriment passes.

3. A zone anterior to, and parallel with, the equator appears also to be active in this respect, though less so than the posterior zone.

4. The posterior pole of the lens also transmits a current of nutriment, though to a less extent than either the anterior or posterior or equatorial zones.

5. No current appears to pass at the anterior pole.

6. The equator is dependent for its nutriment on the currents passing by the zones in front and behind it, but does not itself give entrance to any current.

Magnus's experiments do not give any indication as to the parts at which the nutrient fluid leaves the lens.

With reference to the very interesting question as to how far such experiments throw light on the development of idiopathic cataract, Magnus in the first place draws attention to the fact that in the great majority of cases (in 92.77 per cent. according to a previous investigation of his) senile cataract begins exactly in the same manner as the artificial cataract. This points to senile cataract being essentially a disturbance in the nutrient current, showing itself first at the places where the current enters the lens. While, however, in experimental artificial cataract, the opacity is the result of an altered chemical constitution of the nutrient fluid, this cannot well be assumed in the case of senile cataract. It is more likely that the disturbance is more of a circulatory nature, and probably, too, this is the consequence of the senile sclerosis which takes place in the lens fibres. Further, no doubt there is a diminished power of resistance in the lens fibres of old people which favors the opacity which a stasis in the lymph-current tends to give rise to. In diabetic cataract, of course, it is natural to suppose that the opacity is more directly caused by the altered chemical constitution of the nutrient fluid.

OBSTETRICS.

UNDER THE CHARGE OF

EDWARD P. DAVIS, A.M., M.D.,

PROFESSOR OF OBSTETRICS AND DISEASES OF CHILDREN IN THE PHILADELPHIA POLYCLINIC;
CLINICAL LECTURER ON OBSTETRICS IN THE JEFFERSON MEDICAL COLLEGE ;
VISITING OBSTETRICIAN TO THE PHILADELPHIA HOSPITAL, ETC.

The Porro Operation, with Invagination of the Stump.

Frank's method of performing the Porro operation has been adopted by Beaucamp, who describes five cases so treated (*Archiv für Gynäkologie*, Band xl. Heft 1). Three of the operations were done for contracted rhachitic pelves, with a history of previous confinements with death of the fœtus. Mothers and children recovered.

One case ended fatally from hemorrhage between the membranes and uterine wall. The fifth case was that of a woman, brought to the hospital in a dying condition with ruptured uterus ; the operation consisted of the total extirpation of the uterus after it had been inverted through the vagina. A fatal result followed, but the post-mortem showed the operation to have been successful so far as union was concerned.

Beaucamp describes his method as follows: Patients with contracted pelves are examined in the middle of pregnancy, and the chances afforded by induced labor and the Cæsarean and Porro operations are explained to them, the chances of the two latter being given as equally favorable. Labor is induced at the end of the thirty-third week. If the Porro operation is to be done, the patient enters the hospital in the thirty-ninth week, and is suitably prepared. The operation consists in opening the abdomen and the uterus, and removing the fœtus. The uterus is then inverted, and its attachments to the vagina are sutured. The abdomen is then closed, and the uterus and tubes and ovaries are removed, and the pelvic peritoneum carefully sutured. Simplicity, speed, and safety are claimed for this procedure.

If the elastic ligature is employed, and the uterus resected at the cervix, the pelvic peritoneum is stitched about the stump, which is pushed up into the pelvis and a tampon of iodoform gauze is placed against it. The after-treatment consists in antisepticizing the vagina.

FORCEPS TO THE AFTER-COMING HEAD.

A plea for the forceps to the after-coming head is made by STAEDLER (*Archiv für Gynäkologie*, Band xl. Heft 1). He adduces ten cases from Bischoff's clinic, at Basel, of which no mother died; two children died during labor, and two more after labor. Most of the children were born deeply asphyxiated, but revived. In all, Staedler tabulates fifty cases, showing 72 per cent. of living children. He would first try manual extraction, then forceps, last perforation. His cases were chiefly contracted pelves, complicated by cross position.

THE TREATMENT OF OCCIPITO-POSTERIOR ROTATIONS.

MEYER, of Dorpat, treats posterior rotation of the occiput by combined external and internal manipulation, inserting the whole or portion of the hand within the vagina, while the other hand coöperates by external pressure upon the head. He thus endeavors to rotate the occiput anteriorly, or posteriorly, and holds the head in the most favorable position obtainable until he has applied the forceps. An assistant furthers the endeavors of the operator by pressure upon the trunk through the abdominal walls. Meyer reports three illustrative cases.—*Archiv für Gynäkologie*, Band xl. Heft 1.

PUERPERAL ECLAMPSIA.

At a recent meeting of the Obstetrical Society of London, HERMAN reported five cases, and from these and others previously reported by him, summarized the following observations: (1) Four children out of ten died *in utero*. (2) The cases showed no direct effect of the fits on the temperature. (3) In all the cases observed at the beginning of the disease, except two, the quantity of urine was lessened. Of the two exceptions, one died, and in the other renal disease persisted after childbed. (4) In all the excretion of nitrogenous matter in the urine was absolutely diminished, and in most the percentage was diminished. (5) In all the urine was at one time nearly or quite solid with albumin. In three of the cases the fits appeared to increase the amount of albumin. The two cases in which the albuminous precipitate contained the largest proportion of paraglobulin both recovered. Of three in which the amount of paraglobulin was less than in the rest, two died, and in one renal disease persisted. (6) In all that recovered there was rapid increase in the amount of urine and the quantity of nitrogenous matter contained in it, and diminution in the amount of albumin. This restoration did not, as a rule, take place till some hours after the cessation of the fits, and went on more rapidly after delivery in the cases in which the cessation of fits preceded delivery. This restoration of renal function did not take place in the cases which died. (7) Retinitis was present in only two cases, both of which died.—*British Medical Journal*, 1891, No. 1593, p. 72.

THE HEPATIC LESIONS OF ECLAMPSIA.

An addition to our knowledge of the hepatic lesions in eclampsia, of which so much is due to the report of cases by Pilliet, is made in *Bulletins de la Société Anatomique de Paris*, 1891, vol. vi. p. 353, by PAPILLON and AUDAIN. In the case itself there was nothing of especial rarity among eclamptic cases. Labor was spontaneous; the urine contained albumin, but no bile; the patient died after labor, with icterus and high temperature.

Upon post-mortem examination, multiple ecchymoses of discolored blood were found beneath the capsule of the liver. Microscopic examination of the liver tissue revealed fatty degeneration of the liver-cells with multiple thromboses of the venous radicles, and infiltration with masses of fibrin, the thread-like reticula of which could be traced to the terminations of liver-cells. The hepatic lesions were strongly suggestive of extensive disorganization of the blood.

In discussion, Pilliet confirmed these observations, and added that he had found several sorts of microbes in the livers of eclamptic patients, but none which could be isolated as pathognomonic.

THE POISONOUS PROPERTIES OF THE URINE DURING PREGNANCY.

A curious and interesting corroboration of the belief that during pregnancy the woman excretes more toxic material than when not pregnant, is found in the result of experiments by BLANC (*Annales de Gynécologie*, 1891, Tome xxxvi. p. 15). He injected the urine of the non-pregnant and pregnant woman into rabbits, and observed the effects. Symptoms of ptomaïne intoxication were more marked when the urine of pregnancy was injected, and basing a comparison upon the body weight of the various animals the ratio of toxicity was 115 to 132, the latter expressing the poisonous properties of the urine of pregnancy.

TWIN PREGNANCY IN A PRIMIPARA, FOLLOWED BY ECLAMPSIA; RECOVERY.

LOVIOT (*Bulletins et Mémoires de la Société Obstétricale de Paris*, 1891, No. 8) reports the case of a primipara having albuminuria who was found to be in labor with twins. The first child was safely delivered by the application of forceps to the breech ; the second was a vertex presentation, delivered by forceps. Both children lived.

Several hours after labor the mother had eclampsia ; her paroxysms gradually yielded to treatment. A portion of the vulvo-vaginal tissue became inflamed, and there was high fever. The curette was successfully used to remove the slough, and mercurial solutions were injected into the uterus. Three weeks after labor, the patient suffered from a brief attack of phlebitis. Recovery finally ensued. The most useful measure in the treatment seemed to have been the drainage of the uterus by strips of iodoform gauze.

SECONDARY PERINEORRHAPHY DURING THE PUERPERAL STATE.

VON WEISS has treated five patients who had sustained extensive laceration of the perineum in former labors by perineorrhaphy shortly after a subsequent confinement. One of the cases had prolapse and ulceration of the
cervix. After antiseptic treatment had healed the eroded surfaces, the cervix
was replaced and the laceration successfully repaired. The method employed
was the flap-operation of Sänger, and the time chosen was as soon as abraded
surfaces had healed, and before the patient left her bed. The results were
successful.— *Wiener klinische Wochenschrift*, 1891, No. 29.

ELEVATION OF TEMPERATURE OF OBSCURE ORIGIN IN THE
PUERPERAL STATE.

COE (*American Journal of Obstetrics*, 1891, No. 6) reports, among others, the
case of a patient who had high fever after confinement, without appreciable
cause. A mass was finally discovered in the abdomen, and laparotomy on
the twenty-fourth day after labor revealed an ovarian abscess containing a
drachm of pus, situated deeply among the intestines, shut off by a thick wall
from the peritoneal cavity. The appendix vermiformis could not be found,
and the condition was thought to be an old appendicitis with intestinal adhesions, in which fresh inflammation followed labor. No puerperal sepsis could
be discovered, and nothing abnormal in the pelvis.

TUBAL ABORTION.

In the *Transactions of the Obstetrical Society of London*, vol. xxxii. p. 342,
SUTTON describes a case of tubal pregnancy in which rupture of the fœtal
membranes occurred after examination. On laparotomy the left tube was
found to have been the seat of pregnancy, abortion in the tube having occurred
from apoplexy of the ovum. This apoplexy was attended by pain and slight
shock.

THE INHALATION OF OXYGEN IN TREATING NEWBORN INFANTS.

BONNAIRE (*Bulletins et Mémoires de la Société Obstétricale de Paris*, 1891,
No. 6) has obtained good results, in cases of fœtal asphyxia from imperfect
heart and in infections destroying the red blood-corpuscle, by inhalation of
oxygen.

[In severe broncho-pneumonia of infants with marked cyanosis we have
had a similar experience. The dosage depends entirely upon the effect ;
oxygen may be inhaled until an appreciable result follows, repeated when
needed.—ED.]

CÆSAREAN SECTION.

Successful operations are reported by BAR (*Revue Obstétricale et Gynécolo-
gique*, 1891, No. 4) for cystic enchondroma of the pubis; by PORAK (*Ibid.*)
for cancer of the cervix, the patient and child surviving the operation,
but the cancer steadily progressing to a fatal result. It is worthy of note that
in this case Porak operated before labor began. CAMERON (*British Medical*

Journal, 1891, p. 511) has operated nine times successfully, checking hemorrhage by manual compression, closing the uterine wound with silk, with superficial stitches where required. Cameron had one fatal case, a patient who had fallen and had hemorrhage, who died of fatty, dilated heart. GRANGER (*Ibid.*) operated successfully upon a dwarf, using a drainage-tube through the incision and vagina.

CRIMAIL (*Annales de Gynécologie,* 1891, vol. XXXV.) operated successfully a second time upon a rhachitic woman on whom he operated in 1889. The incision was made at the edge of the first uterine wound. The silk sutures of the first operation had been absorbed, leaving only the knots partially imbedded in the uterine tissue.

GYNECOLOGY.

UNDER THE CHARGE OF

HENRY C. COE, M.D., M.R.C.S.,

OF NEW YORK.

DIVERTICULUM OF THE RECTUM SIMULATING CYST OF THE VAGINAL WALL.

HEYDRICH (*Centralblatt für Gynäkologie,* 1891, No. 21) reports a unique case of this character, in which the correct diagnosis was made before the operation. The patient developed a specific colitis soon after marriage, from which resulted a stricture of the rectum. Ulceration above the point of stricture and inflammation of the cellular tissue between the rectum and vagina followed, and a peri-rectal abscess formed, communicating with the gut; the sac gradually increased in size, causing a protrusion of the posterior vaginal wall, which at length appeared at the vulva, presenting the appearance of an ordinary cyst. The differential diagnosis was extremely difficult, the presence of the stricture being an important aid, as well as the softness and absence of tension noted in the sac. The anterior wall of the sac was incised, a quantity of turbid mucus being evacuated, and its edges were united to those of the vaginal wound. Healing by granulation promptly occurred, after which the stricture was dilated.

PAPILLOMATOUS OVARIAN CYSTOMA.

FRÄNKEL (*Deutsche med. Wochenschrift,* 1891, No. 6) confirms the general opinion that papillomatous ovarian cysts are clinically malignant, since they are prone to metastases, even though anatomically they are not atypical in structure. Their malignancy is shown by the tendency of the papillary masses to penetrate the inner wall of the cyst and spread over its serous covering and thence over the entire surface of the peritoneum. The general thickening of the latter is due to the presence of minute papillary growths, which degenerate to form a viscid fluid. Metastases have been observed in the pleura, and in one rare instance on the aortic valves. The writer believes that, in the case of the former, papillomatous are to be sharply distinguished from simple glandular cystomata, since the prognosis is so much more grave.

ETIOLOGY OF HÆMATO-SALPINX.

WALTHER (abstract of thesis in *Centralblatt für Gynäkologie*, 1891, No. 21), after careful microscopical studies entertains no doubt of the existence of true hæmato-salpinx independent of tubal gestation. Hemorrhage into the tube may be due to primary salpingitis, to retained menstrual blood resulting from atresiæ and malformations, to catarrh of the tube (which may be caused by an ectopic gestation on the opposite side) or to acute congestion from suppression of the menses or infectious diseases. On comparing true hæmato-salpinx with tubal gestation it is evident that in the case of the former there is more evidence of inflammatory thickening of the serous coat of the tube; moreover, symptoms of localized peritonitis are more marked. The contents of a hæmato-salpinx may be absorbed or may remain unchanged; the blood may escape into the uterine cavity or through the distal end of the tube, gradually forming an hæmatocele; or the sac may rupture, with symptoms of internal bleeding and the rapid development of a hæmatocele. Abdominal section is indicated under all circumstances.

VEIT (*Centralblatt für Gynäkologie*, 1891, No. 22) would limit the term hæmato-salpinx to cases in which either the tube is gradually distended by the escape of blood into it, or in which hemorrhage takes place into a previously dilated tube. The latter may be due to torsion of a hydro-salpinx (as in a case reported by Sutton), or more rarely to trauma or neoplasms. An important point in the macroscopical diagnosis of true hæmato-salpinx is the fact that *the distal opening of the tube is closed*, which is not the case in tubal gestation.

[We have called attention to the fact that in true hæmato-salpinx the *entire* tube is apt to be dilated on account of the closure of the distal end, whereas, in tubal gestation the dilatation is confined to a portion of the tube.—H. C. C.]

ANATOMY OF THE TUBES.

COHN (*Med. Monatsschrift*, 1890, Heft ix.), from independent microscopical studies of sections of normal tubes, has arrived at the following conclusions: 1. The folds in the mucous lining of the tube are more numerous at the uterine than at the abdominal end. 2. These folds increase in number with advancing age. 3. In old subjects the ciliated epithelium disappears, being replaced by non-ciliated columnar or squamous epithelia. 4. The columnar epithelium is often replaced by goblet-cells and by cells with branching processes, which seem to possess a sort of contractile power. 5. There is an entire absence of glands.

DIAGNOSIS OF CARCINOMA CORPORIS UTERI.

HOFMEIER introduced a discussion of this subject at the recent meeting of the German Gynecological Society. He called attention to the fact that cancer frequently develops from the superficial epithelium, and that under these circumstances it assumes the alveolar form. The glandular form presents an incipient or adenomatous stage, which persists for some time; later epithelial outgrowths invade and destroy the muscular tissue. The diagnosis of carcinoma can be made microscopically only when the fact of this infiltration of the deeper tissues is established. Hemorrhage (especially after the climacteric) is the initial symptom, sometimes a foul discharge, less frequently colicky pains. The evidence afforded by the bimanual is not positive; the examination of fragments removed by the curette furnishes positive proof of the presence of cancer, and enables the surgeon to decide whether he has to do with the alveolar or glandular variety. It is not sufficient to remove superficial portions of the growth and merely to demonstrate the presence of epithelial clusters in addition to the glandular processes; the invasion of the muscular layers must be noted. The differential diagnosis between carcinoma and malignant adenoma is practically unnecessary. In endometritis there is general and regular hypertrophy of the glands, their columnar epithelium remaining unchanged, while the reverse is the case in carcinoma.

LEOPOLD, continuing the discussion, said that he had examined microscopically seventy-eight cancerous uteri, which had been extirpated *per vaginam*, in twenty-seven the disease being confined to the body. As a result of his studies he had arrived at the following conclusions: 1. Carcinoma uteri, wherever situated, has always an epithelial origin. 2. It is to be described as an atypical epithelial neoplasm. 3. Its most frequent seat is below the level of the os internum, and it originates in the epithelium of the portio, seldom in that lining the cervical canal. 4. Commencing epithelioma of the portio vaginalis is encountered more frequently than has been supposed, and even when apparently springing from the cervical canal its connection with the squamous epithelium of the portio can be demonstrated. 5. In 25 per cent. of the cases of carcinoma of the infra-vaginal cervix the disease extends to the os internum. 6. In cases of carcinoma of the portio the corporeal endometrium is usually hypertrophied. The writer has never observed accompanying sarcomatous degeneration of the endometrium, and rarely adenoma. 7. Isolated cancerous nodules may exist in the corpus uteri in connection with cancer of the cervix. 8. Primary carcinoma of the body of the uterus nearly always assumes the diffuse superficial, seldom the isolated nodular form. The first stage is thickening of the mucosa, followed by glandular proliferation, atypical epithelial outgrowths in the form of tufts and alveoli, and finally invasion and destruction of the muscular layers. 9. The epithelial growth is composed of papillary projections richly supplied with bloodvessels, so that it may be properly described as *carcinoma papillare*. 10. The term "malignant adenoma" is entirely superfluous and misleading, since an adenoma is a benignant neoplasm, and as soon as it becomes atypical—that is, invades the surrounding tissue—it is no longer adenoma, but papillary carcinoma. 11. In the initial stage of the disease the diagnosis may be positively established by the removal of fragments with the curette, in which will be found under the microscope the characteristic glandular proliferation, new formation of vessels, and invasion of the subjacent muscular tissue. When extensive ulceration has occurred, however, the microscopical diagnosis is uncertain, since only necrosed tissue is removed by the curette.

[In this connection *vide* paper on "Adenoma Uteri" in the August number of the JOURNAL.—H. C. C.]

GONORRHŒA IN THE FEMALE.

BUMM (*Centralblatt für Gynäkologie*, 1891, No. 22) thus summarizes the results of his studies of this subject, which extend over a period of ten years:

1. Gonorrhœa in women is a process limited to the superficial layer of the mucosa; the cocci invade the epithelial layer, but are always arrested when they reach the submucosa. The epithelium is originally cast off by reason of the active suppuration, but is quickly renewed, assuming the pavement form; after this change has occurred the active invasion of gonococci is usually arrested, but they continue to grow in the secretion, in which they may persist for months and years.

2. The gonococci have no connection with septic processes; they do indeed cause suppuration of the mucosa, but are destroyed when they reach the subjacent connective tissue. If sepsis develops it must be in consequence of mixed infection; septic germs are frequently present in gonorrhœal pus, and a favorable nidus for the reception of external germs is offered by the purulent genital secretion.

3. The urethra and cervical canal are the favorite seats of gonorrhœal infection; acute gonorrhœa of the cervix gives rise to symptoms only at the outset, but after it has become chronic it may exist for years without causing disturbances, unless it extends to the corpus uteri and thence to the tubes.

The cocci possess no power of spontaneous movement and extend only short distances by proliferation. Extension over larger surfaces must be through the agency of the secretion. Normally the cervical secretion cannot pass the os internum, which also serves as a barrier to the entrance of the specific infection. Menstruation favors the admission of cocci into the uterine cavity, also certain mechanical causes, such as coitus, the introduction of sounds and intra-uterine medication; lastly, this is liable to occur during the puerperium. After they have reached the cavity they again remain stationary, and probably are only carried into the tubes from the causes already mentioned, the puerperium being the most favorable time, as the proximal openings of the tubes are then more patent. In fifty-three patients with gonorrhœa, who were kept under observation for at least five months after the initial symptoms developed, the cervix was infected in 75 per cent., the corpus uteri in 15 per cent., and the tubes in only 3.5 per cent.

WERTHEIM (*Centralblatt für Gynäkologie*, 1891, No. 24) reviews the subject of so called gonococci-peritonitis, the existence of which is denied by Bumm, who affirms that when the cocci come in contact with the peritoneum they are simply encapsulated like any other foreign bodies, the development of peritonitis secondary to gonorrhœa of the tubes being due to mixed infection. Subsequent microscopical studies have shown that the cocci may penetrate the squamous epithelium which covers serous surfaces. Their absence in the exudates of peritonitis is no proof that they may not have originated the inflammatory process prior to their disappearance. After a thorough investigation of the subject, he finds as the result of numerous experiments upon animals that the coccus may, under the same conditions, produce peritonitis the same as the other pyogenic microörganisms.. Now, it may be urged that experiments on animals do not form a reliable basis on which to found a theory as to the development of this form of peritonitis in the human subject; but, as an actual fact, mucous surfaces in the former are less sensitive to the action of the cocci than are those of man, hence in the latter peritonitis would be more likely to occur from contact with them. Not only may the gonococci penetrate squamous epithelium, but they may make their way into the subjacent connective tissue and there enter thē lymph-spaces, extending in the same manner as other pyogenic organisms. This is an important fact, since heretofore all inflammations of the deeper tissues accompanying gonorrhœa have been referred to mixed infection; now, peri-urethral abscesses, suppuration of the glands, parametritis, and even oöphoritis, may be regarded as due directly to the influence of the gonococcus. It is a striking fact that no one has ever found any other pyogenic bacterium except the gonococcus in the contents of a pyosalpinx, even though the condition was complicated with extensive inflammatory changes in the tubes, ovaries and peritoneum.

The writer has found the coccus in the pus from sixteen cases of pyosalpinx, but never succeeded in discovering any other form of microörganism, even after the most careful search; there is no reason to infer from this that other bacteria are supplanted by the cocci, since Menge has shown that the former possess a much greater power of resistance than the latter. The writer has also disproved, by numerous culture experiments, Zweifel's assertion that old gonorrhœal pus forms a particularly favorable nidus for pyogenic and septic organisms; the reverse seems to be the case. It seems only fair to limit the term "mixed infection" to those cases in which, after a distinct preceding gonorrhœal infection, the presence of organisms other than gonococci can be demonstrated; of these the writer has seen but two undoubted examples. Abscesses of the ovary may be divided into two classes, according to their etiology—puerperal and gonorrhœal. The former are not uncommon; the *streptococcus pyogenes* is usually found in the pus. That ovarian abscess may be of gonorrhœal origin is proved by a case cited by the writer in which a girl of sixteen had a double pyosalpinx and abscess of both ovaries; in the contents of the right abscess-sac numerous gonococci were found, while the pus from the left one contained no bacteria whatever.

[We recently operated in private upon a child, aged fifteen years, of good family, who had a condition similar to that in the case cited, for which no cause could be found except exposure to cold at a menstrual period. In this case specific infection and puerperal, or traumatic, influences could be absolutely excluded. The pus was extremely acrid, but, unfortunately, was not examined for microörganisms.—H. C. C.]

ICHTHYOL IN THE TREATMENT OF DISEASES OF WOMEN.

FREUND (*Berliner klin. Wochenschrift*, 1890, No. 45) speaks highly of this drug in the treatment of endometritis. He first tampons the vaginal fornix with pledgets of cotton saturated with ichthyol in glycerin until the cervix is reduced in size, then applies pure ichthyol-ammonium or -sodium to the inflamed mucosa, the patient being directed to use daily a hot astringent

douche. Usually, after a week of such treatment the hypertrophied endometrium is shrunken, and after the astringent injections have been continued
for a short time the affection is entirely cured. In three cases of obstinate
recurring corporeal endometritis, in which no result was obtained by curetting, a rapid cure followed the use of intra-uterine applications of pure
ichthyol-ammonium.

Fissure of the nipple in nursing women is successfully treated by pencilling
the crack with pure ichthyol-zinc after the child has nursed. The pain is
quickly relieved, and a cure may be expected in from two to five days.

The Surgical Treatment of Tuberculous Peritonitis.

Kocks (*Centralblatt für Gynäkologie*, 1891, No. 24) operated upon a patient
with supposed tuberculous ascites, but found no tubercles on the peritoneum.
He raises the question whether ascites may not develop in connection with
extra-peritoneal tuberculosis, the effusion being due either to collateral hyperæmia or to the direct irritation of the secreting surface by atoxine. In like
manner Löffler's diphtheria bacillus has been shown to be the direct cause of
pleural effusions without entering the pleural cavity; also, tuberculous osteitis
may cause synovitis, though the fluid from the joint is free from bacilli.

It is inadvisable to completely close the abdomen after performing laparotomy, as it may be necessary to operate again on account of recurrence;
in one case the writer performed laparotomy three times. He now invariably leaves the lower angle of the wound open, inserting a drain of iodoform
gauze.

Deciduoma.

Under this term, originally suggested by Maier, Sänger (*Centralblatt für
Gynäkologie*, 1891, No. 24) includes true decidual sarcoma and not the ordinary neoplasms which have been loosely described under this head. Several
cases of so called deciduoma have been reported by Maier, Klotz and Küstner, but a careful study of their descriptions shows that only one of these was
a true neoplasm (fibro-adenoma), the other tumors being either mucous
polypi or placental moles; one case turned out to be carcinoma. The writer
first described true "malignant metastatic deciduoma, or decidual sarcoma"
two years ago, since which time Pfeiffer has described one case and referred
to three others reported in 1877 by Chiari, who then regarded the condition
as carcinoma corporis uteri developing immediately after birth. All five
cases presented the same clinical history and terminated fatally within six
or seven months after delivery. Anatomically the writer's case differed from
the others in the following respects: The growth assumed the form of nodules
which originated within the deep muscular tissue and grew inward, forming
fungoid excrescences within the uterine cavity, the mucous lining of which
was entirely wanting, being replaced by a sort of cicatricial tissue containing
small sarcomatous round- and spindle-cells. It thus appeared that while the
decidual remains formed the nidus of the neoplasm, they did not possess the
power of regenerating the endometrium. Sections of the nodules showed
that they were composed of changed decidual cells of a polymorphous char-

acter, imbedded in a well-marked reticulum in which were numerous multi-nucleated giant-cells. The epithelial cells were arranged in pseudo-alveoli, and there were many dilated veins and localized hemorrhages. Metastatic nodules were found in the lungs, which presented an identical structure, undoubted decidual cells being found.

The term "deciduoma" applied to this neoplasm is incorrect, since it is really a sarcoma, the cells of which assume, by reason of the tissue in which it originates, the decidual type. Gusserow has stated that eleven per cent. of the cases of carcinoma corporis uteri are directly traceable to the influence of the puerperal state, so that it is important to distinguish this condition from "sarcoma deciduo cellulare." Probably the majority of the cases of carcino-sarcoma described by Klebs are clinically and anatomically identical with the neoplasms described by the writer.

As regards the etiology of the growth two facts point to its probable infectious origin—its close resemblance to the *mycosis fungoides* of the skin (described by Rindfleisch), and the presence of a preceding septic endometritis in every reported case of decidual sarcoma. It is highly desirable that the condition should be promptly recognized before metastasis has occurred, as early extirpation of the uterus might result in a radical cure.

THE INFLUENCE OF CASTRATION UPON THE CILIATED EPITHELIUM OF THE UTERUS.

KRUKENBERG (*Centralblatt für Gynäkologie*, 1891, No. 22) has made some interesting observations in this direction. While in childhood ciliated epithelium is found only in the tubes and later develops in the uterus, after the climacteric all the ciliated epithelium lining the genital tract is destroyed. As observations upon the living subject are not likely to be conclusive, since the almost constant presence of endometritis before castration would in itself lead to destruction of the cilia, the writer conducted a series of experiments upon rabbits and guinea-pigs, with the following results: Seven months after removal of the ovaries the size of the uterus was not altered and the ciliated epithelium was unchanged; ten months after operation the organ was considerably smaller and the cilia disappeared from the mucous lining of both the uterus and the tubes, showing that there was a direct relation between the uterine atrophy and the disappearance of the cilia. The inference may thus be drawn that castration has precisely the same effect upon the uterus as the climacteric. If the ovaries are removed from a young immature animal the usual development of ciliated epithelium does not occur at all.

DEVELOPMENT OF CARCINOMA IN THE CICATRIX AFTER OVARIOTOMY.

FRANK (*Prager med. Wochenschrift*, 1891, Nos. 21 and 23) reports two cases of this character observed by himself, and has been able to find but three more in the literature, in which, after removal of a simple myxoid cystoma, the cicatrix became cancerous. Olshausen suggests that in these cases either the cyst was of the mixed form, containing malignant portions, or else that fragments of benignant adenoma were left behind or escaped into the peritoneal cavity, sprouted and underwent cancerous degeneration. The writer is inclined to explain his cases according to the latter theory, believing that the cells of adenoma bear a close resemblance to those of carcinoma, and may be inoculated upon the healthy peritoneum in the same way. The occurrence of this complication emphasizes the necessity of preventing the entrance of cyst-contents into the peritoneal cavity during operation, since it may lead to serious results.

[We agree with the writer that these cases are probably not so rare as might be inferred from the small number that have been reported. We recall a typical one at the Woman's Hospital.—H. C. C.]

Torsion of a Fibroid Uterus.

Rick (*Prager med. Wochenschrift*, 1891, No. 19) reports the following interesting case: The patient, aged fifty-six years, had complained for a month of severe pain in the abdomen and obstinate constipation, with moderate elevation of temperature. Two weeks before entering the hospital her bowels had not moved for eight days; four days before entrance she had a small movement, and when admitted her abdomen was greatly distended, so that it was impossible to make out anything definitely. She died suddenly the same night while using the bed-pan.

At the autopsy a subperitoneal fibroid larger than a man's head was found, which had a pedicle that had been twisted about its axis from left to right. Closer investigation showed that this pedicle was composed of the elongated uterus, which had made two entire revolutions on itself, the ovaries and tubes being wound around it. On section the tumor was congested, but nowhere necrotic. Several coils of intestine were adherent to the mass, causing obstruction of the gut. Few similar cases have been recorded and the etiology is obscure. The peristaltic movements of the adherent intestines probably had something to do with the torsion. As is known, torsion of the pregnant uterus is a well-recognized complication in veterinary obstetrics.

Primary Sarcoma of the Cervix Uteri.

Kleinschmidt (*Archiv für Gynäkologie*, Band xxxix., Heft 1) in reporting a case of this affection, refers to Winckel's collection of nine cases published in 1883, some of which were of doubtful character. Winckel reported one case of adeno-myxo-sarcoma and one of round-celled sarcoma of the cervix uteri. The author's patient was thirty-six years of age, and applied at the Munich clinic, in 1888, on account of a sanguineous discharge (with some odor) of two weeks' duration, accompanied with sacral pains. A supposed malignant growth was removed from the cervix with the sharp spoon, and its base was cauterized. She had a recurrence, but became pregnant and had a normal labor; ten weeks after a second operation was performed, a soft tumor about the size of an orange being excised from the posterior lip. Five months later it was necessary to curette and cauterize again. On microscopical examination the neoplasm was found to be a spindle-celled sarcoma, which in spots seemed to be carcinomatous.

Of the fourteen cases on record six patients had borne children. The ages of all varied from ten to sixty years. The symptoms were hemorrhage and foul discharge. Pain was not constant. The symptoms were usually of short duration, seldom over eighteen months. Primary sarcoma is prone to rapid degenerative changes and metastases, especially in the parametric tissues.

The diagnosis is based upon the peculiar whitish, sago-like appearance of the growth and its tendency to break down. It does not tend to extend up into the uterine cavity or to involve the vagina so rapidly as carcinoma of the cervix. The prognosis is bad. As regards treatment, total extirpation of the uterus should be performed if the growth is limited to the cervix, but a recurrence is more apt to occur than with cancer. Temporary relief is afforded by curetting and thorough cauterization.

PÆDIATRICS.

UNDER THE CHARGE OF

JOHN M. KEATING, M.D.,
OF PHILADELPHIA;

A. F. CURRIER, M.D.,   AND   W. A. EDWARDS, M D.,
OF NEW YORK,   OF SAN DIEGO, CAL.

THE IODIDES IN SCROFULOUS CHILDREN.

Iodine and iodoform give better results than the alkaline iodides. To young children tincture of iodine may be given, one drop daily in a little thin porridge made of farina and milk. BESNIER (*Le Bulletin Médical*, 1890, p. 595) prefers the use of iodoform, which may be given continuously for a long time. He prescribes it after the following formula:

$$\text{R.—Iodoform} \quad . \quad . \quad . \quad . \quad . \quad . \quad . \quad . \quad \text{gr. jss.}$$
$$\text{Mellis} \quad . \quad . \quad . \quad . \quad . \quad . \quad . \quad . \quad \text{ʒiv.—M.}$$

ACUTE PEMPHIGUS IN AN INFANT INFECTING THE MOTHER.

An infant three days old had an attack of acute pemphigus, the palms and soles of the feet being the only parts free. Four days before the bullæ ceased to appear several formed on the breast and forearms of the mother, who always wore short sleeves. These bullæ exactly corresponded in form to those on the child, and they ceased to appear after the infant was cured. There was no suspicion of syphilis.—*Lancet*, 1890, p. 850.

DIAGNOSIS OF TUBERCULAR MENINGITIS IN CHILDREN.

At a recent meeting of the American Pædiatric Association, DR. W. P. NORTHRUP read an interesting paper on this subject. He gave four symptoms which, when they existed together, were to him convincing evidence of the disease—persistent vomiting, irregular pulse, irregular breathing, apathy;

there were also other significant symptoms connected with the organs of special sense. Professor Jacobi agreed with Dr. Northrup in the importance of the persistent vomiting as a diagnostic sign; the vomiting is apt to be marked when the meninges of the base of the brain are the seat of the tubercular deposit; if the tubercular deposit is not marked in this region the vomiting is apt to be less pronounced or absent. Distinction must be made between the cerebral type of vomiting, which is projectile and not accompanied by nausea, and that which is merely reflex or of gastric origin. Dr. Northrup traced the infection in one of his reported cases to the use of tuberculous milk.

— —

Pathogenesis and Treatment of Intestinal Catarrh in Children.

ANTIQUEDAD (*Annales de Obstét., Gyn., et Péd.*, 1890) states that the treatment of intestinal catarrh in children is one of the most difficult matters in therapeutics. This is shown by the diversity of methods of treatment, some of which are merely empirical while others are rational. This shows that we must adopt a fixed criterion if we would desire to cure our patients. Treatment has consisted mainly in combating the causes which produce intestinal catarrh and the symptoms which threaten life, without particular reference to the alimentary regimen, which should be adapted to the age and the progressive growth of the child. It should never be forgotten that mothers should be taught that there is no better food for children during the first few months of life than milk, which combines all the elements necessary for growth. The milk must also be of good quality, and if the mother cannot supply it from her own breast it should be supplied by a wet-nurse whose child is of about the same age as the one she is to nurse.

For the fever and the diarrhœa, which constitute the prominent symptoms in intestinal catarrh, the author has found best success in the use of hydrotherapy and sulphate of quinine. For the former he advises general baths once a day, and not more than thirty minutes in duration, of a temperature which shall not be higher than 28° C. nor less than 24° C. The sulphate of quinine is used in sólution, one gramme being dissolved in three hundred grammes of alcohol. It is used in the form of fomentations along the vertebral column. The author also found that the diarrhœa could be satisfactorily treated with chlorate of potash, which is eliminated by the mucous membranes. One part of the potash should be dissolved in one hundred of water and combined with ipecac. Small doses of the mixture should be given every quarter of an hour. If this treatment is not efficient, revulsives in the form of thapsia plasters should be used, the plasters being applied upon the abdomen. The conclusions of the author are embodied in the following propositions:

1. A pathogenesis of intestinal catarrh in children has reference mainly to the use of indigestible food.

2. This catarrh is produced when the milk of the child is of improper quality.

3. Cold is frequently the cause of intestinal catarrh in children by suspending perspiration and producing a fluxion in the place of it.

4. Hydro-therapy, sulphate of quinine, chlorate of potash, and revulsion are the means which will be found most efficient in the treatment of intestinal catarrh in children.

LIGATION OF THE COMMON CAROTID ARTERY, IN A CHILD OF THREE AND A HALF YEARS, FOR HEMORRHAGE FOLLOWING PERITONSILLAR ABSCESS; RECOVERY.

Parenchymatous inflammation of the tonsil is rare in children. In one thousand cases treated by Sir Morell Mackenzie at the Hospital for Diseases of the Throat (*Pharynx, Larynx, and Trachea*, p. 37), there were only thirty-five cases under ten years of age. Dr. Beverley Robinson (Keating's *Cyclopædia of Diseases of Children*, vol. ii. p. 441), in speaking of the age at which deep-seated inflammation of the tonsil occurs in children, says: "I cannot recall a single instance in which I have seen suppurative tonsillitis in a small child." Dr. Goodhart (*Diseases of Children*, p. 105, quoted by Robinson) reports the case of a girl, six years of age, who, when she came under his care, showed a large, deep ulcer, "which could," he thinks, "only have originated in acute suppuration of the tonsil." A case is reported by Norton (*The Throat and Larynx*, 1875) in which the disease in a little girl, four years of age, terminated fatally from hemorrhage, the abscess having ulcerated into the carotid artery.

DUNN's patient (*University Med. Magazine*, 1891) was the offspring of healthy parents, though there was a decided disposition to tuberculosis in the mother's family. No especial tendency to quinsy, rheumatism, or scrofula and no hæmophilia in the family. The child presented an intense right-sided tonsillitis, the inflammation having extended to the adjacent parts of the pharynx and palate.

On the fourth day the tonsillar abscess ruptured, and for the next seven days the child had six severe and prostrating hemorrhages. The blood was seen to flow between the tonsil and upper part of the posterior palatine fold; a lump now appeared in the submaxillary region which rapidly increased and became a pulsating tumor, two and a half inches in length by one and a half in breadth, extending from the mastoid process beyond the angle of the jaw, and with each pulsation the jaw and head were elevated. The temperature at the time was 101° F., pulse 108, feeble and small. The child was in a drowsy condition, and for several hours had refused nourishment. The nature of the tumefaction appeared to be that of false aneurism, and the necessity for the immediate ligation of the artery was impressed upon the parents.

From the uncertainty of the situation of the bleeding-point and the danger of further loss of blood from opening the tumor, ligation of the common carotid above the omo-hyoid was elected. Careful dissection was made, and in a short time the artery was exposed without injury to any important structure. A catgut ligature was used and the ends cut close to the knot. After introducing catgut drainage, the wound was closed with silk sutures and dressed with iodoform and bichloride gauze. The operation was borne well and with but little loss of blood. What did ooze was of a pale wine-color; in fact, it was so watery that the structures could be seen through the little pool which formed in the wound. The pulsating tumor previously described decreased in an hour to one-half its former size and in thirty-six hours was the size of an almond.

Before daylight the child took freely of hot milk and stimulants, and at 8 A. M. the temperature was 99°, pulse 96, respiration normal. No difficulty or pain in turning the head. Recovery was rapid and uninterrupted. The wound united without suppuration, and on the eighth day the stitches were removed.

TETANOID CONVULSIONS IN AN INFANT; OPERATION; RECOVERY.

RONALDSON (*Canadian Practitioner*, 1891) recently reported a case that arose when the child was nine days old. It was considered to be one of tetanus, whose starting-point seemed to be the neglected or badly-taken-care-of umbilicus. At first the convulsions were confined to the left side of the body; restlessness led on to tonic muscular contraction, and that was succeeded by well-marked clonic convulsions. Between the attacks the child was apparently well. The convulsions increased to the number of 204 in the twenty-four hours, while during their occurrence the tongue became blue-black, and at times well-marked opisthotonos supervened. On one occasion they were never absent for one whole hour, and for a period of nine hours the child was unable to suck, in consequence of the frequency of the fits. When they did not come too rapidly, it took its nourishment greedily. They varied in frequency from about 100 to 204 in the twenty-four hours, but not in such a way as to warrant us in believing that treatment, local or general, had any beneficial effect.

Dr. Brakenridge, who saw the child, and subsequently confirmed the diagnosis, gave it as his opinion that the convulsions were not due to any disease originating in the brain, but that they were peripheral in their origin, and probably had the umbilicus as their starting-point.

Excision of the umbilicus was performed, and at once there was improvement, and the fits gradually decreased.

They returned later in a lesser degree, but were controlled by sulpho-carbolate of soda, and the child perfectly recovered. Microscopic examination of the excised umbilicus did not detect any special organism in it.

Note to Contributors.—All contributions intended for insertion in the Original Department of this Journal are only received *with the distinct understanding that they are contributed exclusively to this Journal.*

Contributions from the Continent of Europe and written in the French, German or Italian language, if on examination they are found desirable for this Journal, will be translated at its expense.

Liberal compensation is made for articles used. A limited number of extra copies in pamphlet form, if desired, will be furnished to authors in lieu of compensation, *provided the request for them be written on the manuscript.*

All communications should be addressed to

DR. EDWARD P. DAVIS,
250 South 21st Street, Philadelphia.

THE

AMERICAN JOURNAL

OF THE MEDICAL SCIENCES.

OCTOBER, 1891.

ON THE DISEASES OF THE KIDNEYS POPULARLY CALLED "BRIGHT'S DISEASE."

By Francis Delafield, M.D., LL.D.,

OF NEW YORK.

Our notions concerning the nature of diseases and their treatment are greatly influenced by names and classifications. So, as our knowledge becomes more accurate, it is important, as fast as may be, to modify and change such names and classifications as have become a hindrance instead of a help.

The ordinary history of such names is that during the earlier periods of medicine some man more able than his fellows was able to group together a number of cases of diseases, to describe them plainly and to venture some theory as to their nature. Such a group of diseases then became known by the name of its describer, or by some arbitrary term. As time went on such a name acquired the dignity of use and custom, became generally accepted, and more and more traditions and classical descriptions accumulated about it, until in men's minds were established a name and a clinical picture to which, as to a Procrustean bed, they compelled their cases to correspond. With the further progress of medicine came the fresh study of the old diseases and the discovery that much could be seen and demonstrated which it was difficult to reconcile with the old traditions. Then came an unsatisfactory period during which the old name was retained as expressing a real entity, and the attempt was made to divide and classify the varieties of this entity. Lastly comes the time when the old name is retained as a popular term, but it is recognized that it does not really designate a distinct form of disease. Such has been the history of such names as " cancer," " phthisis," and " Bright's disease."

I believe that the time has fully come to abandon the idea that there is such a disease as Bright's disease, and to cease from the attempt to describe varieties of a disease that does not exist. When we have divested our minds of this tradition we can begin to study the diseases of the kidneys and to try to classify them.

There seem to be three ways in which we can classify kidney diseases—according to their causes, according to the part of the kidney involved, or according to the nature of the morbid process.

The attempt to classify kidney diseases according to their causes is, in the present state of our knowledge, simply impossible.

The attempt to classify them according to the part of the kidney involved, to describe tubal nephritis, glomerulo-nephritis, interstitial nephritis, and arterio sclerosis, has been made many times. It has never given us a classification of any practical use for clinical purposes.

A classification according to the nature of the morbid process is altogether the most promising.

There are three morbid processes which occur in nearly every part of the body, which produce definite anatomical changes, cause regular clinical symptoms, and call for appropriate methods of treatment. These morbid processes are congestion, degeneration, and inflammation.

Congestion, whether acute or chronic, produces an accumulation of blood in the veins and capillaries of the part affected, causes local symptoms and disturbances of function, and is to be relieved by means addressed to the circulation of the blood.

Degeneration, whether acute or chronic, produces changes more or less profound in the parts affected ; is regularly caused by poisons, by disturbances of circulation, and by other diseases ; produces disturbances of function according to its severity ; may be itself a cause of inflammation, and can be but little affected by any treatment.

Inflammation is attended with three essential features, which may occur separately or together—an escape of the elements of the blood from the vessels, a formation of new tissue, and a death of tissue. So we speak of exudative, productive, and necrotic inflammations.

Exudative inflammation is of short duration, leaves behind it no permanent changes in the parts affected, and can be favorably affected by treatment.

Productive inflammation runs an acute, subacute, or chronic course. It effects permanent changes in the inflamed parts. Its acute forms are very apt to become chronic. There is much variety as to the relative quantity of exudation and of new tissue. Treatment is not very satisfactory.

The different forms of kidney disease which are commonly included under the name of Bright's disease can all be conveniently classified under the heads of—

Congestion of the kidney.

Degeneration of the kidney.

Inflammation of the kidney.

Such a classification has the merit of being simple and easily understood, of resting on an anatomical basis, and of being of practical use for clinical purposes.

I. The Congestions of the Kidney.

These are naturally divided into acute and chronic congestions. They must always depend upon causes which affect the circulation and cause an accumulation of venous blood in the kidney.

Acute congestion of the kidney is produced by the ingestion of poisons, by extirpation of one kidney, by injuries, by surgical operations, and by unknown causes.

It may occur in kidneys previously normal, or in those already diseased.

The most marked symptom is the diminution or suppression of the urine, but albumin and casts may be present.

Such an acute congestion is a transitory condition, but when it occurs with injuries and with surgical operations it may apparently be a cause of death.

Chronic congestion of the kidneys is produced by some long-continued mechanical interference with the circulation of the blood, an interference which necessarily causes congestion of other parts of the body as well as of the kidneys.

The characteristic changes in the kidneys are: Swelling or flattening of the epithelium of the cortex tubes, dilatation and thickening of the capillaries of the glomeruli, congestion and dilatation of the pyramid veins.

The urine is more or less diminished in quantity according to the intensity of the congestion.

The specific gravity is from 1.020 to 1.025, but it may for a time fall to 1.010 or rise to 1.035. The excretion of urea is usually ten grains to the ounce; it may rise to twenty-one grains. Albumin and casts are absent, or only present in very small quantities. The bad results of chronic congestion are the diminished production of urine and the liability to the supervention of chronic nephritis.

II. Degeneration of the Kidneys.

Degeneration of the kidney is always a secondary process produced by the introduction into the body of inorganic poisons or of the poisons of the infectious diseases, or by the effect produced on the body by chronic diseases or vicious modes of life, or by disturbances of the circulation.

There are no changes in the kidneys except in the renal epithelium. In these cells are developed a variety of degenerative and necrotic changes.

It may happen that these degenerative changes are developed so rapidly that the bloodvessels are irritated, and there are added congestion and exudation of serum. We include, therefore, in this class both those kidneys the seat of degeneration alone, and those in which both degenerative and exudative inflammation exist, but the inflammation is secondary and subordinate to the degeneration.

Acute degeneration of the kidneys is found almost constantly with the infectious diseases and with poisoning by arsenic, phosphorus and mercury. It occurs in many different degrees of severity, and so we find the renal epithelium : merely swollen and granular, or infiltrated with granules, or broken and disintegrated, or in the condition of coagulation necrosis.

In correspondence with the degree of the degeneration of the renal epithelium is the severity of the clinical symptoms.

The urine is unchanged, or its quantity is diminished, or it contains a little albumin, or the albumin is abundant with casts and red and white blood-cells.

Many of the examples of this lesion are of so mild a type that they have no symptoms except the changes in the urine. The severe forms are dangerous to life ; but dropsy and disturbances of the circulation are not associated with them.

Acute degeneration, therefore, includes a well-defined set of cases, definite in their lesions, their causes, their symptoms, and evidently not likely to be influenced by any treatment.

Chronic degeneration of the kidney is produced by the same mechanical causes as those which produce chronic congestion, by chronic alcoholism and by vicious modes of life. It is, therefore, always a secondary lesion.

The only changes in the kidney are in the epithelium of the tubes, of which the cells are swollen, granular, and infiltrated with fat. But if the degeneration is due to chronic congestion, there will also be changes in the glomeruli.

The quantity of the urine varies at different times in the same case and also in different cases ; it may be abundant, scanty, or suppressed. Albumin and casts in moderate quantities are often present, but the specific gravity is not lowered.

Such a degeneration of the kidneys has a decided effect upon the health and nutrition of the patients. They lose flesh and strength, become anæmic, and finally pass into the typhoid state with delirium and stupor. Dropsy and disturbances of the circulation are not associated with this form of kidney disease. As the kidney lesion is always secondary to some other serious morbid condition, it is often difficult to tell how much of the loss of health is due to the primary disease and how much to the change in the kidneys.

III. The Inflammations of the Kidney.

These are naturally subdivided into—
- A. Acute exudative nephritis.
- B. Acute productive or diffuse nephritis.
- C. Chronic productive or diffuse nephritis with exudation.
- D. Chronic productive or diffuse nephritis without exudation.
  Suppurative nephritis.
  Tubercular nephritis.

A. *Acute Exudative Nephritis.*—This is an acute inflammation of the kidney, characterized by congestion, an exudation of plasma, an emigration of white blood-cells, and a diapedesis of red blood-cells from the vessels; to which may be added swelling or necrosis of the renal epithelium and changes in the glomeruli.

Of such a nephritis we may distinguish three varieties:

1. A mild form, which gives symptoms during life, but leaves no lesions in the kidney after death.

2. A more severe form, in which we find inflammatory changes in the kidney after death.

3. A form characterized by the excessive production of pus-cells.

Lesions. In a nephritis of this type we should expect that the inflammatory products, the serum, white and red blood-cells, and coagulable matter from the blood-plasma, would collect in the Malpighian bodies and tubes or infiltrate the stroma between the tubes; and that of the inflammatory products in the tubes and Malpighian bodies a part would be discharged with the urine and a part found in the kidney after death. We should also expect that the quantity of inflammatory products would be in proportion to the severity of the inflammation, and that an excessive number of pus-cells would belong to the especially severe forms of the disease. Still further it is evident that, with the milder examples of nephritis, with but little exudation, no inflammatory products might be found in the kidney after death, all having been discharged into the urine during life.

As a matter of fact, the kidneys do present just such changes. In the mild cases we find no decided lesions in the kidney after death. In the more severe cases the kidneys are increased in size, their surfaces are smooth, the cortical portion is thick and white, or white mottled with red, or the entire kidney is intensely congested. If the stroma is infiltrated with serum, the kidney is succulent and wet; if the number of pus-cells is very great, there will be little whitish foci in the cortex.

In such kidneys we find the evidences of exudative inflammation in the tubes, the stroma, and the glomeruli, all the changes being most marked in the cortical portion of the kidney.

The epithelium of the convoluted tubes is often simply flattened. As this same appearance is also found in the chronic congestion of heart disease, it seems probable that this change of the shape of the cells is merely due to the inflammatory congestion.

In other cases, not only is the epithelium flattened but there is also a real dilatation of the cortex-tubes. This dilatation does not involve groups of tubes, but all the cortex-tubes uniformly. In other cases, the epithelium of the convoluted tubes is swollen, opaque, degenerated, and detached from the tubes. But in fresh kidneys, properly preserved, this degeneration and desquamation of the epithelium is not nearly as constant or as marked a feature as would be supposed from the descriptions of some English observers. The tubes, whether with flattened epithelium or dilated, may be empty. More frequently, however, they contain coagulated matter in the form of irregular masses and of hyaline cylinders. The irregular masses are found principally in the convoluted tubes; they seem to be formed by a coagulation of substances contained in the exuded blood plasma, and are not to be confounded with the hyaline globules so often found in normal convoluted tubes. The cylinders are more numerous in the straight tubes, but are also found in the convoluted tubes.

They also are evidently formed of matter coagulated from the exuded blood-plasma, and are identical with the casts found in the urine. The tubes may also contain red and white blood-cells.

In the cases in which there is an excessive emigration of white blood-cells, we find these cells in the tubes, in the stroma, or distending the capillary veins. This excessive emigration is not necessarily attended with exudation of the blood-serum, and so the urine of these patients may contain no albumin. The white blood-cells are not usually found equally diffused through the kidneys, but are collected in foci in the cortex. These foci may be very minute, or may attain a considerable size.

In the glomeruli we find changes which, at first sight, seem peculiar, but are really similar to the changes which we find in arteries and capillaries in many inflamed tissues. The cavities of the capsules may contain coagulated matter and white and red blood-cells, just as do the tubes. The capsular epithelium may be swollen, sometimes so much so as to resemble the tubular epithelium, and this change is most marked in the capsular epithelium near the entrance of the tubes.

The most noticeable change, however, is in the capillary tufts of the

glomeruli. These capillaries are normally covered on their outer surfaces by flat, nucleated cells, so that the tuft is not made up of naked
capillaries, but each separate capillary throughout its entire length is
covered over with these cells. There are also flat cells which line the
inner surfaces of the capillaries, although not uniformly, as is the case in
capillaries in other parts of the body. Still, in spite of the presence of
all these cells, the outlines of the walls of the capillaries are fairly
distinct.

In exudative nephritis the swelling and growth of cells on and in the
capillaries change the appearance of the glomeruli. They are larger
more opaque; the outlines of the main divisions of the tuft are visible,
but those of the individual capillaries are lost. It is difficult to tell how
much these changes in the glomeruli interfere with the passage of the
blood through their capillaries. In most cases of exudative nephritis
the patients recover and the glomeruli return to their natural condition

In some examples of exudative nephritis we also find a thickening of
the walls of the branches of the renal artery within the kidney. This
thickening is principally due to a swelling of the muscle-cells in the
walls of these vessels.

Etiology. Acute exudative nephritis is frequently a primary disease, either occurring after exposure to cold, or without discoverable
cause. It complicates scarlatina, measles, diphtheria, typhoid fever,
acute general tuberculosis, pneumonia, acute peritonitis, dysentery, erysipelas, diabetes, and many other of the infectious diseases and severe
inflammations. It is one of the forms of nephritis which complicate
the puerperal condition.

Symptoms. In the milder cases the only symptoms are the changes
in the urine. This is somewhat diminished in quantity, of normal or
high specific gravity ; it contains albumin in moderate quantities, a few
casts, sometimes blood.

In the more severe cases the changes in the urine are more decided.
It is diminished in quantity, or even suppressed ; its specific gravity is
normal or high ; the quantity of albumin is very large ; the casts are
numerous, hyaline, granular, containing white or red blood-cells or epithelium ; there are also free white and red blood-cells and epithelial
cells from the kidney and the bladder. As a rule, the quantity of
albumin and the number of casts are in proportion to the severity of the
nephritis, but this is not always the case. Large quantities of albumin,
numerous casts, and many white and red blood-cells may be found in
the urine of kidneys which, after death, show no structural changes ;
while, on the other hand, small quantities of albumin and a few hyaline
casts are compatible with a severe nephritis. Still further, the number
of casts found in the urine during life is not always in proportion to the

number of casts and quantity of coagulated matter found in the corre-sponding kidneys after death.

In addition to the changes in the quantity and composition of the urine, the patients present constitutional symptoms which vary, in the different cases, as to their number and their severity. A febrile move-ment, with more or less prostration; stupor, headache, sleeplessness, rest-lessness, muscular twitchings, and general convulsions; dyspnœa, loss of appetite, nausea, and vomiting; a pulse of high tension with exaggerated heart-action, or hypertrophy of the left ventricle, dropsy and anæmia—these may be called the characteristic symptoms of acute exudative nephritis. Of these symptoms a certain number—the fever, the prostra-tion, the loss of appetite and nausea, the anæmia, the diminution in the quantity of urine, the albumin and casts in the urine—are such as would naturally accompany an acute inflammation of the kidney, and very often they are the only symptoms which do accompany it.

But with this same kidney lesion a certain number of patients will present, besides the symptoms just mentioned, the additional features of cerebral symptoms, changes in the heart and circulation, and dropsy. We indeed might think that the cerebral symptoms and the dropsy were due to the diminished excretion of urine; but when these conditions occur, as they often do, in patients who are passing large quantities of urine of good specific gravity, and when they are absent, as they often are, in patients who are hardly passing any urine at all, it is evident that these symptoms are not directly due to the nephritis, but constitute a separate, complicating set of symptoms, which may be present or absent in any given case of the disease.

What the complicating lesion is which produces these symptoms we do not fully know; but the changes in the action of the heart and the dropsy naturally direct our attention to the arteries and capillaries, with the expectation of finding in them some morbid condition which will hinder the passage of the blood through them. Whether the morbid condition is of an inflammatory nature, or whether it is only a spasmodic contraction, we are as yet ignorant.

The cases of exudative nephritis, with an excessive production of pus-cells, have a somewhat different clinical history. Such a nephritis occurs both in children and adults; it may be primary, or complicate scarlatina, diphtheria, or measles.

The invasion is sudden, with a high temperature and marked prostra-tion. Restlessness, delirium, headache, and stupor are soon developed and continue throughout the disease. The patients lose flesh and strength and pass into the typhoid state. Dropsy is slight or absent altogether. The urine is not so much diminished in quantity as one would expect; its specific gravity is not changed; albumin, casts, and red and white blood-cells are present in considerable quantities, but not always early in the disease, and may even be absent altogether.

Prognosis. It is a very fatal form of nephritis, and yet one easily misunderstood on account of the resemblance of its symptoms to those of an acute meningitis.

B. *Acute Productive or Diffuse Nephritis.*—This is the most serious and important of all the forms of acute nephritis, not only for the reason that it involves so many of the structures of the kidney, but because its lesions are from the first of a permanent character, and because disturbances of the circulation are so frequently associated with it. It is one of the forms of scarlatinal nephritis; it occurs early and late in the course of diphtheria; it is the most important variety of the nephritis of pregnancy, and it is especially frequent as a primary nephritis with or without a history of exposure to cold.

Lesions. The changes in the kidneys are extensive and well marked.

The kidneys are large, at first smooth, later sometimes a little roughened; the cortical portion is thick, white, or mottled with yellow or red, or congested; the pyramids are red.

In these kidneys we find the same lesions as have been described as belonging to exudative nephritis, but with two additional changes— changes which are found in the earliest stages of the inflammation and which give the characteristic stamp to the lesion; first, a growth of connective tissue in the stroma; second, a growth of the capsule-cells of the Malpighian bodies. Both these changes do not involve the whole kidney, but symmetrical strips or wedges in the cortex, which follow the line of the arteries. These wedges are small or large, few or numerous, regular or irregular, in the different kidneys. But in every wedge we find the same general characters: one or more arteries of which the walls are thickened; the Malpighian bodies belonging to this artery show an enormous growth of capsule-cells, with compression of the tufts; running parallel to these arteries a growth of connective-tissue cells and basement substance in the stroma. Between the wedges we find at first only the changes of exudative nephritis; later, a growth of diffuse connective tissue. Sometimes we find these wedges small, symmetrical, and at considerable distances from each other; more frequently they are much closer together, sometimes even becoming continuous.

If the nephritis is of acute type and recent, the new tissue between the tubes consists largely of cells; if the nephritis is of subacute type and longer duration, the tissue is denser and has more basement substance. Where the growth of new tissue is abundant, the tubes become small and atrophied.

In the wedges the constant change is the growth of new tissue in the stroma between the tubes, not an infiltration of the stroma with pus-cells, as in an exudative nephritis, but a new growth of cells and of

basement substance. The tubes seem to become compressed and atrophied between the new tissue.

In each wedge is one or more of the arteries which run up into the
cortex and give off the little branches ending in glomeruli. The walls
of these arteries are thickened.

The glomeruli belonging to these arteries become the seat of changes
of a permanent character. There is the same growth of the cells covering the vessels, and of the cells within them, as in exudative nephritis,
reaching even a greater development. In addition, there is a growth of
the cells lining the capsules to such a degree as to form a mass of cells
compressing the tuft. The tuft apparently never returns again to its
natural condition, but, as time goes on, the vessels are obliterated, the
capsule-cells are changed into connective tissue, and the glomeruli are
finally transformed into little balls of fibrous tissue.

Symptoms. The urine during the acute periods of the nephritis is
scanty, colored by blood, of high specific gravity. It contains much
albumin, numerous casts of all kinds, and red and white blood-cells.
Exceptionally, the casts are few or absent. Later in the disease, or when
it is of a more subacute type, the urine is more abundant, the specific
gravity falls, the albumin and the casts continue. In the protracted
cases the albumin and casts may for a time diminish or even disappear.

The patients develop all the symptoms which we are accustomed to
associate with Bright's disease—headache, restlessness, neuralgic pains,
delirium, stupor, coma, muscular twitchings and general convulsions,
dyspnœa and cough, loss of appetite, nausea and vomiting, neuro-
retinitis, diarrhœa, increased arterial tension and hypertrophy of the
left ventricle of the heart, anæmia, loss of flesh and strength, and
dropsy, often developed to an extreme degree.

The course of the disease varies with the intensity with which it is
developed and the rapidity with which it proceeds.

The invasion may be sudden, the symptoms marked, and the duration
of the disease short, with a fatal termination ; or, with the same acute
invasion, the disease may be protracted over many months ; or the invasion may be gradual, the course of the disease subacute, the symptoms
not continuous, but with periods of improvement or even apparent
recovery, and the duration of the disease protracted for months and
years.

The *prognosis* of this form of nephritis is bad. The lesion is a permanent and progressive one. It is, indeed, apparently possible to recover
from it, although with damaged kidneys, but this is the exception. The
rule is that, sooner or later, the disease proves fatal, although it may
well happen that periods of improvement give rise to false hopes of
recovery.

c. *Chronic Productive, or Diffuse Nephritis with Exudation.*—Although it is convenient to describe two forms of chronic nephritis—one with exudation and one without—yet it must be remembered that these are not separate lesions of the kidneys, but varieties of the same lesion. For, in all these kidneys, one form of inflammation—productive, with the formation of new tissue—is present. The exudation from the vessels is something which is added to this, but does not change it.

In speaking of the exudation of serum from the vessels and its presence in the urine, we speak of it as it occurs during the whole course of the disease, and not as it occurs for short periods.

We mean that in an exudative chronic nephritis there is usually a large quantity of albumin in the urine, but that in the protracted cases there may be periods during which the albumin diminishes or entirely disappears. In the same way in a non-exudative nephritis there may be periods during which albumin is present in considerable quantities. Generally speaking, the character of the clinical symptoms will vary with the presence or absence of the albumin.

Lesions. In chronic nephritis with exudation the size of the kidney is usually increased; there is a very extensive growth of connective tissue in the cortex; the renal epithelium is swollen, granular, degenerated, fatty, broken, or flattened; the tubes contain coagulated matter, cast matter or blood; the cortex tubes are atrophied in some places, dilated in others.

The glomeruli are changed in several different ways:

1. There is a growth of the capsule-cells in such numbers that they compress the tufts. The cells covering the capillaries are also increased in size and number. The capsule-cells may finally be changed into connective tissue and the tufts become atrophied.

2. The glomeruli are of large size, the cells covering the capillaries are increased in number so that the outlines of the capillaries are lost, but yet the capillaries are not compressed nor the glomeruli atrophied.

3. There is a growth of the cells which cover the capillaries and of the cells within them. Of the cells which cover the capillaries the cell-bodies become very large, the capillaries are compressed, and the glomeruli eventually become atrophied.

4. The walls of the capillary vessels become the seat of waxy degeneration, while the cells which cover them are increased in size and number.

5. If the nephritis follows chronic congestion, the capillaries are dilated and there is an increase in the size and number of the cells which cover the capillaries.

The arteries remain unchanged, or they are the seat of obliterating endarteritis, or there is a symmetrical thickening of all the coats of the artery, or all the coats of the artery are thickened and converted into a uniform mass of dense connective tissue, or there is waxy degeneration of the walls of the artery.

Causes. This form of nephritis occurs very frequently as a primary disease, especially in young adults. It follows acute diffuse nephritis, chronic congestion and chronic degeneration of the kidney. It may complicate syphilis, chronic phthisis, chronic endocarditis, prolonged suppuration, and chronic inflammation of the bones and joints.

Symptoms. The urine varies in quantity at different times. When the nephritis is most quiescent the quantity of urine is normal. During the exacerbations of the nephritis the urine is scanty or suppressed. When the patients are doing badly, often when they are dropsical, the quantity of urine is very much increased.

The specific gravity and the proportion of urea to the ounce of urine slowly diminish. In the cases of shorter duration the specific gravity is apt to run between 1.012 and 1.020. In the very chronic cases it will be between 1.001 and 1.005. Very low specific gravities regularly indicate a large growth of connective tissue in the stroma of the cortex, or waxy degeneration of the capillaries of the glomeruli.

The urine regularly contains albumin and casts. During the active periods of the disease the quantity of albumin is very large; during its quiescent periods it is smaller, and at times may entirely disappear. The number of casts varies in proportion to the quantity of albumin, but occasional exceptions to this rule are seen.

Dropsy may be considered a regular symptom of chronic exudative nephritis. It is rare to find a patient who goes through the disease without exhibiting this symptom. It may be developed at any time in the disease, continue uninterruptedly, or occur only in attacks. A peculiar pallor of the skin and white color of the sclerotic is seldom absent, and is quite characteristic of the disease. It corresponds to a diminution in the quantity of hæmoglobin and in the number of the red blood-cells. These changes in the blood are not, as a rule, far advanced; but sometimes they are, and some cases even die with the symptoms of pernicious anæmia.

Many of the patients are troubled with headache and sleeplessness. Acute uræmic attacks, with contraction of the arteries, convulsions, etc., may occur in the course of a chronic exudative nephritis, but they are of very much more frequent occurrence with the non-exudative form of the disease.

Chronic uræmia, on the contrary, is one of the ordinary ways in which an exudative nephritis proves fatal. The patients pass into a condition of alternating delirium and stupor, with a rapid, feeble, soft pulse.

Simple neuro-retinitis or nephritic retinitis are developed in a moderate number of cases.

Dyspnœa is a nearly constant symptom, but it is not always the same kind of dyspnœa, nor always produced by the same cause. It may be due to hydrothorax, to œdema of the lungs, to contraction of the arteries, or to failure of the heart's action.

In many patients the dyspnœa due to contraction of the arteries, or to failure of the heart's action, is the first symptom which attracts attention. It is a dyspnœa which comes on in attacks, especially at night and in the early morning, and is regularly worse when the patient lies down. It often begins while the patient is apparently in good health, but it is a sure premonition of serious disease.

A catarrhal bronchitis with cough and expectoration is often present.

Loss of appetite, nausea, and vomiting are frequent symptoms.

The heart is often affected. There may be hypertrophy of the left ventricle, dilatation of both ventricles, chronic endocarditis, myocarditis, or a feeble heart.

Course of the disease. There is hardly any limit to the variety of the disease, but the most constant symptoms are anæmia, dropsy, and albumin in the urine.

1. There are cases in which the symptoms are nearly continuous, the patients get steadily worse and die within one or two years. The anæmia, the dropsy, and the albumin are constantly present, and the patients die with dropsy or with chronic uræmia.

2. There are cases in which the anæmia, the dropsy, and the dyspnœa come on in attacks which last for weeks or months. Between the attacks the patients are comparatively well, often able to work, although the urine always contains albumin.

3. There are cases in which a number of years before death the patient has an attack of dropsy, etc, from which he apparently recovers and goes on able to work, but with urine of low specific gravity, which sometimes contains albumin. After an interval of many years comes the fatal attack with all the characteristic symptoms.

4. There are cases which for years have no symptoms but pallor of the skin and urine of low specific gravity containing albumin. These patients often for a long time feel so well that they cannot understand that they have a serious disease.

5. There are cases in which the first symptom is the attack of spasmodic dyspnœa, the patients otherwise feeling well. It may be months or years before the other symptoms are developed.

6. There may be a history of chronic endocarditis lasting for years before the renal symptoms are developed.

7. There are cases which apparently recover from the disease.

The *prognosis* is bad, but life may be prolonged for many years with but few symptoms, and recovery seems to be possible.

D. *Chronic Diffuse Nephritis without Exudation.—Lesions.* The larger number of these kidneys are found after death to be diminished in size; the two kidneys together may not weigh more than two ounces. The capsules are adherent, their surfaces are roughened or nodular, the cortex is thin and of red or gray color. A considerable number of the kidneys do not differ in their size or appearance from normal kidneys, except that the capsules are adherent and the surfaces of the kidneys roughened.

Many examples of chronic non-exudative nephritis follow chronic congestion. The kidneys then remain hard, but the cortex becomes thinned, the capsules adherent, and the surface roughened. Some of the kidneys, instead of becoming atrophied, are increased in size, weighing together from sixteen to thirty-two ounces. The surfaces of these large kidneys may be smooth or nodular; the cortex is thickened, its color is red, gray, or white. There is regularly a growth of new connective tissue in the cortex and also in the pyramids, which becomes more and more marked as the disease goes on. In the cortex the new tissue follows the distribution of the normal subcapsular areas of connective tissue, is in the form of irregular masses, or is distributed diffusely between the tubes. In the pyramids the growth of new connective tissue is diffuse.

The tubes, both in the cortex and pyramids, undergo marked changes. Those included in the masses of connective tissue are diminished in size; their epithelium is flattened, some contain cast matter, many are obliterated. The tubes between the masses of new connective tissue are more or less dilated; their epithelium is flattened, cuboidal, swollen, degenerated, or fatty. The dilatation of the tubes may reach such a point as to form cysts of some size, which contain fluid, or coagulated matter. These cysts follow the lines of groups of tubes, or are situated near the capsules.

Of the glomeruli a certain number remain of normal size, but with the tuft-cells swollen, or multiplied. Many others are found in all stages of atrophy until they are convered into little fibrous balls. The atrophy seems to depend partly on the growth of tuft-cells and intra-capillary cells, partly on the thickening of the capsules, partly on the occlusion of the arteries. If the chronic nephritis follows chronic congestion the glomeruli remain large, but with a marked growth of tuft-cells; or they become atrophied, but with the dilatation of the capillaries still evident. The capillaries of the glomeruli may be the seat of waxy degeneration.

The arteries exhibit the same changes as are found in chronic exudative nephritis.

Complicating lesions. Hypertrophy of the left ventricle of the heart is frequently caused by exudative nephritis, but still more frequently by the non-exudative form; but it must be admitted that such an hypertrophy, although frequent, is not constant, that both with exudative and non-exudative nephritis there may be no change in the wall of the left ventricle. The hypertrophy of the wall of the ventricle may after a time be succeeded by dilatation, or chronic degeneration, or myocarditis.

Chronic endocarditis is very frequently associated with chronic Bright's disease. The valvular lesions may cause chronic congestion, chronic degeneration, or chronic nephritis; or the same patient may suffer from chronic endocarditis, and either form of chronic nephritis, the lesions associated possibly due to the same causes, but not dependent on each other.

Pulmonary emphysema, chronic endocarditis, and cirrhosis of the liver, all of them examples of chronic productive inflammation, frequently accompany chronic nephritis.

With the endarteritis comes the additional danger of cerebral hæmorrhage.

Patients suffering with chronic nephritis are more liable than are other persons to attacks of pericarditis, bronchitis, and gastric catarrh.

Symptoms. The typical urine of chronic non-exudative nephritis is a urine increased in quantity, of a specific gravity of about 1.010, containing a diminished quantity of urea, without albumin or casts, or with a trace of albumin and a very few casts, except during exacerbations of the nephritis, when the quantity of albumin and the number of casts may be considerable. But very important modifications of the urine are of ordinary occurrence. It is quite possible, with nephritis of this type far advanced, to have urine not below 1.020 in specific gravity, and without albumin or casts. In such cases the diagnosis has to be made without reference to the urine. On the other hand, there are cases in which the specific gravity of the urine falls very low, almost to 1.000, either with or without waxy degeneration of the vessels. There are cases in which the quantity of urine is very much increased, several quarts in the twenty-four hours. During the attacks of contraction of the arteries, to which these patients are liable, the urine may be diminished to a few ounces or suppressed.

In a great many of the cases cerebral symptoms are developed at some time in the course of the disease. Headache and sleeplessness are often present, the headache sometimes so severe and continuous that the patient is nearly maniacal; or instead of the headache there are neuralgic pains in the different parts of the body.

Muscular twitchings and general convulsions are much more serious; they may be an early symptom, or not occur until late in the disease.

Hemiplegia, with or without aphasia, may be the first symptom to call attention to the nephritis, or may not occur until late in the disease. The invasion of the hemiplegia is sudden and is usually accompanied by coma. There is loss of motion alone, or of both motion and sensation.

The hemiplegia, coma, and aphasia may continue up to the time of the patient's death, or disappear after a few hours or days. In the latter case the patient may have several such attacks. These attacks have been ascribed to localized œdema of the brain. In the cases which I have seen there were no changes in the brain-tissue, but the cerebral arteries were damaged by chronic endarteritis.

Delirium, mild or violent, stupor, and coma may come on in sudden attacks, or be developed slowly and gradually.

When these cerebral symptoms come on in attacks, the arteries are contracted, the temperature is raised, and the patients are said to suffer from acute uræmia. Very often they recover from a number of these attacks. In the fatal attacks the pulse often loses its tension, but becomes rapid and feeble, and the patients die comatose, with a feeble heart.

Instead of such acute attacks of cerebral symptoms, the symptoms may come gradually in persons already much reduced by the kidney disease. The temperature is then apt to be below the normal, and the pulse is rapid and feeble.

Temporary blindness, neuro-retinitis, or nephritic retinitis, are developed in a moderate number of these patients.

Chronic bronchitis and emphysema very frequently exist, and their symptoms often form a large part of the clinical history.

The left ventricle of the heart is regularly hypertrophied. This by itself gives no symptoms; but if the arteries become contracted, or if the hypertrophied heart becomes feeble, then disturbances of the circulation are established which cause serious symptoms.

In the same way the complicating endocarditis which so often exists gives no trouble until the valves are a good deal changed, or the ventricles dilated, or the heart's action altered, or the arteries contracted; then the circulation is interfered with, and the results of venous congestion of different parts of the body show themselves.

Dyspnœa is a very frequent symptom, often the first symptom noticed by the patient. It is a spasmodic dyspnœa coming on in attacks which last for minutes, hours, or days. It is regularly made worse by mental or bodily exertion, or by the recumbent position. It does not resemble pulmonary asthma. It is apparently due to the association of changes in the arteries and in the heart. With contraction of the arteries alone, or with a feeble heart alone, no dyspnœa may exist; but if the contraction of the arteries is so great that the hypertrophied and laboring heart is unable to overcome the obstruction, or if with the contracted arteries the heart becomes dilated or feeble, then the attacks of dyspnœa begin. At first the attacks are not severe and are of short duration, but if the mechanical conditions which cause them cannot be controlled, they become longer and more distressing.

Perhaps the most striking examples of this dyspnœa are in the patients in whom it is the first symptom of the nephritis. They are apt to be middle-aged or elderly men, often engaged in large financial or commercial enterprises. They profess that they feel quite well and that they can attend to their affairs perfectly, but that they are very much annoyed because early every morning they have an attack of asthma. In spite of their professions of good health, it is evident that they are pale and that they have dyspnœa on exertion. The heart is found to be enlarged, with or without a murmur ; its action is either labored or feeble. The pulse is tense. The urine is of a specific gravity of 1.010 to 1.030 ; it contains no albumin, or only a trace. In the earlier stages of the disease this dyspnœa can be controlled, but later on it is more distressing and difficult to remedy.

The stomach may become the seat of catarrhal gastritis or of spasmodic vomiting. But in some patients it continues to perform its functions fairly well.

Dropsy, as a rule, is absent with non-exudative nephritis, unless it is complicated by chronic endocarditis or cirrhosis of the liver.

Profuse bleeding from atrophied kidneys has been described by Bowlby in three cases.

Regularly, after a time, the nephritis exerts its effect upon the nutrition of the patient, and the flesh and strength are diminished. On the other hand, the patients do not become as pale as they do in exudative nephritis.

Course of the disease. It is characteristic of the chronic productive inflammations of the lungs, the heart, the arteries, the liver, and the kidneys, that, while they often exist as serious and fatal diseases, they also frequently exist as lesions which do not interfere with general good health and long life. This seems to depend, in part at least, on the rapidity with which the inflammatory changes in these different parts of the body are developed. If they are developed slowly enough the functions of the organ continue to be performed, in spite of the new growth of connective tissue in it.

So, with the kidneys, it is common enough to find chronic non-exudative nephritis far advanced in persons who die from accident or intercurrent disease, and have never given symptoms of renal disease.

In the same way we can often observe for years persons who have urine of low specific gravity, an hypertrophied left ventricle of the heart, and occasionally some increase of tension in the arteries, and who yet habitually enjoy very fair health.

But yet these same persons, if they are attacked with pneumonia or pericarditis, or suffer from a severe accident, will often develop serious or even fatal renal symptoms.

A very common form for the disease to take is that of attacks which are repeated a number of times, each attack worse than the preceding, and the general health more and more impaired between the attacks. During the attacks there are cerebral symptoms more or less severe — headache, sleeplessness, delirium, stupor, coma, convulsions. Dyspnœa may be present or absent. The arteries are contracted, with a tense pulse. There is loss of appetite, nausea, and vomiting. The urine is of low specific gravity and usually contains albumin. Between the attacks the patients at first seem to be fairly well, but later they gradually lose flesh and strength. The urine between the attacks is of low specific gravity and contains little or no albumin. They finally die in one of the attacks, feeble and emaciated.

In some of the patients spasmodic dyspnœa is the first symptom. This can often be controlled for months and years, and the patients then seem to be well. But after a time it is more difficult to manage, and other renal symptoms are added.

In some cases there are no symptoms for a long time, so that persons apparently in good health are attacked without warning by convulsions, coma, delirium, or hemiplegia. They may die in the first attacks or live to go through subsequent ones.

In some cases the only symptoms up to the time of the patient's death are gradual loss of flesh and strength and disturbance of digestion, the patient dying feeble and emaciated. These cases are hard to make out, unless the specific gravity of the urine is low and a little albumin present. Otherwise there is nothing to draw attention to the kidneys as the cause of the illness. Loss of eyesight from nephritic neuro-retinitis may be the first symptom.

The patients may suffer from the symptoms of cardiac disease for years before congestion or degeneration of the kidney is succeeded by chronic nephritis.

In many cases the course of the nephritis is modified by the complicating emphysema, phthisis, endocarditis, endarteritis, or cirrhosis of the liver.

TREATMENT.

Such a classification as that above given of kidney diseases brings with it a rational system of therapeutics.

Acute congestion of the kidneys can be relieved by the application of heat to the surface of the body.

Chronic congestion is best managed by the drugs which stimulate the heart and dilate the arteries.

We evidently have no means at our command by which we can influence acute degeneration of the renal epithelium; fortunately the great majority of the cases of acute degeneration are not serious.

Chronic degeneration also seems to be a condition which we are unable to treat.

In acute exudative and in acute diffuse nephritis the main indications for treatment are to diminish the severity of the nephritis and to regulate the circulation.   To diminish the severity of the nephritis we employ cups over the lumbar region, heat over the lumbar region or over the entire body, and the internal use of calomel, sulphate of magnesia, opium, aconite, or digitalis.

The disturbances of the circulation are largely the causes of the cerebral symptoms and of the dropsy. With a laboring heart and contracted arteries we employ the drugs which dilate the arteries—chloral hydrate, opium, nitrate of amyl, and nitro-glycerin—or we diminish the quantity of the blood by venesection, sweating, or purging. With a feeble heart and relaxed arteries we use the cardiac stimulants.

In chronic nephritis climate and mode of life constitute the important parts of the treatment; it is doubtful if drugs exert any effect on the nephritis. A warm, dry climate and an out-of-door life are of the greatest importance. Medical treatment can, however, be employed with advantage for the relief of the anæmia, the dropsy, and the disturbances of circulation.

With the classifications of kidney disease now in common use you are all familiar. You know the number of names employed and the contradictory meanings attached to these names by different authors. Many of you must have experienced the extreme difficulty there has been in teaching students to understand Bright's disease. I leave it to you to determine how far the plan which I have proposed is likely to be of practical use.

CLINICAL OBSERVATIONS ON THE CARDIAC BRUITS OF CHLOROSIS.

By ALFRED G. BARRS, M.D., M.R.C.P.,

SENIOR ASSISTANT PHYSICIAN TO THE GENERAL INFIRMARY AT LEEDS; LECTURER ON MATERIA MEDICA
AND THERAPEUTICS IN THE YORKSHIRE COLLEGE OF THE VICTORIA UNIVERSITY.

IN the medical out-patient department of the Leeds Infirmary, during the last two and a half years, I have been able to record the presence or absence of cardiac bruits in 205 cases of simple chlorosis. Cardiac bruits were present in 115 cases, and absent in 90 cases.

In the 115 cases in which bruits were present, their locality was recorded as follows:

A systolic bruit, audible at the base only,				in	56 cases
"	"	"	apex "	"	13 "
"		"	base and apex	"	24 "
		"	base, apex, and back,	"	22 "

115

So that in 102 cases a bruit, always systolic in time, was heard at the base, wherever else it might be heard, showing the great preponderance of basic bruits over apical bruits pure and simple—a fact in accord with general experience.

The cases in which the systolic bruit was audible at the base, at the apex, and in the back are naturally those which will excite the most interest, and it is to them particularly that I intend the few remarks which follow to apply ; at the same time, it will be perceived that whatever can be said of the chlorotic bruit following, in its locality, rhythm and conduction, all the characters of the mitral regurgitant bruit of organic disease must be applicable *pari passu* to all cardiac bruits arising in the chlorotic state.

I may at once assure the reader that I have no intention of launching into any theoretical disquisition upon the causation of the anæmic murmur beyond the little that is necessary to elucidate the important clinical facts, as they seem to me, which these figures put before us.

It is now about three years ago that I became aware of the fact that in a certain proportion of cases of chlorosis a systolic murmur may be heard, not only at the base and apex, but also at the angle of the left scapula and in its immediate neighborhood, and since then I have been careful to note the locality of all bruits heard in cases of that disease, with the result shown in the figures given above.

The bruits were in all cases clear and distinct, though usually of a soft, blowing character, and audible to the students frequenting the out-patient room, so that there could be no reasonable doubt attaching to the observations. But I am quite sure that now and again the anæmic murmur may be observed to come and go, so that at one time it may be audible and at another not so. Hope noticed this fact, for in his work on *Diseases of the Heart*[1] he says, speaking of the inorganic murmur: "The murmur is not constant, but occasional, coming on whenever the circulation is excited, and for exciting it the most trivial causes, as Laennec has observed, are sufficient."

In the crush and hurry of the out-patient rooms it has been impossible, I am sorry to say, for me to record accurately the concomitant conditions of the heart, but there is no doubt that in the cases presenting a bruit audible at the base, the apex, and in the back, marked changes in the character of the impulse and in the locality of the apex-beat were almost always present, indicating dilatation of the ventricle or ventricles and an increased force of the cardiac contraction. So well marked and constant have these changes been, that I have found myself able, with tolerable certainty, to predict the bruits to be heard after placing the hand upon the præcordium. These changes in the cardiac

---

[1] 1839 ed., p. 106.

chambers, the result of anæmia, were first seriously studied in this country by the late Dr. Pearson Irvine, who made an elaborate communication to the Royal Medical and Chirurgical Society on May 22, 1877,[1] on the subject, in which he stated that "The apex-beat in chlorotics is carried too far outward, is too diffuse, and in this respect corresponds with the general cardiac impulse, which is usually 'slapping' and like that met with in organic disease." This statement is quite in accord with my own observations, the conditions described by Dr. Irvine being most marked in the 22 cases in which the bruit was audible in the back as well as at the apex and base.

Speaking from my own cases, the duration of the cardiac murmur of chlorosis is not long after the patient has been put under efficient treatment by iron. I should say that, *as a rule*, all murmurs have disappeared at the end of three weeks on the average. In the base, apex, and back cases, the order of their disappearance was the reverse of that named, the basic murmur being the last to depart. This seems to suggest what I have no doubt is the fact—that whatever the mechanical conditions giving rise to the bruits may be, the basic bruit is the earliest and mildest result of them, the back bruit the latest and most serious.

In regard to the general conditions attendant upon bruits in chlorosis, I have found it impossible to predict with certainty any cardiac change that may be present from the intensity of the pallor, the duration of the amenorrhœa, or the obstinacy of the constipation—those cases in which the blood-change seemed greatest having sometimes no bruit at all, while those which had a minimum degree of pallor might present bruits audible at the base, apex, and back.

An apex murmur, systolic in time and conducted to the angle of the left scapula, has usually been held to be distinctive of mitral regurgitation; and further, by those who do not agree that mitral regurgitation may take place from functional or recoverable conditions of the mitral orifice and its valve, is also held to be distinctive of organic disease. I well remember that Dr. Fagge always taught that a systolic bruit audible at the apex only might be either organic or inorganic in its origin; but if the murmur was also audible at the angle of the scapula, then there could be no reasonable doubt as to the organic nature of the condition giving rise to the abnormal sound. In his article on "Diseases of the Valves of the Heart,"[2] Dr. Fagge, after quoting Dr. Bristowe, Dr. Austin Flint, and Dr. Andrew, says: "These authorities believe that there are two criteria which may be applied to the determination of the fact that in a particular case a systolic apex murmur is really due to mitral regurgitation. The criteria are: 1. That the murmur

---

[1] Lancet, June 9, 1877, p. 837.
[2] Reynolds' System of Medicine, vol. iv. p. 643.

should be audible in the left side of the back about the inferior angle of the scapula. 2. That the pulmonary second sound should be intensified." He then says, a little later on in the same article: "My own views with regard to the interpretation of systolic apex murmur may be summed up as follows: 1. If such a murmur be audible in the back, it indicates mitral regurgitation. 2. If such a murmur be heard only at the heart's apex, we are unable at the present time to pronounce any positive opinion as to its cause, etc." I think there can be no doubt, from the title and context of Dr. Fagge's article, that he uses the term "mitral regurgitation" as synonymous with "mitral disease."

Walshe,[1] speaking of hæmic murmurs, says: "They are only in exceptional cases audible below the nipple and never within my experience perceptible as far as the left apex or outward toward the axilla." He says also in a note:[2] "I have never yet heard in a purely chlorotic woman a murmur having all the characters of a mitral regurgitant one."

I need not produce further evidence to show how strongly it is held that apical murmurs audible in the back always mean organic disease of the mitral valve. On the other hand, I am able to point to twenty-two cases, in twenty of which murmurs identical with those heard in undoubted examples of mitral disease disappeared under treatment in the course of two or three weeks. Nor am I alone in this observation. Dr. Kingston Fowler[3] says, after reference to the works of Dr. Walshe and Dr. Hoyden: "Is every patient presenting the signs of mitral regurgitation, a systolic apex murmur conducted to the angle of the scapula and audible in the vertebral groove between the sixth and ninth dorsal vertebræ, to be considered the subject of organic disease of the mitral valve? According to Dr. Hoyden and Dr. Walshe this question must be answered in the affirmative. My own experience points to an exactly opposite conclusion. I have within the last three months seen at least fifteen cases of advanced chlorotic anæmia among my out-patients at the Middlesex and Brompton Hospitals, of whose cases I have careful notes, and in whom I have detected a systolic apex murmur, which has been distinctly audible not at the angle of the left scapula only, but in many at the right also, and in most of which cases the bruits have already disappeared under appropriate treatment. I have long taught that the anæmic murmurs obey the same law as to conductions as those of organic origin, and particularly that the conduction of the systolic apex murmur to the angle of the scapula is no sign of disease of the mitral orifice."

[1] Diseases of the Heart, 4th ed., 1873. Page 86.
[2] Op. cit., page 89.
[3] On the Origin of Anæmic Murmurs. London, 1884. Page 35.

Dr. Broadbent also says:[1] "The occurrence of dilatation of the left ventricle and mitral regurgitation is very common as an effect of anæmia."

I do not attempt to reconcile these conflicting statements and experiences. I am content to accept the fact that an apex murmur audible at the angle of the scapula is not unfrequently to be observed in chlorosis, and also that the bruit disappears under treatment directed to the removal of the blood state, and so cannot well be due to structural changes in the mitral valve.

In two of the twenty-two cases the mitral regurgitant murmur has not yet disappeared, and as the cases have now been under observation for seven and nine months respectively, there is great probability that permanent changes in the heart have taken place. I will very briefly relate the chief points in these two cases.

CASE I.—Rhoda H., aged twenty-two years, came under observation January 7, 1891. She presented all the characteristic symptoms of marked chlorosis, except that she was menstruating regularly, and had not constipation. She had not had any rheumatic manifestation nor chorea. The cardiac action was extremely irregular, but no bruit could be heard on this occasion. She was ordered a perchloride of iron mixture. On February 2d she was improving in appearance and general symptoms. The heart's action was still irregular, and a systolic bruit was heard at the apex only. February 17th: Heart's action quite regular, systolic bruit heard at the apex and at angle of the left scapula. She has taken the iron mixture since January 7th. On March 3d I made a note that I thought the bruit was organic, and ordered her a digitalis mixture and sulphate of iron pills. May 26th: Has taken digitalis and iron regularly since March 3d (eleven weeks); cardiac action very irregular, systolic apex bruit heard occasionally. On July 10th she was reported very ill and unable to attend. Saw her ten days ago. Heart regular. Bruit still present.

I have very little doubt that this case ought to be regarded as one of chlorosis in which the bruit has become permanent, unless, as is quite possible, she is the subject of long-standing mitral disease, and had by accident, as it were, become chlorotic. Stokes[1] narrates a precisely similar case, in which mitral disease was found on post-mortem examination, and says that the combination of organic and anæmic murmurs, especially in young females, is not unfrequent, and it is often difficult to say whether the organic or functional disease has had the initiative. "Under these circumstances we have generally with the symptoms of anæmia the physical sign of a mitral murmur unattended by evidence of hypertrophy of the heart."

CASE II.—Ruth A. R., aged fifteen years, came to the out-patient room on November 18, 1890, with a chlorotic aspect and the usual symp-

<hr/>

[1] The Pulse. London, 1890. Page 160.
[2] Diseases of the Heart and Aorta. Dublin, 1854. Pages 150, 151.

toms. She had not menstruated. There was no constipation. She had
not had any rheumatic manifestation nor chorea. A systolic bruit was
heard at the base, apex, and back. She was ordered perchloride of iron
in mixture. December 9th: Bruit still audible in all areas. January
13, 1891: Bruit persists in all areas. I made a note on this date that
the bruit sounded like an organic bruit. February 24th: Bruit very
faint to-day; so much so that I thought it had disappeared, after all.
May 26th: Bruit very loud to-day in all areas and rough in character.
She has been taking iron continuously since November 18, 1890, and has
improved in appearance and has practically no symptoms. (P. S.)
July 17th: Bruit still audible in all areas.

Here, then, are two cases in which a bruit indistinguishable from that
of mitral regurgitation due to organic valvular disease persists in spite
of long-continued treatment directed to the removal of the anæmic state.
The observation of them has called to my mind an important and exceedingly interesting paper by Dr. Goodhart[1] on "Anæmia as a Cause
of Heart Disease," in which he says that anæmia, by leading to dilatation of the left ventricle is a fertile source of valvular disease, and
chiefly of mitral disease. Dr. Goodhart's cases were, I should observe,
not cases of chlorosis, but of secondary anæmia; he nevertheless very
properly applies his conclusions to chlorosis and all other primary
anæmias. Sir Dyce Duckworth, also, writing in 1886,[2] says: "Evidence
is, however, accumulating to show that amongst the results of anæmia
a measure of damage to the mitral and aortic valves occurs."

The chief point I have wished to make in this short paper is that
bruits, indicating mitral regurgitation, occur in a considerable proportion of cases of chlorosis, and that in a small number of such cases the
cardiac condition ends in permanent organic disease.

A CASE OF ELEPHANTIASIS OF THE SCROTUM.

WITH REMARKS ON ITS OPERATIVE TREATMENT.

By CHRISTIAN FENGER, M.D.,
OF CHICAGO.

ELEPHANTIASIS of the scrotum is so rarely met with outside of the
tropics that to us it has little more than a theoretical interest. At the
same time our relations with the surrounding tropical countries where the
disease is endemic are sufficiently intimate now, and are increasing to
such an extent that it is very possible that cases of this disease may be

[1] Lancet, March, 1880, p. 481.
[2] Brit. Med. Journ., July 10th, p. 57

met with here among immigrants from these countries, as, for instance, Barbadoes, Samoa, and China.

J. E., twenty-three years of age, German, was admitted to the German Hospital, Chicago, in January, 1891. He was born in Strasburg, of German parents, both of whom are in good health. He has three brothers and four sisters, all in good health. When he was six years old he came with his parents to Chicago, and a few years later moved to a farm at Rose Hill, one of the suburbs of that city. With the exception of the usual diseases of childhood, and a rather severe attack of typhoid fever three years ago, from which he recovered perfectly, he has always been healthy.

His present ailment, the elephantiasis, commenced eight years ago without any apparent cause, as a slight enlargement of the scrotum, followed later on by thickening of the prepuce. The enlargement increased gradually and uniformly, with no intermission. There was never any pain nor symptoms of inflammation—that is, erysipelatoid attacks in the enlarged scrotum—according to his statement. About four years ago he suffered for some time from frequent micturition and urinary tenesmus, which, after a while, subsided. Two years ago, without any cause so far as he knew, he had swelling and pain in the inguinal glands on both sides above and below Poupart's ligament, accompanied by pain, and followed in a short time by suppuration. This terminated in two or three abscesses on each side, which were permitted to open spontaneously, and after discharging for some time the opening definitely closed.

Several years ago he was obliged to have trousers especially made on account of the scrotal tumor. In spite of the size and weight of the tumor, however, he has been able to work as driver of a wagon for a railroad company with satisfaction up to this time.

On examination he was found to be robust, well nourished, of healthy appearance and color. Thoracic and abdominal organs normal. Muscular strength and development normal (Fig. 1). The scrotum was enlarged and formed a tumor weighing twenty-two pounds, extending down an inch below the knees. The skin was nodular, here and there covered with scales and crusts of dried epithelium. The nodular prominences were somewhat harder than the remainder of the skin. The tumor was of a uniform firm, leathery consistence. Pressure with the fingers did not leave any indentation as in œdema. The skin was thickened so that it could not be lifted up in a fold. On the anterior upper surface of the tumor was seen a second round tumor, about the size of a fist, on the right side of which was a vertical furrow two inches long, through which a probe could be passed upward into the tumor a distance of four inches. This was the opening of the prepuce, through which the patient urinated, the urine dribbling down over the large tumor. The skin over this enlarged prepuce was hard and nodulated, as was the skin of the scrotum. There were no hairs on the scrotum. The pubic hair was sparsely developed. At the junction of the scrotum with the pubic region the skin was softer and not nodulated, but still somewhat thickened and immovable, as if œdematous.

This part of the tumor formed a sort of pedicle six inches wide and three or four inches thick. Neither the testicles nor the penis could be made out.

The inguinal glands on both sides were enlarged to the size of a small walnut, as were also the glands in Scarpa's triangle. On the right side three cicatricial depressions—scars after the old abscesses—could be seen, one below and two above Poupart's ligament; and on the left side two similar scars. There was no enlargement of the deeper glands along the external iliac vessels.

The skin at the upper part of the inside of the thigh and the corresponding skin of the outer part of the tumor was the seat of intertrigo, the surface denuded, red and moist, partially covered with a whitish, fetid smegma. This surface inflammation caused the patient no pain,

Fig. 1.

Fig. 2.

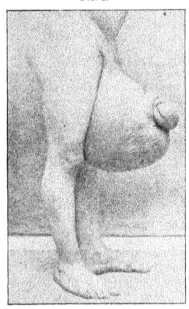
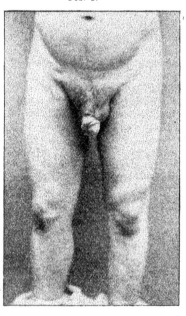

itching, or other inconvenience. There were no enlarged lymph-glands in any other part of the body, and no œdema of the lower limbs, on which, as well as elsewhere on the body, the skin was perfectly normal.

Urine normal. Repeated examinations of the blood at different times of the day and night showed no filaria and nothing abnormal. Appetite good; bowels regular. His mental condition was somewhat abnormal; he was melancholy and morose, did not want to talk with anyone, was not very willing to answer questions, but otherwise appeared to be sufficiently intelligent.

For two weeks previous to the operation antiseptic dressings were applied and local treatment directed to the excoriated surface between the thigh and scrotum, so as to heal the superficial inflammation of the skin at this point and as a further preparation for the operation.

On the day previous to the operation the patient was given a sublimate bath, and on the morning of the operation the tumor was held up in an elevated position for an hour in order to deplete the vessels of blood.

The patient was anæsthetized and the tumor held up by two assistants, and a Turner's clamp, which I had had made to secure bloodless operating, applied over the uppermost part of the pedicle, a careful examination having first been made for inguinal hernia, which showed that no such complication existed.

A grooved director was now introduced into the sinus of the prepuce leading to the glans penis, and the overlying wall of skin divided upon it until the glans penis was exposed about three inches above the peripheral opening.

Flaps of skin were now cut as follows: The anterior surface was divided into three equal parts and three semilunar flaps cut, the median being a little larger than the two lateral flaps—each lateral flap being about two inches long and two inches broad, the median flap of the same breadth but two and one-half inches long. The two lateral flaps were intended to cover the testicles, the median flap to cover the penis. A single posterior flap was then cut through the skin, about two inches long and six inches broad ; that is, the whole width of the posterior surface of the neck of the tumor. The cutaneous flaps were then dissected up to the clamp. The penis was next dissected out of the tumor, leaving about one inch of preputial mucous membrane all around the glans. The skin in this region was somewhat thickened and œdematous, but reasonably movable and pliable. The left testicle was now sought for and found without much difficulty, the tunica vaginalis communis being surrounded by a looser layer of somewhat œdematous tissue, which permitted the isolation of the testicle covered with the tunica vaginalis communis, and the spermatic cord, which was then dissected up to the clamp. The right testicle was now isolated in the same way.

Both testicles and the penis, together with the three anterior flaps, were held up toward the abdomen over the upper arm of the clamp, covered with carbolized gauze, and the neck of the tumor was ablated by a series of cuts. After dividing each portion, all visible vessels were ligated, including a number of veins two to three lines in diameter.

When the ablation of the tumor had been finally completed and all visible vessels ligated, the clamp was loosened a little at one end, whereupon a number of bleeding vessels appeared, which were taken up and ligated one by one. In all, more than sixty ligatures to large and small vessels were applied. All bleeding-points in each portion cut were ligated before the next portion was divided.

The clamp was then removed, and the hemorrhage having entirely ceased, the wound was irrigated with two and a half per cent. solution of carbolic acid and the flaps united in the following way :

The two lateral flaps were united to the lateral portion of the posterior flap over each of the testicles, and the median anterior flap and the middle portion of the posterior flap made to cover the penis by stitching the lower end to the prepuce above the glans penis. The glans penis was uncovered, and although there was no tension in the covering of the body of the penis when not in a state of erection, I should in a future case like to make the median anterior flap and the middle portion of the posterior flap about an inch longer, because the skin and the prepuce were here somewhat thickened and stiff, and thus not as mobile and flexible as in the normal condition.

Three short drainage-tubes, one for the penis and one for each testicle, were inserted and stitched to the border of the wound, and a dry iodoform dressing applied.

The wounds healed without suppuration, pain, or rise in temperature. After a week the drainage-tubes were removed, and in four weeks the granulating surfaces at the point of insertion of the drainage-tube and at one side of the penis, where the union between the skin and prepuce had reopened a little, were entirely healed over. As will be seen from a photograph taken six weeks after the operation (see Fig. 2), the shape of the external genitals is comparatively normal, and the following condition is now present:

The glans penis is plainly visible, protruding below the scrotum. On the left side the skin of the penis is normal; on the right, above the glans penis, there is an œdematous fold which is rapidly decreasing in size and becoming softer. The left half of the scrotum is of almost natural shape and size; the right half not so much so, but both testicles can easily be palpated in the normal position, behind the penis. The skin at the root of the penis in the pubic region is a little thicker than normal, and is still a little more voluminous than normal, but nearly approximates the natural shape. Both inguinal regions are somewhat enlarged on account of the swelling of the subjacent lymph-glands, as will be seen in Fig. 2, where the depressions due to the somewhat retracted scars over the openings from the glandular abscesses of two years ago are plainly visible.

Urination normal. As to the sexual function, I know nothing at present. His mental condition is widely different as compared with his condition prior to the operation. Instead of his former morose and non-communicative behavior, he shows now a bright and smiling countenance, and, without being invited to do so, states that his present condition is one of great happiness as compared with the period before the operation.

Microscopical examination of the structure of the tumor from the skin downward shows thickening of the epidermis and papillary layer, but the epithelial cells are of normal shape and size. There is no line of demarcation between the cutis and the subcutaneous tissue, the entire tumor consisting of a wide, semi-solid, elastic mass of tissue, which shows under the microscope the following characteristics:

Large areas of thick bundles of non-fibrillar connective tissue: the bundles in some locations running parallel to each other, and in other places interwoven and cut obliquely or transversely. Between the bundles may be seen occasional and rare connective-tissue corpuscles of normal size and shape. The vessels, arteries as well as veins, but especially veins, show an enormous thickening of the walls, the smaller veins having walls five to ten times the normal thickness. This thickening is mainly an enlargement of the external coat, the endothelium not participating at all in the thickening of the wall. In the perivascular spaces are seen here and there conglomerations of leucocytes; in other places no young cells are to be seen at all. Islands of young granulation tissue, consisting of embryonal cells densely packed together and having the same appearance as the cells in ordinary young granulation tissue, are spread all over the connective tissue. These islands differ greatly in size. I was unable to find anywhere enlarged lymph-spaces or lymphatics, but am inclined to believe that some of the islands occupied by embryonal cells, in which no bloodvessels could be seen, are lymph-vessels or lymph-spaces in a state of plastic inflammation.

Elephantiasis of the scrotum (elephantiasis Arabum) is anatomically identical with elephantiasis of other parts of the body, whether affecting the scrotum, prepuce, labia majora or the lower extremities. We find in all cases, irrespective of the etiology, an increase in all the constituent elements of the skin and subcutaneous tissue, with the exception of the hair and the glands. Thus we find thickened epidermis and inter-papillary spaces of the epithelium, enlarged papillæ and connective tissue of the cutis. The enlargement here and in the subcutaneous tissue is due to a universal formation of new connective tissue. This new formation of connective tissue in the vessel wall, chiefly in the external coat, produces the characteristic thickening of the vessels to five or ten times their normal size. It also produces a thickening of the nerves by a similar increase of interstitial tissue between the nerve bundles.

We find in the lymphatics in the later stages of elephantiasis, as in the case reported, no very characteristic dilatation. It is different in the earlier stage of elephantiasis of the scrotum, the so-called " lymph scrotum," where the tissue is still soft and œdematous. Here we find lymph-vessels and lymph-spaces dilated, sometimes to such an extent that when situated at the surface of the skin they may form thin-walled, transparent bullæ on the surface of the tumor, which may burst and empty a clear or milky lymphatic fluid, which sometimes escapes in great quantity and may cause a temporary decrease in the size of the tumor.

The condition of the lymph-glands is important. It is common to find, as in the above case, a considerable enlargement of the glands, an inflammatory enlargement, which, when due to invasion of pus microbes from an abraded surface on the scrotal tumor, may terminate in suppuration.

The etiology of elephantiasis is still shrouded in mystery; this is especially true in the non-parasitic forms of the disease. Etiologically there is a great difference between the elephantiasis found in tropical countries and the variety of the disease seen in temperate and cold regions. In tropical countries the disease is uniformly ascribed to a parasite belonging to the class of nematodes, namely, the *Filaria Bancrofti*.[1] This filaria, a thin, white worm, three to four inches in length, and as thick as a human hair, is found in the lymph-vessels of the area of the elephantiasis. Here it deposits its thousands of eggs, out of each

[1] B. Scheube : " Die Filaria-krankheit." Volkmann's Sammlung klin. Vorträge, 1833, No. 232.

of which is developed an embryonal worm small enough to pass through the capillaries. This worm is periodically found in the blood of patients suffering from this disease, and is the so-called *Filaria sanguinis hominis.* It is supposed that the mature animal, as well as the ova and embryos, may cause on the one hand, by accumulation in the lymph-vessels and glands, stoppage of the lymph-current and consequent œdema in the corresponding distal territory; and on the other hand, by chemical products of their excretions, they may cause inflammation of the lymph-vessels, a plastic lymphangitis, which naturally would tend to further obstruct the lymph circulation. This may, perhaps, account for the repeated attacks of erysipelatoid inflammation in the territory of the elephantiasis.

This parasite, also, whose life history and relation to elephantiasis have been studied so carefully by Wucherer in Brazil, Lewis in Calcutta, and especially by Manson, father and son, and Myers in Amoy, and whose method of entering the human body has been studied by the last-named authors and by my friend of former years, Prospero Sonsino, of Egypt, is commonly found in our Gulf States, as has been shown in an excellent paper by Mastin, of Mobile, and confirmed by Matas, of New Orleans, and others.

It is natural, then, to find elephantiasis a common, and in some places an endemic, disease in tropical countries, to which the filaria of Bancroft is geographically limited. In some localities, as for instance Samoa, the disease is so common that, according to Turner, 50 per cent. of the adult population will, sooner or later in life, have the disease. The filaria and elephantiasis have probably been imported into islands comparatively near our coast by coolies from China, as, for instance, Barbadoes, where the disease has become endemic.

But the filaria Bancrofti is not the only cause of elephantiasis, for sporadic cases of this disease in the scrotum, as well as in the lower extremities, are found in temperate and cold countries where the filaria does not exist, and are found in patients, as in the case here reported, who have never been in places where they could have been exposed to the invasion of the parasite. As would naturally be expected, the parasite is never found in these patients. Cases of this kind have been reported in England by Fergusson, in France by Velpeau, in Germany by Graefe, in Switzerland by Bircher, and also by other observers.

Clinically and anatomically there seems to be no difference between the elephantiasis of the tropics due to the filaria, and the elephantiasis in the temperate zone where no filaria is found. The changes in the lymphatic system, erysipelatoid inflammations in the lymph-spaces of the skin, and swelling of the lymph-glands, are characteristic of both classes of the disease. This swelling of the lymph-glands does not necessarily mean obliteration of the lymph-current, as stated by Kocher in his excellent monograph on diseases of the male genital organs,[1] for in a case of elephantiasis published by Bryk, the enlarged lymph-glands were permeable and the lymph-vessels dilated, even as far as the thoracic duct. Swelling of the lymph-glands, according to Kocher, often precedes the development of elephantiasis, and is supposed to play an important part in the etiology of the disease, both within and outside of the tropics. But it is entirely unknown why so common an affection as enlargement of the lymph-glands should result in elephantiasis in such exceedingly exceptional instances as we find to be the case.

Symptoms.—Elephantiasis of the scrotum is usually of a softer consistence than when the disease exists in the legs, but the swelling increases more rapidly. Soft and œdematous at first, the so-called lymph-scrotum, it gradually becomes harder. The unequal thickening of the epidermis causes the surface, which was originally smooth, to become nodular and irregularly corrugated. The increase is not uniform, but intermittent, following the repeated inflammatory attacks. These attacks are characterized by redness and swelling, but are attended by very little pain, the skin over the tumor being to a greater or less extent anæsthetic. Atrophy of the sebaceous glands and hair-bulbs is followed by falling out of the hair. Here and there scales of thickened epidermis and crusts of dried secretion from abraded surfaces or from ruptured dilated lymph-vessels cover smaller or larger areas over the tumor.

By the increase in the size of the tumor the testicles are buried, so that after a while their location cannot be detected except when hydrocele coexists. The increase in size of the prepuce, together with the increase in the skin of the scrotum, makes the penis disappear, the skin being drawn downward and forward in front of the glans, forming a sinus sometimes several inches long leading up to the urethra, surrounded by a separate tumor like a smaller appendix on the anterior surface of the large tumor. A deep furrow is usually seen on the end or on one of the sides of the transformed prepuce, which forms the entrance to the urinary sinus through which the urine dribbles down during micturition over the tumor, which probably helps in the causation of the maceration of the epidermis and the surface inflammation.

As the elephantiasis is on the whole painless, the chief inconvenience to the patient is caused by its weight. Tumors of thirty to fifty pounds in weight are commonly seen, and a tumor weighing one hundred pounds has exceptionally been observed. This, however, does not influence the general health of the patient, who is, as a rule, as in the case cited above, able to do manual labor, notwithstanding the presence of the large tumor.

---

[1] Theodor Kocher. "Die Krankheiten der männlichen Geschlechtsorgane." Deutsche Chirurgie, von Billroth und Luecke, 1887.

The *prognosis* is good, and it is only in exceptional cases that danger arises from septic inflammation on the surface of the tumor, with gangrenous destruction of a portion of the inflamed area and resultant general sepsis.

Treatment.—Elevation of the tumor, compression, warm, moist applications, local mercurial inunctions, in connection with the internal use of the iodides, iron, chlorate of potassium, and bichloride of mercury, have proved successful in exceptional cases only, and then in the earlier stages alone.

Non-radical treatment is, of course, of far more importance in elephantiasis of the lower extremities, where amputation should be deferred as long as possible, than in elephantiasis of the scrotum, where early operation is so much the more admissible, as no mutilation of the genital organs is caused by it.

The dangers of the operation in elephantiasis of the scrotum are hemorrhage and sepsis. For this reason, in former times, partial excisions and operations with the écraseur or galvano-cautery were resorted to, but these procedures have now become entirely obsolete.

The prognosis of the operation, which in pre-antiseptic times was comparatively grave, has gradually lost its dangers. Thus we see, from Kocher's statistics, an early mortality of twenty-seven per cent. in sixty-one cases reported by Fayrer; of nine and one-half per cent. in twenty-one cases reported by Ballingall; of five per cent. in one hundred and sixty-one cases reported by Esdaile; of three and three-tenths per cent. in sixty-one cases reported by Manson ; and more recently one and one-half per cent. in one hundred and thirty-eight cases reported by Turner. The better prognosis of the operation in Turner's cases is due to asepsis as well as to the great improvement in the technique of the operation. Therefore, in the case above reported I adhered strictly to the method of operating as laid down by Turner. Hæmostasis is made absolute by the use of Turner's clamp, which has been already mentioned.

Perfect covering of the penis and testicles is secured by the flaps as devised by Turner and described in my operation, thereby avoiding sepsis from non-union of a large wound surface, as in the older operations, in which for fear of hemorrhage the tumor was cut off transversely, or in which sometimes the penis and testicles were removed with the tumor and the large wound surface left to heal by granulation.

The bloodless operation, by means of the clamp or elastic constriction, gives the operator time to carefully dissect out the penis, testicles, and spermatic cord, and to open and radically operate upon hydrocele, if present. The clamp is preferable to an elastic constrictor, because the latter is, as stated by Kocher, very liable to slip off during the separation of the tumor, while the clamp can be gradually loosened one end at a time, admitting ligation of the smaller vessels step by step. This makes the operation with the clamp, notwithstanding the numerous and very large vessels, almost entirely bloodless.

The removal of the penis and testicles can in all probability be always avoided by Turner's operation, and should at least be always attempted, although Esdaile regards it as dangerous not to remove these organs in tumors which weigh more than fifty pounds. In two cases reported by Lloyd, tumors of sixty-five and sixty-one pounds in weight, respectively, were successfully removed with preservation of the penis and testicles. In these operations soft twisted ropes were used as constrictors and the flaps made according to the method of Turner.

The preservation of the penis and testicles is the more important because the genital functions remain undisturbed in the case of patients suffering from elephantiasis.

RESPONSES TO THE ALTERNATING GALVANIC CURRENT IN NORMAL AND DEGENERATE MUSCLES.

By M. Allen Starr, M.D.,

OF NEW YORK,

AND

Charles I. Young, A.B.,

THE OBSERVATORY, PRINCETON, NEW JERSEY.

I.

By Dr. Starr.

The following article presents in a concise form the results of a scientific investigation upon the effects of an alternating galvanic current of electricity upon normal and degenerate muscles. The research has been made by one who is thoroughly conversant with all recent advances in the knowledge of electricity and of all its mechanical appliances, and who has had exceptional facilities at Princeton for the prosecution of careful experiments by the aid of the best apparatus. Mr. Young is a practical electrician, who has been for three years recovering from a condition of acute anterior poliomyelitis of considerable extent, produced by the passage of an alternating current through his entire spinal cord. His treatment· has been partly mechanical, various devices for exercising paralyzed muscles having been made and used by him with success; partly electrical, the muscles being daily stimulated by alternating currents of moderate strength in the manner described by him; partly medicinal, by arsenic and strychnine, with results whose effects have been objectively proven by electrical tests in the manner presented in this paper. The results reached appear to be of importance in confirming Neumann's statements regarding the physiology of muscular response to electrical stimulation; in presenting a series of facts regarding the effect of the application of alternating currents to muscles, not as yet investigated; in determining the possibility of reaching prognostic facts of great value in doubtful cases by electrical tests with the alternating current; and, finally, in demonstrating the effect of strychnine and arsenic on the nervous functions.

Erb says (Ziemssen's *Cyclopœdia*, Amer. edit., vol. xi. p. 433), " the extraordinary fact that in the reaction of degeneration the muscle fails for a long time to react to the stimulus of the faradic current while it readily responds to the galvanic stimulus has been explained by Neumann in the following satisfactory manner: 'Muscles,' he says, 'that have undergone this pathological change have simply lost the power of responding to currents of momentarily short duration, while they react in an increased and qualitatively altered manner to currents of longer duration. But inasmuch as faradic currents are, without exception, currents of only momentary duration, the muscles do not react to them. . . . The value of the change by which the muscular tissue loses its normal power of reacting to currents of short duration is a question the solution of which must be left to physiologists.' "

Mr. Young has shown that the length of duration of stimulus required to cause contraction in a paralyzed muscle varies in accordance with the degree of progress toward recovery; varies also in accordance with the subjective feeling of strength; varies also in dependence upon the use of strychnine in interrupted or continuous dosage.

The practical result of his investigation is to enable a physician by careful measurement to construct a prognostic curve which will enable him to give certain hope of recovery to a patient completely paralyzed, or will establish the unfortunate fact of a permanent loss of power. It also makes it evident that in using arsenic or strychnine as a stimulus to the spinal cord it is better to give the drug for short periods with intermissions than continuously.

The accuracy and care of the investigation and the importance of the conclusions arrived at should attract the attention of physiologists, and especially of neurologists, to this contribution to medical science.

II.

By Mr. Young.

Certain nervous diseases are followed by a loss of voluntary contraction in the muscles, and in such muscles we sometimes notice electrical reactions which present a marked contrast to those of muscles in their normal condition.

A normally healthy muscle responds to the rapidly interrupted current from the faradic coils, and the muscle remains permanently contracted as long as the current is applied.

On applying the perfectly steady current of a galvanic battery we find the following effects: With the negative electrode on the muscle, and the positive anywhere on the body remote from the muscle, we get a contraction at the moment the circuit is completed ; but this contraction, unlike that produced by faradism, is not tetanic. If we now interchange the electrodes we find that the muscle responds also to the positive pole of the battery, but not so strongly as to the negative. We again notice that, during the interval between making and breaking the circuit, the muscle tends to return to a state of rest.

On applying the above tests to a degenerated muscle we find, first, no response whatever to the faradic current. In the second place we find the responses to a galvanic current appearing in reverse order ; viz., while a healthy muscle responds more vigorously to the negative than to the positive electrode, on completing the circuit, the degenerated muscle responds more vigorously to the positive; and these reactions, in the case of a degenerated muscle, are again reversed on breaking the circuit.

If we now examine a muscle which is regaining its power after being paralyzed, we may find the response to the positive pole of a galvanic battery the stronger ; the responses to positive and negative may be equal ; or that to the negative may be the stronger, as in the case of a normally healthy muscle. On applying the faradic current we may find no response, a response to but one of the electrodes, or a response to both, according to the condition of the muscle and the strength of the current applied.

It is well known that the faradic coil does not give a true alternating current. The current is strong in one direction and weak in the other, so that one electrode is a strong positive and weak negative, while the other is a strong negative and weak positive.

The writer, who has been able to supply the muscles for testing in his own person, has at different times found all the responses referred to above. Where a muscle has responded to but one electrode of the faradic coil it has invariably been to the strongly positive; but in such a case it has sometimes been possible to obtain a response to the strongly negative by increasing the strength of the current. As might be supposed, that muscle has shown a stronger response to the positive pole of a galvanic battery than to the negative.

Dr. Starr, in his article on "Therapeutic Uses of Electricity,"[1] says: "The difference of response to the faradic current from that of

[1] The Medical News, March 30, 1889.

voltaic alternatives, in conditions known as the reaction of degeneration, is not to be ascribed to any difference in the nature of the current, but only to the fact that the degenerated muscle will not respond to changes of state so rapidly produced.''

There must be a certain amount of lag in the response of any muscle to an applied electro-motive force, though in the case of a healthy muscle it must be very small, and probably would have to be measured in thousandths of a second, if not in some smaller unit. But in a degenerated muscle it would appear that this lag amounts to something appreciable. If, by means of a suitable commutating device, we apply voltaic alternatives to such a muscle, and have some means of measuring . the rate of alternation at which the muscle ceases to respond to a given current, we can ascertain the lag of that muscle's response behind the applied electro-motive force.

It has occurred to the writer that this test might possibly give some knowledge of the condition of a degenerated muscle, and with this end in view the following apparatus was assembled:

First, a rotary commutator (Figs. 1 and 2) to give voltaic alternatives. For every revolution of this commutator the current is reversed six

FIG. 1.

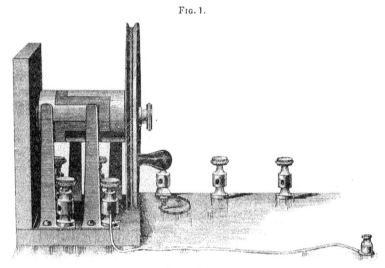

Commutator.

times. The pulley wheel of the commutator is four inches in diameter and is driven from a half-inch pulley on a small electric motor (Fig. 3) Current is supplied to the motor from a storage battery; and by means of a variable resistance the motor can be made to run at any speed from about 500 to over 6000 revolutions per minute.

The speed of the commutator is recorded automatically on a chrono-graph, which may be thrown in and out of circuit at pleasure by a switch placed within easy reach (see Fig. 3, near the base of the motor).

FIG. 2.

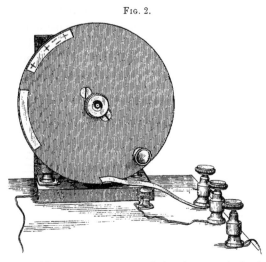

Commutator, with arrangement for completing chronograph circuit at every revolution of wheel.

FIG. 3.

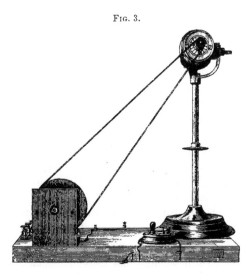

Commutator and motor.

The chronograph (which is near at hand in the astronomical obser-vatory of Princeton) records every other second from a standard clock.

The recording of the commutator revolutions is effected in the following manner:

On referring to Fig. 2 there will be seen, at the base of the commutator, a projecting tongue of brass, so placed that at every revolution a little knob on the commutator wheel strikes it and depresses it, causing it to come in contact with the head of a screw placed beneath. This, when the switch (referred to above in Fig. 3) is closed, completes the chronograph circuit, so that each revolution of the commutator wheel is recorded.

Fig. 4 shows the appearance of a record made by the chronograph. The first five lines show the clock record alone. In the lines below each .

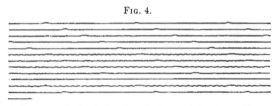

FIG. 4.

Fragment of chronograph sheet showing clock record, together with records made by commutator when run at different speeds.

little tooth stands for one revolution of the commutator. Now, as there are six reversals of the current for every revolution of the commutator, it is a simple thing to compute the number of reversals per second from the chronograph record.

The current which we apply to the muscle in our test is supplied by a battery of Leclanchè cells giving about 40 volts, is regulated by a liquid resistance which we can vary at pleasure from about 30,000 ohms to less than 1 ohm, and is measured by a milliampère-meter. In connection with the milliampère-meter is a switch to cut it out of circuit when the commutator is turning. It may be well to mention the fact that the resistance of the milliampère-meter is so small compared with the total resistance of the circuit that our cutting it out changes the value of the current by only an inappreciable amount.

In the following tests the electrode placed on the muscle we wished to examine was circular in shape and about three-fourths of an inch in diameter.

Test on biceps of right arm. This muscle has lost all power of voluntary contraction. In it we find the usual phenomena which accompany degeneration, viz., no response to faradism, and with the galvanic current a stronger response to the positive than to the negative pole. We apply the small electrode to the muscle at the motor point, the other electrode, a sponge, being placed on the left arm near the shoulder. On adjusting the variable resistance to give a current of about ten milliampères through the muscle, and setting the commutator in motion, we find the effect of the voltaic alternatives is as follows:

(*a*) We start at a low rate of speed and find the muscle responds separately to each reversal of the current.

(*b*) At a higher rate of speed the muscle becomes permanently con- tracted and begins to lift the forearm, and the arm is held up as we increase the speed up to a certain point.

(*c*) We still increase the speed, little by little, and we now observe the muscle gradually relax; the arm sinks down; and at last we attain such a speed that, on breaking and making the circuit by means of a suitable key, we find the muscle refuses to make the slightest response to the current alternating at such a rate.

To show that the sinking down of the arm, observed at *c*, was not due to fatigue of the muscle, we have the circuit closed and gradually reduce the speed of the commutator. The muscle begins to contract as the rate of alternation grows less; the forearm is again lifted and held up for a while; the muscle begins to relax, and the arm gradually sinks down again; and, at the end, the muscle contracts separately for each reversal of the current. In short, the phenomena *a, b* and *c* appear again, but in reverse order.

On making the above test with currents of different strength, we find that the rate of alternation at which the muscle ceases to respond varies

FIG. 5.

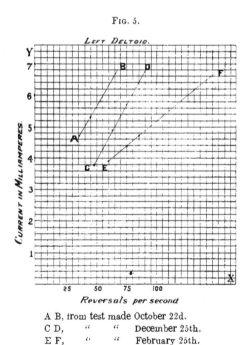

A B, from test made October 22d.
C D,   "   "   December 25th.
E F,   "   "   February 25th.

with the strength of the current used. This being so, by making three or more tests on a muscle for disappearance of contraction, with different strengths of current, we can plot the whole result on cross-section paper, and draw a line which may, perhaps, tell us something about the condition of the muscle at the time the test was made. Fig. 5 shows three such lines drawn from tests made respectively October 22d, December 25, 1890, and February 25, 1891, on the left deltoid. The condition of that muscle was practically the same as that of the biceps of right arm. As will be seen, the current, in milliampères, is plotted on the axis of Y, and the rate of alternation (reversals of current per second) on the axis of X. The lines A B, C D, and E F, represent respectively the October 22d, December 25th, and February 25th tests, and demonstrate an increasing power of response in this muscle to the alternating current.

Let us, for brevity, call the rate of alternation at which the muscle ceases to respond to a given current, the *critical rate* for that current. On referring to Fig. 5 it will be seen that, in the line A B, the critical rate for a current of 5 milliampères is about 41 ; in C D, for the same current, it is about 64 ; and in E F about 93. Of course the critical rates for any other current can also be compared by a glance at the three lines given in the figure.

In a series of tests made on the right and left deltoids, and covering a period of about five months, the changes in the critical rates have been anything but uniform, and the two muscles have not always varied alike. But the writer has noticed that on days when he felt energetic and "full of snap," so to speak, the critical rates were generally higher than those of the preceding tests ; and on days when there was a feeling of lassitude the critical rates were generally no higher than those of previous tests, and they were often lower.

Now, to combine a series of tests in a single line, suppose, for example, we measure off time, in days, on the axis of Y, and the critical rates for some given current on the axis of X. The line we get may be called a graphic representation of changes in the condition of the muscle tested, with respect to electrical reaction, during the interval between the first and last test. If the line incline to the right there has been a gain ; if it be vertical, no gain ; and if it incline to the left it indicates a loss. In Fig. 6 we have drawn such a line from tests made on the left deltoid. The line demonstrates the progress toward recovery in that muscle.

After the experience gained in following up a large number of muscles by the critical rate test, it seems evident that it might be possible to draw what could be called, in general, a prognostic line of a given muscle, after a certain number of tests had been made on that muscle at stated intervals.

While the tests given here are merely tentative, and have been made without any former experience to guide us, they seem to make it obvious that, given a degenerated muscle which will not respond to faradism, but will respond to a current alternating at a much slower rate, we can ascertain the rate of alternation at which the muscle first ceases to respond to a given current, by beginning at a slow rate and gradually

FIG. 6.

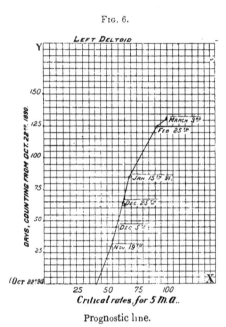

Prognostic line.

increasing. It is also clear that this rate varies with the strength of current applied, being higher for a stronger current and lower for a weaker; and the fact that the different points in each test in Fig. 5 lie so nearly in the same straight line makes it look as if this rate varied *directly* with the strength of current, at least within the limits of these tests.

We, moreover, think we are justified in assuming that if, with a given current, a healthy muscle will respond to a rate of alternation which will not affect a degenerated one, an increase in the rate to which the degenerated muscle will respond shows increased susceptibility in that muscle, and a tendency to approach, in some way, the condition of a healthy one.

We have noticed incidentally a coincidence between a change in the electrical response and the use of medicine (acid. arsen. $\frac{1}{80}$, strych. $\frac{1}{50}$, t. i. d.). It has seemed that we got a better response of the muscles from about the third day after beginning the medicine and that this improvement continued about a week; after which time the response seemed to be less vigorous.   This can be seen by a study of the follow-ing table.   This also shows that the cessation of the medicine after it had been taken for a month continuously was followed by an increase in the response.   It seemed, therefore, that better results were secured by taking the medicine for ten days and intermitting for ten days than by taking it continuously.

Responses of the Left Deltoid Muscle.

Critical rates.

	With 3.8 milliampères.	With 4 7 milliampères	
October 22,	22	36	No medicine.
November 13,	38	48	Medicine from November 5th to
" 19,	47	53	December 3d.
December 5,	36	53	Medicine stopped.
" 10,	45	58	
17,	38	52	
" 25,	48	62	
January 2,	53	62	
" 8,	33	47	Medicine from January 6th to
15,	60	76	February 2d.
" 26,	47	51	
February 2,	57	78	
" 9,	53	69	Medicine stopped.
19,	62	95	
23,	53	80	
" 25,	54	84	Medicine from February 24th to
March 3,	63	95	March 10th.
" 10,	52	83	Medicine stopped.
16,	60	87	
18,	54	77	

The writer, making no claim to medical knowledge, feels some diffi-dence in approaching the medical profession with an article upon a subject which lies within their peculiar province.   But having good reason to be interested in the subject of degenerated muscles, and being also more or less familiar with the handling of electrical apparatus, and having the chronograph and most of the other appliances at hand, he undertook to test his own muscles by this method.   The results ob-tained seemed so interesting that, at the suggestion of Dr. Starr, the method is here given.

THE POSSIBLE RESULTS OF CÆSAREAN DELIVERY,

As Shown by the Marvellous Record of Leipzig, Germany, for
the Years 1880 to 1891, under Seven Operators, and as
the Result of Improved Methods, Timely
Resorted to.

By Robert P. Harris, A.M., M.D.,

of Philadelphia.

No one living writer has done so much to disseminate a knowledge of the past in puerperal cœlio-hysterotomy in all countries and to reduce the mortality of the operation itself by improved methods as Dr. Max Sänger, of Leipzig, who, upon August 20, 1880, inaugurated with success, in a very unfavorable case, the "New Cæsarean operation," as it is usually performed to-day. It is not generally known that he was led to prepare his monograph, *Der Kaiserschnitt bei Uterusfibromen nebst vergleichender Methodik der Sectio Cæsarea und der Porro-operation*, in 1881, because of an experience with a then novel plan of treating the uterine wound, by which he became one of seven operators out of forty-one who each saved a case in a list of forty-three, where the Cæsarean operation became a necessity because of an obstruction due to a uterine fibroid. This valuable paper of two hundred pages is a mine of wealth to anyone who wishes to compare the present with the past of Cæsarean surgery, and no one can better appreciate the labor bestowed upon it than the writer of this present paper, who has himself had some experience in the same line of arduous research. In this monograph Dr. Sänger devotes over ten pages to a full report of his first Cæsarean case, from which we learn that he introduced six strong carbolized silk sutures at equal distances nearly through the uterine walls and then intermediately four superficial ones, taking in a portion of muscular tissue, the serous coat being applied to serous coat all along the wound ("Serosa lag überall an Serosa"); these being tied, there was no gaping between them and no escape of blood.

Fearing that this mode of closure might not be sufficient in all cases to prevent the escape of fluid from the uterus, Dr. Sänger proposed to use a much larger number of stitches, to exsect a portion of the muscular edges of the wound, and to welt in the peritoneal coat in tying the superficial sutures. This plan, proving a great success in the hands of Leopold and others, was given, out of compliment to its proposer, the name of the "Sänger operation." In time it became evident that the resection of the muscularis and the dissecting up and welting in of the peritoneum were not absolutely essential to success, and the operation was simplified by leaving them out—first the resection, and then, in ordinary cases, the welting in. These changes, in the view of many, eliminated from obstetric surgery the Sänger operation ; but has it changed his title to his original method of treating the uterine wound ? We are not partial to calling operations by the names of their originators, but are satisfied that there is still a *Cæsarean operation after the method of Sänger*. We may call all the operations " new Cæsarean" in which asepsis, multiple suturing in two rows, with careful adjustment of the serosa, and the use of carbolized silk, silver wire, or chromic catgut, is employed. But who did the most to bring these steps into use and to make known their value to the world? Everyone is supposed to know what the "old Cæsarean operation" was, and what a frightful mortality it had, except where it happened to have been performed early and upon healthy women. Suturing the uterine wound was a grand step—but how timid men were in doing it! One stitch, sometimes two or three, and very rarely five. They were apparently more afraid of doing it than leaving a gaping wound as an exit for poisoning fluid to escape through into the peritoneal cavity. It will be of interest to examine our American suture record down to August 20, 1880, and see what material was used, how many stitches were taken, and how the case terminated :

Here we have an array of cases, some of which might be placed in contrast with that of Dr. Sänger of the year 1880. The first to use as many as ten uterine sutures was Dr. T. A. Foster, of Portland, Maine, on May 23, 1870; but these stitches were all deep and their ends were brought out of the abdominal wound. Then we have the operation of Dr. R. O. Engram, of Montezuma, Georgia, following a craniotomy, on September 18, 1874, but not reported until October, 1885. In this case carbolized silk sutures to the number of ten were used in the uterine wound, of which three were deep, three semi-deep, and four peritoneal. This operation saved the woman, but lost its value to the profession in the fact that the process was not reported until there had been twenty-six operations founded upon the example of Sänger, with sixteen women and twenty children saved. A claim to precedence now made would amount to very little in view of the advances gained under the teachings of Leipzig and Dresden. And then we have a third case, which has been really heralded as a prior claim, in which after a labor of seven hours a woman and child were saved, on May 8, 1875, under a disciple of Hahnemann, in Toledo, Ohio, five deep sutures of silver wire being used and "care being taken to approximate the peritoneal edges." [1] This word "edges" was subsequently altered to "surfaces," with a pen ; but we take the original text as we have it, which is the old surgical

---

[1] Silver-wire Sutures in the Cæsarean Section. By S. S. Lungren, M.D , Toledo, Ohio, 1876. Pamphlet, 13 pages.

direction of "edge to edge" in the closure of incised wounds.[1] But with only five sutures in a five-inch wound we should have little control over gaping and leakage in a Cæsarean operation following a long or exhausting labor.

Year.	Time in labor.	Material used.	Number of sutures.	Cause of death in woman.	Time of survival in woman.	Result to woman.	Result to child.
1828	15 months at intervals.	Silk.	2 or 3	Peritonitis.	To second week	Died.	Dead.
1851	4 days.	"	?	Exhaustion.	24 hours.	"	"
1852	40 hours.	Silver.	?	R.		Recovered	"
1867	62½ hours.	Hemp.	3	R.	......	"	Living in 1883.
1867	10 days.	Silver.	6		......	"	Dead.
1870	44 hours.	"	1		42 hours.	Died.	Living.
1870	2 weeks.	Silk.	10 with the ends left out.	....	60 "	"	Living; died in a few days.
1871	3 days.	Silver.	2	Peritonitis	72 "	..	Dead.
1872	Long.	Silk.	1	Hemorrhage and exhaustion.	Short time after operation	"	"
1874[2]	....	Carb. silk.	3 deep, 3, ½ deep, 4 peritoneal	R.	......	Recovered.	"
1875	7 hours.	Silver.	5	R.	......	"	Living in 1889.
1875	38 hours. Membranes entire.	Silk.	1	R.	......	"	Living.
1875	6 hours. In bad health.	"	5	Exhaustion, 15 yrs. old.	2 days	Died.	Lived 13 days.
1876	Early.	Silver.	3	Peritonitis.	5 "	"	Dead
1877	Almost died of exhaustion in operation.	"	1	Exhaustion.	15 "	"	Lived 2 days.
1877	7 days.	"	4	R.	......	Recovered.	Dead.
1878	Not in labor.	Silk.	7	R.		"	"
1878	24 hours.	Carb. catgut	7	Heart-clot.	7 days.	Died.	"
1879	2½ days.	Silk.	3	Probably hemorrhage	36–40 hours	"	Moribund.
1879	30 hours.	?	1	Septicæmia.	33½ "	"	Dead.
1880	3 hours.	Horsehair, silk.	9 horsehair 3 silk.	R	......	Recovered.	Living in 1889.
1880	30 hours.	Silver.	2	R.	......	"	Dead.

| | | Silk, 11 Recov. 5 Silver. 9 Recov. 5 | Average, 4 $\frac{7}{20}$ | .... | | Recov. 10 Died 12 | Dead 13 Lived 6 Soon died 3 |

From ten silk sutures used by Sänger in 1880, the number gradually grew to a maximum of sixteen deep and thirty-five superficial, under Döderlein, of Leipzig, in 1887, since which time a desire to simplify has largely decreased the number without any apparent increase of risk, until Murdoch Cameron, of Glasgow, has saved nine women out of ten by the use of seven to twelve deep sutures and superficial intermediates as may be required. And Dr. Kelly, of Baltimore, saved his fourth patient, on January 16, 1891, by the use of seven deep and eight semi-deep silk sutures, going back almost to the number used in Sänger's

---

[1] Archives de Tocologie, Paris, Jan. 1877: "En ayant soin d'affronter les bords péritonéaux."   [2] Reported in 1885.

first case, and using them as he did. We may call this method the "new Cæsarean," the "improved Cæsarean," or, if the sexual power o the woman remains intact, the "conservative Cæsarean" operation; but it is Sänger's method in its original form notwithstanding, and antedates the first improvement by him under Leopold by twenty-one months. It will, no doubt, surprise many to learn that Prof. Sänger still has a claim to the "improved Cæsarean operation," although his main additions to the technique have disappeared from general use.

We now present the very remarkable Cæsarean record of the city of Leipzig, as furnished, under a request, by Prof. Max Sänger:

No.	Date	Operator	Hospital or private.	Age	Number of pregnancy.	Cause of difficulty.	C. V.	Result to woman.	Res to chi
1	Aug.20, 1880	Dr. Sänger,	Private	30	2d	Retro-uterine fibroid.	..	Recovered	Dea mon
2	May 25, 1882	" Leopold,	Private clinic.	29	2d	Contracted pelvis.	6 cm	"	Livi
3	Nov.16, 1884	" Sänger,	University clinic,	21	1st	" "	6–6.5	"	
4	July 3, 1885	" "	" "	32	4th relative indication.		...	..	
5	Aug 2, "	" Obermann	" "	42	♦ 1st	Contracted pelvis.	...		
6	Oct. 20, "	" Sänger,	" "	38	4th	" "	...	..	
7	Dec. 9, "	" "	" "	35	4th	" "	...	..	
8	Nov.13, 1886	" Donat,	" "	34	4th	" "	...	"	
9	Nov.18, "	" Weber,	" "	36	5th	" "	...	"	
10	Apr 12, 1887	" "	" "	33	4th	" "	7.5	Died of sept peritonitis.	
11	May 1, "	Prof Zweifel,	" "	41	5th	" "	6.5	Recovered	
12	May 3, "	" "	" "	32	7th	" "	7–7.5	"	
13	June22, "	" "	" "	30	7th	" "	7.5	"	
14	Aug.22, "	Dr. Döderlein,	" "	31	2d	" "	8	"	
15	Sep.23, "	" Obermann	" "	28	4th	" "	7.5	"	
16	Dec.17, "	" Sänger,	Private clinic.	30	5th	" "	6	"	
17	Feb. 8, 1888	Prof. Zweifel,	University clinic.	21	1st	" "	6	"	
18	Nov. 2, "	" "	" "	25	......	" "	7	"	
19	Dec.17, "	" "	" "	31	8th	" "	7–7.5	"	
20	Dec.29, "	" "	" "	26	......	" "	6.6	"	
21	Jan.13, 1889	" "	" "	25	......	" "	9.5	"	
22	Jan.26, "	" "	" "	23	......	" "	7.6	"	
23	Feb.12, "	" "	" "	26	......	" "	7.5	"	
24	July 2, "	" "	" "	29	......	" "	7.5	"	
25	Dec 21, "	Dr. Sänger,	Private clinic.	36	1st	Contracted pelvis and rupture of lower uterine segment.	8–8.5	"	
26	Oct. 14, "	Prof. Zweifel,	University clinic,	41	......	Osteomalacia.	5	"	Der
27	Dec.31, "	" "	" "	34	8th	Second Cæsarean of Case 12.	7–7.5	"	Livi
28	June 2, 1890	" "	" "	28	1st	Contracted pelvis and eclampsia.	7	Died of uræmia.	
29	July 9, "	" "	" "	30	1st	Contracted pelvis.	...	Recovered	
30	Aug 14, "	Dr Hertzsch,	" "	37	3d	" "	...	"	
31	Sep 14, "	Prof Zweifel,	" "	23	2d	" "	8	"	
32	Nov 17, "	" "	" "	36	2d	" "	8.5	"	
33	Nov 30, "	Dr. Döderlein,	" "	32	3d	" "	7.75	"	
34	Dec. 9, "	Prof Zweifel,	" "	27	1st	" "	8.5	"	
35	Apr. 16, 1891	Dr. Sänger,	Private clinic.	21	1st	" "	6.5	"	

Prof. Paul Zweifel now stands at the head of the Cæsarean operators of the world, having lost but one woman and one child in eighteen cases. He is a rapid operator, still uses a large number of sutures, and is partial to chromic-acid catgut as a material. He has completed an operation in twenty-four minutes. The woman lost was hopelessly ill with diseased kidneys, and had convulsions before the operation ; she died of uræmia in four days, during which time the wounds had nearly healed.

Dresden, under six operators, furnishes a longer list of cases than Leipzig, but with a somewhat greater mortality, from the fact that a larger proportion of the women were operated upon under desperate circumstances. Prof. Leopold has had more Cæsarean deliveries than any man living ; he had lost three women when he reached the present number of Prof. Zweifel. I cannot give the full record, but the percentage of loss has been smaller than the best Porro-Cæsarean work in Europe. The Porro record of all countries for the years 1885, 1886, 1887, 1888, and 1889 amounts to 157 cases, with 48 deaths, and 25 children lost. In the year of the lowest mortality (1888) there was a loss of 15⅗ per cent., or 5 out of 37 ; but in the following year it rose to 32¼ per cent., or 10 out of 31.

The best Porro record in Europe taken from its beginning, is that of Milan, under eight operators. The mortality in 31 cases has been 9, with only two children lost; this makes the percentage 29 against 5⅘ per cent. in Leipzig under cœlio-hysterotomy. Vienna has had many more Porro operations than Milan, but lost 15 women out of her first 31. For the past four years, her unpublished record will show a much diminished death-rate ; that of Milan, during the same period, being far higher. We may safely rate this operation as having therefore a general average mortality of 28 per cent. In the year 1887 there were 53 "new Cæsarean" operations, with 11 women and 4 children lost, or a mortality of 20¾ per cent.; and in 1888, 79 operations, losing 18 women and 3 children, or 24 per cent. The Cæsarean record shows a decidedly lower average mortality in both the women and children than that of the Porro operation. Both are capable of a considerable reduction in the death-rate, but the exsection of the uterus must always add to the gravity of a Cæsarean delivery in cases where this organ is sound and the child living. Where the child is dead and putrid, where the body of the uterus is the seat of fibroids, or where there are septic symptoms due to the condition of the uterus, the Porro-Cæsarean method is to be preferred. In exceptional tumor cases, where exsection is not advisable, the tumor should not be removed.

The "conservative Cæsarean" operation is preferred by Prof. Sänger and by many Continental operators, who are opposed to removing the ovaries or tying the Fallopian tubes, especially in a married woman, who becomes thereby not only sterile, but, in some few instances under the former, sexually changed.[1] If the danger of Cæsarean delivery can

[1] This point is in dispute, but there are certainly instances in which this occurs.

be reduced to 6 per cent.—and this ought to be reached in women previously operated upon—then the question of sexual mutilation becomes one to be very seriously weighed.

I have heard it claimed that the children of rhachitic women were of so little value that their mothers ought not to be allowed to generate. This has certainly not been the experience of this country, where rhachitic women have in many instances given birth to exceptionally fine children, some of whom are now living as adults and others as very robust babies or little children. When a rhachitic dwarf bears a fourteen-pound baby or one of twenty-two inches in length and perfect in proportion, as has happened in our country, we cannot see any evidence of inferiority. Rhachitic children are rarely such by inheritance, and if those born to rhachitic women become themselves rhachitic the disease generally arises in some defective hygienic conditions such as the parent was forced into through poverty. In the rhachitic unmarried pauper, or in the same even when married, the condition of extreme poverty may be considered in deciding the question of tubal ligation. One rhachitic woman of Ohio, whose tubes were ligated in 1880, has certainly had two fine Cæsarean children—a girl, now sixteen, and a boy, eleven—as their photographs in my possession attest. With a death-risk reduced to 6 per cent., why should such a mother not continue to bear children ? This is a question also to be considered.

The two vital questions for consideration in regard to the Cæsarean operation are those of *time* and the *technique,* and these two must go hand-in-hand if the death-rate is to reach a low percentage. The woman must be in the best possible condition and the child vigorously alive, or the technique will be a weak dependence for success. We learn a positive lesson on this point from the fact that nine women out of thirteen, or $69\frac{3}{13}$ per cent., recovered after that frightful casualty, a Cæsarean horn-rip, of which we shall have more to say at a future time. What saved these women was certainly not the surgical skill, nor even the technique, for in not one was the uterus sutured. It must have been the condition of unexhausted strength and of health in the subjects. I have for twenty years been engaged in trying to prove that the operation of "puerperal cœlio-hysterotomy" is not in itself one of excessive danger, but becomes such when performed upon a woman made unfit for it by bad obstetrical management; and I believe this has been well established by the work in Leipzig, Dresden, Vienna, and in the hands of certain private operators, as also by my researches in the abdominal and uterine lacerations under casualties in pregnant women, amounting to over twenty cases.

329 S. TWELFTH ST., PHILADELPHIA.

CONTRIBUTIONS TO THE NORMAL AND PATHOLOGICAL HISTOLOGY OF THE FALLOPIAN TUBES.

By J. Whitridge Williams, M.D.,

ASSISTANT IN GYNECOLOGY, JOHNS HOPKINS HOSPITAL, BALTIMORE.

For convenience of description I will divide the tube into three portions (Henle[1]): The isthmus, or the straight, narrow portion extending directly outward from the uterus; the ampulla, or the enlarged curved lateral part of the tube; and the infundibulum, or the fimbriated end of the tube. The isthmus is usually about 2 to 3 mm. in diameter, and the ampulla 6 to 10 mm. or more.

Roughly speaking, the tube may be said to consist of three coats: the serous (or, more properly speaking, the subserous), the muscular, and the mucous coats. Of these, the muscular and mucous coats are by far the most important.

The Serous Coat.—As the tube lies within the folds of the broad ligament at its upper margin, it is consequently almost entirely covered by peritoneum, except below where the two layers of the broad ligament converge and the tissues of the tube and broad ligament become continuous. Beneath the peritoneal covering is a thicker or thinner layer of connective tissue, the subserous coat. This layer is most rich in bloodvessels, and in its inferior portion—that is, the part not covered by peritoneum—run most of the large vessels that supply the tube.

The Muscular Coat.—As the uterus and tubes were originally the same canal—Müller's ducts—and as in adult life they are continuous, it would appear only natural to suppose that their muscle layers would be continuous, and that the tube, like the uterus, would contain three distinct layers of non-striated muscle, as is really the case. This fact was known to Henle,[2] whose description of the tube is certainly far superior to any yet written; but it has apparently been lost sight of by all the later writers on the subject, such as Martin,[3] Orthmann and Coe,[4] for they mention only two coats. The greater part of the thickness of the tube is due to its muscular layer, which can only be studied properly in serial sections of the same tube, for the arrangement differs considerably in different tubes and even in different parts of the same tube.

The greater part of the muscular wall consists of a thick band of circular fibres which is usually quite distinct, except at the lateral end

---

[1] Henle: Handbuch der Anatomie, Bd. 2, p. 485.   [2] Ibid.

[3] Martin, A.: Handbuch der Frauenkrankheiten, 2 Auf., p. 378.

[4] Coe, H. C.: "Anatomy of the Female Pelvic Organs," Mann's System of Gynecology, vol. i. p. 161.

of the tube, where it fuses with the other layers and forms an irregular meshwork of muscle fibres, with the fibres running in all directions.

Outside of this comes a thinner layer of longitudinal muscle, which is also very distinct; and upon this follows the subserous connective tissue.

These are the two layers usually described by writers upon the subject, for they are readily seen on section from any part of the tube, except near the fimbriated extremity, where all the layers fuse together.

In some cases, however, the two layers become so blended throughout the entire length of the tube that it is impossible to separate them. (Fig. 4.)

These two layers correspond to the outer and middle coats of the uterus, and constitute almost the entire thickness of the wall of the tube.

Beside these two layers there is a third, corresponding to the third or inner muscular coat of the uterus. On cutting sections of the tube just at the cornu uteri (Fig. 1) one sees, just within the circular layer, a

FIG. 1.

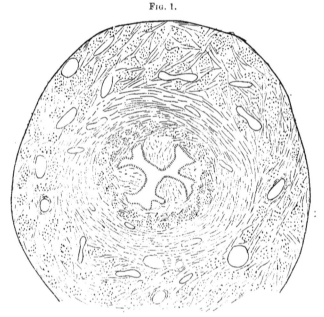

Cross-section of tube at cornu uteri, showing the four primary folds of the mucous membrane and the three layers of muscle forming the tube wall.

well-marked but thin layer of longitudinal muscular fibres. This can be traced as a distinct layer for some little distance, but it gradually becomes thinner and thinner, and, fusing with the circular coat, finally disappears.

Fig. 2 represents a section from the same tube about one inch nearer the fimbriated extremity than Fig. 1; and even at this distance from the uterus, the inner longitudinal layer has completely disappeared. It is apparently due to this fact that it is not mentioned by most writers, for sections from the middle portion of the tube show no trace of it.

FIG. 2.

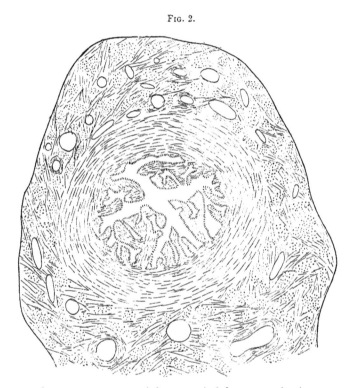

Cross-section of the same tube at isthmus, one inch from Fig. 1, showing a more complicated arrangement of the mucous membrane and the disappearance of the inner longitudinal muscular layer.

THE MUCOUS MEMBRANE.—The most important and characteristic portion of the tube is the mucous membrane. Its arrangement is most remarkable, and in none of the English works is any adequate idea given of its complexity. The figure from Luschka,[1] which is usually given in the text-books, cannot pretend to represent a section from any part of the tube with any degree of accuracy.

It is only by the study of serial sections that the true arrangement of the mucous membrane can be appreciated, for in no other way can one

[1] Luschka: Anatomie.

follow the wonderful changes from the simple, irregular canal at the uterine end of the tube to the wonderfully complicated structure at the ampulla.

Like all mucous membranes, that of the tube has its epithelial lining, its membrana propria, and its connective-tissue framework into which muscle fibres frequently penetrate.

The mucous membrane is arranged in longitudinal folds, which vary in appearance according to the portion of the tube under examination.

Sections at the cornu uteri (Fig. 1) show a star-like lumen, which is formed by a few folds of the mucous membrane, usually four in number, though the number may vary from three to six. This is the arrangement of the entire tube at an early period of fœtal life, and is the permanent arrangement throughout life in the bat and monkey. We may designate these folds as primary folds.

A short distance from the cornu uteri, secondary folds develop from the sides of the primary folds and thus produce a more complicated picture, as shown in Fig. 2, a section through the isthmus, one inch from the cornu uteri. This represents the general arrangement throughout the isthmus.

From these secondary folds, other folds may develop until at last each primary fold presents the most complicated appearance, so that the lumen of the tube is almost entirely filled with dendritic processes, as shown in Fig. 3.

This formation of folds attains its greatest development in the thickest part of the ampulla, and becomes less marked as one approaches the fimbriated extremity, where the original folded condition becomes once more apparent on the surface of the fimbriæ.

If one only examined cross-sections of the tube, one could readily suppose that the mucous membrane was provided with villi with glands between them, similar to the follicles of Lieberkühn.

Longitudinal sections, however, show that these processes are not villi at all, but simply cross-sections of longitudinal folds, which increase in number as one approaches the fimbriated extremity.

These folds are composed mostly of connective tissue, though they may contain a considerable amount of muscular tissue. The larger folds contain bloodvessels of considerable size and frequently large empty spaces corresponding to lymph-vessels.

The entire lumen of the tube is covered by a single layer of high columnar ciliated epithelium, under which comes an imperfectly developed propria.

All the cells are ciliated, and cilia can be seen in motion several hours after death ; they are frequently as long or longer than the cells themselves. My statement that the epithelium is disposed in a single layer is supported by the statements of Henle,[1] Frommel,[2] and Orthmann.[3] On the other hand, Hennig[4] and others state that it is composed of several layers of cells; this statement was evidently made on the strength of observations made on sections which had been cut obliquely; for in that case one might readily suppose that the epithelium was composed of several layers.

FIG. 3.

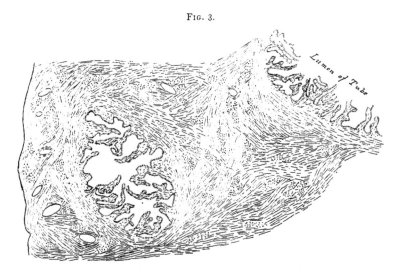

Cross-section of the same tube through the thickest part of the ampulla, one inch from Fig. 2, showing the extremely complicated arrangement of the mucous membrane and the two layers of muscle composing the wall.

These three sections are from a tube which was obtained at the autopsy of a nineteen-year-old virgin dead of typhoid fever.

They are all drawn under the same power of a Winckel microscope with a Zeiss camera lucida, and so represent with tolerable accuracy the absolute increase in the size and complexity of arrangement of the tube from its uterine extremity to the ampulla.

The statements of Hennig,[5] Bland Sutton[6] and others that the tube contains glands is also based upon false observations, as was conclusively

[1] Handbuch der Anatomie.

[2] Frommel: "Beiträge zur Histologie des Eileiters," Verhandlungen der Deutsch. Gesellschaft f. Gynäkologie, 1886, p. 95.

[3] Orthmann: "Beiträge zur normalen Histologie und zur Pathologie der Tuben," Virchow's Archiv, Bd. cviii. p. 165.

[4] Hennig: Katarrh der weiblichen Genitalien.

[5] Hennig: "Ueber die Blindgänge der Eileiter," Arch. f. Gyn., Bd. xiii. p. 156.

[6] Sutton: "Glands of the Fallopian Tube and their Function," Trans. of the London Obstetrical Society, 1888, vol. ii.

shown by Frommel,[1] who, after tying both ends of the tube, injected it with Flemming's solution, and when it was hardened, cut sections. "The effect was that all the folds which were in contact were separated from each other, and the rounded lumen of the tube was lined by branching, tree-like processes, but no trace of glands could be found." The blood-supply of the tube is most abundant, especially on its lower margin, where bloodvessels, sometimes three to four mm. in diameter, are found.

An interesting condition which I have observed in the arteries of the tubes of multiparous women and which I have not observed in nulli-parous women, is that they are often the seat of a marked endarteritis, similar to that found in the vessels of the uterus and attributed to a secondary growth of connective tissue, consequent upon the increase in size of the vessels produced by pregnancy—its object being to narrow the lumen according to the needs of the parts.

This is the only change that persists after pregnancy, for Thomson[2] has lately shown that the only change that takes place in the tubes of pregnant rabbits is an increase of the muscle cells to double their size, but that they return to their normal size within twelve days after labor, and show no trace of the past pregnancy.

The tube has three layers of muscle, corresponding to the three layers in the uterus, and not two, as usually stated.

Its mucous membrane is arranged in longitudinal folds, not villi.

Its epithelium is arranged in a single layer and contains no glands.

The arteries of parous women frequently show marked endarteritis.

DIVERTICULA OF THE TUBE.—In connection with the normal anatomy of the tube, I desire to call attention to an abnormality in its de-velopment which may bear a causal relation to the production of extra-uterine pregnancy. I refer to diverticula extending from the lumen into the wall of the tube, reaching almost to its peritoneal cover-ing. They are lined by the typical single layer of ciliated epithelium, and correspond in all respects to the structure of the normal lumen of the tube.

They should not be confounded with the so-called accessory ostia of the tube; for, unlike them, they do not open on the outer surface of the tube, and, on simple inspection, give no evidence of their existence.

I have observed this anomaly on two occasions, one as follows :

The specimen was obtained from a laparotomy performed by Dr. Kelly for a papillomatous cyst of the left ovary and a small corpus

---

[1] Loc. cit.

[2] Thomson : "Ueber Veraenderungen der Tuben und Ovarien in der Schwangerschaft und im Puerperium," Zeitschrift f. Gyn., Bd. xviii. p. 273.

luteum cyst of the right ovary. Both Fallopian tubes appeared perfectly normal and it was only on cutting sections of the right tube that this condition was discovered.

The sections were made from the ampulla of the tube and presented the following appearance: The lumen of the tube presented the characteristic normal appearance, but was situated excentrically in the tube, the anterior wall being at least twice as thick as the posterior. The

Fig. 4.

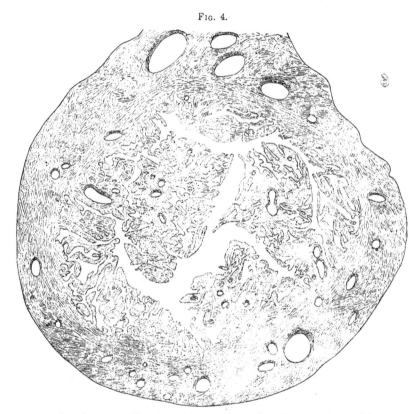

A portion of a cross-section of the tube at the ampulla. It represents the thickened anterior wall, containing a cross-section of the diverticulum from the lumen. It also shows how the layers of muscle may become blended together.

normal arrangement of the muscular layers was not observed, the entire wall being composed of fibres interlacing in all directions; otherwise it presented nothing abnormal.

In the thickened anterior muscular wall, somewhat below the level of the lumen and near the peritoneal covering, a small duct about one mm. in diameter was observed, separated from the lumen by a mass of muscular tissue about two mm. thick.

This "duct" presented the characteristic appearance of the tube, and was lined by a single layer of ciliated columnar epithelium, as represented in Fig. 4.

On cutting serial sections, it was found to communicate with the lumen of the tube, and was consequently a diverticulum from it. The diverticulum at its point of departure from the lumen of the tube was about two mm. in diameter. In its further course it was surrounded by a narrow layer of circular fibres, outside of which came the inter-lacing network of muscular tissue.

A glance at Fig. 4 will show that the diverticulum ran obliquely through the thickened anterior muscular wall, and for a certain distance constituted a canal distinct from the lumen of the tube.

How often similar formations occur I am unable to state, for I have only found them twice, and the only reference to them in the literature was made last year by Landau and Rheinstein,[1] who found a similar case.

They bear some resemblance to the accessory tubal ostia of Richard.[2] Rokitansky[3] and Klob,[4] but do not open on the surface as they do.

They also bear a marked resemblance to the sieve-like epithelial struc-tures found in the tube in tubal pregnancies, as described by Werth.[5] As the tubes in my cases were not pregnant, we in all probability do not have to deal with the same formation, for I regard the structures men-tioned by Werth as secondary to the changes produced by the tubal pregnancy.

Whether they be connected with these formations or not, I consider that they may hold a causal relation to tubal pregnancy. For what could be simpler than for the fertilized ovum to be driven by the action of the cilia into such a cul-de-sac, and to remain there and develop.

Such an origin would also explain the early rupture in these cases; for the ovum would only be separated from the peritoneal cavity by a thin layer of muscle, instead of the whole thickness of the tube wall.

In this opinion I am supported by a case of Landau and Rhein-stein's:[6] In a six weeks' tubal pregnancy, and in which the woman died from hemorrhage, on cutting sections of the pregnant tube they found the embryo in the upper part of the tube close under the peritoneum; while in the lower part of the tube, and separated from the ovum by a thick mass of muscular tissue, they found the almost unchanged lumen of the tube. From this observation they concluded that the pregnancy

[1] Landau und Rheinstein: "Beiträge zur path. Anatomie der Tuben," Arch f. Gyn., Bd. xxxix, p. 273.
[2] Richard: "Pavill. multipliés, etc.," Gaz. Méd. de Paris, 1851, No. 26.
[3] Rokitansky: "Ueber accessorische Tubarostien und ueber Tubaranhänge," Allg. Wiener med. Zeitung, 1859, No. 32.
[4] Klob: Die path. Anatomie der weiblichen Sexualorgane, Wien, 1864. "Accessor-ische Tubarostien," p. 279.
[5] Werth: Beiträge zur Anatomie der Extra-uterinschwangerschaft. 1887.
[6] Loc. cit.

developed in a diverticulum from the lumen, similar to the one just described.

The proof is not absolute, but the facts are extremely suggestive.

TWISTINGS OF THE FALLOPIAN TUBE.—I also desire to direct attention to a twisted condition of the tube, and will attempt to show that it may help to explain some conditions which were previously inexplicable.

Freund,[1] of Strasburg, and one of his pupils, Schober,[2] were the first to direct our attention to the significance of this condition, and my observations tend to substantiate their statements.

A peculiar and inexplicable fact in the development of the Fallopian tubes is that at an early period they undergo a process of twisting which begins at the uterine end of the tube and extends outward until at last the entire tube presents a corkscrew-like appearance.

What causes this twisting is absolutely unknown, unless we suppose it to be due to the resistance offered to its growth by the surrounding parts, as in the case of the sweat-glands.

In a fœtus of five months this process is quite marked (Fig. 5, A), and it gradually increases until the eighth month, when it has reached its highest development.

At this period it presents a corkscrew-like appearance with from six and a half to seven and a half twists, beginning at the uterine end. (Fig. 5, B.)

This condition I have noticed in several cases.

In the period between birth and puberty the tube is gradually untwisted, beginning at the uterine end and extending outward, until at puberty the twists have entirely disappeared or are only represented by a mild curve in the course of the tube.

This process is represented in Fig. 5, C, from a three-year-old child, and Fig. 5, D, which represents the normal tube at the time of puberty.

What significance this process may have in the development of the tube I am unable to state; though even during childhood it may become so marked as to cause the tube to be twisted apart, as has been observed by Rokitansky.

Owing to lack of development or some unknown cause, the twisted condition of the tube may persist throughout life. Most of the cases in which this has been noticed are in women who are poorly developed sexually.

It will be readily understood that such a condition in an adult woman may lead to serious consequences.

---

[1] Freund: "Ueber die Indicationen zur operativen Behandlung der erkranken Tuben," Volkmann's Sammlung klinischer Vorträge, 1888, No. 323.

[2] Paul Schober: "Ueber Erkrankungen gewundener Tuben." Inaug. Dissert., Strasburg. 1889.

FIG. 5.

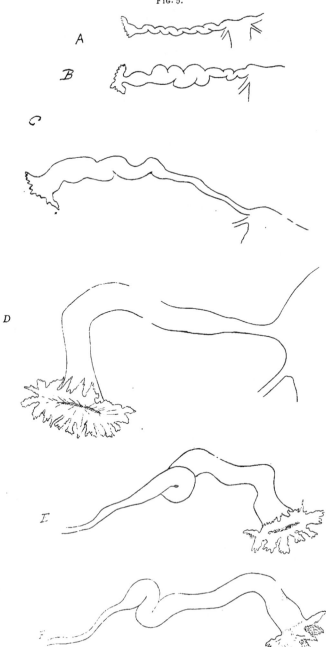

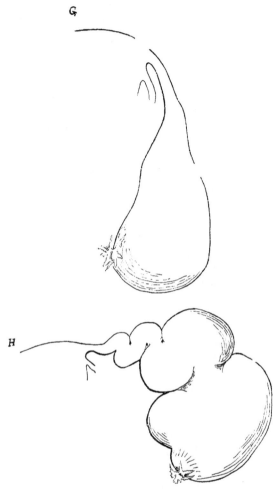

A represents the tube of a five-months' fœtus, with the twisting well marked. *B,* the tube of an eight-months' fœtus with the twisted condition at its highest develop-ment. *C,* the tube of a three-year-old child, showing the gradual obliteration of the twists. *D,* the tube of a well-developed girl at puberty. *E* and *F,* the tubes of a sterile married woman, aged thirty-nine years, who was otherwise perfectly healthy. *G* represents a hydrosalpinx developed in a normally arranged tube, and *H* a hydro-salpinx developed in a twisted tube.

In the first place, one or more of the twists may be so marked as to cause a total occlusion of the lumen, just as one may do with a rubber tube. The consequence of such an occlusion would be that the woman would be sterile, for the ova could not pass beyond it on their passage to the uterus, nor the spermatozoa above it on their way to the ovary; and if the condition were the same on both sides, the woman would be perfectly sterile. Fig. 5, *E* and *F*, represent both tubes from a sterile woman aged thirty-nine years, who was otherwise perfectly healthy.

A similar condition of the tube may cause retention of the normal secretions and so give rise to a hydrosalpinx, which may be lobulated or not, according to the number of twists by which the lumen is occluded. Fig. 5, *G*, represents a hydrosalpinx in a normal non-twisted tube, and Fig. 5, *H*, in a twisted tube.

I desire to record the following case of hydrosalpinx, which I believe was caused in this way. I will quote from my records—" January 26, 1891: Tube and ovary from left side. Tube . converted into a lobulated hydrosalpinx, immensely distended, and wound around the ovary; 19 cm. long, 6 cm. in widest and ½ cm. in thinnest part. For a distance of 7 cm. from uterus the tube is apparently unchanged and about 5 mm. in diameter, then it suddenly expands into the lobulated hydrosalpinx, which was densely adherent to the ovary. The median end of the tube is perfectly pervious, but it is impossible to pass a fine probe from it into the hydrosalpinx, for it appears to pass into a cul-de-sac and go no further. On cutting open the dilated end of the tube and probing toward the uterus, on giving a slight twist the probe readily passed into the undilated part, thereby giving the impression that the constriction was caused by a twist in the tube."

This certainly appears to be a rational explanation for some cases of hydrosalpinx. In other cases the twisting may not totally occlude the tube, but only cause a narrowing of its lumen, and this also may lead to serious consequences.

If, for example, the tube becomes inflamed, the swelling of the mucous membrane may be sufficient to cause total occlusion or to so narrow the lumen that the secretions collect and greatly interfere with healing by preventing drainage of the parts.

If we have a purulent salpingitis, nothing is simpler than for the apposed surfaces of the twisted portion, which have lost their epithelium, to become adherent and thus produce a total and permanent occlusion and rapidly form a pus cavity. And according as one or more twists become imperforate, we get a more or less lobulated mass.

These twistings, of course, cannot be diagnosed during life, except in cases in which they lead to the formation of lobulated tumors, when the lobulated form will distinguish them from the more rounded or pear-shaped tumors, which develop from the normally shaped tube.

This abnormality, however, deserves consideration, for it may explain many cases of sterility, some cases of obstinate catarrhal salpingitis, and many cases of hydro- and pyosalpinx.

REVIEWS.

A PRACTICAL TREATISE ON DISEASES OF THE SKIN. By HENRY G. PIF-
FARD, A.M., M.D., Clinical Professor of Dermatology, University of the
City of New York; Surgeon-in-charge of the New York Dispensary for
Diseases of the Skin, etc.; assisted by ROBERT M. FULLER, M.D. With
fifty full-page original plates and thirty-three illustrations in the text. New
York: D. Appleton & Co., 1891.

THIS is an *édition de luxe* of a work covering not the whole but a
large and essential part of the great field of cutaneous medicine, with
numerous illustrations of disease, chiefly reproductions of photographs
taken by the author, many of which are so good as to constitute the
chief element of value in the book. The whole is a striking evidence of
the courage and ability of the author.

Only a fearless contributor to science would venture upon questions
in the discussion of which the schoolmen have produced ponderous
tomes, and dismiss the same in as many pages. For example, in touching the enormous group of the syphilodermata, to whose peculiar symptoms such writers as Duhring, Crocker, and Keyes have devoted from
two to three score of folios, and the mere references for which, in the
treatises of such authors as Jullien and Fournier, would alone furnish
a good-sized volume, Dr. Piffard contents himself with ten pages merely
of the work before us and the ten portraits which serve to explain
the text. Let not the reader of these lines think that in commenting thus upon the fruit of our author's labor the contrast suggested is
designed to convey a sarcastic reproach. Far from it. There is no more
constant mark of the man of genius than his power to compass this particular end. Where others toil with infinite pains over the obstacles
in a tortuous road, the mind of the explorer traverses the direct and
smoother path which he soon pursues as a pioneer. Louis XIV. could
express the whole of his autocracy in an epigram. Haden has por-
trayed a landscape with a few touches of his burin. Certainly no
observant physician can study these pictures of disease without gaining
some insight into the problems which other writers have required so
much space even to adequately propose to the understanding. The best
of the illustrations are: Fig. 1 (erythematous eczema of the hand),
Plate II. (symmetrical eczema of the knees), Plate IV. (psoriasis of the
sole), Plate XIV. (dactylitis syphilitica), Plate XXV. (elephantiasis),
Plate XXVI. ("seborrhœa kerativa"), Fig. 19 (an admirable portrait
of the pediculus pubis, the best thus far exhibited by any contributor to
the subject), Plate XLVIII. (ichthyosis), and Plate L. ("psorospermosis"). The portraits of psoriasis of the general surface of the body
are some of them good, but not superior to those which have been before

published. The hand represented on the upper portion of Plate III., described as the seat of an eczema, looks suspiciously like those displaying a palmar syphiloderm, an appearance which would doubtless be dispelled if the original colors of the exanthem could have been reproduced. Indeed, allowance must be made in studying all of these interesting plates and figures for the absence of color-effects, upon which the diagnostician relies, in part at least, for his conclusions. But it is excellent practice to dispense at times even with the aid of vision in making some investigations of disease.

Perhaps the gravest charge that can be brought against our author in the production of this really creditable work is one which he must bear with many of his clan—that of burdening dermatology with new names. There was a day of joy in medicine when the senior Hebra with unsparing hand swept into the street the dust of dermatology, the rubbish of its meaningless names which had accumulated during the centuries. For a brief time thereafter it was a reproach to give a new title to a disease of the skin, a name likely to share the fate of "rupia," "lichen eczematodes," "porrigo larvalis," and the like. But as time passed the temptation grew great, opportunities multiplied, and men "rose up which knew not Joseph." The greatest sinner on this score is one of the most prolific contributors to cutaneous medicine, and not a few of his peers in the late Congress at Paris besprinkled their discussion of diseases of the skin by distinguishing that upon which they engrafted their own names from another to which they did not refuse to give the name of a colleague. Even the newborn "eczema seborrhoicum" of Unna, Dr. Piffard designates as "sudolorrhœa," a faulty term if employed to suggest the characteristic picture of the process, though our author accurately describes the malady in the text of his work. "Seborrhœa kerativa" and "mammillitis maligna" are novelties in name if not as to the process they represent. No reader of these pages familiar with the text-books on diseases of the skin written by the first ten authors in dermatology of America and Great Britain, would recognize, without some study, the classical and well-named tinea versicolor in "chromophytosis." There is no law binding upon any writer to observe strictly the nomenclature of the American Dermatological Association. That nomenclature is unquestionably defective and can doubtless be revised with enormous advantage. But with all its defects it has in this country done more in the direction of systematizing a knowledge of diseases of the skin than an entire edition of the most valuable treatise on the subject that has yet appeared. It would have been a gracious and valuable concession if the man who once filled the honored position of president of that Association had at least given the American titles of diseases of the skin in brackets after those of his own preference. The reason he has not done this has already been shown. In all seriousness, it is admitted that his is the mind of a genius impatient of barriers and disdainful of routine.

But let not the soul of the average professional man searching for the truth in cutaneous disease despair of finding his facts beneath this enormous and accumulating rubbish of names, many of them with the cards of their proprietors affixed to each. There is no evil under the sun but carries within it the germ whose development is its doom. When the burden becomes at last too heavy, and the shoulders beneath sufficiently impatient, the hour strikes for rebellion, and lo! the reformer is at hand for the relief of the victim of oppression. He that will do this great thing for dermatology is probably living to-day. He will almost surely be an American, but he will know all that is worth knowing of the lore of the schoolmen and of the dicta of the masters. He will have scanned all the fields that have been opened to the eye by the microscope, but he will be broader than a bacterium and not mensurable with a micrometer. And he, too, shall sweep into oblivion heaps upon heaps of idle names whose chief value is to furnish the landmarks dear to the historian, showing how laboriously and by how many devious roads man climbs to the light. He will, however, do more than this. He will show that it is indeed quite rare for a man to suffer from a disease of the skin whose morbid products intoxicate his liver, his spleen, or his kidney, and that it is quite as rare for any one of these organs to generate a poison that induces a disease of the skin.

The chapter of special interest in this volume, one in fact of such importance in the mind of the author, that he specially refers to it in his preface, is that which concludes the list, touching upon psorospermosis. The opinions here stated are those already published over Dr. Piffard's signature in the *Journal of Cutaneous and Venereal Diseases*, issue with which was speedily taken by Dr. Lustgarten in the same periodical. The facts are nearly these:

In the year 1889 Darier and Wickham exhibited to the members of the Congress of Dermatology and Syphilography in Paris, a patient displaying the symptoms of a disease termed by them "psorospermose folliculaire végétante," illustrating the results of invasion of the skin by psorosperms or coccidiæ (also termed pseudo-naviculæ), parasites classed by some zoölogists among the protozoa; and considered by others as algæ. They are not rarely found parasitic in the viscera of the vertebrata, particularly in the livers of ill-fed rabbits.

Soon after appeared Wickham's monograph,[1] practically exhausting the subject to that date, claiming not only for the disease exhibited in the Paris patient, but also for Paget's disease of the nipple, molluscum sebaceum, and possibly other maladies, an origin due to parasitic invasion by psorosperms. Dr. White, of Boston, had already described one patient in this country (another since that date) exhibiting all the symptoms of the so-called psorospermosis of Darier and Wickham. The bodies figured by Wickham in his work are those recognized in London by Delépine, Bowlby, and Hutchinson, Jr., who failed to get definite reactions by which to identify the coccidiæ and to distinguish them clearly from altered epithelial cells. The parasites appear as oval, roundish, or spindle-shaped bodies which later elongate and become in turn pyriform or fusiform, eventually showing long, coiled, sickle-shaped filaments within a capsule not unlike spermatozoa.

Dr. Piffard, after employing polarized light by transmission through sections of tissue containing the so-called psorosperms, concludes that they are rete cells undergoing a species of corneous degeneration; and it must be confessed that the evidence in favor of this view is slowly accumulating. Thin, of London, under date of May 16, 1891, reports that in cases of Paget's disease he had found an "immense number" of these bodies, "psorosperms," and believes that "they were nothing else

---

[1] Contribution a l'étude des Psorospermoses Cutanées et de certaines formes de Cancer; Maladie de la peau dite "Maladie de Paget," par le Dr. Louis Wickham. Paris, 1890.

than epithelial cells in various stages of transformation." Lastly, Messrs.
Shattock and Ballance, of London, taking psorospermial material from
the livers of rabbits, have inoculated therewith other rabbits, monkeys,
dogs, and rats with negative results, the injections into the jugular vein,
" vaccination " experiments, etc., producing merely hyperplastic products
at the site of injury.   These authors claim that Darier's views must be
tested according to Koch's postulates, experimental infection of a human
being or lower animal being produced by fluids obtained from culture of
the products of a carcinomatous lesion, or from the "psorospermose
folliculaire végétante " of the French writers.

Dr. Piffard's style is clear and attractive ; at times the philosophical
amplitude of even his shortest sentences is highly suggestive.   He has
made here a valuable contribution to the clinical resources of the student
of dermatology, and deserves great credit for the manner in which he has
produced both text and portraits.   There are a few errors in the book,
the most conspicuous of which occurs in describing " chromophytosis "
as due to the " microsporon Audouini " (P. 113), as this fungus was first
named by Eichstedt, of Greifswald, in 1846, as the microsporon furfur.
The microsporon Audouini was named by Gruby after Audouin, and was
the fungus supposed to be effective in the production of alopecia areata;
but it has since shared the fate of the impostor who claimed to have first
discovered the parasite productive of scabies, and whose name survives
only among the French, by whom that disease is still called " Gale."

                                                   J. N. H.

DIABETES: ITS CAUSES, SYMPTOMS AND TREATMENT. BY CHARLES W.
PURDY, M.D. With Clinical Illustrations. Pp. viii., 184. Philadelphia
and London : F. A. Davis, 1890.   .

DR. PURDY'S little volume is a meritorious effort to set forth the
present status of our knowledge on the subject of diabetes, "in such
practical and concise form as shall best meet the daily requirements of
practice," and is based upon "a careful study and recorded observation
of the disease, extending over a period of twenty-one years."   He has
"endeavored to bring out prominently the leading features of diabetes
as it occurs in the United States, together with the natural resources of
the country best suited to the disease, as the waters, foods. and climate,
since the very extensive range of these entitles them to rank in point of
efficiency for the relief of the diabetic patient as at least equal to those
in any other land or clime."

The first section is devoted to Historical, Geographical, and Climato-
logical Considerations of Diabetes Mellitus from the data afforded by
mortality statistics of the census of 1880, not including States and Territories furnishing a total death-list of less than 5000.   The author has
compiled a number of tables illustrative of the comparative mortality from
diabetes in different portions of the United States and the relations of
the mortality to temperature, rainfall, elevation, population and urban
and rural residence.   By these tables he apparently demonstrates that,
in the United States at least, cold and altitude are the chief climatic
features which determine high mortality from diabetes.   Thus, for instance, in the State of Vermont we have 6.36 per thousand deaths

attributed to this disease; according to the author, the highest ratio of any place in the world. Vermont is noted for its long continued and severe winters. Maine, the climate of which is very nearly the same as Vermont, gives the next highest mortality in diabetes in the United States, 4.41 per thousand. The difference between Maine and Vermont is attributed to the greater altitude of the latter. A striking contrast is afforded by Alabama, where the mean annual temperature is about 75° F., and the elevation above the sea in considerable. The mortality from diabetes sinks to the lowest ratio in the country, 0.55 per 1000 deaths.

With Dickinson, and against Sir William Roberts, Purdy finds a mortality from diabetes among the rural population greater than among the dwellers in cities. In the North Atlantic coast region the mortality among the rural population is 3.55 per 1000 deaths, and among urban dwellers 1.76. In the Gulf coast region, on the contrary, the rural mortality is 0.49, the urban 1.56. The author advances the following explanation of these facts:

" Cold greatly increases the mortality from diabetes. In cold climates those who are best sheltered from climate suffer least from disease. This fact is brought out in strong contrast in the United States, because there the houses are constructed with a view to greater warmth and comfort than in Europe. In the warm climates of the South the evil effects of cold no longer appear, and the atmospheric conditions affecting the disease are chiefly those of purity. The country people are able to live in the open air the year round without exposure to cold or chill, and oxidation obtains its greatest activity. In the cities more or less confinement and impurity of atmosphere is inevitable, which tends to impede oxidation and give greater impetus to the disease."

The mortality reports of the United States census for 1880 record no death from diabetes among either the Indian or the Chinese population of the country. The Indians are spare eaters and subsist almost exclusively on nitrogenous foods, leading at the same time an active out-of-door life. The exemption from the disease enjoyed by the Chinese bears out the record from their native land, and appears to be due to a race peculiarity. One of the most important features, and the most deplorable one of the careful statistical investigations of the author, is that the relative mortality from diabetes in this country has been very decidedly on the increase during the last forty years. In 1850 it was 0.72 per 1000 deaths, and in 1880 it was 1.91 per 1000 deaths. The most marked increase was between 1860 and 1870—nearly 100 per cent.; from 0.98 to 1.70. The author rationally attributes this to the decided change in the habits of the nation consequent upon the Civil War. Previous to 1860 we were "a frugal and economical people, enjoying but moderate luxuries in living." The inflation of the currency; speculation; political and social demoralization, with its concomitants of luxurious living and extravagance; excessive labor and widespread dissipation, have inevitably increased the morbidity and the mortality of neuroses in general and diabetes among the number.

The sections devoted to Physiological and Pathological Considerations, to Etiology, Morbid Anatomy and Symptomatology, are clear, sufficiently full for the purpose of the work, and on the whole, reliable.

Treatment is considered under three divisions: Dietetic, Medicinal and Hygienic. After varied and laborious experiments with substitutes for bread the author found the following method most satisfactory. The patient is permitted to use his own regular table bread, but the allowance is limited to half the usual amount. If sugar still appears in the urine the bread is further reduced by one-half, and if the sugar still persists bread is prohibited absolutely. According to the author's experience, if the patient cannot assimilate two to three ounces of bread daily without excreting sugar in the urine he cannot assimilate any substitute therefor, and under such circumstances the sooner all bread is stricken from the diet list the better. The author has never seen good results from an exclusive milk diet, and seems rather inclined to limit the amount of milk allowed to the patient. He gives a useful list of wines which may be permitted and those which should be prohibited, on the basis of analysis for sugar. All mineral waters are permissible as beverages and some of the alkaline waters he considers as curative. Among medicinal agents he discusses opium, antipyrine, the bromides, ergot, arsenic, iodoform, jambul, oxygen, and the alkalies. He finds limited use for opium, codeine being preferable in cases showing a continued high percentage of sugar in the urine despite the institution of strict dietetic measures; but he believes that sooner or later the drug has to be abandoned on account of its damaging effects on nutrition. Antipyrine is unsuitable for lengthy periods of administration in doses of forty-five grains a day, and in smaller doses is not claimed to modify the disease. Moreover, it is likely to cause albuminuria, and therefore cannot be considered a safe agent for use in these cases. Ergot has a useful influence over mild cases in which the patient retains good digestive powers. He has seen little benefit from either Giliford's or Clemens' solution of arsenic bromide, even when combined with Martineau's lithium treatment. The chief benefits he has obtained from arsenical preparations in diabetes have been from arsenite of iron in cases complicated with anæmia or malaria. Iodoform, if used carefully in doses of from one to three grains repeated three times a day or in sufficient doses at bedtime, continued for two weeks and resumed after an interruption of two weeks, seems to cause a diminution of thirst, of polyuria and of the amount of sugar excreted. The use of oxygen by inhalation is highly lauded, from three to five gallons of a freshly made gas being administered twice daily. Hydrogen dioxide water (one to two drachms, largely diluted with water) may he used, but is less efficacious. The alkalies are believed to increase the oxygen-holding powers of the blood. Stress is laid upon the avoidance of constipation, of mental emotion and of fatigue, as these are likely to lead to the production of coma. In addition to avoidance of fatigue, the points to be attended to in the hygienic treatment are proper aëration, proper clothing, and proper temperature. Besides hygienic clothing, in order to preserve the warmth of the body, warm baths followed by thorough rubbing of the skin are recommended. A moderate degree of exercise in the open air is necessary, and habits of regularity must be observed in eating, drinking and sleeping. A number of illustrative cases are recounted. A section is devoted to diabetes insipidus. A short but well-selected bibliography is appended.   S. S. C.

TEXT-BOOK OF OPHTHALMOSCOPY. By EDWARD G. LORING, M.D. Edited by FRANCIS B. LORING, M.D. Part II. Diseases of the Retina, Optic Nerve, and Choroid: Their Varieties and Complications. New York: D. Appleton & Co., 1891.

THE reviewer's task is an agreeable one when he can praise without qualification; when the material presented to his critical analysis is of such real value as to justify him in commending the work to fellow-students; and when he feels that the knowledge gained from it better equips him for his daily work.

Dr. Loring's work is original and practical; it is a record of thorough and painstaking care in the observation of abundant clinical material. Not satisfied with the description of the coarse lesions so often exclusively given in text-books, his investigations have included subjects slighted or altogether neglected by other writers, subjects which to careful practitioners are matters of the highest importance. His studies, for example, of the minute changes in the light-reflex, color, pulsation, etc., of the retinal vessels taught him, and through his book teaches us, the grave systemic disturbances of which they are the forerunners. By diligent care in the use of the mirror, changes of diagnostic and prognostic significance are detected which escape the superficial and routine observer. Thus the field of ophthalmology is broadened by Dr. Loring's work. He teaches us how to diagnose by the mirror heart and blood irregularities, valvular disease, splenic, kidney, cerebral, and spinal affections in their incipiency, and proves the ophthalmoscope to be indispensable to the physician. The ophthalmic surgeon who absorbs the knowledge contained in this book is something more than an "eye doctor"—recognizing, as he must, that the eye is a connected part of the whole organism, he becomes an expert in the observation and interpretation of its signs. The fine distinctions between the healthy and unhealthy appearances of the eye-ground are especially noticed and emphasized, and it is in this particular that the eminently original studies of Dr. Loring are of great value.

The book contains 253 pp., divided into seven chapters. The first considers the vascular disturbances in the retina, such as changes in the length, breadth, and walls of the arteries and veins; vessels of new formation, aneurism, embolus, thrombus, stasis, hemorrhage, and anæmia, and of their causative relation to general disease. Chapter II. deals with an intermediate stage between purely vascular changes and those associated with signs of inflammation, designated by Jaeger as "irritation" of the retina. The importance of this chapter is well expressed in its opening paragraph. "This form of congestion, although chiefly distinguished from hyperæmia by the presence of functional disturbances, has yet some physical characteristics and features of its own which it is important to notice, especially in these days when all symptoms of asthenopia are referred to an error of refraction, should any chance to exist, even of an infinitesimal degree." Chapter III. treats generally of the characteristics of retinal inflammation, while Chapter IV. classifies and describes minutely the specific forms of inflammation. Particularly clear and instructive are the sections devoted to a description of albuminuric retinitis, retinitis pigmentosa, and detached retina. A classical account of diseases of the optic nerve, which leaves nothing unsaid, is

396 REVIEWS.

given in Chapters V. and VI. Chapter VII. concludes the book with original observations in diseases of the choroid. It will be noticed that the author has not adhered to that generally accepted classification of retinal and choroidal diseases which would seem to have been based largely upon the changes in the pigment coat. He has noticed alterations in the pigment in both retinal and choroidal disease, as they seemed to him dependent upon coexisting inflammation of one or the other membrane, and has described specific changes—hypertrophy and atrophy—of the pigment layer in separate sections.

The illustrations are numerous and well executed. Many are after Dr. Loring's own sketches and others are reproductions from Jaeger and Liebreich. In addition to the black-and-white prints in the body of the book there are at the end six plates, each containing two chromolithographs. The fault common to most attempts to portray diseases of the fundus—exaggeration of the abnormal conditions showing too great a contrast between healthy and unhealthy structures—is found in many of these illustrations.

The editor has done well to limit his duties chiefly to the arrangement and classification of the material of the author, and as he says in the preface, " I found there was so much original matter in it, so much that from its very nature must provoke discussion and argument, that I determined to publish it as it stood, without addition or correction." The wording throughout clearly conveys the author's meaning, and the ideas are purposely clothed in a conversational rather than a polished literary garb. Indeed, in his effort to be concise, the author has in a few instances fallen into the error of colloquial expression. Thus on p. 105 he uses the following language: "Not a single case of the slightest retinitis or neuro-retinitis can I find in all the literature of these cases, *let alone* a choked disc."

The type is of good size, the paper white and thick, typographical errors are few ; in short, the book is in all respects admirably printed.

The reviewer earnestly commends the work to students of ophthalmoscopy as the best treatise in the English language on the subject.

H. F. H.

HYPNOTISME ET CROYANCES ANCIENNES. Par le DR. L. R. REGNIER, Lauréat de l'Académie de Médecine, etc. Avec 46 figures et 4 planches. Paris, 1891.

HYPNOTISM AND ANCIENT BELIEFS. By DR. L R. REGNIER, Laureate of the Academy of Medicine.

THIS book has a distinct and special value. It differs from the common run of works on hypnotism, and has a literary merit which few of them possess. This is partly because it leaves the beaten track. It does not deal altogether with the modern " craze " called hypnotism, but pursues its subject in the distant past. It introduces us to the mysterie of the Rig-Veda of the Hindoos and of the Zend-Avesta of the ancient Persians. It culls little items of interest from a papyrus found under the ruins of Thebes and from the cuneiform inscriptions of the ancient

Turanians. The Hebrew, Greek and Latin literatures are searched to prove the wonderful sameness of human weakness and gullibility through all the ages. Truly a wonderful book—fascinating and instructive. "One touch of nature makes the whole world kin." Dr. Regnier has given this touch, with grace and learning, to a subject which was quite worn out until reanimated by the magnetism of his pen.

The book is evidently inspired, however, by a preconceived idea. The author is an advocate and uses his stores of learning sometimes in the manner of a special pleader. For him hypnotism did not exist in the past. It is a modern product, almost as much as the steam-engine or the telegraph. He finds little, if any, evidence of hypnotism in the religious ecstacy of the ancient fakirs, the impostures of the magi, the serpent-worship of the Egyptians and the hysterical contortions of the Grecian pythoness on her tripod. To establish his thesis he gives minute and interesting details of the various usages and rites of these different mystic sects, and accompanies his narrative with penetrating and instructive criticism. He is more bent, however, upon making distinctions than upon finding analogies. It is here, perhaps, that the philosophic student of hypnotism will take issue with him. He defines hypnotism as a special state of the nervous system, artificially produced, the characteristic of which is a complete or partial unconsciousness, with total forgetfulness of all that transpires during its continuance. This artificial sleep was not known until after Puysegur, and was first described by the Englishman, Braid.

It is not for us to combat here the author's views. Far from it, we agree with him that hypnotism is quite a modern cult, and nowhere so much at home as in his own France. There the practice has been made perfect; the ritual is complete. We nevertheless think, in the author's own concise words: "L'humanité, depuis que nous la connaissons par l'histoire, n'a guère changé." Man has not changed—and the essential facts of hypnotism were in him at the beginning. Only this has happened—a new method is in vogue: the fakir and the pythoness have given place to the trained comédienne of the modern hypnotic séance. The induced sleep is no sleep at all, but only the inhibition of a weaker brain by the suggestion of a stronger one, and the adjuncts of time and place. This *suggestion* is the vital fact in hypnotism, and not, as Dr. Regnier would have us believe, the artificial sleep. From our point of view we can see very many striking analogies between the modern practice and the mystic rites which the author describes. From the time when Moses elevated on a pole the brazen serpent in the wilderness; or when the ancient Egyptians cast a spell over the faithful with the cabalistic triangles; or when the Hindoo seer went into an ecstasy with gazing on his own navel, down to the recent day when an aged priest in Pennsylvania cured by faith the credulous and devout—humanity has changed but little.

Hence Dr. Regnier's book may raise an issue in the minds of some students; who will not fail, however, to accord to it the high praise which its historic value and literary excellence abundantly deserve. The book contains many illustrations, some of them quaint, and many of them unknown to us before. It has also a very long and useful list of references.   J. H. L.

ŒUVRES COMPLÈTES DE J. M. CHARCOT. HÉMORRHAGIE ET RAMALLISSE-
MENT DU CERVEAU, MÉTALLOTHÉRAPIE ET HYPNOTISME, ELECTRO-
THÉRAPIE. Tome IX. Paris, 1890.
COMPLETE WORKS OF J. M. CHARCOT. CEREBRAL HEMORRHAGE AND
SOFTENING, METALLOTHERAPY AND HYPNOTISM, ELECTROTHERAPY.

As we are told in the preface by the editor, Bourneville, this volume
comprises three parts of unequal importance. The first is devoted to
diseases of the brain, especially to cerebral hemorrhage, and some of its
complications, immediate and remote. In the second part have been
collected the numerous papers of Charcot on metalloscopy, metallo-
therapy and hypnotism. Scattered everywhere in the medical journals
or in the transactions of the learned societies, it was very difficult for
physicians to have recourse to the original publications, or to gain an
exact idea of the work of the chief of the school of the Salpêtrière on
these subjects.

It is further pointed out with what circumspection Charcot undertook
the study of hypnotism—neglected, discredited for many years, and
regarded as difficult by the best minds. On this point, as on all others,
the learning of Charcot rests on a most solid basis, on facts submitted
to the severest tests, especially as the most pronounced scepticism prevailed at the time. His facts are to-day definitely accepted by the great
majority of physicians who are seriously occupied with this department
of neurology.

In the third part is reproduced a lecture by Charcot on static electricity, and which to some extent is related to the other subjects.

Among the more important papers in the first part is the admirable
research of Charcot on the Pathogenesis of Cerebral Hemorrhage, published originally in 1868 ; on Hemorrhage into the Posterior Third of the
Internal Capsule, published in 1875 ; on Neo-membranes of the Dura
Mater, 1860 ; and on Arthropathies depending on Lesions of the Brain
and of the Cord, 1868. The last mentioned is especially interesting.

In the second part the more important are, Hints and Observations
on Metalloscopy and Metallotherapy, embracing among other things a
consideration of the action of magnets, and published in 1877 ; and
another on the same subject, in which the phenomena of transfer are considered ; others on Catalepsy and Somnambulism follow. The most interesting of all, however, are his studies on Hypnotism among Hysterical
Subjects, published in 1881, and on which subject one of his pupils, Paul
Richer, afterward published a volume. Surely the collection of papers
before us shows how much we owe the knowledge we possess of these
obscure subjects to Charcot and his school.

Thus far nine volumes of Charcot's works have been published, and a
tenth is to follow. All of them relate to neurological subjects except
three—the fifth, sixth and seventh—which respectively embrace Charcot's
productions in the field of diseases of the lungs and vascular apparatus,
diseases of the liver and kidneys, and diseases of the aged, gout and
rheumatism. They form an imposing monument of the life-work of this
industrious man, and in their present shape the papers, properly collected and arranged, form an indispensable source of reference.

F. X. D.

PROGRESS

OF

MEDICAL SCIENCE.

THERAPEUTICS.

UNDER THE CHARGE OF

FRANCIS H. WILLIAMS, M.D.,

ASSISTANT PROFESSOR OF THERAPEUTICS IN HARVARD ·UNIVERSITY.

ON THE PREPARATION AND USE OF OINTMENTS IN DISEASES OF THE SKIN.

DR. L. DUNCAN BULKLEY has published a practical and suggestive article on the above subject and gives many hints of value to practitioners. The application of ointments constitutes such a large element in the treatment of diseases of the skin, by the profession at large, that it seems desirable to present a few words of caution concerning their preparation and employment, for want of success often results from the improper compounding or application of one or another of this class of remedies.

It is better not to trust to any artificial means for preserving the freshness of ointments, but to secure sweet and good material and always to reject that which is at all old, or ointments which have been long prepared. It is important to avoid the slightest rancidity in ointments, and it is better to order ointments to be freshly compounded of the strength desired, rather than to take those officinally prepared and kept in stock.

Among cerates, which are in some respects more valuable for ointments for most skin affections than lard, we have two, *ceratum simplex*, consisting of white wax 30 parts, lard 70 parts; *ceratum cetacei*, which is composed of spermaceti 10 parts, white wax 35 parts, and olive oil 55 parts. To these should be added *unguentum cetacei*, which is very like the latter, only somewhat softer. These all have considerable body, and when spread on the skin form a protective coating, more suitable for many conditions than lard alone; but the first mentioned, or simple cerate, is far too hard for easy application in most diseases of the skin. The *glyceritum amyli*, composed of starch 10 parts and glycerin 90 parts, is a good basis for ointments when fatty substances are not well borne, or when it is desirable to remove the application frequently with water. Combined with oil of cade 25 parts, sapo viridis 15 parts, and glycerite of starch 60 parts, it makes a most valuable application in psoriasis, which can be well rubbed in at night and washed off completely in the morning.

The *oleum theobromæ* is ordinarily but little used in compounding ointments. It is particularly useful when added, in about a quarter part, to ointments for use on the hairy scalp, to give them a low melting-point and to aid in forming a protective coating over the skin; when employed in too large a proportion it will prove irritating to many skins.

Under the head of "ointments" we find but two preparations in the Pharmacopœia—the *unguentum simplex*, composed of lard 80 parts and yellow wax 20 parts, and the *unguentum aquæ rosæ*, of expressed almond oil 50 parts, spermaceti 10, white wax 10, and rose-water 30 parts. The *unguentum simplex* is a good combination—much better for general use than simple lard; but, on the other hand, it is often found to be too hard, and ointments made with it will often be difficult of application, and when made up for some time with other ingredients, will become too stiff for ready use; as ordinarily kept in drug-stores it has not infrequently been found quite rancid.

The best ointment of all, when fresh and properly made, is the *unguentum aquæ rosæ*, the cold-cream of the Pharmacopœia. But some judgment and skill is necessary in its preparation, for unless very perfectly compounded, with prolonged rubbing together of the ingredients, the ointment will not be perfect; in summer, also, it will require rather a larger proportion of the spermaceti and white wax in order to have the proper consistency for a perfect application. Very frequently, when the skin tends to be too dry, a portion of the water may be replaced by glycerin. Occasionally the odor of the rose-water is not agreeable to the patient, and simple distilled water may be used in its place. The water held in this ointment is undoubtedly an important element in its remarkable effects on the skin, for the *ceratum cetacei* and *unguentum cetacei* have quite a similar composition, but are by no means agreeable to most skins.

When the various products of petroleum, known in the Pharmacopœia by the general name of *petrolatum*, were introduced, it was thought they would furnish the best possible bases for ointments, and that they would rapidly supersede all other excipients; in Dr. Bulkley's opinion they will never supplant those already mentioned and others of recognized value. They are by no means always agreeable and non-irritating to the skin; indeed, many individuals are found who cannot bear them on the skin at all. Most of them have not body enough to form good ointments, although for simple inunction, as a lubricant, or for the application of carbolic acid to the skin as an antipruritic, vaseline serves the purpose very well.

Recently, when lanolin, and subsequently agnine, were presented to the profession, it was expected that this substance would replace other ingredients as an excipient for ointments. But again we have been disappointed, and lanolin forms but a very small portion of the base of ointments used by those especially occupied with diseases of the skin. It is too sticky and not easy of application, and, moreover, it will often prove irritating to a delicate skin. While it was thought to afford a means for the more ready absorption of medicaments, more experience has shown it to be questionable if this is the case. Indeed, in some experiments by Brooke, it was shown that the substances incorporated with lanolin were the slowest in entering the system. Lanolin, is, however, useful as an addition to certain ointments, in the proportion of about 20 per cent., to give an adhesive quality to them, thus securing a firmer and more adherent coating for affected parts.

Of some forty officinal ointments, very few can be prescribed as they are with advantage in diseases of the skin. Thus the carbolic ointment is made of a strength of 10 per cent., which is far too strong for most skins; whereas the tannin ointment of the same strength is too weak to be of real service. The belladonna ointment is also of the same strength, and is capable, if used at all freely, of producing serious constitutional effects. Also, the officinal ointment of chrysarobin should be diluted for most skins.

Eight ointments are officinal containing preparations of mercury. Of these the blue ointment, containing 50 per cent. of metallic mercury, is well known and of great value; but for inunction on most skins it requires dilution by one-half, in order not to excite too much local irritation. White precipitate ointment has commonly to be diluted two or three times, even in psoriasis and seborrhœic eczema. The red iodide ointment is of fair strength, but to be effective in lupus, or where its corrosive power is required, it should be employed much stronger. Citrine ointment, one of the best known of the mercurial applications, is far too strong to be freely used. When diluted two to four times, it often serves a good purpose in reducing infiltrations of the skin. The yellow and the red oxide of mercury require to be very greatly diluted for use about the eyes.

The single ointment of iodine is a good preparation, containing a trifle of iodide of potassium. A prescription which is of great service in reducing glandular enlargements in syphilis, is a mixture of iodine ointment with the ordinary mercurial ointment in equal parts. When well rubbed together an ointment of the green iodide of mercury is made, which acts much more quickly than either of the ointments alone. For delicate skins it may require some dilution, but generally it is well borne. It is useful as a parasiticide in ringworm and favus of the scalp.

The *unguentum picis liquidæ* is an excellent remedy, composed of equal parts of tar and suet; but it is far too strong for general use undiluted. When combined with oxide of zinc and rose ointment it forms one of the most perfect applications known for a large share of cases of subacute eczema, both in children and in adults:

R.—Ung. picis . . . . 3ij.
Ung. zinci oxidi . . . . 3ss.
Ung. aquæ rosæ . . . . ℥iv.—M.

The ointments of the carbonate of lead and iodide of lead, each 10 per cent., are also good combinations.

The latter is certainly an excellent means for causing absorption of enlarged strumous glands. The stramonium ointment, containing 10 per cent. of the extract of stramonium, is likewise a good application, and forms a most valuable base for combination with acetate of lead and opium in the treatment of hæmorrhoids.

There are four ointments containing sulphur, only one of which, the *unguentum sulphuris*, containing 30 per cent. of sublimed sulphur, is well known or much used. This is also too strong for direct application to most skins; diluted two or three times with a little storax, and perhaps a little tar ointment, it forms an excellent treatment for scabies, although the more agreeable applications of naphthol and resorcin have largely taken its place in dermatological practice.

The oxide of zinc ointment of our Pharmacopœia is a fairly good preparation. It is made with benzoinated lard, which is not agreeable to all skins; it is sometimes rancid and irritating in cases in which a freshly prepared zinc ointment in cold-cream is grateful and healing.

Diachylon ointment, when freshly and properly made, is one of the most valuable means of local therapy known for many diseases of the skin. The preparation made according to the original formula of Hebra, and given in the German Pharmacopœia, is a soft, buttery ointment, easily spread, and of a delightfully soothing character to most skins, and is decidedly superior to the ointment made according to the U. S. Pharmacopœia.

A few words may now be added in regard to the actual preparation or compounding of ointments, a feature which continually requires the attention of the physician, if he would have success in the treatment of skin diseases. It is desirable for the physician to frequently inspect the ointments or other preparations which are being employed, and to test them by smelling, feeling, rubbing on the skin, etc.

More harm is commonly done by too strong ointments than is usually supposed. The skin is a sensitive and irritable organ, and more often wants to be treated considerately and soothed into good action than it does to be stimulated and irritated. It is well to begin with a mild preparation, increasing the strength as circumstances seem to demand.

It is also well to remember that the average patient, who has not heretofore been instructed, or who has not had special experience, knows nothing in regard to the best mode of application of an ointment, and if the highest degree of success is to attend the use of any particular remedy, it must be only by its proper employment. Careful directions should, therefore, always be given to patients exactly how to apply ointments.

Where it is desired to keep a part continually under the effect of an ointment, it should be soaked in it, if it were possible, as completely as though the part were immersed in a very large mass of the same; but as this is not possible, we have recourse to lint, and the ointment, which should always have considerable body, is spread to a very thick layer on the woolly side of the lint, and then firmly bound on the part.

An excellent illustration of the necessity for minute directions in regard to all these data is found in connection with eczema of the scrotum. When treated carelessly, or when the patient merely smears on an ointment, the disease will prove most distressing and rebellious; but when, on the other hand, very minute directions are given in regard to the sudden and brief application of hot water once daily, at bedtime, and when the part is quickly dried and enclosed in a piece of lint spread with the tar and zinc ointment previously alluded to, and covered by a suspensory bandage, the patient has complete relief, and with proper accompanying treatment can surely be cured, and that with reasonable speed.

The demand in dermatology is not so much for new drugs, applications, or methods of treatment, as it is for the diffused knowledge of what is already known to be of service, and the faithful carrying out of methods which experience and observation have proved to be useful.—*Therapeutic Gazette*, August 15, 1891.

THE TOXICITY OF SALOL.

Although salol has been very freely used, both among children and among adults, and although it has come to be regarded as one of the least dangerous of the new remedies having antiseptic and antithermic properties, there are not wanting clinical testimonies which tend to show that, under certain circumstances at least, its use may be attended with a fatal result. Two cases of fatal result attending its use have been reported, one in which a fifteen-grain dose of salol was used. In this latter case the patient was suffering from severe gastric symptoms, and was under examination according to Ewald's method. After taking the dose the patient became restless and unconscious, the pupils were dilated, the pulse was irregular, there was constant vomiting, and the urine became dark and contained salicylic acid. Death occurred twelve days later. At the autopsy there were found gastritis and hemorrhagic enteritis, a gastric ulcer cicatrized at the cardiac end, chronic endometritis, and a cyst of the ovary. No doubt was entertained that the salol had been the cause of the symptoms of poisoning.

NAPHTHALINE AS A VERMIFUGE.

DR. MIROVITCH, in the *Mercredi Médical*, speaks of naphthaline as the best agent for expelling tænia. In his opinion it is superior to all other remedies, because of the certainty of its action and the absence of all toxic effect, for it is absorbed in but very minute amount by the gastro-intestinal mucous membrane. The dose for adults is fifteen grains, given when the stomach is empty and followed immediately by two tablespoonfuls of castor oil. Children may take from four to eight grains, and at the same time a tablespoonful of castor oil, flavored with a few drops of essence of bergamot. During the two days preceding the administration of the drug the patient is to eat freely of salted, acid, and spiced foods. In all of the cases one dose of naphthaline was sufficient to expel the tapeworm, the head included, even in cases in which other drugs had failed. He has also found the drug most effective in the treatment of patients with ascarides.

USE OF PURE BENZOLE IN WHOOPING COUGH.

DR. W. ROBERTSON, after some years' experience with the use of benzole in whooping-cough, is satisfied that it effects better results than all the other remedies recognized as useful in this affection. In adult and child it is of equal benefit. In an infant just now under treatment the attacks have been reduced from twenty or thirty in the night to two or three, and whereas when the treatment was begun evidences of bronchitis were present, now the chest is clear, and the child able to be taken out of doors daily. All this improvement was brought about in less than ten days. In cases where convulsions and other complications were fast reducing all chances of recovery, its use was attended with perfect success within a few days. In adults, where pertussis assumes often serious aspects, benzole has proved equally efficacious. Two minims in mucilage are sufficient for a child six months old, and five minims in mucilage on sugar or in capsule, for adults. Whenever the benzole odor is observed in the breath of the patient, then all anxiety as to the result may be allayed.—*Lancet*, vol. ii., No. 6, 1891.

ANTIPYRINE AS A HÆMOSTATIC.

PROFESSOR G. CESARI, of Modena, finds that antipyrine applied to an injured bloodvessel or to living tissues, whether in the form of fine powder or watery solution, does not irritate or dry or produce any caustic effect on the tissues or cause pain. It gives rise to local anæmia more or less marked according to the length of time the agent is applied. A fifty to one hundred per cent. watery solution produces no change in the calibre of the capillaries; but made to bathe the veins of the mesentery of a frog, or the jugular or femoral vein of a rabbit, more or less perceptible narrowing of these vessels can be observed. When applied in solutions containing at least fifty per cent. of antipyrine, or in the form of powder, in both cases the application should be made on plugs of cotton-wool; it arrests hemorrhage more or less speedily.

Antipyrine, if placed in contact with blood at its normal temperature, thickens and condenses it, and, without causing coagulation, prevents it from escaping from the vessels. It stops secondary hemorrhage.—*British Medical Journal*, 1891.

REMOVAL OF SUPERFLUOUS HAIR.

DR. E. O. LEBERMAN offers the following formulæ, which, in his hands, have proved quite successful. (This formula is recommended by McCall Anderson):

R.—Barii sulphidi . . . . ℥iss.
    Zinci oxidi . . . . ʒvj.

Mix with sufficient water to form a paste, apply for three minutes, and then wash off.

For the removal of stiff, coarse hair, the formula of Neumann is serviceable:

R.—Calc. hydrat. . . . . ℥iss.
    Orpiment. . . . . ʒiij.
    Amyli . . . . ʒj.
    Aq. calcis . . . . q. s.
Ft. pasta.

The paste should be spread over the parts from which the hair is to be removed as thick as the blade of a knife. The softened hairs should be scraped from the skin with a dull knife or ivory spatula, the parts washed with warm water and afterward thoroughly dried. A bland ointment should then be applied to the reddened surface. The length of time these pastes should remain upon the skin is best determined by the severity of their action. They both cause slight itching, which sensation is followed by an intense burning; when the latter begins the paste had best be removed. The effect of chemical depilatories can scarcely be more than temporary, as their action can extend no deeper than the epidermis; the hair-bulbs remaining, a new growth will soon appear. Great care should be exercised in their application, and their effects should be carefully watched, for sometimes deep and painful ulcerations occur by their incautious use. However, they serve a purpose, and if properly applied will often leave the skin free from hirsute appendages which disfigure it.

For Corns and Warts.

A mixture of one part each of lactic acid and salicylic acid in eight parts of collodion is recommended as an excellent application to warts or corns, effecting their removal in a short time.

Menthol in Hay Fever.

Dr. Lennox Wainwright has found menthol of great service in hay fever. It acts best when mixed with carbonate of ammonium, and used as smelling-salts. Patients state that all irritability disappears, and in many cases they get no return of the symptoms.—*Medical Record*, vol. xl., No. 9, 1891.

Common Thyme in Whooping-cough.

Common thyme, which was recommended in whooping-cough three or four years ago by Dr. S. B. Johnson, is regarded by Dr. Neovius, who writes a paper on the subject in a Finnish medical journal, as almost worthy of the title of a specific. During an epidemic of whooping-cough he had ample opportunities of observing its effects, and he came to the conclusion that if it is given early and constantly it invariably cuts short the disease in a fortnight, the symptoms generally vanishing in two or three days. They are liable to return if the thyme is not taken regularly for at least two or three weeks. He gives from one ounce and a half to six ounces per diem, combined with a little marshmallow syrup. It may produce a slight diarrhoea. It is important that the drug should be used quite fresh.

Hypodermatic Injections of Strychnine in Ten Cases of Chronic Alcoholism.

Dr. Ergloski has published an account of ten cases of chronic alcoholism among his patients. They had the habit of taking brandy. They were given subcutaneous injections of nitrate of strychnine, one-sixtieth to one-twentieth of a grain at each injection.

After a dozen injections the results were remarkable, as they all acquired a distaste for brandy. In such cases as are desirous of being cured this treatment may prove to be of assistance.—*Bulletin Général de Thérapeutique*, No. 20, 1891.

MEDICINE.

UNDER THE CHARGE OF

W. PASTEUR, M.D. Lond., M.R.C.P.,

ASSISTANT PHYSICIAN TO THE MIDDLESEX HOSPITAL; PHYSICIAN TO THE NORTHWESTERN HOSPITAL FOR CHILDREN;

AND

SOLOMON SOLIS-COHEN, A.M., M.D.,

PROFESSOR OF CLINICAL MEDICINE AND APPLIED THERAPEUTICS IN THE PHILADELPHIA POLYCLINIC; PHYSICIAN TO THE PHILADELPHIA HOSPITAL.

THE NATURE, ACTION, AND THERAPEUTIC VALUE OF THE ACTIVE PRINCIPLES OF TUBERCULIN.

DR. WILLIAM HUNTER (*British Medical Journal*, 1891, No. 1595) writes that Koch's remedy for tuberculosis is a glycerin extract of pure cultivations of tubercle bacilli.

"The only substance capable of fulfilling, although still with difficulty, all the conditions laid down by Koch for his active principle would, in Hunter's opinion, be one of crystalloidal nature—presumably a toxine. Such a body might (1) be in sufficiently close association with one of proteid nature as to be carried down when the latter was precipitated by absolute alcohol, and yet (2) at the same time sufficiently loosely attached to be dialyzable away. Further, it might (3) be able to resist the action of high temperature without losing its poisonous properties. On the other hand, a protein substance which would readily fulfil the first and third conditions could not possibly fulfil the intermediate one of dialyzing easily through the parchment membrane. And, lastly, a poisonous peptone which could fulfil the condition as regards precipitation by alcohol, and might also fulfil the one as regards easy diffusibility, could with difficulty fulfil the third one of being unaffected by heat."

Hunter's observations, commenced in January of the present year, have had for their object:

1. To isolate the constituents of tuberculin, and to determine their chemical nature.

2. To ascertain their action with special reference to their power of inducing the two most characteristic effects of tuberculin—namely, local inflammation and fever.

3. To ascertain how far it was possible to eliminate all substances having an injurious action, and thus to obtain its remedial, without any of its injurious, effects.

"SUMMARY OF RESULTS.—In their order of importance, as well as of amount, the chief substances present in tuberculin are, according to these observations:

"1. Albumoses; chiefly proto-albumose and deutero-albumose, along with hetero-albumose, and occasionally a trace of dysalbumose.

"2· Alkaloidal substances; two of which can be obtained in the form of the platinum compounds of their hydrochlorate salts.

"3. Extractives; small in quantity, and of unrecognized nature.

"4. Mucin.

"5. Inorganic salts.

"6. Glycerin and coloring matter.

"So far as the observations go, the following substances are absent from tuberculin, namely, serum-albumin, globulin, peptones."

With the view of ascertaining to which of these bodies or groups of bodies tuberculin owed its characteristic properties, observations were made first on animals—mice and guinea-pigs—and subsequently on tuberculous patients. The following modifications of tuberculin were employed:

Modification A: This contained the total precipitate thrown down from tuberculin by the action of absolute alcohol. The solutions of this precipitate were found to contain every constituent of tuberculin; but the proportion of albumoses was relatively increased, that of salts relatively diminished.

Modification C was the counterpart of A, the salts and other soluble substances being relatively in excess, while the amount of albumose was relatively small.

"The most interesting contrast was afforded by the action of these ·two modifications, A and C. Both of them had remedial properties, causing absorption and disappearance of tuberculous tissue; but while in the case of A this was attended by decided and occasionally severe local inflammatory reaction, even with small doses, accompanied by comparatively little, sometimes no fever, in the case of C the improvement was attended with no local inflammation, and nevertheless high fever."

Modification B: In this the whole of the albumoses of tuberculin were precipitated by means of ammonium sulphate, so far at least as that was possible without the aid of heat or acetic acid. The precipitate was then taken up in distilled water and dialyzed.

"The solution thus prepared was found to possess in an eminent degree the power of inducing local reaction, followed by healing change around tuberculous lesions, unaccompanied by any constitutional disturbance whatever."

A fourth modification, C B, prepared from C, yielded a solution which gave all the reactions characteristic of albumoses (the salts having been separated by dialysis) and proved to be capable of inducing very distinct local improvement, unattended with fever (in most cases) and still more markedly accompanied by scarcely noticeable inflammatory reaction.

Dr. Hunter summarizes his conclusions as follows:

"1. Tuberculin owes its activity not to one principle, but to at least three, and probably more, different substances.

"2. Its action in producing local inflammation, fever, and general constitutional disturbance is not a simple but an extremely complex one.

"3. Its active ingredients are of the nature of albumoses, alkaloidal substances, and extractives. The action of these is in certain instances antagonistic.

"4. Its remedial and inflammatory actions are connected with the presence of certain of its albumoses, while its fever-producing properties are chiefly associated with substances of non-albuminous nature.

"5. The albumoses are not lost by dialysis, the latter are. By the adoption of suitable methods it is thus possible to remove the substances which cause the fever, while retaining those which are beneficial in their action.

"6. The fever produced by tuberculin is thus absolutely unessential to its remedial action.

"7. The same holds true, I would fain believe, with regard to the inflammation produced by it. Inflammation is certainly not absolutely necessary for the manifestation of its remedial action. It is in some cases, however; beneficial, and helps, under certain circumstances, the action of the remedial substance.

"8. The difference between the substance which causes the inflammation and the one which possesses the remedial properties as regards their action is not merely one of degree. The local reaction which occurs with small doses of the former is much greater than that producible by large doses of the latter.

"9. Nevertheless the remedial substance has as truly a local action as the one which tends to produce inflammation. This is evidenced in two ways— first, by distinct and obvious shrinking of the tuberculous tissues; and, secondly, increased scaling, pointing to the existence of a certain amount of deep local congestion. In some cases this congestion becomes obvious by slight superficial reddening.

"10. The power of favoring recurrence, which tuberculin possesses, is connected partly with the non-albuminous substances removable by dialysis, possibly also with a portion of the albumoses present.

"11. The remedial substance resists the action of high temperatures. Its action is, however, lessened if exposed to a temperature above 70° C. in a dry condition. Its properties, moreover, can be altered in other ways, sometimes, for example, materially by dialysis. This change is not due to the passage of the substance through the membrane, but to changes occurring in it within the dialyzator. Its sensitiveness in this respect I regard as one of its chief features, and causes its preparation to be attended with special difficulties.

"12. Both it and the albumoses present probably belong to the class of proteins—albuminous substances derived from the plasma of the bacilli themselves, and not merely formed by the action of these bacilli on the surrounding tissues."

As regards the therapeutic value of the above modifications of tuberculin, Dr. Hunter speaks in very guarded terms.

To justify the claim to be classed as a remedial agent, every substance must fulfil the following simple requirements: 1. It action must in a suitable proportion of cases be beneficial. 2. In competent hands its action must not at the time produce any immediate ill effects. 3. Its action must not be followed by remote ill consequences directly traceable to it, still less by consequences which may endanger the life of the patient.

Judged by this standard, tuberculin cannot be regarded a safe remedy, and any modification of tuberculin must be subjected to the same test and fulfil the same requirements before it can be regarded as a safe remedial agent.

Modification A and modification C are not recommended for use.

Modification C B fulfils the first condition, and so far also the second. It contains the remedial agent present in C without the fever-producing qualities of the latter. The absence of local reaction other than a very slight reddening gives it great advantages if it be employed for internal tuberculosis.

Modification B contains the remedial properties of C B, with the additional property of inducing local inflammation. It fulfils the first condition, and so far the second, with the exception of producing local reaction. The crucial condition to be fulfilled is, however, the third, and time alone can decide this.

The author is of opinion that the action of the various substances has been materially intensified by the process of purification.

OSTEOMALACIA IN INSANE PATIENTS.

DR. DAVID WALSH (*Lancet*, 1891, No. 3543) records four cases occurring among a population of 1300 women in Wakefield Asylum. A post-mortem examination was made in three cases, the fourth was still living. One woman had borne " several," another three, the third two, whilst the fourth was childless. The average age at which the disease was first noted was sixty-eight. (Cf. the conclusions arrived at by Durham in Heath's *Dictionary of Surgery* from the analysis of 145 collected cases, " that the great majority began to suffer between twenty-five and thirty-five years of age.")

In three of the author's cases chronic rheumatism was suspected; in three fractures took place from trifling causes, and though not absolutely proved, fracture was probably present in the fourth.

In all four cases there was aortic valvular disease.

One of the patients showed epilepsy of many years' duration, winding up with a rapid final development of osteomalacia and of phthisis.

The life history of the patient who is still alive is remarkable. Springing from a mentally affected family, she first came under treatment for delusional insanity at the age of sixty-six, and was readmitted at seventy for a similar complaint. An aortic murmur was noted at seventy-one, and fractured hip occurred one year later with well-marked osteomalacia at seventy-five, and, lastly, a scirrhus of the mamma at seventy-nine.

The author lays especial stress on the advanced age, absence of frequent child-bearing, and the coincidence of aortic disease with recurrent attacks of delusional insanity.

LOCAL MILIARY TUBERCULOSIS IN THE COURSE OF TREATMENT WITH TUBERCULIN.

TANGL (*Deutsche medicin. Wochenschr.*, 1891, No. 19) reports the fatal case of a man, twenty-five years old, admitted to the wards of A. Fränkel, in the Berlin Urban City Hospital, with pulmonary and laryngeal tuberculosis, in whom, in the course of treatment with tuberculin, tuberculosis of the tongue developed. The case had been demonstrated by Fränkel to the Berlin Medical Society. When admitted to the hospital the patient presented the evidences of pulmonary and laryngeal tuberculosis of moderate degree, without excavation, or more than slight superficial ulceration respectively. At the end of six weeks, during which he was treated with injections of menthol, gaining weight, and the disease not progressing, injections of tuberculin were begun. Two weeks later, after 0.1 gramme of tuberculin had been given in fourteen injections, there appeared at the anterior margin of the right side of the tongue, which hitherto had not shown the slightest evidence of involvement, a number of small, whitish vesicles, some of which ruptured, leaving superficial, painful, aphthous ulcers. The tongue now became reddened and indurated ; small nodules appeared, while the ulceration extended. In the pus removed from the ulcers tubercle bacilli were found. Subsequently there developed in the right half of the tongue a large mass, at the periphery of which ulceration took place, while in the area beyond the ulceration numerous miliary and submiliary nodules developed. A bit of the callous margin of the ulcer and three nodules were excised for histological examination. A week later numerous new nodules had developed, while some of the older appeared grayish-white. Of the latter, a number were excised for histological examination. In this way the condition of the tongue progressively advanced. Deglutition became difficult, the vital forces rapidly failed, dyspnœa increased, and death ensued three months after the treatment with tuberculin had been begun. Diarrhœa was present during the last three weeks of life, the stools containing tubercle bacilli.

The autopsy was made twelve hours after death. The lungs were extensively involved in the tuberculous process; the left lung contained a cavity as large as a fist, lined with cheesy matter. The larynx was the seat of profound ulceration and advanced perichondritis. The large and small intestine were involved in extensive and profound ulceration. The mesenteric and bronchial glands were enlarged and cheesy. The liver, spleen, and kidneys contained numerous gray, translucent, miliary tubercles. The tongue presented the conditions indicated during life.

The treatment with tuberculin, which was withdrawn eighteen days before death occurred, covered in all seventy-eight days, forty-eight injections, a total of 1.165 grammes being given; the initial dose was 0.001 gramme, the final dose 0.06 gramme. Examination, by approved methods, of the tissues excised clearly demonstrated the tuberculous nature of the ulceration, established that the gray nodules that were constantly forming were true miliary tubercles of recent origin, and failed to disclose any evidence of unusual necrosis or unusual inflammatory small-celled infiltration.

In a discussion of the origin of the tuberculosis of the tongue, two possibilities may be considered : either the bacilli were present in the tongue before the injections were begun, or they were carried thither in the course of the treatment. If the bacilli were primarily present they must have been few in number; they could not have been abundant without giving rise to evident changes. Granting that bacilli were present, it follows that treatment with tuberculin did not prevent their rapid multiplication; on the contrary, the nodules that appeared afresh from time to time could only have been developed as a result of renewed deposition. It is more probable, however, that the bacilli reached the tongue during the course of treatment. This they may have done either through the blood or lymph, or through the sputum. Unfortunately, the primary ulceration was not examined for tubercle bacilli. It is known that aphthous ulcerations heal notwithstanding the presence of tubercle bacilli in the sputum ; while, according to the experiments of Koch, local inoculations in tuberculous animals are not progressive. The actual mode of infection of the tongue cannot therefore be definitely determined. There can be no doubt, however, that the tubercles developed adjacent to the ulceration were of local origin, the largest in size and number being nearest the area of ulceration, around which they were clustered in a corona. The histological examination, in conjunction with the clinical course of the case, makes it apparent that some of the nodules examined could have been but a few days old, having developed in the course of treatment. The conclusion forces itself upon one that in the case reported tuberculin failed both to prevent the development of new tuberculous masses and to exert any curative influence upon the processes that existed.

Tangl disclaims any wish to make general deductions as to the utility of tuberculin. He rather considers the case as one of a number in which, for reasons not yet known, tuberculin fails to exert any beneficial influence. A careful study of such cases may lead to a knowledge of the conditions that interfere with the favorable action of the remedy, or contraindicate its application. At the same time, the cases must not be ignored in which tuberculin undoubtedly exercises a favorable influence.

ALLOCHIRIA.

WEISS (*Prager medicin. Wochenschr.*, 1891, No. 24) reports the case of a woman, fifty-four years old, with a neuropathic heredity, who had for a number of years presented typical symptoms of locomotor ataxia. In addition, the patient was hysterical and a victim of morphinism. Beside the ordinary manifestations of tabes, she presented bilateral ptosis, bilateral temporal hemianopsia, decided salivation, tachycardia, laryngeal and gastric crises, and an excessive (trophoneurotic) formation of callus at the seat of an old fracture of the tibia; a tendency to melancholia, an impairment of memory and a pseudo-paralysis of the lower extremities that existed, were ascribed to the hysteria. On testing sensation, it was found that impressions made upon one side of the body were referred to the corresponding point on the opposite side : stroking the skin of the lower extremity, the prick of a needle, the application of a hot sponge and of a bit of ice, the passive fixation of the great toe, of the foot, and of the knee, were all recognized, but referred to the opposite extremity. There thus existed allochiria of tactile sensibility of the pain, of the temperature, and of the muscle-sense.

Weiss considers as plausible Hammond's explanation of the occurrence of allochiria : an obstruction in the cord that diverts a sensory impression made upon one side of the body to the same side of the brain, as a result of which the impression is referred to the opposite side of the body. The disappearance of the symptom that commonly occurs may depend upon structural removal of the sensory obstruction. Weiss believes that the phenomenon would be more commonly encountered if careful sensory examinations were habitually made.

ALBUMINATURIA.

In a communication presented to the Société de Biologie, GAUBE (*La Méde-cine Moderne*, 1881, No. 23) described as albuminaturia a condition character-ized by the presence in the urine of a small quantity of albumin in association with carbonates, or especially with earthy phosphates. Albuminaturia may be physiological, pathological, or experimental. Physiological albuminaturia is transitory; it accompanies pregnancy; in both sexes it follows coitus; in the female it follows menstruation. Pathological albuminaturia is protracted in duration and of grave prognosis; it appears in the course of extensive suppuration, or associated with changes in the nervous system. Experimental albuminaturia is a result of the stomachal ingestion of an excess of phos-phates soluble in the urine, of which the excess is eliminated as albumino-phosphates. Calcic albumino-phosphate, the most abundant in the urine during the existence of albuminaturia, is a combination of albumin with the bibasic calcium phosphate, and has a rotatory constant of —92°. The urine of albuminaturia is scanty; it contains but a small proportion of urea, of mineral matters, and of phosphoric acid; it is scarcely acid; filtered, not acidulated and heated, a precipitate of the bibasic calcium phosphate is thrown down, soluble by the addition of one or two drops of acetic acid; the solution of the precipitate is followed by a cloudiness of the urine, dependent upon precipitation of albumin, insoluble by heat or acids, but soluble in alkalies. Albuminaturia is distinguished from ordinary albuminuria or serumuria, in addition to other physico-chemical characteristics, by the pre-ponderance in the urine of the mineral over the proteid matters; in serumuria proteids predominate over mineral constituents.

DANGER OF BREAKING-DOWN CAPSULES ABOUT COLONIES OF BACILLI.

In an address made before the Medical Society of Hanover, in March, 1890, BRUNN-LIPPSPRINGE (*Deutsche med. Wochenschr.*, Jan. 22, 1891) re-ferred to the irregularity of the nasal surfaces, the tortuous course and pro-gressively narrowing lumen of the air-passages, with their ciliated epithelium and constant outward current of mucus, as natural protections against the invasion of infection and the entrance of bacilli into the deeper respiratory passages. In the event of infection taking place, the bacilli passing the pul-monary portals and gaining entrance into the alveoli, where they find the conditions for the development of their activities, the organism makes a final effort to rid itself of the invaders; failing in this, it endeavors to prevent their entrance into the blood. The colony of bacilli is surrounded by a wall of living cells; the latter destroy or isolate the former, cutting off their nutrition and preventing general infection. As a result of mechanical or chem-ical irritation a connective-tissue capsule is formed. The slow development of the tubercle bacillus accounts for the long period of incubation of tubercu-losis, and affords abundant time for the formation of a surrounding capsule. In this way the prolonged localization and the slow extension of the disease find explanation. In the absence of a specific remedy for tuberculosis, the therapeutics must be so directed as to supplement the efforts of Nature, by favor-ing the development of the protecting capsule, an end best accomplished by elevating the nutrition, improving the general condition, and regenerating the blood and bodily fluids. If this view be correct, any procedure which causes destruction of the surrounding capsule, with setting free of the bacilli, carries with it the danger of dissemination. This is illustrated in the general infection following operative treatment of tuberculous bone disease and of fistula-in-ano of tuberculous character.

SURGERY.

UNDER THE CHARGE OF

J. WILLIAM WHITE, M.D.,

PROFESSOR OF CLINICAL SURGERY IN THE UNIVERSITY OF PENNSYLVANIA; SURGEON TO THE UNIVERSITY AND GERMAN HOSPITALS ;

ASSISTED BY

EDWARD MARTIN, M.D.,

CLINICAL PROFESSOR OF GENITO-URINARY SURGERY IN THE UNIVERSITY OF PENNSYLVANIA ; SURGEON TO THE HOWARD HOSPITAL AND ASSISTANT SURGEON TO THE UNIVERSITY HOSPITAL.

THE SUPPOSED CURATIVE EFFECT OF OPERATIONS, PER SE.

Under this title, DR. J. WILLIAM WHITE, of Philadelphia, contributes a paper to the *Annals of Surgery* for August, 1891, which, not only from its subject, but from the great number of authorities quoted and from the peculiarly rich experience of the writer, makes an article of unusual interest and importance to both surgeon and physician. The author's attention was first directed to this subject by reason of his experience with the operation of trephining for so-called traumatic epilepsy.

During the past five years, with Dr. D. Hayes Agnew, he has trephined in fifteen cases of supposed traumatic epilepsy. All but one recovered from the operation. The patient who perished was an imbecile and a confirmed drunkard, as well as an epileptic. Death occurred from suppression of urine, probably secondary to etherization.

In one case a bullet was found imbedded in the brain substance ; in another an irregular portion of the internal table was dissected out from beneath the dura mater, to which it was attached by cicatricial adhesions. In another there were projecting spicules of bone on the internal surface of the button removed and the adjacent portions of the skull. In two, marked sclerosis and thickening of the cranium were observed about the field of operation. In the remaining cases nothing abnormal was seen. Although this was the case, they were, without exception, markedly improved by trephining, in two instances even to the point of apparent cure, no return of symptoms having been observed for eighteen months and for two years after the operation. In the other seven the results were strikingly favorable, convulsions disappearing for weeks or months, although previously of more than daily occurrence.

The author has, in so far as this is possible, classified the cases in which operation *per se* seemed to be the main factor in bringing about a cure. These cases are divided into three groups, in accordance with the anatomical seat of the symptoms or of the supposed disease. This brings them under the following heads:

1. Operations for the relief of nervous phenomena, as epilepsy, insanity, paralysis, etc.

2. Operations for abdominal and pelvic disorders, as peritonitis, tumors, etc.

3. Miscellaneous operations.

This classification is further carried out by grouping together (*a*) those cases in which nothing whatever was found explanatory of the symptoms; (*b*) those in which some departure from normal conditions was observed, but was so slight as to be apparently inadequate to explain the symptoms; (*c*) those cases in which an apparently grave and irremediable condition was disclosed by an exploratory operation, but notably improved or altogether disappeared after mere inspection and handling, no further surgical interference having been thought justifiable.

Under the heading of " Operations for the Relief of Nervous Phenomena," Dr. White has tabulated, including his own service, 154 cases. Many of these are given in detail, and coming as they do from recognized authorities, are of exceeding great interest.

In 56 cases of trephining for epilepsy nothing abnormal was found to account for the symptoms. Nineteen cases were reported in six months or less after operation; 11 cases were reported from one to two years after operation; 1 was reported eight years after operation.

Of these cases 25 were reported as cured; 18 as improved; in 3 it was mentioned that a relapse occurred later.

In 30 cases of ligation of bloodvessels for epilepsy 14 were reported as cured; 15 as improved; 1 died seven days after operation. In the fatal case the right common carotid artery was tied. No fit occurred after the operation.

In 10 cases of castration for epilepsy all were reported as cured. One case was reported four months after operation; 4 cases were reported more than two years after operation; in 5 the time when reported is not mentioned.

In 9 cases of tracheotomy for epilepsy 2 were reported as cured; 6 as improved; 1 as much improved, though death in this case followed in two months after the operation.

In 24 cases of removal of the superior cervical ganglia of the sympathetic nerves 6 remained well at the end of three years; 10 were improved; 5 remained unimproved; 2 died soon after the operation, but not from its direct effect.

In 6 cases of incision of the scalp for epilepsy nothing was found to account for the symptoms. Three of these cases were reported as cured at the end of one year; 2 were reported as cured at the end of two years; 2 other cases, almost similar, were reported as cured.

Twelve cases of epilepsy are reported as cured by such operations as stretching of the sciatic nerve, excision of the musculo-cutaneous nerve, cauterization of the larynx, circumcision, application of a seton to the back of the neck, tenotomy of the external recti muscles, burning of the scalp, puncture of the heart, etc.

Thirteen cases of spontaneous or accidental cures of epilepsy are also reported, at a time varying from two months to five years after the traumatism, which was a fall, a burn, a wound, an amputation for intercurrent injury or disease, etc.

Passing from the cerebral to the spinal region, Dr. White cites an illustrative case of his own. A man aged fifty-five years was attacked on December 25, 1887, with severe pains in his arms and shoulders. ¯A few days later there was weakness of the thighs, spreading rapidly down the legs to the feet, and upward on the body to the nipple line. In eight days there was absolute paralysis of the parts involved, including both sphincters, while at the same time the paralyzed parts became the seat of profound anæsthesia. Girdle pains developed, bedsores made their appearance, percussion of the spine over the third and fourth vertebræ became painful. The reflexes were exaggerated, and light blows on the head in the direction of the spinal axis gave rise to frightful exacerbations of the girdle pains. In spite of every remedial measure these symptoms increased in severity for ten months. An exploratory operation was then undertaken. Dr. White removed the spines and laminæ of the first five dorsal vertebræ, opened the slightly thickened dura, separated some firm adhesions to the subjacent pia mater, explored the cord, and having failed to discover any serious pathological changes, closed the wounds in the dura and soft parts.

The girdle pains had entirely disappeared by the following day, sensation began to return in the feet the day after, voluntary motion in the toes after the eighth day, and so one symptom after another disappeared until the patient completely recovered, and is now earning his living by manual labor.

In the list of abdominal and pelvic disorders apparently cured by operation *per se* a number of extraordinary cases are cited. The experience of Tait, who has more than once drawn attention to the astonishing disappearance of tumors, often of large size, after a mere exploratory incision, and the corroborative testimony of Von Mosetig, are cited at length. Koenig's analysis of 131 cases of tubercular peritonitis treated by abdominal incision is carefully discussed.

In response to letters of inquiry upon the subject, Dr. White received many communicatians from prominent operators, the great majority of them containing notes of cases not previously published.

Among the signers of these letters are to be found the names of Goodell, Hirst, Battey, Roswell Park, Lusk, Cheever, Chas. T. Parkes, Cabot, Hunter McGuire, Nancrede, Weir, Stimson, and many others of equal note.

Under the heading of Miscellaneous Operations the author has given several of very diverse character. ·

First are quoted cases of osteomalacia, cured, after weeks or months of confinement in bed, by either oöphorectomy or Cæsarean section.

Passing to another subject, the question of graduated tenotomy of the eye muscles for the relief of severe nervous symptoms is carefully discussed. The author freely acknowledges the value of tenotomies, both complete and graduated, in the restoration of equilibrium in badly balanced ocular muscles, but he is none the less convinced that in numbers of instances of reported cures of chronic chorea, *petit mal*, and even delusional insanity, the effect of the operation *per se* is in large measure the potent cause of the supposed cure. This belief is founded not alone on theory but upon the fact that in certain cases of reflex nervous troubles a cessation of the symptoms has followed the tenotomy, although this has not produced perfect equilibrium. Again, the relapses which may take place after a perfectly successful series of tenotomies would indicate that the nervous phenomena attributed to the insufficiency, for the relief of which the operations were made, were not correctly so attributed, and that the temporary relief must be ascribed to some cause other than the restoration of an imperfect balance of the external ocular muscles.

In seeking for a reasonable explanation of the phenomena observed in the above cases, the author has formulated the conditions which are common to nearly all of them. These are:

1. Anæsthesia.
2. Psychical influence, or so-called mental impression.
3. Relief of tension.
4. Reflex, action or the "reaction of traumatism."

These influences were operative in the majority of cases, although not one of them, except the last, applies to the whole list.

With the idea that it was conceivable that a disease of the nerve centres not reached by ordinary drugs might be affected by agents of such volatility and diffusibility as ether and chloroform, the author instituted a series of observations upon a number of epileptics in various stages of the disease. All other treatment was withdrawn, ether was given to the production of full anæsthesia at intervals of from forty-eight to seventy-two hours. The results were either entirely negative, or in consequence of the withdrawal of their bromides the patients grew worse.

Since in the great majority of cases upon which Dr. White bases his paper there were either undoubted symptoms, such as are habitually associated with organic disease, or there was demonstrable and unmistakable evidence of such disease, it is necessary to believe, in considering the psychical influence of operation, that powerful impressions acting upon the emotional or intellectual nature may affect the organic processes of secretion, nutrition, etc., and may arrest pathological changes and bring about reparative or recuperative action. Cases are cited in which such influences are clearly set forth.

The author holds that the normal equilibrium which we witness between the cerebro-spinal and the sympathetic systems as respects their influence upon the bloodvessels is obviously more or less interfered with when the brain transmits a more than wonted impulse, allowing the unrestrained action or paralyzing the influence of the sympathetic vasomotor nerve. In this relation the author narrates some remarkable cases of hypnotism, and quotes some striking examples of the influence of the central nervous system upon the body.

Belief is expressed that in many of the cases described there can be little doubt that relief of tension is an important factor in amelioration or cure. If it is assumed that preternatural tension exists in the cranial cavity, this would be relieved to an extent by trephining, and there would be but few exceptions to the rule, that in each case something was done which lessened tension in the cavity or organ of the body. There are other cases, however, in which no such relief was obtained, and yet cure resulted from operation. A diminution of the tension would manifestly alter the blood-supply to any important organ in the body, and with it the nutritive processes, local and general. Beyond this nothing definite can be said except as it applies to cases of ascites, in which, as in cases of hydrarthrosis, one tapping may prove permanently curative because the original source of irritation and hypersecretion has already disappeared.

Under the head of Reflex Action, the author includes the "reaction of traumatism," as well as the effects of revulsion and counter-irritation.

Verneuil has long since shown that very slight traumatism sometimes excites in the entire economy a general perturbation, and sometimes, by selection of the weak point, a sudden aggravation of lesions that are only slight or have slumbered. This same excitement, usually prejudicial, may occasionally be curative. In the case of spinal surgery above detailed, Dr. White believes that the local shock of the operation was promptly followed by a corresponding reaction in which the vitality of the tissues was raised sufficiently high to determine a return to the normal state. In this relation the reciprocal influence of one portion of the body on another is briefly discussed.

In considering abdominal tumors, attention is called to the possibility of the spontaneous disappearance of such tumors, the relation of this disappearance to the operation being coincidental; cases are cited in point. As to the cure or amelioration of growths thought to be malignant by merely exploratory operation, a long search through the literature of the subject has met with but little success.

The cure of tuberculosis of the peritoneum as the result of exploratory incision is explained on the ground that the removal of ascitic fluid allows the peritoneal surfaces to fall together and to acquire adhesions. The tubercles are then shut in between the coils of intestine, the omentum, and the abdominal wall. They are thus surrounded by tissues in a high degree of activity, which can now throw around them the limiting zone of young cells and eventually fibrous tissue, which, if the tuberculous process is not too far advanced, may effectually resist it and may cause it to retrograde, the process being analogous to that which we see imperfectly going on around a cancerous growth.

As a result of a study of the subject, the author believes the following conclusions are warranted :

1. There are large numbers of cases of different grades of severity and varying character which seem to be benefited by operation alone, some of them by almost any operation.

2. These cases include chiefly epilepsy, certain abdominal tumors, and peritoneal effusions and tubercle, though the improvement in the latter is, perhaps, to be explained on general principles.

3. Of the possible factors which, by reason of their constancy, must be considered, anæsthesia seems least likely to have been effective. The other three—viz., psychical influence, relief of tension, and reflex action—may enter in varying degrees into the therapeutics of these cases, and taken together, serve to render the occurrence of occasional cures less mysterious.

4. The theory of accident or coincidence scarcely explains the facts satisfactorily.

———

DEEP URETHRAL MEDICATION IN THE TREAMENT OF URETHRAL CATARRH.

Some practical suggestions for deep urethral medication in the treatment of posterior urethral catarrh are made by KEYES (*Medical Record*, vol. xv., No. 4), whose position as a genito-urinary surgeon is such as to entitle any of his writings to careful consideration.

He again calls attention to the fact that it is impossible to say exactly what a stricture is, since every natural undulation of the canal may be so classed by the physician who is properly impregnated with the large-calibre-stricture idea, and hence he is sure to find what he looks for in every case of gleet.

Keyes states that the vast majority of chronic gleet cases have already been cut anteriorly in the urethra from one to eleven times, and that very few of them have been tested to ascertain whether they have posterior urethritis or not. He states that one may easily learn how to cure many, and diagnosticate all, cases. Where the trouble is due to anterior urethral catarrh, caused by stricture, granulations, or what not, the source of the pus may be demonstrated without the endoscope by gentle, thorough, hot irrigation of the anterior urethra by means of a soft catheter passed into the sinus of the bulb, and the immediate subsequent use of the simple metallic bulbous bougie, provided the meatus be reasonably large; for if the pus comes from granular or strictured portions of the pendulous urethra, the irrigation will only wash away what lies loose in the canal, and the bulb will subsequently bring forth upon its shoulder soft muco-purulent clots, generally tinged with blood, which have been scraped off the excoriated areas from around which the inflamed mucous membrane secretes whatever free pus exists. There may be tight areas, which the bulb will detect; but if there be not a granulating surface upon the tight area or behind it, which the bloody muco-purulent clots on the shoulder of the bulb will demonstrate, or their absence disprove, then the cutting of such tight areas will not favorably modify gleet in most instances. Even though there may be some tight areas and a moderate condition of granulation, if there is also posterior urethritis the cutting of the tight areas, although it may greatly moderate, will not cure the gleet; and this should be told a patient before such operation is undertaken.

When there is posterior urethritis the quantity of pus lying in the urethra behind the bulbo-membranous junction is disproportionately great when compared with the amount of gleety discharge that appears at the meatus. This may be readily demonstrated. If the urethra be milked by firm pressure with the finger, from the perineum forward, until all the pus that will come be squeezed out, and then the patient be instructed to urinate in two parts, into separate glasses, if he have even moderate posterior urethritis the quantity of pus mixed with the first urinary gush, representing the washing out of the deep urethra, will be disproportionately great when compared with what has flowed out spontaneously from the meatus or been milked out by the physieian before the urinary act, as shown by gross inspection of the specimen. And if the grade of posterior urethritis be intenso, not only will the first urinary gush be purulent, but also the entire secondary flow will be turbid with pus. In case of doubt, the anterior urethra may be irrigated before the urinary test is applied. The pus may, of course, come from the prostate gland or the seminal vesicles; but this may be demonstrated by milking of these organs by means of a finger in the rectum, between the first and second urinary flows, urine being retained in the bladder to be ejected in a third urinary discharge, and the specimens to be examined microscopically after settling.

The clinical picture of posterior urethritis is fairly typical. After the subsidence of an acute attack of gonorrhœa, which has, perhaps, been complicated by cystitis or vesical irritability, there follows a mild gleet. So long as the patient uses an injection, his urethra remains dry and he thinks himself cured. On leaving off this treatment, however, the discharge reappears, sometimes accompanied by discomforting sensations in the anterior urethra near the meatus, or referred to the perineum, and sometimes accompanied by urinary urgency and precipitancy. Wines, spirits, or indulgence in sexual intercourse promptly aggravate the gleet. Most of these cases have the anterior urethra widely cut for a close stricture of large calibre, and are subsequently treated by large sounds, often with much benefit; frequently, however, the passage of these instruments aggravates the discharge and lights up either cystitis, prostatitis, or epididymitis. Most of these cases ultimately get well, and without local treatment.

Rest, balsams, alkalies, demulcent drinks, counter-irritations, change of air, treating of the anterior urethra, iron in chronic cases, all of these are potential, and most of these can be happily combined with local posterior treatment. Some few cases are positively unsuited to local treatment and get worse under it. Most tubercular cases, and some simple inflammatory and some ordinary gonorrhœal cases, can be classed in this group. When the treatment disagrees, symptoms become so promptly and obviously aggravated that the futility of repeating applications is at once clear. There is no danger of producing cystitis or epididymitis if instruments are used carefully and not inserted too far; the risk incurred of occasioning these symptoms is vastly less than in treating the disease with anterior injections or sounds and internal medication. The instrument employed is founded upon Ultzmann's model, differing from the latter in being made in one piece. The syringe has only one minute opening at the tip. The latter may be inserted just within the hole in the triangular ligament, that is a trifle beyond the bulbo-membranous junction. The membranous urethra grasps the tip of the instrument, and the contents of the syringe, twenty minims, or more, may be gently thrown in ; the entire injection will flow backward along the membranous urethra, through the prostate, and into the bladder, with as little violence as possible, not one drop escaping at the meatus upon the withdrawal of the syringe. Instead of using a few drops of strong solution it is better to use a larger quantity of a mild solution. The entire contents of the syringe should be used in every instance, excepting when nitrate of silver is employed in a strength greater than ten grains to the ounce, The strength of a given substance is increased gradually after establishing tolerance to milder strengths. When the source of the flow of pus is reasonably well forward in the urethra the injection may be made before the patient urinates; when the inflamma-tion extends further backward, and the supply of pus is considerable, the patient should urinate just before making the injection, so that the fluid will flow into the bladder and become thoroughly applied to the mucous mem-brane at the internal prostatic urethral orifice, without being diluted or neu-tralized by coming in contact with urine in the bladder at this point.

In suitable cases the free pus disappears from the second urinary flow, then it disappears entirely from the urine, some shreds still remaining. These are attacked by increasing the strength of the injected fluid, or if there be some stricture in the membranous urethra by the use of sounds, after the catarrhal surface has been modified by the previous employment of injections, com-bined often with anterior astringent injections, which the patient himself administers.

After an extensive use of the various remedies which have the repute of controlling the flow of pus from mucous membranes, Keyes relies almost ex-clusively upon four substances—sulphate of thallin, sulphate of copper, glyce-role of tannin, and nitrate of silver.

The sulphate of thallin is bland and practically unirritating, and may be used up to a saturated solution, which is about twenty-four per cent. It is suitable in all the acuter forms of inflammation (except cases of acute frank, recent gonorrhœal cystitis, in which the nitrate of silver has the preference), and is the substance which should first be used in a watery solution of about three per cent., increasing at each injection up to six, nine, and even twelve per cent. The last-named strength will usually accomplish all that this drug can do in reducing the free secretion of pus. The intervals between injec-tion should be two, three, or four days, according to the effect. The treat-ment causes practically no discomfort, and the injection may be retained as long as the patient chooses.

The sulphate of copper is used in the strength of one per cent. in pure glycerin. This solution is given in water, commencing with about one grain to the ounce and working up rapidly to full strength. This drug is markedly astringent in suitable cases.

Where a more astringent effect is aimed at than that produced by copper, the glycero-tannin may be employed. This substance is too thick to be sucked readily into a syringe. It is thinned by the addition of water.

Nitrate of silver is exceedingly valuable in gonorrhœal cystitis, and is most useful when copper and tannin prove inefficient. The first injection should be of the strength of about one grain to the ounce. The applications are made from three to eight days apart, and are increased in strength to ten grains to the ounce. This is the harshest of the applications, but carefully used is free from danger of producing complication, and is very efficient. Thallin and nitrate of silver should not be used in the same syringe, as a black solution is made which is difficult to wash out.

OTOLOGY.

UNDER THE CHARGE OF

CHARLES H. BURNETT, M.D.,
AURAL SURGEON, PRESBYTERIAN HOSPITAL, ETC., PHILADELPHIA.

OPERATION FOR THE RELIEF OF DEAFNESS, NOISES IN THE HEAD AND EARS, AND VERTIGO, DUE TO CHRONIC CATARRH OF THE DRUM OF THE EAR.

In this brochure of fourteen pages (*Archives of Otology*, 1891, Part 2), DR. SAMUEL SEXTON, of New York, gives the results of the operation of excision of the membrana and the two larger ossicula as carried out by him. Very interesting notes of seven cases are given, and Dr. Sexton then says that the list of cases might be extended if space permitted him. He offers the following conclusions:

"In certain cases the advance of progressive sclerosis, and consequent deafness, tinnitus, etc., cannot be arrested, nor, indeed, can any permanent improvement in hearing be made by means of any known local medication, directed either to the ear itself or the throat. On the contrary, valuable time may be frittered away in useless experimentation until the disease has become more and more firmly seated. This is the more lamentable in younger patients, when deafness is but beginning and is therefore amenable to an operation. The deafness due to progressive ankylosis of the ossicula may be arrested in most cases, and where the operation does not improve hearing the further increase of deafness is thus prevented. . . . . All the manipulations in performing the operation are carried on in the ear through the ordinary ear speculum, introduced into the external auditory meatus." The operation is carried on under narcosis, is not attended, therefore, with pain, and there is seldom any reaction or feeling of soreness in the ear afterward. If regeneration of the membrana tympani occur, the new membrane may be cut away after the application of a 10 per cent. solution of cocaine. Regenerative processes are lessened, in Dr. Sexton's opinion, by abstaining from eating meat, both before and after the operation. The aim of the operation, of course, is to maintain an opening into the drum-cavity. An immediate result of the operation is generally an improvement in hearing high tones.

For a few hours after the operation the patient should maintain a recumbent position, and remain in the house a day or two. On the fourth day the patient may go out of doors.

If a new membrana form, the improved hearing may disappear, though this is not invariably the case, as observed by Lucae and by C. H. Burnett.

A NEW MODIFICATION IN BORIC ACID TREATMENT OF CHRONIC SUPPURATIVE OTITIS MEDIA.

This, according to SCHEIBE (*Münchener med. Wochenschrift*, 1891, No. 14), consists in the direct insufflation of boric acid powder into the drum-cavity through small perforations. It is to be accomplished by means of a powder-blower with very fine nozzle. All such manœuvres must be regarded as interfering with drainage and liable to induce damming of pus and septi-cæmic symptoms. [There can be no cure in such cases until perfect drainage is obtained and maintained. This can be accomplished but by excision of the membrana tympani and the two larger ossicula or their remnants.—REV.]

MÉNIÈRE'S VERTIGO AND THE SEMICIRCULAR CANALS.

The experiments of Flourens, which seemed to attribute to the semicircular canals the rôle of maintaining the equilibrium of the body, have been contro-verted by others to such an extent as to make it appear doubtful whether that part of the labyrinth is the seat of the lesion which determines the so-called vertigo of Ménière. The peculiar character of the vomiting, the fact that the latter symptom may occur suddenly without nausea, after irritation of the membrana tympani, the intimate connections between the pneumogastric and the auditory nerve at their origin, renders it more probable that the vertigo and cardiac symptoms are due to a reflex action in the pneumogastric dependent upon a lesion in some portion of the auditory nerve. The term Ménière's disease serves more frequently to mark ignorance of the lesion which occasions a series of symptoms often analogous but which are under the influence of very different causes.—(SIR WM. B. DALBY, Brit. Med. Journal, and Annales des Maladies de l'Oreille, etc., vol. xvii.)

AUDITORY AFFECTIONS IN TABES DORSALIS.

E. MORPURGO made a careful examination of fifty-three ataxic patients, and found that only ten possessed normal auditory apparatus.—Annales des Maladies de l'Oreille, etc., vol. xvii., 1891.

USE OF COLLODION IN RELAXATION OF THE MEMBRANA TYMPANI.

DR. LANNOIS, of Lyons, France, calls attention (Annales des Maladies de l'Oreille, etc., vol. xvii., No. 1) to the above-named treatment, first suggested, he says, by McKeown, of Belfast, in 1879. Employment of collodion has no inconveniences nor dangers, and the author thinks that it not only holds the relaxed membrana in proper position, by its contractive and extracting power, but also that it possesses a truly curative effect, as the patients con-tinue to hear better after the collodion film is removed from the ear.

Two cases are then told in detail illustrative of the good results of this treatment in relaxed conditions of the membrana tympani. McKeown recommended to paint the collodion on the membrana, but Lannois prefers to drop into the ear a few drops of the collodion after the membrana tympani has been pushed into the normal position by inflation of the tympanic cavity.

FORMS OF OTITIS MEDIA PURULENTA IN TUBERCULOUS SUBJECTS.

According to DR. T. BOBONE, there are two principal forms of otitis media purulenta occurring in tuberculous subjects, viz.:

1. A very characteristic form: The membrana tympani presents neither

thickening nor hyperæmia, but at most only a slight rosy blush. In its inferior portion, a perforation is found the edges of which are smooth and sharp. Beyond this perforation is seen the mucous membrane of the drum-cavity, smooth, without granulations or exudation. Hearing is found considerably diminished—even to one-fifth of its normal distance.

2. The second form is seen in those far advanced in phthisis. The membrana tympani is entirely destroyed. An upper arc of the membrana is found in the middle of which the malleus is suspended. The tympanic cavity is lined with a diphtheroid membrane, grayish-white in color, not to be removed by syringing. Later in this affection caries of the petrous bone and of the mastoid apophysis are found. In this advanced form the disease, which appeared first as an indolent otorrhœa, may cause acute pain. Suppuration is slight, but the hearing is greatly diminished.

Of these two forms the first is sometimes curable, or rather arrested *in situ*. The second is incurable, and it is difficult to allay the pain it causes.— *Annales des Maladies de l' Oreille*, etc., vol. xvii., No. 1.

————

HEMORRHAGES INTO THE LABYRINTH, IN CONSEQUENCE OF PERNICIOUS ANÆMIA.

DR. J. HABERMANN, of Prague, has reported a case of the above nature (*Prager med. Wochenschrift*). The patient was a young woman, twenty-one years old, who, with other symptoms of anæmia, became deaf a short time before death. The post-mortem examination revealed cicatrices in the stomach from peptic ulceration, follicular enteritis of the large intestine, intense anæmia, with hemorrhages into the meninges, the brain, the pharynx, pericardium, and small intestine, and also in the retina. Fatty degeneration of the myocardium. The right organ of hearing was examined by Habermann, and the middle ear was found entirely normal. Microscopic sections of the decalcified internal ear showed a normal internal auditory canal and auditory nerve. Numerous minute hemorrhages were seen in the cochlea; otherwise the cochlea was normal. Extensive hemorrhages were found in the vestibule and in the semicircular canals. The symptoms, deafness and roaring in the ears, shown in this case before death, are to be explained probably by the hemorrhages in the labyrinth. The vertigo, which was also marked, may be referred, perhaps, to the hemorrhage in the semicircular canals, or to the simultaneous lesions in the brain.

————

THE IMPORTANCE OF SURGICAL MEANS APPLIED TO THE NASO-PHARYNX IN THE RELIEF OF NASO-PHARYNGEAL AND MIDDLE EAR DISEASE.

DR. C. W. RICHARDSON, of Washington, D. C. (*Journal of the American Medical Association*), writes, among many valuable things, the following: " In showing how inadequate the ordinary treatment of ear affections under the care of the auro-ophthalmologist is, I do not wish it to be understood that I am to any extent an aural nihilist. I am afraid a great many of my medical *confrères* are claiming too much for the independent use of the forceps, cautery, snare, drills and saw (in nose and throat). I doubt very much of their curing all the ills to which the ear is subject, unless they at the same

time resort to a judicious use of aural therapeutic measures. Firmly convinced as I am of the value of naso-pharyngeal surgical methods, I have not
thrown away the leech, douche, paracentesis knife, Politzer bag, nor catheter
(for the ear); our only safeguard is the judicious use of these means, and the
acknowledgment of their just therapeutic value. On the other hand, we must
acknowledge the increased successfulness, or aid to success, in otological work
rendered by rhinal surgeons; but while acknowledging their achievements
one must remember that there are a vast number of aural cases falling under
our observation thoroughly independent of any change within the naso-
pharyngeal cavity, the relief of the one not arresting the retrogressive progress
of the other." The author alludes to sclerotic cases with patulous Eustachian
tubes. In these cases, if the patient is to have relief, he "must get it through
aural therapeutic measures employed in the hands of the skilled otologist."
It is nonsense for one to agitate ideas having in view the condemnation of
otological therapeutic methods—they have a vast field of usefulness. What
is desirable is that the aurist should become more of a rhinologist, and the
rhinologist more of an aurist. Unfortunately, "one does not find in aural
clinics that careful examination and treatment of the naso-pharyngeal cavity
as is carried out in rhinal clinics, nor in rhinal clinics that same care and
attention to the ears that one finds in aural clinics; and an appreciation of
the inadequacy of the routine treatment of the case as resorted to by the auro-
ophthalmologist."

DISEASES OF THE LARYNX AND CONTIGUOUS STRUCTURES.

UNDER THE CHARGE OF

J. SOLIS-COHEN, M.D.,

OF PHILADELPHIA.

MORBID GROWTHS OF THE LARYNX.

A globular laryngeal tumor, about twelve millimetres in diameter, removed
by DR. F. H. HOOPER, of Boston, from the anterior portion of the left vocal
band and ventricle of a man fifty-three years of age (*Medical Record*, March
7, 1891, illustrated), was found on microscopical investigation to be a telangi-
ectatic myxofibroma in a state of amyloid degeneration.

M. GAREL, of Lyon, reports (*Arch. Internat. de Lar.*, etc., 1891, No. 3) the
spontaneous recession, after tracheotomy, of a papilloma occupying the entire
left vocal band and the inter-arytenoid commissure of a child, four years of
age, and occurring as a result of laryngitis contracted in sequence to an attack
of influenza.

At the last meeting of the Pathological Society of London, DR. F. SEMON
and MR. SHATTOCK (*Medical Press and Circular*, May 27, 1891) showed a
papillomatous tumor which had been removed by the former from the left
ary-epiglottidean fold of a man, forty-four years of age, and which, prior to

its examination after being taken from the throat, was thought to be an angioma. It was completely surrounded by a shell of blood-clot, and this, together with the unusual position of the growth and the spontaneous hemorrhage occasioned by its presence, were the chief features of interest presented in connection with it.

DR. LUC reports (*Arch. Internat. de Lar.*, etc., March-April, 1891) an instance of multiple or diffuse fibro-adenoma of the laryngeal and pharyngeal mucous membrane. A soldier, twenty-six years of age, had some difficulty in glutition in the summer of 1889, for which he was subjected to nine months' active treatment with iodides without effect. When seen by Luc, in June, 1890, a rounded reddish-gray tumor the size of a nut was observed behind the right palatine fold. The larynx was obstructed by a number of similar tumors of varying size, in front of the arytenoid cartilages and along the posterior and lateral walls of the larynx. They were removed after protracted operative procedures with the incandescent electric snare, the electric cautery, and cutting forceps. Subsequently a similar tumor of large size was discovered on the superior surface of the soft palate, whence it was excised with cutting forceps. Adenoid vegetations existed in abundance, which were removed with Gottstein's knife. These growths were found by Dr. Dubar to be formed in great part of fibrous tissue, with well-developed glandular acini at various portions.

An instance of a very large myxoma of the larynx is recorded by M. AD. DUDEFOY from the laryngological clinic of the Hôpital Lariboisière (*Annales des Mal. de l'Oreille, du Larynx*, etc., April, 1891). A male cook, forty-six years of age, had been treated for some time as a subject of laryngeal tuberculosis. Personal and antecedent history was good. Inspiration was easily accomplished, but expiration was difficult. Exertion exaggerated the dyspnœa and produced temporary cyanosis. The respiratory difficulty had begun about six months previously, and had steadily increased. The intense dyspnœa, unfitting the patient for work, was of some three or four weeks' duration. There was hardly any cough. For some two months the voice had begun to be hoarse at moments, and, if persistently used, temporary aphonia ensued, subsiding after repose of the voice. For two days the voice had been permanently and totally veiled, being, in fact, almost indistinct.

On laryngoscopic inspection, the epiglottis was found normal. The arytenoid region and the arytenoid folds were normal, unswollen, and a little vascularized. There was some vascularization of the vestibule of the larynx, which did not appear tumefied. The glottis was completely obstructed, save for a minute passage posteriorly, by a voluminous rounded tumor, as large as the seed of an apricot, intensely red at some points and clearer at others. There was a slight evidence of hemorrhage at the most salient part of its surface. It appeared adherent to the left side of the larynx, in part to the ventricle, in part to the glottis. Being removed in fragments with forceps by Dr. Gouguenheim, it was found on histological examination by Dr. Latteux to be a characteristic myxoma, corneous exteriorly. The laryngoscopic aspect of the tumor and its microscopic characteristics are illustrated in the paper.

DR. GEORGE STOKER reports (*Journ. of Lar. and Rhin.*, 1891, No. 5) an instance of pedunculated malignant growth removed in fragments by electro-caustic snare from the vocal cord of a gentleman sixty-seven years of age, with subsequent electro-cauterization of the site of attachment. By one histologist it was pronounced a horny carcinoma, by the other an epitheliomatous growth. Success was complete as to voice and comfort of the patient, and there had been no recurrence nine months after the operation, although the affected vocal band remained deeply congested and somewhat thickened.

An inter-arytenoidal sarcoma, the size of a chestnut, was removed from the larynx of a woman, fifty-eight years of age, by M. GEVAERT six years ago (*Annales des Mal. de l'Oreille, du Larynx,* etc., June, 1891), and there has been no recurrence.

FOREIGN BODIES IN THE LARYNX, ETC.

DR. SCHOYLER, of Berlin, extracted (*Journ. of Lar. and Rhin.*, August, 1890) from the trachea of a girl of nineteen a needle attached to a feather. It had been aspirated, and could not be removed by traction on the feather. Laryngoscopic examination showed that it was fixed with one end in the bifurcation of the trachea and with the other on a tracheal ring. The needle was liberated by the aid of a probe introduced between it and the trachea.

A case of sudden death from escape of milk into the air-passages is reported by DR. EMILE MÜLLER (*Gaz. Méd. de Strasbourg,* April 5, 1890). A child, five months of age, had no other indisposition than slightly difficult respiration when lying on its back. One morning, after having been nursed and laid down, it made a grimace as though sick at the stomach, became blue, and died in a few moments. At the autopsy the thymus gland was found larger than is usual, and the larynx, trachea, right bronchus, and all its divisions were found filled with milk. The size of the thymus explained the difficulty of respiration alluded to.

MR. LENNOX BROWNE reports (*The Medical Press,* December 17, 1890) an instance of supposed laryngeal cancer or phthisis in a lady thirty-five years of age, from whose larynx he had removed an impacted plate of artificial teeth which, from the history, had been aspirated into the larynx twenty-three months previously, probably during an epileptic seizure. Six weeks after its removal the patient had regained twenty-three pounds of her lost weight. It is remarkable that laryngoscopic inspections had been made by four gentlemen who had failed to detect the presence of a foreign body.

DR. WILLIAM MACEWEN reports (*Glasgow Med. Journ.,* December, 1889) a case in which a nutshell lodged in the trachea for thirteen days was removed by tracheotomy during impending suffocation. It was found buried in the posterior wall of the trachea just under the cricoid cartilage, lying obliquely, and covered to a great extent with granulative tissue, one thin layer of which was spread over the surface of the nutshell. When removed with forceps its concave surface was found to contain a mass of granulation tissue surrounding a portion of the kernel.

An interesting case from the practice of PROF. SONNENBURG is reported by HERMES (*Deut. med. Ztg.,* June 23, 1890). A girl, aged seventeen years, had swallowed a needle the September previous, and had since suffered with intense gastric pains, compelling her to keep the body bent forward. The parts were cut down upon and a projecting point was found in the posterior edge of the transverse fascia. The peritoneum was incised at this point and the needle was found in a mass of connective tissue in which it had become engaged after having perforated the stomach.

WOUNDS OF THE LARYNX.

A gunshot wound of the larynx is reported by DR. G. FABIANI (*Arch. Ital. di Lar.*, July, 1890). A ball from a revolver penetrated the right wing of the thyroid cartilage. Tracheotomy became necessary the following day. Death by septicæmia ensued a few days later. The ball was found to have passed through the left ventricular and vocal bands and to have fractured the base of the left arytenoid cartilage.

FRACTURE OF THE LARYNX.

DR. UBERT CLARAC reports (*Gaz. des Hôp.*, September 25, 1890) an instance in a man, due to sudden contact against an iron plate which was projecting from a wagon, and which knocked him over backward. Although the symptoms were marked and cutaneous emphysema extensive, tracheotomy was not performed. Sudden dyspnœa and cyanosis occurred on the fourth day, and although tracheotomy was then performed, the patient expired as the trachea was opened. The cricoid cartilage was found to have suffered a double fracture one centimetre to each side of the middle line, and there was nearly complete rupture of the crico-tracheal membrane. The fracture to the right was complete, the fragment separated and the mucous membrane torn. The fracture to the left was in the form of a Y, the lower portion of which was vertical and inferior, and the fragments were in contact. The vocal bands and the ventricles were ecchymosed. The ary-epiglottic folds were the seat of considerable emphysema. Emphysema was extensive in the connective tissue of the mediastinum, the whole cellular tissue protruding hernia-like, when the thoracic covering was removed. The emphysema had invaded the entire trunk and the upper part of the hips. Both lungs were engorged. A little blood was in the trachea.

[It need hardly be said that the issue in this case exemplifies the importance of immediate tracheotomy in all cases of fracture of the larynx, even if performed only as a prophylactic measure; although it must be admitted that severe injury to the cricoid cartilage is fatal in the great majority of instances despite the most judicious management.—ED.]

SURGEON E. JEAUMAIRE reports (*Arch. de Med. et de Pharm. Militaire*, January, 1890) a case of multiple fracture of the larynx and of the hyoid bone in an artileryman. While engaged in helping to move an engine formed of two beams connected by a transverse bar of iron, he slipped and fell backward, the bar of iron striking the anterior portion of his neck violently. He expectorated considerable blood, was unable to swallow, and was aphonic. Palpation increased a violent pain felt in the swollen neck, chiefly over the hyoid bone and the thyroid cartilage. At each inspiration a slight depression was noted over the region of the greater horn of the left wing of the thyroid cartilage. There was no emphysema, and there was no crepitation. Death ensued on the seventh day. The hyoid bone was found to have sustained an incomplete fracture or fissure six millimetres in length directed vertically from the upper border of the bone to a point of union of the right horn with the body of the bone. The large horn of the right wing of the thyroid cartilage was completely fractured some millimetres above its union with the lateral face of the cartilage. A vertical fracture in the middle line separated the cartilage into two portions for its entire length, the edges being turned outward, especially on the left side. There were two symmetrical perpendicular fractures of the cricoid a little within the facets where the cricoid cartilage is articulated with the smaller horn of the thyroid cartilage, that on the right side being a centimetre in length, and that on the left being a little less extensive.

DERMATOLOGY.

UNDER THE CHARGE OF

LOUIS A. DUHRING, M.D.,

PROFESSOR OF DERMATOLOGY IN THE UNIVERSITY OF PENNSYLVANIA ;

AND

HENRY W. STELWAGON, M.D.,

CLINICAL LECTURER ON DERMATOLOGY IN THE JEFFERSON AND WOMAN'S MEDICAL COLLEGES.

PSOROSPERMOSE FOLLICULAIRE VÉGÉTANTE (DARIER).

A. R. ROBINSON, of New York (Canadian Practitioner, vol. xvi.), gives an admirable exposition of this subject, which is now attracting so much attention. According to Darier there exists in man a group of cutaneous diseases which merit the name of psorospermosis, being due to the presence in the epidermis of parasites of the order sporozaires, of the group psorosperms, or coccidia. In one of these diseases the coccidia of a particular species invade the follicular orifices of a greater portion of the cutaneous surface, where they appear in the form of round bodies, generally encysted and contained in the epithelial cells, or as refracting granules, the accumulation of which forms a plug which projects from the orifice of the follicle. This is the disease described by J. C. White as keratosis follicularis, and by Darier and Thibault under the name psorospermose folliculaire végétante. Darier adds, that " the presence of these bodies enables one to make a diagnosis of the disease, as they are not met with in any analogous clinical affection. The neck of the follicles invaded become secondarily the seat of papillomatous vegetations, which can develop to a great degree and form real tumors. The affection. from an etiological point of view, should be placed with Paget's disease of the nipple, and probably with molluscum contagiosum."

Neisser, of Breslau, regards molluscum contagiosum as caused by psorosperms, but this view is not as yet generally accepted—many pathologists, like Robinson and others, regarding the molluscum bodies as chemically changed epithelial cells and not organisms, although believing the disease to be a communicable one and parasitic in nature. In epithelioma, especially that clinical form known as Paget's disease of the nipple, which was generally considered to commence as an eczematous process, Wickham has endeavored to show that psorosperms are very abundant, and argues that they are essential factors of the disease and the cause of the anatomical changes which occur.

Robinson quotes the cases of J.C. White and of Darier, and gives the notes of a case observed by himself, Weiss and Lustgarten, of New York. All these cases represent the same affection. Dr. Robinson's microscopical studies upon his case show the disease to be a "para-typical" keratosis. Darier and Bowen (in White's case) came to similar conclusions.

APPLICATION OF DRYING-IN LINIMENTS (LINIMENTA EXSICCANTIA) IN THE TREATMENT OF SKIN DISEASES.

PROFESSOR PICK, of Prague (*Prager medicin. Wochenschr.*, Jahrgang xvi.), after referring to the gelatin preparations brought forward by him some years ago, calls attention to a new remedy with which he has been experimenting, namely, bassorin (obtained from tragacanth). This kind of gum differs from gum arabic in being almost insoluble, but swells up with water into a syrupy mass which permits of being smeared over and rubbed into the skin in a remarkably satisfactory manner, and drying-in as a thin and delicate covering or film. The formula given consists of tragacanth 5 parts, glycerin 2 parts, water 100 parts, which makes the best consistence. It may be prepared hot or cold. According to the latter method, the finely powdered tragacanth is rubbed with water, the mass taking on a smooth syrupy or lanolin-like character. The application is, when first used, cooling to inflamed skin. As it dries in, a fine, smooth, dry covering forms, with, in the case of inflamed skin, a feeling of tension, which however is not painful, and in its results is beneficial.

A variety of medicaments, both soluble and insoluble, may be added to the base, as in the case of the gelatin preparations and pastes.

BASSORIN PASTE: A NEW·BASE FOR DERMATOLOGICAL PREPARATIONS.

This paste, proposed by ELLIOTT (*Journal of Cutaneous and Genito-urinary Diseases*, vol. ix,) is composed of bassorin, glycerin, water and dextrin. The author's experience permits the following conclusions: 1. Bassorin paste is a perfectly neutral substance, which of itself produces no irritation whatever, and when used alone simply acts as a protective to the skin. It does not become rancid, or decompose, or undergo changes when kept for a length of time, unless it be exposed in an open vessel. When this is done it becomes dry and hard, but even then rubbing it up with a little water renders it again as serviceable as at first. 2. It is easy and simple in application, requiring only to be spread upon the skin with the finger or a brush. It dries in the space of a few minutes if so applied, adheres closely, does not rub off and soil the linen, but forms a flexible coat, which does not interfere with the movements of the body. When its removal is desired, the preparation can be washed off with a little water or a damp cloth or sponge. It remains *in situ* without change for a variable length of time, depending upon the condition of the surface on which it has been applied. 3. With the bassorin paste almost any drug can be incorporated: those which exist in the form of powders or in solid form in any amount desired; the tars, ichthyol, and oily substances in smaller percentages, but sufficient for all practical purposes. 4. The action of drugs incorporated with it and their effect upon disease appears to be as good as when such are used in other excipients—or perhaps better in some cases. 5. It is of wide applicability and of value in both acute and chronic forms of disease, its use being limited only by the degree of moisture on the surface being treated, or to which it may be exposed.

The exact proportions of the various constituents of this paste are not given by the writer, it being added that the chief one is bassorin.

REPORT OF A CASE OF LUPUS VULGARIS TREATED WITH KOCH'S TUBERCULIN.

LOOMIS and FULLER report (*Journal of Cutaneous and Genito-urinary Diseases*, 1891) a case of long-standing lupus treated successfully by Koch's method. The disease was complicated by an epitheliomatous growth. The case was under treatment twelve weeks, receiving in all twenty-two injections. Five weeks after the beginning of the treatment the disease appeared to be cured. Marked local changes and constitutional reaction occurred during the first two weeks, since which time fever reactions were noted but twice; local disturbances continued during the first month, becoming less and less perceptible. The epithelioma has shown no reparative changes, although the injections were followed by evidences of local reaction. The highest dose was 0.015 c.c. As to the permanency of the cure time must decide. An interesting feature was the fact that the lymph rendered apparent foci of disease before unrecognized.

LUPUS VULGARIS TREATED WITH TUBERCULIN: DEATH RESULTS.

A case of long-standing lupus of face treated with tuberculin, in which death followed thirty-six hours after an injection of two milligrammes, is reported (*Wien. klin. Wochenschrift*, iii. p. 972) by GARISCH. The patient was otherwise healthy. At the same time several other patients were being treated by the same fluid, but showed nothing more than the usual reactions. Following the injection the patient became somnolent; the next day heart action was so frequent that the pulse could not be counted. Patient failed to respond to stimulation and died of heart failure that evening.

At the autopsy were noted: pneumonic infiltration and œdema of the lungs, œdema of the brain and spinal cord, acute swelling of an already enlarged spleen, and slight parenchymatous swelling of liver and kidneys. The pleura, pericardium and spinal cord were the seats of capillary hemorrhages. The local disturbances in the lupus tissue were typical.

AN EXTENSIVE CASE OF FAVUS.

MORRIS places on record (*British Journal of Dermatology*, vol. iii.) an extremely unusual and extensive case of favus. The patient, a female, aged thirty-seven years, when coming under observation was suffering with acute phthisis, of which she soon died. Upon examination the scalp, trunk, arms were found to be the seat of favus crusts; the scalp completely covered, the trunk to a great extent, and the arms to a less degree. The finger-nails were also invaded. The disease, according to the statement of the patient, began on the scalp fourteen years previously, gradually involving the whole of that region; two months before coming under the writer's observation the back became affected, and from that time the disease had rapidly invaded other parts of the trunk and arms. The several points of interest in this case are: the extensive area involved, the late age (twenty-three years) at which disease first began, the involvement of the nails, and its rapid spread during the last stage of phthisis.

A CLINICAL STUDY OF PRURITUS HIEMALIS.

CORLETT reports (*Journal of Cutaneous and Genito-urinary Diseases*, vol. ix.) several cases of this disease—the so-called frost or winter itch. The author's observations as summarized are in the main the experience of others: " 1. That the state of the general health has no (?) appreciable effect upon the pruritus. 2. The local irritation of the clothing, although capable of aggravating the malady, is not of itself able to produce it. 3. Meteorological conditions appear to furnish the main etiological factor. These were most potent with a low temperature, low humidity and the wind blowing from the northwest. The greater the velocity of the wind, *cæteris paribus*, the more severe the itching. 4. Pruritus hiemalis is not infrequently associated with other neuroses of the skin."

The author places little reliance upon internal treatment, inasmuch as, with the possible exception of ichthyol, it proved negative. The most efficient local measures employed, which are in the main necessarily palliative, consisted of resorcin, ichthyol and menthol lotions, the first named being usually of greatest benefit. Change to a warm and humid climate, where also the temperature variations are but slight, is curative.

OBSERVATIONS ON TWO CASES OF LUPUS TREATED BY KOCH'S TUBERCULIN.

These two cases, reported by LESLIE PHILLIPS (*British Journal of Dermatology*, vol. iii.), represent deep-seated and superficial types of the disease. In the former case the patient, a male, aged twenty-six years, exhibited the disease, of eight years' duration, on the cheek and ear. In the other—superficial case—the patient, a female child, aged three and a half years, presented two patches, one on the centre of the cheek, and the other on the dorsum of the hand; this latter was secondary, and was, the writer believed, due to auto-infection, the child having the habit of sleeping with this part of the hand curled under and applied to the cheek. Both cases were perseveringly treated by injections of tuberculin in increasing doses, with characteristic reaction. The result in the deep-seated variety was negative; in the superficial type—the child—the result was satisfactory, the two patches " were smooth, pale-red in color, homogeneous in appearance, and entirely free from nodules, either in the cicatrix or in the margin." Six weeks later, " The scar on the back of the hand is paler, and no suspicion of lupus present; but the periphery of the patch on the cheek is redder, and at one or two points are seen spots which suggest the return of lupous foci."

OBSTETRICS.

UNDER THE CHARGE OF

EDWARD P. DAVIS, A.M., M.D.,

PROFESSOR OF OBSTETRICS AND DISEASES OF CHILDREN IN THE PHILADELPHIA POLYCLINIC;
CLINICAL LECTURER ON OBSTETRICS IN THE JEFFERSON MEDICAL COLLEGE;
VISITING OBSTETRICIAN TO THE PHILADELPHIA HOSPITAL, ETC.

PERFORATION OF THE UTERUS FOLLOWING AN INTRA-UTERINE DOUCHE; SUBLIMATE POISONING.

GEBHARD (*Zeitschrift für Geburtshülfe und Gynäkologie*, Band xxi., Heft 2) reports an interesting case in which intra-uterine douches were given to a multipara in the treatment of gonorrhœa. The patient was not pregnant at the time. While the third douche was being given the patient complained of pain in the abdomen, followed by giddiness, vomiting, and unconsciousness. Rapid pulse, with pallid features and perspiration, followed her recovery from the shock of the injection. Symptoms of mercurial intoxication, with bloody, mucous diarrhœa supervened; the patient dying eight days after the injection. On post-mortem examination two perforations of the uterus were found, admitting a uterine sound readily. The sublimate solution, 1 : 5000, had been absorbed by the peritoneum. Microscopic examination of the kidneys showed the epithelium of the tubules infiltrated with an amorphous substance from which calcium crystals were readily produced by treating with sulphuric acid.

PUERPERAL PSYCHOSES, WITH REFERENCE TO ECLAMPSIA.

OLSHAUSEN (*Ibid.*) reviews the literature of the puerperal psychoses with especial reference to the relation between them and eclampsia. He concludes that psychoses are not rare after eclampsia, developing usually from two to four days after the eclamptic outbreak. Hallucinations are constant, the derangement proceeds rapidly, without fever, and usually tends to eventuate in recovery. Mental derangement persisting for several months is rare after eclampsia. It is as yet impossible to say what cases of eclampsia especially predispose to psychoses; mental derangement follows various intoxications, and among these are affections following chronic kidney lesions and uræmia.

Olshausen divides puerperal psychoses into: 1. Those following fever—infection psychoses. 2. Idiopathic, without fever or constitutional cause; under this head are included the greater part of the psychoses of the puer-

peral state, that accompanying lactation and following hemorrhage at labor.
3. Intoxication psychoses, following eclampsia, or exceptionally with uræmia
without eclampsia.

KNOTS IN THE CORD IN TWIN PREGNANCIES.

An instance of this rare complication of pregnancy is reported by HERR-
MANN (*Archiv für Gynäkologie*, Band xl. Heft 2). But sixteen cases could be
recorded, and as this complication can only arise when the twins occupy the
same fœtal sac, its occurrence is rare.

Herrmann's case was one of twin abortion in a multipara, following a fall.
The cords seemed fused together in an ovoid mass, which on careful examination was found to be two intertwined figure-of-eight knots. Such inter-
twining of cords has been observed to follow violent fœtal movements, and
also sudden exertion on the mother's part. In the great majority of cases
fœtal death and premature labor follow.

PREGNANCY COMPLICATED BY FIBRO-CYST OF THE OVARIAN LIGAMENT; ECTOPIC PREGNANCY, TREATED BY LAPAROTOMY.

DOLÉRIS (*Nouvelles Archives d'Obstétrique et de Gynécologie*, No. 7, 1891)
reports the case of a woman who bore a dead child after a protracted labor
complicated by the presence of a fibro-cyst of the ovarian ligament. Recovering from this labor she became again pregnant and bore a living child at
term. When lactation ceased, her menstruation became deranged, and she
consented to laparotomy for the removal of the tumor. This was readily
accomplished, the mass proving to be what had been diagnosticated. Uninterrupted recovery followed.

Doléris also reports the case of a woman, married eight years without conception. After amenorrhœa of two months' duration, she expelled a membranous mass from the uterus, with great pain. On examination the uterus
was found slightly enlarged. A small tumor could be felt on the left side,
behind the uterus. A diagnosis of salpingitis with hæmato-salpinx was
made and the uterus was curetted and disinfected. Three days later laparotomy was performed, when tubal pregnancy was found on the left side,
and upon the right a sclerosed ovary. The patient made an uninterrupted
recovery after the removal of both.

THE PROTECTION OF THE PERINEUM DURING THE PASSAGE OF THE SHOULDERS.

COUDER (*Archives de Tocologie et de Gynécologie*, No. 7, 1891) has found it
of advantage to unfold an arm when the shoulders present with folded arms
after the expulsion of the head. When a hand presents before the shoulders,
it should be drawn down and the arm entirely delivered. When this is not
possible, the hips of the mother should be raised, and when the head has
rotated externally, the head must be pulled down and the anterior arm
freed to the elbow. The elbow is then to be flexed toward the back of the
fœtus and the anterior arm entirely extracted. The head is then to be raised
and the trunk allowed to emerge slowly.

THE DEVELOPMENT OF THE PLACENTA.

A possible explanation of some clinical facts is afforded by YOUNG, in a summary, the results of investigations upon the development of the placenta. It seems probable that the fœtal epiblast extends over the greater part of the placental area, replacing the maternal decidua and resembling in its growth the formation of epithelial tumors. This mass of epithelium is tunnelled by blood spaces communicating with maternal bloodvessels into which fœtal capillaries, free from epithelial investment, project.

These facts explain the ready passage of micrococci from mother to fœtus. Fœtal nutrition results from ready diffusion through the walls of the capillaries. After abortion, retained placental epithelium and continued development of fœtal epithelium may result in carcinoma.—*The Medical Chronicle*, No. 4, 1891.

———

MATERNAL IMPRESSION FOLLOWED BY THE PRODUCTION OF A MONSTER.

An interesting example of the direct association of maternal impression and the production of monsters is given by GROUND (*Northwestern Lancet*, No. 15, 1891). A primipara, illegitimately pregnant, gave birth to a seven-months' fœtus in which the arch of the skull was absent, and other malformations existed, giving the fœtus an especially horrible appearance. Shortly after, a pregnant patient saw the monster in a jar in a physician's office, and was deeply impressed by its appearance. Six weeks after seeing the monster, she aborted at four months with a monster closely resembling the first.

———

GYNECOLOGY.

———

UNDER THE CHARGE OF

HENRY C. COE, M.D., M.R.C.S.,
OF NEW YORK.

———

THE ACTION OF THE GALVANIC CURRENT UPON UTERINE FIBROIDS.

BÄCKER (*Centralblatt für Gynäkologie*, No. 28, 1891) reports a case in which intra-uterine galvanization was employed for five months at intervals of two or three days, the strength of the current varying from 50 to 140 milliampères. At the end of this period the tumor had decreased in size one-half, several necrosed fragments having been discharged *per vaginam*. From a careful analysis of similar recorded cases it appears that whenever a fibroid tumor is positively reduced in size by the action of galvanism, this is due to softening of the deeper parts of the neoplasm, with subsequent contraction of the surrounding tissue. There is probably an actual formation of thrombi in the vessels of the tumor. The process of electrolysis does not consist so much in a decomposition of the albumins; the current follows principally the course of the vessels and secondarily decomposes the interstitial fluid. The necrotic process which follows is aseptic and is unaccompanied with fever or other evidences of inflammation, as in cases reported by Gusserow. This is a strong argument in favor of the powerful antiseptic action of the positive pole, as claimed by Apostoli.

FIBROMA OF THE OVARY.

At a recent meeting of the Vienna Obstetrical Society, LIHOTZSKY presented a fibrous tumor of the ovary, weighing six pounds, which had been complicated with ascites. It was removed successfully from a patient twenty-three years of age. Chrobak stated that he had removed a similar neoplasm of smaller size, which was also attended with ascites. The latter complication, which was usually present only with malignant growths, he believed was due to excessive dilatation of the vessels, although Olshausen ascribed it to irritation of the parietal peritoneum. Hofmokl held that in the ascites accompanying ovarian fibromata the fluid was clear, whereas in cases of malignant disease it possessed a characteristic turbidity. [No satisfactory explanation has yet been offered for the presence of ascites in connection with ovarian fibromata. The accumulation of fluid is entirely out of proportion to the size of the tumor, which would seem to disprove the theory of peritoneal irritation. Moreover, the smaller fibromata are often hard and non-vascular; the vessels in the pedicle are of average size, and there is no evidence of venous obstruction and dilatation. It is well known that these tumors have usually long pedicles and are seldom adherent, so that they are freely movable. This fact would seem to suggest the possibility of the ascites being due to direct pressure upon large veins, were it not for the absence of œdema of the lower extremities. Torsion of the pedicle may exist without ascites. We have discussed this interesting class of neoplasms at length in the *American Journal of Obstetrics*, vol. xv. p. 561.—H. C. C.]

ABDOMINAL EXTIRPATION OF THE FIBROID UTERUS.

LIHOTZSKY (*Wiener klin. Wochenschrift*, No. 27, 1891) reports ten cases of abdominal hysterectomy in Chrobak's clinic with only one death, from causes independent of the operation.

Chrobak's technique is briefly as follows: After ligating the broad ligaments, the operator dissects off the peritoneum anteriorly and posteriorly, and separates the bladder as low as the vaginal fornix. The cervix is then constricted with a rubber cord, the tumor is removed, and the cavity of the stump is packed with iodoform gauze (after being thoroughly cauterized), which is closed in with temporary sutures. The vaginal fornix is then opened, a sound being introduced from below as a guide; the uterine arteries are tied, and the stump is removed. After tamponing the wound from above, the edges of the peritoneum are united in such a way as to cover in the stumps of the broad ligaments, and the abdominal wound is closed, drainage being maintained *per vaginam*. The advantages of this method over supra-vaginal amputation are not only the avoidance of the danger of sloughing of the stump, but the shortening of the period of convalescence, and the doing away with repeated dressing of the wound. The operation is practically reduced to the level of a simple ovariotomy, and there is no unsightly and painful cicatrix, or risk of hernia. The patients are free from the discomfort incident to traction of the stump.

[This would appear to be the ideal operation for fibroids, although the technique is not new, as the writer admits the closure of the peritoneum to be the essential improvement. When the patient is placed in Trendelenburg's posture, as recommended by Dr. Krug, of New York, we have found that total extirpation of the uterus can, in an ordinary case, be performed with the expenditure of but little more time or labor than supra-vaginal amputation. Whether the removal of the stump seriously weakens the pelvic floor, and leads to subsequent prolapse of the vagina and bladder, is a point to be settled only after a number of patients have been kept under prolonged observation.—H. C. C.]

The Ultimate Results of Vaginal Hysterectomy for Cancer.

Leisse (*Archiv für Gynäkologie*, Band xl., Heft 2) replies to the criticisms of the statistics of the Dresden clinic by presenting a tabulated statement of the histories of all the patients, so far as they could be obtained. These are compiled with great care. Of eighty patients who were heard from upwards of two years after the operation, 56.25 per cent. were still living. Since eight of the deaths were not due to a recurrence of the disease, this leaves the actual mortality only 17.8 per cent. Thirty-seven of the forty-five surviving patients were examined at the clinic, so that there was no question as to their local condition, and in the other cases reports were received from competent physicians. The following are the facts: Of eighty patients examined over two years after operation, forty-five were free from recurrence; 58.6 per cent. (out of fifty-eight patients examined) were well after three years; 59.5 per cent. (out of forty-two) after four years; 60 per cent. (out of thirty) after five years; 66.6 per cent. (out of nine) after six years; and the two patients who had survived the operation seven years were both perfectly well. [The writer properly makes no comment on these statistics. They need none. So conscientiously have they been compiled that no room is left for scepticism. The opponents of vaginal hysterectomy will find in them food for reflexion.—H. C. C.]

The Results of High Amputation of the Cervix Uteri for Cancer.

Winter (*Ibid.*) commends the operation in cases of commencing epithelioma of the portio vaginalis. Subsequent observation of patients on whom high amputation has been performed has shown that not only is conception possible, but that parturition may occur normally. Obstructive dysmenorrhœa is rare after the operation, and is easily overcome; neither has the writer observed the development of marked endometritis, as claimed by Schauta. The principal argument in favor of high amputation, in incipient cases, as compared with total extirpation, is the less danger attending the former operation. At the Berlin clinic 35.7 per cent. of the patients were free from recurrence upward of two years after operation.

[The relative claims of the two operations could be more accurately determined if operators would only state clearly the exact anatomical condition in every case of total extirpation. It goes without saying that when the disease is limited to the portio, the chances of recurrence after either operation are vastly less than when it has extended along the cervical canal as high as the os internum. We may safely assume that, in the hands of an expert operator, recurrence within six months after total extirpation means that the case was not a proper one for the radical operation. Every honest surgeon ought to be willing to frankly acknowledge this. Americans will never succeed in settling this vital question until they lay aside personal, and what might be termed national, prejudices and discuss it in a broad scientific spirit.—H.C.C.]

THE AFTER-TREATMENT OF LAPAROTOMY.

KEHRER (*Ibid.*) read a paper on this subject at the recent meeting of the German Gynecological Society, in which he referred to the fact that the diminution in the mortality was due to the simplification of the technique. In a considerable proportion of the fatal cases death was due to heart-failure, pneumonia, and chloroform. The greatest danger from the operation, he believed, was due to the escape into the cavity of septic fluids, especially pus, fecal matter and portions of malignant growths. The usual practice was to remove these by sponging and irrigation, but the reader believed that it was better to prevent them from escaping by surrounding the pedicle of the tumor with a rubber cloth in the form of a sleeve and packing its cavity with gauze, so that any fluid which escaped would at once be absorbed. The pedicle could then be tied and the entire mass be removed without exposing the tumor.

In order to prevent the formation of adhesions no antiseptic fluids should be brought in contact with the peritoneum, nor should any strong antiseptic be applied to the stump. Early evacuation of the bowels was correct both in theory and practice, since after every abdominal section the intestines were in a state of atony. Finally, it was highly important that there should be a firm cicatrix in the line of the incision in order to prevent the subsequent development of hernia. If the linea alba was much relaxed it was better, he thought, to excise sufficient tissue to obtain firm union.

THE CONDITION OF THE OVARIES IN CASES OF FIBRO-MYOMA.

HOFMEIER (*Ibid.*) calls attention to Hegar's theory that after castration not only is the influence of the ovarian nisus eliminated, but a diminished amount of blood is supplied to the tumor. He believes that in the majority of the cases the latter fact alone explains the cure. In two instances he found the ovaries atrophied, with few or no traces of ovisacs, yet hemorrhage ceased after their removal. He asks if the same result might not be obtained by simply ligating the ovarian arteries.

BULIUS (*Ibid.*) has examined the ovaries in fifty cases of uterine fibro-myoma, and finds that anatomical changes are the rule. He makes the following deductions: 1. In cases of fibro-myoma the ovaries undergo changes. 2. The stroma is the seat of both hyperplasia and hypertrophy. 3. The vessels are the seat of marked changes. 4. Cystic degeneration of the Graafian follicles is common. 5. The primordial follicles are destroyed.

[Every pathologist will be inclined to agree with the latter writer. Hofmeier's deductions are clearly founded on insufficient anatomical evidence.— H. C. C.]

THE INFLUENCE OF THE CLIMACTERIC UPON FIBRO-MYOMATA.

MÜLLER (*Ibid.*) has made a careful study of this subject, based upon 109 cases. He found that while in many cases the tumor evidently diminished in size after the menopause, in nine instances it was clearly proved that the neoplasm continued to grow; such an increase in size was noted in women aged fifty-six and seventy-nine respectively. He infers that it is not safe to trust too much to the curative influence of the menopause.

In opening the discussion Werth took occasion to differ from Hofmeier regarding the effect of castration. The removal of the ovaries had, he believed, a direct atrophic influence upon the tumor. When menstruation ceases its vascular supply is diminished, but if the hemorrhages continue atrophy does not take place. Tait's statements on this question were valueless.

Benckiser stated that in examining a fibroid uterus removed three months after castration had been performed, he found the same atheromatous changes in the vessel walls which were so often observed after the climacteric. This was a form of obliterating endarteritis which Thoma had described as a result of extensive arrest of the capillary circulation of an organ.

Veit said that he had seen large myomata increase in size in elderly women. He did not expect retrograde changes to take place in the tumor before the age of fifty or fifty-four. Progressive increase of the neoplasm after the climacteric must be due to some unusual source of blood-supply.

Fritsch had found that the occurrence of both the artificial and the natural climacteric arrested the growth of the tumor. If it continued to grow, it was usually due to cystic degeneration of the neoplasm.

Note to Contributors.—All contributions intended for insertion in the Original Department of this Journal are only received *with the distinct understanding that they are contributed exclusively to this Journal.*

Contributions from the Continent of Europe and written in the French, German or Italian language, if on examination they are found desirable for this Journal, will be translated at its expense.

Liberal compensation is made for articles used. A limited number of extra copies in pamphlet form, if desired, will be furnished to authors in lieu of compensation, *provided the request for them be written on the manuscript.*

All communications should be addressed to

DR. EDWARD P. DAVIS,
250 South 21st Street, Philadelphia.

THE

AMERICAN JOURNAL

OF THE MEDICAL SCIENCES.

NOVEMBER, 1891.

CONDITIONS UNDERLYING THE INFECTION OF WOUNDS.[1]

By William H. Welch, M.D.,

PROFESSOR OF PATHOLOGY, JOHNS HOPKINS UNIVERSITY.

THAT the presence of certain kinds of bacteria is an essential condition of wound infection is a fact so well established, and so generally recognized, that no discussion as to this point is likely to arise in this assembly. The practical results of the application of this doctrine to the management of wounds are the most eloquent testimony to its life-saving truth. The recognition of this truth, even before its complete demonstration, and the introduction of methods of wound treatment based upon it, will remain the immortal merit of Lister, even although every detail of his treatment be replaced by measures found by riper experience to be better suited to the purpose.

The simple conception which was the basis of early antiseptic procedures in surgery—that a wound to which bacteria gain access becomes infected in the same way as a sterilized infusion of meat undergoes putrefaction when a single suitable germ enters—has been greatly modified. Furthermore, it is found that the traumatic infections present their own peculiar problems, which must be studied by themselves, and

---

[1] Paper of the Referee, read at the meeting of the Second Congress of American Physicians and Surgeons in Washington, D. C., September 22, 1891.

The full title of the subject proposed for discussion was: "Conditions Underlying the Infection of Wounds: including a Discussion of Disinfection with Reference to Treatment of Wounds, of the Relation of Bacteria to Suppuration, of the Resistance of Tissues to the Multiplication of Bacteria, and of the Effects of Antiseptic Agents on Wounds."

cannot be solved by analogies drawn from observations of other specific infections, such as anthrax and the septicæmias of the lower animals. The study of wound infections involves the consideration of many varying and often complicated factors, relating both to the agents of infection and to the individual exposed to infection.

Without consuming time with any historical review, I shall proceed at once to indicate some of the questions which are of especial importance, and which may be profitably considered in this discussion.

What are the microörganisms concerned in the infection of wounds, and how do they act?

How are we to explain the great differences in the effects produced by the pyogenic bacteria, their apparent harmlessness under some conditions, their fatal virulence in others?

What are the ways by which bacteria gain access to a wound?

How often are bacteria to be found in wounds treated antiseptically or aseptically? What are the characters of these bacteria and whence do they come?

What are the best means of surgical disinfection?

No attempt can be made on this occasion to treat exhaustively a single one of these questions. My aim will be to present a brief survey of our knowledge, as well as of the defects in our knowledge, concerning some of the more important questions; to offer some results of personal observation and experiment, and to indicate in conjunction with the Co-referee the lines which this discussion may follow. It does not seem necessary, indeed it would be presumptious before this audience, to dwell in detail upon established facts which are the common property of all who are interested in the subject.

So far as personal observations and experiments are concerned, I may say that these have been made in the Johns Hopkins Hospital and Pathological Laboratory, and that I am indebted to several of my colleagues and co-workers there for work which they have done either independently or under my supervision. I take this opportunity of acknowledging especially the assistance of Drs. Halsted, Abbott, Ghriskey, Robb, and Howard.

This paper will relate only to the ordinary inflammatory and suppurative traumatic affections, and not to specific wound infections, like tetanus, diphtheria, and hospital gangrene.

It would be wearisome on this occasion to consider or even enumerate all the bacteria which have been found in suppurative and other traumatic inflammatory processes, so that in this connection I shall touch only upon a few points drawn chiefly from our own experience.

We have found the staphylococcus pyogenes aureus far more frequently than any other species of bacteria in furuncles, abscesses, osteomyelitis, and other forms of suppuration. The prevalence in Strassburg, according to Levy, of the staphylococcus pyogenes albus in all kinds of suppurative inflammation (excepting furuncles), raises the question whether there may not be differences in different regions as regards the relative frequency of the various kinds of pyogenic cocci.

We have, however, met a white staphylococcus in a certain class of cases with great frequency, viz., in small stitch abscesses, and in the slighter grades of inflammatory disturbance of wounds treated antiseptically or aseptically. This coccus has been often seen by Bossowski and others in the same class of wounds, and has been hitherto identified with the staphylococcus pyogenes albus of Rosenbach, but we have some hesitation in so regarding the micrococcus which we have found in the cases mentioned. The staphylococcus pyogenes albus is generally described as not differing essentially from the aureus, except by the absence of the yellow color in the cultures. This coccus, however, differs from the staphylococcus pyogenes aureus in much greater slowness of liquefaction of gelatin and of coagulation of milk, and in far less virulence when inoculated into the circulation of rabbits. It may be an attenuated form of the staphylococcus pyogenes albus. Until this is settled I propose to call it the staphylococcus epidermidis albus, as it is an almost constant inhabitant of the epidermis, as will be apparent when I come to speak of the bacteria in aseptic wounds. I shall only add here that this coccus may be present in graver suppurative inflammations, but then it has been nearly always associated with some other pyogenic organism, or has assumed the form of the typical staphylococcus pyogenes albus.

It is, perhaps, not out of place to remark that the diagnosis of the staphylococcus pyogenes albus in cultures from abscesses and other suppurations should not be made too hastily. It may require several days before colonies of the aureus assume a distinct yellow color. Cultures upon potato are particularly favorable for the speedy development of this color. There may be marked differences in the rapidity with which different colonies of the aureus from the same source and in the same plate or roll cultures turn yellow.

The efforts to differentiate into distinct species the pathogenic streptococci have thus far met with little success, so that the weight of opinion favors the view that the streptococci of erysipelas, of phlegmonous inflammations, of septicæmia, of puerperal fever, and of various forms of angina, belong to one and the same species. In conformity with the results of most investigators I have been unable to determine any decisive differences between the streptococcus erysipelatus and the streptococcus pyogenes. Von Lingelsheim has recently divided the streptococci into two groups: one non-pathogenic, called the streptococcus brevis, and the other pathogenic, the streptococcus longus. Among the points of distinction which he gives there is one which I have not found constant, viz., the invisible growth of all pathogenic streptococci upon potato. The behavior is usually as stated by Von Lingelsheim, but I have isolated from a case of phlegmonous cellulitis, and from one of septicæmia, a streptococcus presenting a distinct grayish-white growth upon potato. Von Lingelsheim made no use of one of our most valuable differentiating media, viz., sterilized milk colored with litmus. In this medium the common streptococcus pyogenes produces a very firm coagulum with separation of nearly colorless serum, as has been pointed out by E. Fränkel. I have from different sources isolated pathogenic streptococci which do not coagulate milk, although they change the color of the litmus to a lilac pink, indicating the production of a certain amount of acid.

While we must admit that all inflammatory affections caused by the pyogenic staphylococci may be produced also by streptococci, and, with the probable exception of erysipelas, the reverse also holds true, nevertheless we are not prepared to accept the statements of Levy and some other recent writers that the character of the microörganisms, whether staphylococci or streptococci, has no influence upon the symptomatology of the disease. In conformity with most investigators, we have found the staphylococci prone to form circumscribed areas of suppuration, whereas the pyogenic streptococci have a tendency to produce spreading phlegmons with lymphangitis and a wide zone of surrounding redness and inflammatory œdema. It is the custom in our gynecological wards to isolate the operative cases in which streptococci are found at the time of the operation in the seat of the disease, or subsequently in the wound.

Of other pyogenic cocci we have found the staphylococcus pyogenes citreus twice in abscesses, the staphylococcus cereus albus three times in combination with other bacteria in suppurating wounds, the diplococcus pneumoniæ once in a fibrinous peritonitis, and the micrococcus tetragenus once, together with the staphylococcus aureus in an abscess of the lung.

The list of bacilli which may be concerned in suppurative and other inflammatory affections is much longer than was formerly supposed, and is likely to be still further extended. Those which we have chanced to encounter are: the bacillus pyogenes fœtidus, twice in abscesses containing bad-smelling pus; the proteus Zenkeri, once in pure culture in an ovarian abscess with purulent salpingitis; a bacillus apparently identical with the bacillus emphysematis maligni of Wicklein, once in an emphysematous cellulitis of the arm; a bacillus apparently identical with the bacillus enteritidis of Gärtner, in the brain and other organs of an infant three months old with cerebral abscess and meningitis following operation for imperforate anus; the typhoid bacillus, once in pure culture in an osteomyelitis of the ribs following typhoid fever: a hitherto undescribed bacillus, rapidly liquefying gelatin and characterized by rapid solution or peptonization of milk, without coagulation, once in peritonitis; bacilli which could not be cultivated in our ordinary culture media, in three cases of suppurative inflammation; and the bacillus coli communis, fifteen times.

As these bacillary infections are far less common than those caused by micrococci, I shall take some other occasion to describe them, and here shall ask your attention only to one group, viz., those associated with the bacillus coli communis, as they have been relatively common in our experience and present some points of especial interest.

The first observation of the bacillus coli communis in connection with wound infection was made by Tavel, in 1889. This has been followed by a few isolated observations of this organism either in the unchanged organs of the body or in abscesses, until recently A. Fränkel reports its presence in nine out of thirty-one cases of peritonitis. I first came across this bacillus in the organs of the body in 1889, in a case of multiple fat-necrosis with pancreatitis, which I reported to the Association of American Physicians. As in this case diphtheritic colitis existed, it seemed probable that the lesion of the intestine opened the way for the entrance into the circulation of this inhabitant of the healthy intestinal canal. This view subsequent experience has confirmed, for I have already isolated in pure culture from the internal organs the bacillus coli communis in twenty-five autopsies where some distinct lesion of the intestinal mucous membrane existed, such as ulceration, diphtheritis, hemorrhage, traumatic injury, and I have almost uniformly failed to find it outside of the intestine when no demonstrable lesion of the mucous membrane existed. I am therefore prepared to say that this bacillus is an extremely frequent invader in intestinal disease, although I have no evidence to offer that it does any harm except under certain especial conditions. The autopsies were in nearly every case made within three or four hours after death, once in less than one hour. Moreover, the colon bacillus does not invade the blood and organs in the process of post-mortem decomposition.

The cases in which we have found the colon bacillus under circumstances pointing to its pathogenic action have been as follows: perforative peritonitis, four cases; peritonitis secondary to intestinal disease without perforation, two cases; circumscribed abscess, three cases; and laparotomy wounds, six cases.

Its presence, several times in pure culture, in laparotomy wounds treated aseptically, although apparently not a source of serious trouble, was not a matter of indifference. It was generally accompanied with moderate fever and a thin, brownish, slightly purulent discharge, of somewhat offensive, but not putrefactive odor. The smooth and rapid healing of the wound was interfered with. In some of the cases there was evidence of intestinal disorder; in others this was not apparent, and infection from without could not be excluded.

For the purposes of the present discussion, perhaps the chief interest of our observations concerning the colon bacillus is that they furnish an illustration of the possible predisposition to infection afforded by intestinal lesions, and also give an example of the much-disputed auto-infection.

Of suppurative inflammations which we have examined bacteriologically with negative result, may be mentioned abscesses in which the bacteria were presumably dead, several hepatic abscesses caused by the amœba dysenteriæ, and many cases of suppurating buboes and of pyosalpinx, doubtless caused by the gonococcus.

From the foregoing brief summary, mainly of our own limited experience, it is clear that the bacteria which may be concerned in surgical infections are many, but the pyogenic cocci of Ogston, Rosenbach, and Passet far out-rank in frequency, and therefore in importance, all other bacteria combined.

In view of the more practical matters to be considered, we cannot tarry long over the theories of suppuration, interesting as just this part of the subject is at the present time.

There are very good reasons to believe that the process of suppuration serves a useful purpose, and is one of the most important and efficient weapons employed by Nature in combating invading microöganisms. Man is not subject to those forms of septicæmia, common in many lower animals, in which enormous numbers of bacteria are present in the blood; but, on the other hand, he is particularly subject to suppurations and other localized inflammations. The same microörganism, for instance the diplococcus pneumoniæ and the bacillus anthracis, which produces in many of the lower animals the form of septicæmia mentioned, causes in man localized inflammations. In the experimental septicæmias of lower animals there is an unmistakable relation between the extent of the local reaction at the point of inoculation on the one hand, and the duration of life and number of organisms present in the blood on the other. The more extensive and intense the local reaction, the fewer, as a rule, are the bacteria found in the blood and the longer the duration of life. There are two varieties of the swine-plague bacillus, the one kills rabbits in twelve to eighteen hours with trifling local reaction and a large number of bacilli in the blood, the other produces extensive purulent infiltration around the site of subcutaneous inoculation and permits the animals to live for several days, and at the autopsy very few bacteria are found in the blood. In a susceptible animal the virulent anthrax bacillus produces an acute septicæmia, the attenuated bacillus a local abscess. There is even experimental evidence that if inoculation of a susceptible animal with the virulent anthrax bacillus be speedily followed by inoculation at the same point with a pyogenic organism so that suppuration soon ensues, the development of anthrax septicæmia may be warded off and the animal recover. It seems reasonable to infer, when the same organism produces in one animal a rapidly fatal septicæmia without local reaction and in another species only a local abscess, that the latter animal is protected by the barrier of suppuration. As is well known, the fatal infections from wounds received at post-mortem examinations are not generally those where marked local reaction with suppuration appears at the seat of the often trifling injury.

Exactly how abscess formation checks the invasion of bacteria we do not know. That bacteria may die, often in a short time, in pus both within and outside of the body, has been demonstrated. The leading theories are these: leucocytes and other cells act as phagocytes, taking into their bodies the bacteria and killing them; the wall of leucocytes and other cells at the margin of an abscess acts as an obstacle to the passage of the bacteria into the surrounding tissues; pus contains chemical substances injurious to bacteria or antidotal to their toxic products; the bacteria starve in pus, not being able to assimilate such concentrated food. Something can be said in favor of each of these theories, more in favor of some than of others, but none is proven and we cannot stop to discuss them here.

That pyogenic bacteria set up suppuration by chemical substances produced by them, seems to be proven. The zone of necrosis around these bacteria which can be demonstrated as the first effect of their lodgment in the tissues points to such chemical action. Moreover, from cultures of pyogenic cocci several chemical products have been obtained capable of causing suppuration. The most interesting observations here are the recent ones of Buchner and his pupils, who have found the proteid constituents of many bacteria capable of producing suppuration. These bacterio-proteïns of Buchner possess in a remarkable degree the property of positive chemotaxis, that wonderful quality by which certain chemical substances influence the leucocytes to migrate from the vessels and move actively toward them. A flood of unexpected light seems destined to come from the studies of chemotaxis to illumine many dark problems in pathology.

Since we know that the chemical products and constituents of certain bacteria are the direct agencies in the production of suppuration, it is less surprising to find that various other chemical substances are likewise able to cause suppuration. But important as this fact is for the theory of suppuration, the demonstration that these other chemical irritants, such as turpentine, nitrate of silver, etc., can cause suppuration has no especial bearing upon the ordinary suppurations in human beings.

We come now to the consideration of a division of our subject beset with difficulties at every turn, but one no less interesting to the surgeon than to the bacteriologist.

How are we to explain the extraordinary variability in the effects produced by the pyogenic cocci ? The specific infectious agents with which
we first became familiar, the bacteria of the natural and of the experimental septicæmias of lower animals, are nearly constant in the effects
which they produce when inoculated in small quantity into susceptible
animals.   Not so with the pyogenic cocci.   Here we meet the most
puzzling differences.   We find the same coccus in the most insignificant
epidermal pustule which we find in a dangerous phlegmon, in osteomyelitis, in pyæmia, in septicæmia, in acute ulcerative endocarditis.
The manifold varieties of puerperal fever, which we now know to be a
typical wound infection, may be caused by apparently the same streptococcus, producing a mild endometritis, a pelvic abscess, localized or
general peritonitis, pyæmia or the most virulent and rapidly fatal septicæmia.

If we seek an explanation of these things by experimentation upon
animals, we find that in order to get any positive effects at all it is often
necessary to introduce enormous quantities of our cultures, containing
vastly more bacteria than we can suppose to be concerned in the primary infection in human beings.   If we inoculate smaller quantities,
these can often be disposed of by the animal without any manifest
symptoms.

It must be confessed that we stand here before problems many of
which still await solution, but it will not do to pass them by on this
occasion without some discussion, although time will permit me to touch
upon only some of the salient points.

It is well to bear in mind that the inflammatory infections of wounds
do not represent specific morbid entities in the same sense as do anthrax
and typhoid fever, for example.   The latter diseases are caused by a
single specific germ and no other, and present a definite and characteristic clinical and anatomical picture, whereas the former correspond to
the reaction of the body toward a great variety of noxæ and offer
manifold variations in symptoms and lesions.

The quantity of a culture of the staphylococcus aureus required to
produce suppuration is not the same for all tissues and all parts of the
body.   A mere trace, a fraction of a drop, of a dilute suspension of the
yellow staphylococcus in salt solution when injected into the rabbit's
eye will set up a suppurative inflammation.   It takes a larger amount
of such a suspension to produce an abscess in the loose subcutaneous
tissue of the back than in the dense tissue of the ear of a rabbit.
Enormous quantities, five to ten cubic centimetres and more, of the
suspension can be injected often without effect into the normal peritoneal cavity of rabbits and dogs, as has been shown by the well-known
experiments of Grawitz and his pupils, confirmed by several other investigators.

It is probable, as claimed by Grawitz, that this difference in the be-havior of different tissues depends in large part upon the rapidity with which the injected material, more particularly the toxic substances, are absorbed. But we must also reckon with a predisposition apart from this in the normal tissues, for the introduction even of very large num-bers of staphylococci into the circulation of rabbits is followed by the formation of abscesses only in certain situations, mainly the kidneys, heart and certain muscles, although we must suppose that the cocci have been carried to all parts of the body.

That there are variations in the virulence of different cultures of the pyogenic cocci is admitted by most writers and may be inferred from the discrepant results of various experimenters as regards the amount of the culture required to produce suppuration. These discrepancies can-not be explained wholly by different conditions of the experiments. We have found no especial difference in the result, for example, whether we introduced into the peritoneal cavity of dogs cultures of the staphy-lococcus aureus according to Grawitz's method, or according to Paw-lowsky's method, or by a small laparotomy wound. By one as well as by another method we were able to inject 5 c.c. and often more of a suspension in salt solution of the yellow staphylococcus without any appreciable effect.

In order to test this matter of varying virulence, I have injected into the ear-veins of rabbits bouillon cultures, forty-eight hours old, of the staphylococcus aureus obtained from many different sources. Consider-able variations in virulence were found to exist both in the original cultures and in the successive generations of the same culture. The most virulent culture was one from a beginning furuncle. The injection of 0.1 c.c. of this culture caused the death of the rabbit in twenty-four hours with a large number of staphylococci in the blood and many necrotic foci in the kidneys. After the second generation the virulence was lessened. From a case of hypertrophic cirrhosis of the liver with-out suppurative complications a moderate number of colonies of the staphylococcus pyogenes aureus were found in cultures made from the liver. 1.5 c.c. of bouillon cultures, forty-eight hours old, of this staphy-lococcus were injected without any effect into the ear-veins of two rab-bits, the animals being still alive eight months after the injection. These extremes are met only exceptionally. In the great majority of cases we have found the injection of 0.2 to 0.3 c.c. of bouillon cultures sufficient to kill the animal in four to seven days with the usual abscesses in the kidneys and heart and occasionally elsewhere. As a rule there was no material change in the degree of virulence for many successive generations, but sometimes without any apparent cause there would occur a marked weakening of the virulence either after a few generations or after many.

Our conclusions from these experiments are that while variations in virulence occur and may explain in large part the varying results of different experimenters operating upon animals under similar conditions, they are not sufficient in degree or in frequency to afford adequate explanation of the great differences in the effects of the pyogenic cocci upon human beings, or at least can do so only in part.

How far can we apply to human beings the experiments showing the great tolerance of animals toward the pyogenic cocci? The experimental evidence upon this point is naturally scanty, but such as we possess indicates that man is not equally tolerant, that his tissues respond more readily by suppuration to inoculation of pyogenic cocci. The experiments upon this point of Garré, Bumm, Bockhart, Fehleisen, Waterhouse—and these names should not be mentioned without expressing the debt of gratitude which science owes to them—are too well known to necessitate here any statement of their results. But while these experiments appear to indicate less immunity on the part of human beings toward the ordinary staphylococci of suppuration—a matter, however, which cannot be considered absolutely certain—they have also demonstrated that the difference, if it exists, is only one of degree, and that large numbers of the pyogenic cocci may be inoculated into human tissues without effect. Waterhouse, for example, injected under the skin of the abdomen and of the scrotum 0.25 c.c. of a suspension of the staphylococcus aureus, made by mixing one loopful from an agar culture with 5 c.c. of water, and the result was completely negative.

It is true that undue emphasis should not be laid upon the negative results, for there are equally trustworthy experiments with positive result, showing that even small quantities of suspensions of the pus organisms may cause suppuration, both in animals and in human beings.

That there exist bacteria capable of producing abscesses regularly, even when inoculated in very small quantity into animals, is proven by the discovery by Dr. Bolton of a hitherto undescribed bacillus in garden earth. This bacillus, for cultures of which I am indebted to Dr. Bolton, who will hereafter publish its description, produces with certainty localized abscesses when inoculated in small amount into the subcutaneous tissues of rats, mice, and rabbits. When injected into the circulation it causes multiple abscesses in the kidneys, joints, bones, and other situations.

Inasmuch as it is by their toxic products that the pyogenic bacteria do injury, it is not surprising to find that it makes a great difference in the result whether these bacteria enter the tissues already equipped with a reserve force of this poisonous material, or must begin the fight unarmed. There is abundant experimental evidence to show that even in very small number the pus-producing micrococci will cause suppuration if they are accompanied, or soon preceded or followed, in sufficient amount and concentration by various toxic substances which are present in pure cultures of the cocci, and the extent of the inflammation bears a relation to the quality and quantity of these substances. The experiments and researches of many investigators, such as Hankin, Brieger and Fränkel, Buchner, Dirckinck-Holmfeld, Grawitz, Leber, Dubler, Kronacher, Ribbert, have shed light upon this subject. It would seem as if the issues of the battle between the invading micrococci and the tissues depend often upon the first blow; and if the invader can strike this with the aid of powerful weapons which he has forged before he enters, the victory, for the time at least, is with him.

This matter of accompanying toxic substances is probably of great importance in our understanding of the potentialities of the living agents of wound infection as they occur under natural conditions. Here we have to do, not with pure cultures of the pyogenic cocci, still less with those that have been washed in sterilized salt solution or water, but with pus-producing organisms which have come from all sorts of sources, which have been engaged in very different activities, which have been growing under various conditions or have been long dormant, and which are mixed with many kinds of bacteria. There is proof that under some of these conditions the infectious material may possess a degree of virulence with which we are not familiar in our artificial cultures. When a strong, healthy man (I have now in mind such a case in a medical student) dies in a few days from septicæmia caused by the inoculation of a mere scratch on the finger with fluid from a puerperal peritonitis, it is the quality of the infectious material which brought about the fatal result, and not any especial predisposition of the individual. When we find, as has been done, that the peritoneal fluid contains in pure culture the streptococcus pyogenes, and that the same organism is present in pure culture in the patient accidentally infected with this fluid, the observation is just as convincing and clear in its interpretation as if the experiment had been made intentionally upon an animal. No number of experiments showing that millions of apparently the same species of micrococcus can be injected in artificial cultures into the peritoneal cavity of dogs and rabbits can do away with the force of such an observation. No surgeon, no obstetrician, however strong may be his trust in the germicidal power of the animal tissues and fluids, would willingly permit the smallest particle of that peritoneal fluid to come into contact with a fresh wound or the uterus after childbirth.

The differences in virulence which have been found to exist between inflammatory exudates from various sources containing pyogenic bacteria are much greater than those observed in the cultures of the same bacteria on artificial media. To explain this, some assume that the differences in virulence pertain to the pyogenic cocci as such, that they are specifically endowed with different biological attributes; while others think that the varying virulence relates not so much to the bacteria as to the character of the toxic substances with which they are associated. In favor of the latter view, which is the one advocated by Bumm, Fehleisen, Chantemesse, and others, may be cited such observations as that of Bumm, who found that the injection into the peritoneal cavity of a rabbit of a quarter of a drop of fluid from a case of acute septic puerperal peritonitis quickly killed the animal with peritonitis, whereas the streptococci artificially cultivated from the same fluid were much less virulent; or the experiment of Fehleisen, showing that a minimal quantity of an artificial culture of the staphylococcus aureus added to a little of the clear serum obtained from the germ-free zone of inflammatory œdema around a spreading cellulitis was capable of producing extensive abscesses, whereas the mixture of the same organism with water had no such effect. The question is still an open one, and very likely both factors are concerned.

We have thus far confined our attention to the microörganisms of infection, and have said nothing concerning the conditions predisposing to infection in the exposed individual. Everybody believes in the doctrine of predisposition, some more than others. The tendency at the present time is certainly not to minimize its importance. Predisposition is a term to conjure with. It is often made to explain in a vague sort of way things which we do not understand. Nevertheless it is a very real thing, and we cannot pass it by here without notice, even if this must necessarily be very brief. Every surgeon knows that wounds in some persons do much better than in others, and that some kinds of wounds are much more prone to suppurate than others.

The interesting studies upon immunity which have shed so much light upon the nature of predisposition toward some infectious diseases have not as yet cleared up the question of immunity against the pyogenic cocci. We know that the healthy tissues can dispose of a certain number of these cocci under ordinary circumstances, but how they do it we do not know.

An experiment of Roger is suggestive. He found that the streptococcus of erysipelas grew as well in the blood-serum of rabbits rendered immune as in the blood-serum of other animals, but that in the former they lost their virulence. As we now know that the protective influence of the blood-serum of immune animals consists quite as much in the power to destroy the poisons produced by bacteria as in the power to kill the bacteria directly—already demonstrated examples of this are diphtheria, tetanus, and septicæmia produced by the diplococcus pneumoniæ—it is not unreasonable to suppose, in the light of Roger's experiments, that this antidotal capacity of the blood and animal fluids may be one of the means employed by Nature in disposing of the pyogenic cocci. That these cocci are not directly killed by the extra-vascular blood-serum of rabbits, dogs, swine, and human beings, or if at all in very small number, we know. On the other hand, this serum is an excellent medium for their growth. But if the toxic products of the bacteria are destroyed by the fluids of the body, the bacteria can do no harm, and are at the mercy of the tissues, as has been shown by the recent brilliant researches of G. and F. Klemperer on the diplococcus of pneumonia. When we have a clearer insight into the nature of immunity against the pyogenic bacteria, our understanding of the conditions underlying the infection of wounds will be greatly advanced.

I cannot undertake to discuss all the general conditions of the body, such as diabetes, syphilis, alcoholism, anæmia, obesity, typhoid and other fevers, Bright's disease, etc., which have been regarded as predisposing causes of infection with the pyogenic cocci, some of these diseases upon most conclusive clinical evidence. Gärtner has recently brought forward evidence derived from experiments on animals showing that general anæmia and hydræmia render easier the infection with small quantities of the staphylococcus aureus, and Ribbert has demonstrated that the presence of toxic products of the same microörganism in the circulating blood favors the development of foci of suppuration, a fact which evidently bears upon the pathology of pyæmia and of some cases of furunculosis, as well as upon the importance of evacuating pus. An instance has already been given of the predisposition to infection afforded by intestinal lesions. In dismissing thus hastily the matter of general predisposition to suppuration, it will not be understood that these few words are a measure of the importance of the subject. I believe that the surgeon cannot be too thorough in the examination, before contemplated operations, of all the important organs and functions of the body, and that, wherever possible, he should endeavor to put the patient into the best possible condition of health before undertaking a severe operation.

Of very immediate practical interest to the surgeon is a knowledge of the various conditions in and about a wound which favor the lodgment and development of pyogenic bacteria. In a general way it may be said that anything which interferes with the integrity of the living tissues in a wound is a predisposing cause of suppuration, in case suitable microorganisms gain entrance. Experiments have shown that the necroses produced by chemical irritants, such as carbolic acid and corrosive sublimate, favor the multiplication of the microörganisms of suppuration. Dr. Halsted has shown that the irrigation of fresh wounds by a solution of corrosive sublimate as weak as 1 to 10,000 is followed by a distinct line of superficial necrosis demonstrable under the microscope.

We are not so well informed as to the influence exerted by blood in a wound. On the one hand, Von Bergmann and most modern surgeons lay the greatest stress upon prompt and careful hæmostasis in surgical operations ; on the other hand, Schede has revived and more fully developed an old method of treatment, by which a certain class of wounds are permitted to fill with a blood-blot, and he and other surgeons have obtained rapid and aseptic healing by this method. Is this blood-clot, as such, a source of danger in the same sense as dead tissue is ? As has already been mentioned, fresh blood-serum does not possess any such germicidal power over the pyogenic cocci as it does over the typhoid bacillus and many other bacteria. Not being able to find any direct experimental evidence upon the point, I have, with the assistance of Dr. Howard, made a large number of experiments upon dogs. The operations were done with strict antiseptic or aseptic precautions. In most of the experiments a cavity was chiselled out of bone, and this and the rest of the wound were allowed to fill with a coagulum of blood, the conditions pertaining to similar operations in human beings being observed. The blood-clot, after its formation, was inoculated with a culture of the staphylococcus aureus, either by injecting into it a few drops of a fresh bouillon culture or by inserting a platinum loop carrying a bit of the growth on agar. The outcome of the experiments was that the so-called organization of the blood-clot went on as it does in human beings, and the wounds did not suppurate. The staphylococci survived, at least for many days, in the clot, but they did not appear to multiply. This result is in conformity with the experience of Grawitz, who found that the aureus lives for a long time, although it does not multiply, in blood-coagula outside of the body, and that no development of this organism takes place in a solidified mixture of equal parts of nutrient gelatin and blood.

It is not my province to consider the extent of application of the method advocated by Schede to human surgery, nor the advantages of retaining the material employed by Nature in filling up cavities and pockets in fresh wounds as against the insertion of sterilized extraneous material and the obliteration of the dead spaces by deep stitches, which, without great care, are liable to strangulate tissue, produce undue tension, and interfere with the circulation.

Where the healing of the wound by the blood-clot method is not directly purposed, undoubtedly it is important for its aseptic course to check the oozing of blood and to prevent the unintended formation and retention of blood-coagula whose presence is not arranged for by the surgeon in the management of the wound. That loss of blood, as such, predisposes to suppuration has already been mentioned.

In contrast with the negative results of the experiments just mentioned stands a series of positive ones which illustrate the readiness and uniformity with which suppuration of an infected wound ensues which contains masses of tissue strangulated by ligature. These wounds were .

inoculated with the same cultures which yielded negative results as regards the infection of the blood-clot.

We have made also a large number of experiments upon dogs by ligating portions of the omentum and then injecting cultures of the staphylococcus aureus, peritoneum. In most of these cases general peritonitis developed, in some localized peritonitis, and in some no peritonitis followed the inoculation.

In order to demonstrate the influence of foreign bodies in favoring suppuration, we inserted into the peritoneal cavity of nine dogs pieces of potato presenting a growth of the staphylococcus aureus, and in every instance general peritonitis developed, although in no case was the insertion of similar pieces of sterilized potato followed by peritonitis; and the injection of 1 c.c. bouillon culture of the staphylococcus aureus into the peritoneal cavity of twenty-three dogs was not followed in a single instance by peritonitis.

There is a gratifying harmony between the views entertained by bacteriologists concerning the power of the living tissues to overcome a certain number of pyogenic bacteria, and the tendency of the modern surgeon to respect these tissues more and more, not to destroy their vital capacities by the unnecessary application of strong chemical disinfectants, not to bruise them, not to make them too tense, not to strangle them, not to suffer the presence in wounds of spaces and foreign bodies, which remove bacteria from the influence of the living tissues and fluids.

From this necessarily hasty and imperfect survey of this division of our subject, it is apparent that, while there is no reason to doubt that the pyogenic cocci are specific agents of infection, the effects which they produce depend upon a variety of conditions, such as the source, the number, and the virulence of the micrococci, the accompanying toxic substances, the part of the body invaded, the readiness of absorption, the presence of foreign bodies and of pathological products, the general state of the patient, and the condition and handling of the wounded tissues.

In giving due weight to each of these factors one should not forget that the infectious material may exist under natural conditions, in a state capable of causing traumatic infections just as directly, just as certainly, just as independently of predisposition, as infection of a susceptible animal takes place with the anthrax bacillus.

As to the various ways by which pathogenic bacteria may gain access to wounds, there is at the present time general agreement of opinion that the greatest danger is from contact with infected hands, instruments, and other objects. The danger of infection by contact is a lesson which has been learned no less by bacteriological workers in the laboratory than by practical surgeons and obstetricians.

The possibility of infection from the air, insignificant as it may be in comparison with contact infection, cannot be ignored quite as much as some seem inclined to do. The staphylococcus pyogenes aureus has been repeatedly found in the dust floating in the air, particularly of surgical wards where there are suppurating cases. The streptococcus erysipelatus was found by Von Eiselsberg in the air of a ward containing cases of erysipelas and the streptococci found by Prudden in the air of hospital wards were probably identical with this. When we had more confidence than we now have in the power of chemical disinfectants to destroy all bacteria which might accidentally get into a wound during a surgical operation, it seemed proper to disregard the air as a source of infection, and no less a surgeon than von Volkmann could say, " Auch auf einem Abtritte würde ich dreist operiren wenn die Hände rein wären." A privy, by the way, is not the most dangerous place which he could have selected.

Now that our trust in chemical disinfectants for the purpose named is shaken, and that what is called aseptic surgery is the watchword of the day, I believe that a surgeon who aims at the best will try to have the air of his operating-room as free from germs as possible, and will have it so constructed that the floor and walls and all that is in it can be readily cleaned and disinfected. He will regard the influence of currents of air and of commotion in the room in stirring up dust, and will not ignore the value of moisture in laying dust and in keeping it in its place. These suggestions may seem pedantic when the whole tendency of surgery now is to simplify technique and to throw overboard unnecessary ballast, but they appear to me to rest upon bacteriological facts which should not be ignored.

An example has already been given in this paper of auto-infection from the intestinal canal by the bacillus coli communis. The not infrequent invasion of the pyogenic cocci in typhoid fever, diphtheria, scarlet fever, and other diseases with lesions of the alimentary tract, are probably explicable partly by these lesions opening a passage for the bacteria into the circulation, and partly by the predisposition afforded by the presence in the body of toxic substances belonging to the primary disease. It is known that the pyogenic cocci are often present in the alimentary canal. For instance, in a case of perforative peritonitis from typhoid fever, recently examined in my laboratory, there were isolated from the peritoneal exudate, not in single but in many colonies on the roll cultures, the staphylococcus aureus and the streptococcus pyogenes, in addition to the typhoid bacillus, the colon bacillus, and an unidentified bacillus liquefying the gelatin.

Rinne observed in his experiments on dogs that the injection of sterilized putrid fluids together with staphylococci into the peritoneal cavity was followed by suppuration of all open wounds, which otherwise healed kindly, but that subcutaneous wounds were unaffected. The bacteria found in the suppurating open wounds, however, were not those injected, but were derived from the air. This is unquestionably an interesting and important observation, but he goes too far in supposing that such wounds, as well as other loci minoris resistentiæ, may not become infected from pyogenic cocci in the circulation, as has been demonstrated by the experiments of De Wildt, Waterhouse, and others.

That even under the most unfavorable conditions of general infection a wound may heal by first intention is known to surgeons. In one of our cases, for example, the patient soon after an extensive operation for removal of a cancer of the breast, developed diphtheritic ulcerative dysentery; and at the post-mortem examination were found, in addition to the dysentery, pneumonia, abscess of the lung, and fresh pleurisy, with wide distribution of the staphylococcus aureus; nevertheless, the operation wound had remained perfectly healthy without a trace of suppuration.

Into the burning question of auto-infection from the genital tract in puerperal women I cannot enter, save to say that the pyogenic cocci seem to be present only very exceptionally in the normal tract and do not thrive there if intentionally put in, but that they are found in pathological utero-vaginal secretions, when, of course, they may become a source of puerperal infection. The question is a difficult one and requires further investigation. This passing mention is only intended to indicate that the subject belongs to our theme and may appropriately enter into the discussion.

I must beg permission to defer for a few moments the question of infection from the skin of the operator and of the patient.

That an aseptic wound is not necessarily one free from bacteria has been known since the early days of antiseptic surgery, the subject having been investigated by Ranke, Demarquay, Fischer, Schüller, Watson Cheyne, and others. Kümmell found that pieces of muscle, adipose tissue, or connective tissue taken from fresh wounds immediately after irrigation during the entire operation with corrosive sublimate solution 1 : 10,000, contained bacteria, and the same result was obtained after frequent washing with sublimate solution 1 : 1000.

The most recent investigation of the bacteria in fresh wounds treated antiseptically is by Bossowski, who found, of 50 cases, 10 with negative and 40 with positive result from the bacteriological examination. He found the staphylococcus albus 26 times, the staphylococcus aureus 9 times, the streptococcus pyogenes 2 times, and other organisms, non-pathogenic, 8 times. He several times found a coccus, liquefying gelatin after several days, growing at first white and then slowly turning yellow, and incapable of producing suppuration in rabbits or in wounds. This he proposes to call staphylococcus gilvus. In every case in which the staphylococcus aureus or the streptococcus pyogenes, with or without other organisms,

was present, suppuration occurred. On the other hand the staphylococcus
albus produced generally no interference with the healing of the wound,
but sometimes it caused a little suppuration of the drain canal or a stitch
abscess. In the majority of cases there was absolute *prima intentio*.
The small number of the colonies indicated meagre development in the
wound.

Drs. Ghriskey and Robb have made under my observation the bacteriological examination of 45 laparotomy wounds treated with strict
antiseptic precautions in the gynecological wards of the Johns Hopkins
Hospital. The method of treatment and the technique adopted for obtaining the cultures have already been published by Dr. Robb, in the
Bulletin of the Johns Hopkins Hospital, July, 1891.

Of these 45 cases the result was negative in 14, positive in 31, or
nearly 69 per cent. of the cases. The organisms found were the staphylococcus albus 19 times, the staphylococcus aureus 5 times, the bacillus
coli communis 6 times, the streptococcus pyogenes 3 times, once alone
and twice in combination with the albus. Of the cases with the aureus
in only two was there reason to suspect infection from without; in the
others this organism was present in the seat of disease for which the operation was performed. In the first case with streptococcus pyogenes the
operation was performed for an ovarian abscess which contained streptococci in large numbers; the other two cases probably became infected in
some way from the first patient.

In all of the cases presenting the staphylococcus aureus or the streptococcus pyogenes the wound suppurated, and, as a rule, the general condition of the patient was bad.

In many of the cases where the white staphylococcus was found there
was no disturbance in the healing of the wound. This was true especially
when the organism was found in small number, and when it made its
first appearance subsequent to the first dressing, which took place usually
twenty-four to forty-eight hours after the operation. In many cases,
however, the white coccus was the cause of more or less trouble, although
rarely of a serious nature. It was found to travel down to the bottom
of the wound along the side of the drainage-tube, and any purulent discharge attributable to its presence was usually confined to the tract occupied by the drainage-tube, so that the drainage-tube distinctly favored
the invasion and growth of the coccus. Sometimes fever without suppuration seemed attributable to the presence of this coccus. That this
organism is the most frequent cause of the ordinary stitch abscesses has
already been mentioned.

Under especially favorable circumstances this white staphylococcus
may cause peritonitis, as is shown by a fatal case of hystero-myomectomy
where at the autopsy a volvulus of the ileum was found. The stump
and the laparotomy wound both looked healthy, but there was a fresh

fibrino-purulent peritonitis clearly starting from that part of the peritoneum agglutinated to the inner edge of the laparotomy wound. This part corresponded to the peritoneum covering the twisted ileum. The twist was not so tight as to have produced gangrene or even a marked hemorrhagic condition; but it had interfered sufficiently with the circulation and the nutrition of the peritoneum to have rendered this a favorable soil for the growth of an otherwise comparatively innocent bacterium, our white staphylococcus having been found in pure culture in the inflamed peritoneum.

The efforts to find out the origin of this very common inhabitant of wounds, treated aseptically or antiseptically, have led us to some interesting and new observations concerning the bacteria of the skin.

The skin may have all sorts of bacteria upon its surface, but, like the mouth and the intestine, in addition to these it has its own distinctive bacterial flora.

If the hands be thoroughly scrubbed with soap and hot water with a sterilized brush, or if this be followed by washing the hands in sublimate solution and the mercury be precipitated by sulphide of ammonium, the cultures obtained from scrapings of the skin so treated will generally be found to contain, as the prevailing organism, the white staphylococcus, and often this will appear in nearly or quite pure culture.

But the most important point is that this coccus is very often present in parts of the epidermis deeper than can be reached by any known means of cutaneous disinfection save the application of heat. We were directed to this conclusion first by experiments on animals. Then the observation of the same white coccus in pure culture time after time in wounds where every possible antiseptic precaution had been taken, pointed to the same deduction. More conclusive evidence was afforded by the examination of skin stitches in cases where at the time of the operation it was proven that the silk used for stitches was sterile and that the surface of the skin after thorough disinfection was sterile. The silk sutures when removed were proven both by microscopical examination and by roll or plate cultures to contain with great regularity the white staphylococcus, often in considerable number, often enclosed within leucocytes, and this not only where a stitch abscess had formed but also where there was not a trace of suppuration or visible reaction around the stitch.

A crucial experiment is the following: The skin is thoroughly disinfected, in the manner to be presently described, so that culture-tubes of nutrient agar or gelatin inoculated by scrapings from its surface remain sterile. A silk thread, sterilized by steam and proven by culture methods to be sterile, is passed one or more times by means of a sterilized instrument through the skin, is withdrawn, and at once a tube of melted nutrient agar is inoculated with the thread and rolled. This amounts to a ready

means of making cultures directly from the deeper layers of the epidermis and the skin, and is a method applicable for many purposes to
the bacteriological examination of the skin. By this method the presence
of the white staphylococcus, often in pure culture, has been repeatedly
demonstrated in parts of the epidermis deeper than were acted upon by
any methods of disinfection of the surface of the skin. So far as our
observations extend, and already they amount to a large number, this
coccus may be regarded as a nearly, if not quite, constant inhabitant of
the epidermis. It is now clear why I have proposed to call it the
staphylococcus epidermidis albus. It possesses such feeble pyogenic
capacity, as is shown by its behavior in wounds as well as by experiments on rabbits, that the designation staphylococcus pyogenes albus
does not seem appropriate. Still, I am not inclined to insist too much
upon this point, as very probably this coccus, which has hitherto been
unquestionably identified by Bossowski and others with the ordinary
staphylococcus pyogenes albus of Rosenbach, is an attenuated or modified form of the latter organism, although, as already mentioned, it presents some points of difference from the classical description of the white
pyogenic coccus.

We can now understand how, without any flaw in the antiseptic technique of the surgeon, this microörganism may be present in wounds,
and we have a satisfactory explanation of the frequent occurrence of
stitch abscesses, although, of course, the inference should not be drawn
that the white staphylococcus is the only bacterium which may be concerned in the production of these annoying complications.

How much practical importance attaches to the demonstration of this
coccus in the deeper layers of the epidermis I am not prepared to say.
The surgeon with good technique who does not bother himself about it
is not likely to be severely punished by the behavior of his wounds.
Those who put drainage-tubes and other extraneous substances into their
wounds I think will have to consider it. Dr. Halsted, on the basis of
researches on the bacteria of the skin and the difficulties of complete disinfection of the skin of the patient, has abandoned for nearly all wounds
the use of skin stitches, the edges of the wound being brought together
with admirable coaptation by subcutaneous sutures. The results, both
as regards the scar and the aseptic healing of the wound, have been most
gratifying. Stitch abscesses are, of course, avoided by this procedure.

Another coccus which we have found, although less frequently than
the white coccus, on the surface and in the deeper layers of the epidermis,
is one already referred to which corresponds to that called by Bossowski
staphylococcus gilvus. This organism seems to bear about the same
relation to the pyogenic yellow staphylococcus which our epidermal white
coccus does to the typical pyogenic white staphylococcus.

The staphylococcus pyogenes aureus we have found very frequently on the hands of surgeons and their assistants who have to do with suppurating cases of any kind. It may be present in this situation at least for several days after contact with surgical cases. It was met only exceptionally upon the hands of other persons.

The demonstration of microörganisms in layers of the epidermis deeper than can be disinfected by present methods suggests that more attention than seems now to be customary should be paid to the skin of the patient as a source of traumatic infections. It also admonishes us to receive with caution the statements recently made concerning the elimination in suppurative diseases of staphylococci by the sweat.

A considerable part of our work has been devoted to the subject of surgical antisepsis, and particularly to the disinfection of the skin. Dr. Abbott has conducted in my laboratory careful experiments regarding corrosive sublimate as a disinfectant against the staphylococcus pyogenes aureus, in which many fallacies in previous work on the same subject have been pointed out. In view of the time already consumed, I must ask permission simply to refer to Dr. Abbott's paper on this subject, already published in the *Bulletin of the Johns Hopkins Hospital* for April, 1891.

The conditions for the efficient action of chemical disinfectants have been found to be far more complicated and less easily controlled than was formerly supposed, and the substitution, wherever applicable, of the simple and certain methods of disinfection by heat, such as have been long employed in bacteriological laboratories, is to be commended. Chemical disinfectants still have their place for many purposes in the operating-room, but their place is not in fresh, healthy wounds.

Thorough scrubbing of the skin with soap and warm water by a sterilized brush removes many bacteria, but not all, and it cannot be regarded as a satisfactory means of cutaneous disinfection.

The fallacy in previous work on disinfection of the skin with corrosive sublimate has been that in testing its efficiency the sublimate was not first precipitated by sulphide of ammonium. If this precaution, to which attention was first directed by Geppert, be observed, it will be found that corrosive sublimate accomplishes much less than is generally supposed. Our revision of the work relating to cutaneous disinfection with sublimate has led to some curious and interesting observations, and to results which at first seemed paradoxical.

By examining the hands of surgeons who are in the habit of washing them daily in solutions of corrosive sublimate, it was found that the mercury becomes so intimately incorporated with the epidermis that its presence there can be demonstrated by means of sulphide of ammonium at least six weeks after any contact with mercurial solutions has taken place. Micrococci in the epidermis which have not been killed by washing in sublimate solutions, but which have been brought into such relation to the sublimate that even after prolonged washing of the skin with alcohol and water they will not grow on culture media until the skin is washed with sulphide of ammonium, may also remain a long time in the epidermis. Hence it may happen that prolonged scrubbing of the hands of such persons simply with soap and warm water may remove so many superficial bacteria that the cultures from the scrapings of the epidermis may show very few, occasionally even no, colonies; whereas, when this is followed by washing in sublimate and then in sulphide of ammonium, a much larger number of colonies appear in the cultures. This apparently paradoxical result, which is obtained only from the hands of those who have previously washed them in sublimate solution, has no reference to the application of the sublimate immediately after the soap and water, but is to be explained by the liberation, by means of sulphide of ammonium, of the bacteria held in check by the mercury used, it may be, several days before the experiment. The same result is, of course, obtained if the sulphide of ammonium be applied immediately after the scrubbing with soap and water. These observations upon the persistence of mercury in the epidermis and its long-continued inhibition of the growth of bacteria, make it necessary in all work upon disinfection of the hands to first precipitate the mercury with sulphide of ammonium whenever the experiments are to be made upon hands which have been washed in sublimate solutions, even if this has occurred a long time previously. Exactly what relation the mercury in the epidermis holds to the bacteria which it does not destroy, but whose growth in our nutrient media it prevents, we cannot say. We may, perhaps, think of these bacteria as enveloped in an albuminous combination of mercury. One thing is certain—that, when the sublimate has been as thoroughly washed off from the skin as possible with water, or has been applied days before, the nutrient gelatin or agar is not rendered unfit for the growth of bacteria by the mere presence of the small quantity of mercury carried into it with scrapings from the epidermis, for the bacteria which have reached the epidermis after the application of the sublimate—and these are often identical with those inhibited by the mercury—develop as usual. It is only those bacteria which were originally brought into contact with the sublimate in some such manner as that suggested which will not grow until after the application of sulphide of ammonium, and it is not—as has been usually supposed in other observations of a similar kind in disinfectant experiments with sublimate—the alteration of the nutrient medium by the presence of a trace of sublimate which inhibits the growth of the colonies.

As to the practical efficiency of disinfection of the skin with solutions of corrosive sublimate, it is to be said that this agent, when properly applied, kills most of the bacteria upon the surface of the skin. The washing of the skin with alcohol immediately before the use of the sublimate increases its efficiency to a marked degree. If Fürbringer's method be carried out according to the strict letter of his directions it yields fair results, but it is not certain. If the mercury after employment of this method be precipitated by washing the hands in sulphide of ammonium, it will be found that the results are much less favorable than would appear by cultures made from the skin and under the nails, without the use of ammonium sulphide. It is especially the scrapings under the nails and around the matrix of the nails which yield positive results when ammonium sulphide is used, but often negative ones without this precaution. It need hardly be said that in our experiments all of the well-known, although often neglected, precautions to insure the full strength of the sublimate solutions were observed.

It may be urged that it is not necessary actually to kill the bacteria upon the skin; it is sufficient if they are rendered incapable of growth, and as most of those which are not killed by the sublimate do not grow upon our ordinary nutrient media, it is reasonable to infer that they will not grow in wounds. This line of argument certainly deserves consideration; nevertheless, there is no positive proof that these bacteria will not grow in wounds under some conditions, and surely one will feel safer with a method of disinfection which actually kills the bacteria.

I shall not detain you with the results of our experiments with other disinfectant agents. These will be published in a short time elsewhere. I shall simply state here that we have thus far obtained the best results in disinfection of the skin by the following method:

1. The nails are kept short and clean.

2. The hands are washed thoroughly for several minutes with soap and water, the water being as warm as can be comfortably borne, and being frequently changed. A brush, sterilized by steam, is used. The excess of soap is washed off with water.

3. The hands are immersed for one to two minutes in a warm saturated solution of permanganate of potash and are rubbed over thoroughly with a sterilized swab.

4. They are then placed in a warm saturated solution of oxalic acid, where they remain until complete decolorization of the permanganate occurs.

5. They are then washed off with sterilized salt solution or water.

6. They are immersed for two minutes in sublimate solution, 1 : 500.

The bacteriological examination of skin thus treated yields almost uniformly negative results, the material for the cultures being taken from underneath and around the nails. This is the procedure now employed in the gynecological and surgical wards of the hospital.

The principal conclusions of this paper may be summarized as follows:

The number of different species of bacteria, particularly of bacilli, revealed by the systematic study of traumatic infections is much greater than was formerly supposed. The pyogenic staphylococci and streptococci, however, are by far the most common causes of suppurative affections of wounds.

A coccus, which may appropriately be called the staphylococcus epidermidis albus, is a nearly, if not quite, constant inhabitant of the epidermis, lying both superficially and also deeper than can be reached by present methods of disinfection of the skin. This coccus is found frequently in aseptic wounds. It may be the cause of disturbances, usually of a relatively slight degree, in the healing of the wound, especially when drainage-tubes are inserted. It is the most common cause of stitch abscesses in wounds treated antiseptically or aseptically.

The bacillus coli communis is a frequent invader of various organs of the body in cases with ulcerative or other lesions of the intestinal mucous membrane. In such cases its presence is usually unattended by evidence of pathogenic action, but this bacillus may be associated with inflammatory affections of wounds, with peritonitis, and with abscesses.

There are many reasons for believing that the process of suppuration serves a useful purpose in combating bacteria and preventing their invasion of the circulating fluids and the tissues of the body.

The pyogenic bacteria set up suppuration by means of chemical substances produced by them and entering into their composition. The studies of chemotaxis have shed much light upon the mode of action of these substances.

The effects produced in the animal body by the pyogenic cocci are determined by many factors relating to the infectious agents and to the individual exposed to infection. There are differences in these effects depending upon the species of animal, upon the tissues and part of the body infected, upon the readiness of absorption from the infected part; upon the source, the number, and the virulence of the organisms; upon the nature and amount of the toxic substances accompanying and produced by the bacteria, upon general predisposing conditions of the body, and upon local conditions in a wound such as the presence of foreign bodies, of pathological products, of dead spaces, of bruised, necrotic, and strangulated tissues.

Infectious agents, as they occur under natural conditions, may possess greater virulence than the same bacteria in artificial cultures, and this probably depends upon accompanying toxic substances.

Results of experiments on animals explain clinical experience concerning the aseptic healing of wounds by the so-called organization of a blood-clot.

The tissues of a wound should be handled so as to interfere as little as possible with their vital capacity to overcome bacteria.

Although the greatest danger of infection of a wound from without is by direct contact, nevertheless the possibility of infection from the air should not be disregarded.

Auto-infection may take place by the entrance into the circulation and tissues of pyogenic bacteria from the alimentary and the genital canals, but there is no evidence that this can occur when these tracts are in a healthy condition. Moreover, with the requisite lesions of these tracts other general and local conditions of the body are important, if not essential, factors in bringing about pyogenic or septic infection.

The presence in the circulating blood and tissues of certain chemical products of pyogenic and of putrefactive bacteria, as well as that of various other injurious substances, favors the growth in wounds of septic and pyogenic bacteria, both of those which may be carried to the part by the circulating fluids and those which may enter from outside of the body.

Whenever we have been able to demonstrate the presence in wounds in human beings of the staphylococcus pyogenes aureus or of the streptococcus pyogenes the wound either was suppurating or subsequently it suppurated.

Only in the minority of cases were the aseptic wounds which we examined free from bacteria. By far the most common organism in these wounds pursuing an aseptic course is the staphylococcus epidermidis albus, which without the presence of a drainage-tube or other foreign body rarely causes suppuration in the wound.

The presence of microörganisms in layers of the epidermis deeper than can be reached by existing methods of cutaneous disinfection points to the skin, especially to that of the patient, as a source of infection to be carefully guarded against.

The substitution so far as possible of subcutaneous for cutaneous sutures lessens the chances of infection from this source, and particularly those of stitch abscesses.

Wherever applicable in surgical antisepsis, disinfection by heat should be preferred to that by chemical agents.

Previous experiments to determine the efficacy of disinfection of the skin with corrosive sublimate are vitiated to a considerable extent by the failure to precipitate the mercury with ammonium sulphide before testing by culture methods its germicidal power on the skin.

The mercury remains for days and weeks intimately incorporated with the epidermis.

Epidermal bacteria not killed by the sublimate may be brought into such relation with it that they will not grow in ordinary culture media until the mercury is precipitated by ammonium sulphide, and such bacteria may remain for days and weeks in the epidermis.

The results of Fürbringer's method of disinfection of the skin are found to be less favorable when they are tested after precipitation of the mercury with ammonium sulphide than without this precaution.

The best results in cutaneous disinfection we obtained by a method in which permanganate of potash followed by oxalic acid plays the principal disinfectant rôle.[1]

References to authors mentioned in the text, arranged according to order of citation.

Levy: Archiv für exp. Path. u. Pharmakologie, 1891, Bd. xxix. p. 135.
Bossowski: Wiener med Wochenschr., 1887, Nos. 8 and 9.
Von Lingelsheim: Zeitschrift für Hygiene, 1891, Bd. x. p. 331.
E. Fränkel: Centralbl. f. Bakteriologie, 1889, Bd. vi. p. 692.
Wicklein: Virchow's Archiv, Bd. cxxv. p. 75.
Gärtner: Correspondenzbl. d allg. ärztl. Vereins von Thüringen, 1888, Heft 9.
Tavel: Correspondenzbl. f. Schweizer Aerzte, 1889, No. 13.
A. Fränkel: Wiener klin. Wochenschrift, 1891, Nos. 13-15.
Welch: The Medical News, May 24, 1890, p. 566.
Ogston: Arch. f. klin. Chirurgie, Bd. xxv. 1880, and Brit. Med. Journ., 1881, p. 369.
Rosenbach: Die Mikroörganismen der Wundinfectionskrankheiten des Menschen, Wiesbaden, 1884.
Passet: Untersuch. über d. Aetiologie d. eiterigen Phlegmone des Menschen, Berlin, 1885.
Buchner: Berliner klin. Wochenschrift, 1890, Bd. xxvii. pp. 673 and 1084.
Grawitz: Charité Annalen, 1886, Jahrg. xi. Virchow's Archiv, 1889, Bd. cxvi.
Grawitz and De Bary: Virchow's Archiv, 1887, Bd. cviii.
Pawlowsky: Virchow's Archiv, 1889, Bd. cxvii.
Garré: Fortschr. d. Med., 1885, No. 6.
Bumm: Sitzungsber. d. phys.-med. Gesellsch. zu Würzburg, 1885, No. 1.
Bockhart: Monatshefte f prakt. Dermat , 1887, No. 10.
Fehleisen: Aetiologie d. Erysipels, Berlin, 1883.
Waterhouse: Virchow's Archiv, 1890, Bd. cxix. p. 342.
Hankin: British Med. Journ., July, 1890. Centralbl. f. Bakteriologie, 1891, Bd. ix. p. 336.
Brieger and *Fränkel:* Berliner klin. Wochenschr., 1890, p. 270.
Buchner: Loc. cit.
Dirckinck-Holmfeld: Annales de l'Institut Pasteur, 1888, p. 469.
Grawitz: Virchow's Archiv, 1887, Bd. cx.
Leber: Fortschr. d. Med., 1888, p. 460.
Dubler: Ein Beitrag zur Lehre von der Eiterung, Basel, 1890.
Kronacher: Die Aetiologie und das Wesen der acuten eitrigen Entzündung, 1891.
Ribbert: Die path. Anat. u. die Heilung der durch den Staph. pyog. aur. hervorgerufenen Erkrankungen, Bonn, 1891.
Bumm: Münchener med. Wochenschrift, 1889, No. 42, and Arch. für Gynäkologie, 1889, Bd. xxxiv. p. 325.
Fehleisen: Arch. f. klin. Chir., 1886, Bd. xxxvi. p. 966.
Chantemesse: Progrès méd., 1890, Nos. 13 and 19.
Roger: Le Bulletin méd., 1890, p. 966.
G. and *F. Klemperer:* Berliner klin. Wochenschr., 1891, Nos. 34 and 35.
Gärtner: Ziegler's Beiträge zur path. Anat., etc., 1891, Bd. ix. p. 276.
Ribbert: Op. cit.
Halsted: "The Treatment of Wounds, with Especial Reference to the Value of the Blood-clot in the Management of Dead Spaces," The Johns Hopkins Hospital Reports, vol. ii. No 5, 1891.
Von Bergmann: Klinisches Jahrb., Bd. i. 1889.
Schede: Arch. f. klin. Chir., 1886, Bd. xxxiv. p. 245.
Grawitz: Virchow's Archiv, 1889, Bd. cxvi.
Von Eiselsberg: Arch. f. klin. Chir., 1887, Bd. xxxv.

---

[1] Cultures were exhibited showing various species of bacteria mentioned in the paper, the white staphylococci and other bacteria isolated from the epidermis, the growths from skin sutures, and illustrating the results of different methods of disinfection of the skin, and the importance of precipitation of the mercury with ammonium sulphide when testing the germicide action of corrosive sublimate on the skin.

Prudden: THE AMERICAN JOURNAL OF THE MEDICAL SCIENCES, May, 1889, p. 452.
Von Volkmann: Quoted from an article by *Fritsch* in Deutsche med. Wochenschrift, 1890, No. 19, p. 397.
Rinne: Ueber den Eiterungsprocess und seine Metastasen, Berlin, 1889, p. 61.
De Wildt: Abstract in Centralbl. für path. Anat., 1890, Bd. i. p. 9.
Waterhouse: Loc. cit.
Ranke, Demarquay, Fischer, Schüller, quoted from references in *Watson Cheyne,* Antiseptic Surgery, London, 1882.
Watson Cheyne: Op. cit., and Brit. Med. Journ., Sept. 20, 1884.
Kümmell: Verhandl d. Deutschen Gesellschaft für Chirurgie, XIV. Congress, 1885.
Bossowski: Loc. cit.
Halsted: The Johns Hopkins Hospital Bulletins, 1889, vol. i. p. 13.
Geppert: Berliner klin. Wochenschrift, 1889, Nos. 36 and 37.
Fürbringer: Untersuchungen und Vorschriften über die Disinfection der Hände des Arztes, Wiesbaden, 1888.

WOUND INFECTION: THE CAUSES WHICH PREDISPOSE TO ITS PRODUCTION, OR FAVOR IMMUNITY, AND THE ROLE OF ANTISEPTIC AGENTS.[1]

BY ROSWELL PARK, A.M., M.D.,

PROFESSOR OF SURGERY IN THE MEDICAL DEPARTMENT OF THE UNIVERSITY OF BUFFALO, ETC.

THE study of wound infection is inseparable from that of immunity from the same, and when we have learned that which constitutes or favors immunity, we shall approach nearer that which is now a *terra incognita.* As Brunton has well said, in his recent address before the British Medical Association, "immunity is a complex condition not dependent upon any single factor," and from pathological interest, as well as from clinical importance, our endeavor now must be to analyze the main question, of what constitutes or confers immunity, and try to first recognize and then solve its various subordinate queries.

This statement, too, is inseparable from another, which is to the effect that the surgery of to-day should aim to be *aseptic,* strictly speaking, and not merely *antiseptic;* in other words, we should abolish sepsis, and not merely aim to antidote it or conquer it when present.

The only excuse for surgery which is not strictly aseptic should be met with in cases of injuries where sepsis in some form has already occurred, or those where continuous aseptic precautions are impossible; as, for example, in the mouth, rectum, etc., or in military practice, where the exigencies of the occasion do not permit that which we would ordinarily carry out with precision.

The condition of sepsis itself is a most complicated one, consisting, as far as we now see, of a condition of poisoning by ptomaines, toxines, and albumoses having widely varying strength and properties, some of which are so antagonistic in physiological action to others, that one may

---

[1] An address delivered before the Second Triennial Congress of American Physicians and Surgeons, at Washington, D. C., September 22, 1891.

neutralize another, as it is well known often occurs. Some of these sub-stances are perfectly harmless in their proper places, but deadly in others. The chemical processes going on within our bodies are as complex and as difficult of appreciation as are those mental processes which so bewilder us when sometimes we endeavor to study and read the character of various individuals. Virchow, in his address before the Tenth Inter-national Congress, voiced the general sentiment when he said: "The scientific problems of medicine are, for the most part, centred about the determination of the biological peculiarities of animal and vegetable cells." (*Vide* paper by Braatz, *Deutsche med. Wochenschrift*, 1891, No. 22.) "Lépine has lately shown that while the pancreas is pouring into the digestive channel the ferment which will form sugar, it is at the same time emptying into the system another ferment which will destroy it." (Brunton.)

But this is no more than is constantly happening in the alimentary canal, into which the intestinal glands are constantly pouring fluids which shall assist in the digestion of ingesta, while the intestinal absorb-ents may be taking up poisons produced by their mutual reactions. I esteem the proper realization of this fact as of great importance to the surgeon, as well as a due recognition of the organ through which these various poisonous substances are filtered out before reaching the sys-temic circulation. The physiologists have shown us that the organ by which this is accomplished is the liver, by virtue of its so-called depura-tive action. This is but one of its multiple functions. I have upon another occasion endeavored to show that it is by virtue of this hepatic function that many cases of septic intoxication in surgical patients are avoided, and that when this function is interfered with, the most promising surgical case may go wrong or even terminate fatally.[1] I have also there endeavored to show that in the division of the general subject of blood-poisoning a condition which we will call, if you please, intestinal toxæmia, or entero-sepsis, deserves a distinct place; that it occurs not infrequently; that by a continuation of it the condition may be merged into one of sapræmia, septicæmia, or pyæmia, and that when promptly antidoted or checked there is a speedy return to a desirable condition, both of wound and of the patient.

All of which leads to a statement upon which I desire to lay all the stress it may bear, which is to this effect—that when we have apparently commencing sepsis we are altogether too prone to look first to the wound itself for an explanation of its origin. I claim—basing this claim upon observation and laboratory study—that by no means all cases of surgical sepsis have their origin in or about the wound, no matter

[1] " Mütter Lectures on Surgical Pathology." Annals of Surgery, vol. xiii., June, 1891, p. 446.

how soon the wound may begin to show changes. To this statement I shall recur after a little.

As bearing on what has already been said, however, I wish to appeal to the personal experience of all those who have done general or special surgery. The very facts that careful surgeons prepare their patients for operation and that those who institute the most careful measures in this direction enjoy the greatest success, are, of themselves, proofs of the strength of this position. And the practice which has obtained from time immemorial in such septic conditions as puerperal fever, and many others, of giving a purgative, by which the alimentary canal is freed of toxic materials and the action of the liver stimulated, is additional evidence in the same direction. However others may interpret these conditions, the individuality of a condition of entero-sepsis is for me too apparent to be contested.

We have learned a little, and have yet much to learn, with reference to the antagonisms of different bacteria and the poisons which they produce. If a microbe can enter the system and produce a proteid or albuminoid poisonous to the animal harboring it, it may there thrive and produce such poison, while the injection or the introduction of some other substance may neutralize this poison and save the animal. The principle involved herein is the same whether the antidotal poison be injected as such, or whether a second species be inoculated by which it may be produced. The study of proteid materials is even yet so occult that we know but little about them. Were the truth concerning all the details of our body chemistry known, we should see in every human being a laboratory in which are going on more processes of manufacture and destruction than can be witnessed even in a World's Fair.

Brunton has suggested that blisters do good in this way, not merely by affecting the circulation, but by an endermic administration of proteids derived, of course, from the blood, but so altered in passage from the vessels as to have a different effect, and probably also, as will be seen, by their chemotactic properties. He also suggests that bleeding may be of benefit in a similar way, since experiments have shown that by abstraction of venous blood there is caused absorption of proteid matters from the tissues, and that these proteids may have an action of their own on tissues with which they may come in contact. The indisputable benefits, in many cases, of free purgation probably finds here also its proper explanation.

I have already introduced a term implying a condition but recently recognized, to which it seems necessary to ask your attention for a few moments. It is known under the name, given it by Pfeffer, of *chemotaxis*, and refers to that faculty possessed by all motile bacteria of moving toward or away from certain substances which seem to attract or repel them. This faculty is, however, by no means confined to the bacteria,

since Stahl has shown that the same power is inherent in the plasmodia
of myxo-mycetes, as well as in various other unicellular organisms; and
what especially concerns us here is the fact that the leucocytes at least,
if not various other cells of our own bodies, possess the same property.
As yet a general recognition of this fact hardly obtains among the profession, although an elaborate article on the subject has been published
recently by Prudden;[1] but it seems to me a matter of common importance to all who study inflammation and its results. Observers in this
direction have shown that bacteria, for instance, move toward nutritive
material, and this power has been utilized by Ali Cohen to separate
motile from immotile bacteria. He filled capillary tubes with positive
chemotactic material, like potato-juice, and with this could attract
typhoid and cholera bacteria from fæces, and thus make their pure cultivation much easier.

The chemotactic properties of leucocytes remind one very much of the
so-called tactile sensibilities which the amœbæ possess, only they enjoy
them in perhaps higher degree.   Lactic acid, 10 per cent. salt solution,
quinine 0.5 per cent., 10 per cent. alcohol, chloroform, glycerin, and bile
produce in leucocytes chemotactic activity by which they are repelled.
It must be said here that chemotaxis is spoken of as positive or negative,
according as there appears to be attraction or repulsion. Among the
most actively positive chemotactic substances are cultures of bacteria.
These are powerfully attracted by the leucocytes.   Hence it appears
that bacteria and leucocytes are mutually attractive, and the effect is
the same whether the cultures are alive or have been killed by boiling;
but it is not the culture medium itself by which this activity is manifested, but by some product of the life and growth of the bacteria.

It has been Buchner's happy lot to widely extend our knowledge of
the function and importance of the leucocyte in its chemotactic relations.
He has demonstrated that its phagocytic action is but a part of that
general power which it possesses of responding to chemotactic attraction
and incorporating into itself whatever there is of foreign, dead, or offending material, and then removing it.   It matters not that it often per-
ishes in this attempt, that is, it matters not in a logical sense, although
a quantity of leucocytes which have thus perished constitute a mass of
pus, their dead bodies remaining in this form to show the violence of the
conflict, and, as it were, their heroism in the engagement.   In other
words, it follows from Buchner's researches that the process of resolution is in large measure, or for so much as concerns the solid material
resorbed, a matter of chemotactic attraction and its results. Furthermore, that of all substances, that which seems to offer the most attraction
for leucocytes is the albuminoid material furnished by bacterial cells

---

[1] New York Med. Journ., June 6, 1891, p. 637.

It is this that attracts leuco:ytes, which are brought to the infected area by a magnetism, so to speak, which they cannot resist. This statement is especially true of proteid or albuminoid materials without reference to alkaloids, etc., produced as special products of individual forms. This is the explanation of those cases of that anomalous and clinically unimportant condition known as non-bacterial suppuration, sometimes produced in the laboratory. It is evidenced in such results as those of Wyssokowitsch, who filtered the fluid off from anthrax cultures and found that the filtrate was not pyogenic, while the solid material was.

By ingenious use of Councilman's tubes Buchner proved for the pneumo-bacillus of Friedländer that its free albuminoid material has a marked pyogenic action, and so with numerous others, especially the staphylococci, the bacillus pyocyaneus, and the typhoid bacillus.

It appears thus that the chemotactic activity of bacteria may be exerted by them whether living or dead. In either case they seem to attract toward them leucocytes which then and thus act as scavengers for the surrounding tissues. Buchner has further shown how vegetable caseins and alkali-albumins possess the same chemotactic possibilities.

I would not detain you with a rehearsal of these facts, interesting and important as they are, were it not that they appear to have a most important bearing upon questions which vitally concern the surgeon. First of all, I do not see how in the light of such researches the possibility of phagocytosis can be denied, and the importance of this process looms up in a flood of light when one discusses the phenomena of suppuration, or of other kinds of infection as well as of recovery or immunity therefrom. In suppuration and in absorption, it is proteid material which attracts the leucocytes, the same being furnished either by bacteria or by disintegrating tissue suffering from other infection. Metschnikoff, assuming the truth of his own theory of phagocytosis, invokes that of chemotaxis to explain immunity and freedom after one attack of a contagious disease. He claims that the variety of chemotaxis is variable, and that positive may be converted into negative, or vice versa, and that cells may be attracted to substances in mild form, which in strong form they repel, so that by inoculating with attenuated virus chemotaxis at first negative will change slowly to positive, and the phagocyte will at last be induced to attract and attack the invading element of disease. Whatever may be the final outcome of this perhaps fanciful development of his original theory, it is at least the result of laborious research and patient watching.

Those interested in the phagocyte explanation of conferred immunity will find choice reading in the *Transactions* of the recent International Congress of Hygiene and Demography, where, for instance, Roux, Buchner, Kitasato, and Metschnikoff himself, expounded the views which have set students the world over to thinking and to renewed investiga-

tion, and which have made their originators famous. Let it be enough
for our present purpose to say that the theory of phagocytosis appears
to be more strongly grounded than ever, and that were we deprived
of the theory, though acquainted with the facts which corroborate it,
we should be at great loss for any rational explanation of the same.

Support of the phagocyte theory has also come from another source,
namely, from Hankin's recent work on *Defensive Proteids*. From the
spleens and livers of various animals he has isolated the proteid which
has. the power of killing bacteria, and he has found that this, though
absent from normal blood, could be obtained from that of febrile animals.
There follow from these facts, if true, various deductions as to the im-
politic course of too strenuous efforts to reduce fever in septic cases, upon
which, if there were time, one might wish to dwell. This also agrees
with Hankin's suggestion that phagocytes not only kill microbes which
they have taken in, but can also, by liberating their contents, exert a
bactericidal action. It also makes plausible the view that animals that
are refractory to particular diseases have the power of producing some
particular variety of defensive proteid. There is here opened a most
attractive though difficult field for study.

The next important bearing of these views is with reference to the
absorption and separation of dead or dying materials, such as large
sloughs after extensive burns. These, of course, are loosened by physiological processes in which the formation of proteid material figures
largely. By the positive chemotactic properties already alluded to, this
attracts leucocytes in large quantities and brings them in numbers
where they are needed for tissue repair, and at the same time explains,
perhaps, the poisoning with which in these cases we have to deal.

A third not less important bearing is on the use of so-called antiseptic
agents. The ideal antiseptic is probably blood serum ; its parasiticide
properties being, in all probability, connected with the existence in it
of a globulin which is only soluble in a weak solution of common salt.
This, by the way, may explain the well-known antiseptic action of common salt, and, as Spencer Wells has said, may strengthen the belief that
we have in dilute saline solutions a safe and useful fluid for surgical
irrigation, preferable to water which has been sterilized simply by boiling, and to various other solutions which may irritate the tissues.

I am not aware that as yet any systematic study of the various antiseptic materials now in general use by surgeons, with reference to their
chemotactic activities, has been made. It strikes me, however, that
such a study offers the greatest promise of aid in the decision as to what
antiseptic to use. But it will be easily seen that once having appreciated this peculiar attraction or repulsion between organized or unorganized materials, we shall have reason to hesitate and reflect before we
apply to fresh, raw surfaces, which are supposed to be free from infec-

tion, materials, *i. e.*, antiseptic agents, of a character which may disturb
the ordinary physiological course of events by begetting such inordinate
excitement, serous outpour, and gathering of the leucocytes, as we have
seen may occur.

Although it be here a digression, I cannot avoid for a moment stopping to epitomize some of Hankin's recent work, as well as that of
Behring and Kitasato, concerning blood serum and its properties.

The work of Buchner and Nissen showed that the bactericidal action
of pure blood serum is an important factor in the conflict between the
microbe and the animal organism. This has been further confirmed by
Bouchard, who showed that the serum of a rabbit will serve as a culture medium for the bacillus pyocyaneus; but if a rabbit be made
immune against the diseases caused by this bacillus, the bacillus can no
longer be cultivated on the serum of that particular animal. In other
words, by making an animal immune against a disease the bactericidal
action of its serum is greatly increased. This is true also in the case of
cholera, anthrax, hog-cholera, and other diseases. The investigations
of Behring and Kitasato have yielded astonishing results. They found
that the serum of a rabbit which had been made immune to diphtheria
or to tetanus exerts no bactericidal action on the bacilli of these diseases;
but that it does possess the remarkable power of destroying the poisons
produced by these microbes. In other words, that such serum has *anti-
toxic* and *not bactericidal* power, and by taking advantage of such power
Behring has cured mice of tetanus in which the disease had so far progressed that two or three limbs were in a condition of spasm. Hankin,
in a very recent address (*Lancet,* August 15, 1891, p. 339), in discussing this topic, gives the following definition of immunity in the light of
recent study: "Immunity, whether natural or acquired, is due to the
presence of substances which are formed by the metabolism of the animal rather than by that of the microbe, and which have the power of
destroying either the microbe against which immunity is possible, or the
products on which their pathogenetic action depends." In giving this
definition he expressly states that it is not comprehensive for all instances, and that in some animals immunity against certain diseases
depends wholly or in part upon their causes.

He then goes on to briefly describe how he was able to separate from
serum the particular compound which conferred this power. He finally
narrowed it down to and isolated a particular ferment-like proteid,
known as cell-globulin B. And he further showed how this and other
defensive proteids in animals, and we may conclude also in man, can be
altered in amount by various conditions of diet, environment, etc.

For these defensive proteids Buchner has suggested the name *alexine;*
but Hankin would discriminate between them more carefully, and has
divided them into those which occur naturally in normal animals, which

he proposes to call *sozins,* and those occurring in animals that have been articially made immune—these he would term *phylaxins.* The former he has found in all animals yet examined.   He further shows how each of these classes can be subdivided into those that act on bacteria and those that act on the poisons they generate.   These sub-classes he would denote by the prefixes *myco-* and *toxo-;* thus *mycosozins* are proteids of the normal animal which have the power of destroying various bacteria, and *toxosozins* are proteids occurring also in the normal animal, which destroy or antagonize the poisons of bacterial origin.   Similarly *myco-phylaxins* and *toxophylaxins* will denote the classes of the phylaxins.

It has already been stated that by no means all the sources of sepsis concern the wound itself.   It is necessary now to classify and briefly allude to the principal reasons why a wound, or a patient who suffers from it, may not be able to resist infection from other sources; or, in other words, to mention the principal other sources of infection possible. These I would classify as follows:

1. Previous long-existent toxæmia (*e. g.*, syphilis, diabetes, acetonæmia, lithæmia, alcoholism, malaria).

2. Previous anatomical changes which reduce vitality (*e. g.*, inherited diatheses, old age, amyloid change, chronic and acute nephritis).

3. Recent or acute toxæmia (uræmia, typhoid, intestinal toxæmia, stercoral toxæmia).

4. Other acute conditions (starvation, scurvy, anæmia).

5. Conditions of environment (bad hygienic surroundings).

6. Effect of anæsthetics.

7. Effect of antiseptics.

1. *Previous long-existent toxæmia.*   The disastrous results of operating upon diabetic patients, as well as those presenting active manifestations of syphilis, have long been recognized by surgeons.   Nor does one deliberately operate on patients suffering from chronic alcoholism or malaria, if he can avoid it.   Other conditions which deserve to be mentioned here as having an occasional yet distinct bearing in this direction are lithæmia, cholæmia, acetonæmia, and the various conditions which are represented by the presence of the oxalates, uric acid, acetone and peptone in the urine.

2. *Previous anatomical changes which lower vitality.*   Old age, with its accompanying arterial sclerosis, its cardiac debility, and other well-known tissue alterations, favors sluggishness of wound repair, leads not infrequently to sloughing or to bedsore, and predisposes toward sepsis. Amyloid changes betoken impaired vitality, and chronic or acute nephritis implies that excretion may be interfered with, and some form of toxæmia thereby induced.   The inherited diatheses, including tuberculosis and syphilis, may or may not be factors of considerable importance in this respect.

3. *Recent toxæmia.* To illustrate this class of cases a little better, let me mention an illustrative case: A middle-aged woman, of healthy antecedents, recently convalescent from typhoid, which had run an average course, presented a rapidly growing tumor (sarcoma) in one breast. So rapid was its growth that operation could not be delayed. It was made with every aseptic precaution. Nevertheless the skin flaps, which would ordinarily have united without pus, necrosed completely, and left a large surface to heal by granulation.

No one would wittingly operate on a patient suffering from uræmia save in dire emergency. To the condition of entero-sepsis, intestinal toxæmia, or fæcal or stercoral intoxication, I have already alluded. My own studies and experience with this condition have led me to profound conviction, since time and again I have seen commencing septic wound disturbance aborted by the institution of measures calculated to clear out the alimentary canal, this being true of wounds in all parts of the body. The same is true, also, of the toxæmia produced in puerperal, diphtheritic and scarlatinal cases, in which, as is well known, we operate only when compelled to in the interest of life.

One form of entero-sepsis upon which but little has been written, and yet which furnishes a clue to many fatal cases, especially those connected with abdominal surgery, is that produced by the bacillus coli commune. This, as is well known, is a regular inhabitant of the alimentary canal, and its presence there is presumably connected with the chemistry of digestion. Yet, under certain circumstances, it either escapes or is carried beyond its normal limits, and, entering the portal circulation, perhaps the lymphatics also, appears to set up septic disturbances which are typified by the production of septic peritonitis, and possibly other forms of septicæmia in which the peritoneum does not primarily figure. The subject is an inviting one for further research; the condition has hardly yet been dignified by a proper and distinctive name, though Drs. Welch and Councilman, who should be credited with its discovery, term it " colon infection." It is mentioned here only as one variety of enterosepsis, and as one in which, perhaps, good results are obtained in such cases as those which the gynecologists often meet with, namely, of incipient septic peritonitis, in which the administration of a large dose of magnesium sulphate appears to provoke not merely catharsis, but absorption of septic fluid from within the peritoneal cavity.

4. *Other acute conditions.* As representatives of this group should be mentioned starvation, scurvy, acute anæmia such as follows the post-febrile and post-puerperal state. By all of these conditions vital resistance is so lowered that infection from within or without is greatly favored.[1]

---

[1] Concerning the influence of hunger upon immunity and infection, vide Caualis u. Morpurgo, Fortschritte der Medicin, viii. pp. 693, 729.

5. *Conditions of environment.* Emergency is the only justifiable reason for surgical operation where the hygienic surroundings are bad. Universal experience justifies this statement, but experimental proof of the same is not lacking. The experiments of Trudeau beautifully exemplify this. He inoculated a number of rabbits with tuberculosis, isolated them upon a small island in the Adirondack region, fed them well, gave them every benefit of fresh air and sunlight, and, upon killing them four months later, only one was found to present the slightest evidence of tubercular disease. The same number of rabbits in another group were inoculated in the same way and confined in a dark cellar, amidst damp air with poor ventilation. These became rapidly diseased, and without exception all were notably tubercular. (The American Journal of the Medical Sciences, vol. xciv., July, 1887, p. 119.)

The popularity of fresh-air missions, the benefit of removal of the poor and ill-fed to good hospitals for operation, and numerous other well-known facts, attest the importance of the matter of environment.

6. *Effect of anæsthetics.* There is good reason to think that chloroform and ether administered for some time may produce such changes in the blood and tissues that vital processes of repair, cell resistance, and chemotaxis may be so far interfered with as to facilitate subsequent infection. In making this statement I feel assured of the corroboration of surgeons generally. Yet I know of no particular researches bearing upon it, and would suggest it as offering a fine field for orginal research.

7. *Effect of antiseptics.* Upon first blush the idea that an antiseptic may favor infection would seem to be essentially opposed to facts. Yet the fact is made clear, both by clinical experience and by experiment. Such an event may happen in more than one way. Mercurial and iodoform poisoning are by no means unknown to the surgeon as arising from the use of these drugs for antiseptic purposes. When this condition is established the case becomes at once one of recent toxæmia, to which I have already alluded. That wounds will fail to unite, and that suppuration will occur in these toxæmic conditions, is well known. The individual is so poisoned that his cell-resistance is diminished or destroyed, and in consequence there is little or no opposition to infection.

The other method is by such chemical reaction between vital fluid and antiseptic agent that decomposition of one or both ensues, the antiseptic itself being decomposed, its properties as such lost, while the tissues upon which it acts may have their constitution so changed as to favor rather than resist infection. The best experimental proof of this statement that I know of has been furnished by Abbott (*Johns Hopkins Hospital Bulletin*, April, 1891). Without rehearsing his experiments with mercuric chloride, let me simply remind you of his conclusions:

1. That under the most favorable conditions a given amount of sublimate has the property of rendering inert only a certain number of

individual organisms, since there is a definite chemical reaction between the bacterial protoplasm and the mercuric salt.

2. That the disinfecting activity of sublimate against organisms is profoundly influenced by the proportion of albuminous material contained in the medium in which the bacteria are present.

3. That the relation between staphylococci and sublimate is not a constant one, since organisms from different sources and of different ages behave differently when exposed to the same amount of the salt for the same length of time.

4. That the organisms which survive exposure may experience a temporary attenuation, which, however, may disappear by successive cultivation. (His other conclusions enumerated are irrelevant here.)

From these studies he justifies the statement which has been frequently made, that to the employment of sublimate solutions upon wound surfaces it is plain that there exist at least two serious objections:

First, that the albumin of the tissues and fluids of the body tends to diminish the strength of, or render entirely inert, the solution employed. Since the surgeon possesses no means by which he can determine the amount of such material with which his solutions are to come in contact, he is therefore never in position to say à priori that his efforts at disinfection of a wound are or are not successful.

The second objection is that the integrity of tissues is materially disturbed by the application of solutions of this sort.

There is abundance of evidence to lead to the belief that normal tissues and fluids of the body possess the power of rendering inert many kinds of organisms which may have gained access to them. This function must therefore be diminished or destroyed by agents which bring about alterations in the constitution of these tissues. Such changes are known to follow the application of sublimate solutions, which may cause a condition of superficial necrosis, by which the inroads of infectious organisms are not resisted as they would have been had the tissues been left in their natural condition.

From all of which it would appear best to keep not only those, but all other antiseptic agents away, from absolutely clean flesh surfaces. The experiments of Nuttall, Lubarsch, Von Fodor, Bonome, Springfeld, and others have shown the value of blood serum as an antiseptic, while the experience of all laboratory workers points in the same direction. Such serum will always be poured out, it is presumable, in quantity sufficient to serve not only as a cohesive but as an antiseptic agent.

Just here in passing the query is provoked, What agent can best be used as an antiseptic? We are learning every day that, providing everything else be clean and fresh, wounds such as made by the surgeon will also be clean, and that the dry method of operating is, per-

haps, the best of all; but inasmuch as the surgeon is often compelled
to disinfect an area which has already become infected, he must per-
force employ some actively antiseptic agent. It would appear that for
most purposes we find the ideal in peroxide of hydrogen, which not
merely destroys living organisms, but by oxidation of all undesirable
and infected material acts as a scavenger of the tissues, and, in one
phrase, when it can be efficiently employed locally, is the conqueror of
sepsis.

While such artificial agents as the peroxide must rank as among the
highest of their class, it seems to me that we have yet to learn how to
utilize to fullest advantage the properties of blood serum. To be sure,
this varies among the different animals, and by the limitations of experimental study we are less familiar with such as are possessed by the
serum of the human blood than with those enjoyed by that of various
animals. For instance, it is well known that a mouse will die of inoculated anthrax, while a rat will not. Also that if the inoculated mouse
receive a few drops of rat blood serum it recovers. Practical advantage has been taken of this principle, and it has been proposed, and even
carried out, to inject into consumptive patients blood serum of the goat
or dog, which are known to be almost immune from tuberculosis.
Bonome has found that staphylococci thrown directly into the blood of
young animals are there destroyed much more quickly than in that of
old animals, namely, in from ten to twenty-five minutes. (This has a
bearing on the effect of old age already alluded to.) This bactericidal
action of the blood is enhanced if the poisonous extract of empyemic
or rather of any old pus be injected into the animal before the experiment, while the extract of recent or acute pus has no such effect. On
the other hand the latter, i. c., the extract from acute pus, appears to
diminish the chemotactic or phagocytic power of the cell elements.
Water also diminishes this bactericidal power of the blood, and an
important inference may be drawn from this with reference to the
advisability of infusion of saline or other solutions for the relief of
acute traumatic anæmia.

Having discussed immunity and conditions which predispose to infection, let us consider how direct infection may be brought about.
Infection may be divided into two varieties: Self- or auto-infection and
contact infection, including that from the skin and wound, from the
air, and from ingesta. And yet, while making these two varieties,
namely, infection from without and from within, it must be stated
that infection as such is presumably due to the same organisms in either
case, and that such varieties are arbitrary and not founded upon essential differences. The causes which lead to auto-infection have been
already alluded to, as well as those cases of contact infection which
originate from the air and from improper food. To be sure, the experi-

ments of Kocher, and of others, in the direction of feeding animals with putrid or putrifying material, and then insulting the thyroid or bone-marrow, in the endeavor to provoke acute sepsis by infection from the alimentary canal, have not been sufficient to completely satisfy one that by improper food alone sepsis may be caused. But I would make a sharp distinction between such experiments and their results, and the condition of entero sepsis, which includes only a condition of toxæmia arising from presumably proper food, undergoing perverted chemical changes within the alimentary canal, and there producing poisons as the result of such changes, which, when absorbed, give rise to deleterious effects.

But contact infection, as it usually occurs, arises from the air or from some other unclean foreign substance which comes in contact with exposed raw surfaces. Air contact, is, on first thought, a most fertile source of trouble. Pasteur and Lister first made us fear the air as the most dangerous medium of all, but we have gradually learned that its dangers in any proper operation locality are so small as scarcely to deserve consideration in comparison with the others to be mentioned. Not that germs may not be deposited from the air just as they are in an improperly protected culture-tube, but that nearly all of these are non-pathogenic, and that they, with the pathogenic forms, are nearly always either washed or wiped away, or are destroyed by the blood serum or the phagocytic action of the cells.

The principal sources of contact infection are to be enumerated as follows :

1. Skin and hair.
2. Instruments.
3. Sponges or their substitutes.
4. Suture materials.
5. The hands of the surgeon and his assistants.
6. Drainage materials.
7. Dressing materials.
8. Miscellaneous, *e. g.*, drops of perspiration, an unclean irrigator-nozzle, the nail-brush, the clothing of the operator or the bystanders, etc.

1. *Skin and hair.* The danger here comes not so much from what may be on the surface as from that which may be contained within the hair-follicles and sebaceous and sudoriparous glands. The prevention of infection from this source, therefore, requires more than ordinary shaving of the surface or superficial application of soap and water. Lister claimed for carbolic solutions that they had the power of impregnating greasy material with their antiseptic virtues, though as the latter are very questionable we must doubt the former. But it is vitally necessary that, by whatever means we may, we should make our pre-

cautions reach into these crypts, for the possibility of the hibernation of infectious organisms in the crypts or even the tissues of the skin has been experimentally proven.   This is especially true of the streptococci of erysipelas, which have been found latent, but alive, within the skin long after the subsidence of active manifestations of the disease, the skin having become apparently, at least temporarily, tolerant.

What then are the best means of sterilizing the skin ?   These must depend upon whether time is afforded for careful preparation or not. When we deliberately do a craniotomy or laparotomy we have ample time for such measures, but when an amputation for injury, time and means are both limited.

In the former instance, there should first of all be a careful shaving of the skin, the razor being, as some Frenchman has described it, an admirable dermal curette. I would prefer, then, to use for a day or two some antiseptic ointment, properly prepared (see No. 8), such as one made with resorcin or lysol, and lanolin, by whose use we may hope to bring about absorption into the skin of the antiseptic employed.   After one or two days' use of this, the skin should be again thoroughly washed, and for this purpose the best soap is the sapo viride of the German Pharmacopœia, with 5 per cent. of lysol or hydro-naphthol.   Now for an equal period there should be worn over the part a compress kept moist with some liquid, non-irritating antiseptic. For this purpose creolin or lysol, 5 per cent., or hydro-naphthol in saturated cold aqueous solution, perhaps with a little glycerin added, should be worn until the time of operation.   Now everything being ready and the patient being anæsthetized, a final scrubbing with hydro-naphthol soap with shaving should be practised, and then the skin washed with equal parts of alcohol and ether or alcohol and turpentine.   By this means the operator may feel confident that the surface has been thoroughly disinfected.

In cases of the other class, where time for this programme is not afforded, we must content ourselves with the thorough use of the nail-brush, the razor, and antiseptic soap, with the subsequent use of alcohol and ether upon the skin.

2. *Instruments.* Aside from the information which has long been at hand with regard to the necessity of having clean instruments, I know of nothing so significant as the experience of Thiriar, who had several cases of tetanus following his operations, and whose disastrous experience ceased as soon as he sterilized his instruments by heat. That instruments should be in some way sterilized is now everywhere accepted. The question is now solely with regard to the best method, whether with dry heat, in steam, or by boiling.   It appears that the method of dry sterilization injures the instruments, especially those with keen edges, less than any other. For my own part, I prefer a dry sterilizer in which they are subjected for half an hour to a temperature of 140° or 150° C.,

although I prefer to content myself with passing a delicate cutting instrument two or three times through the flame. Long immersion in hot water certainly does injure all edged instruments, as does also superheated steam or hot air.

3. *Sponges.* There appears to be nothing to add in this connection to the well-known directions for cleaning and sterilizing sponges. It is important, however, to know whether a sponge which has once been used can be employed again. A careful series of experiments has convinced me, at all events, that sponges which have been used in non-septic cases, and have been carefully cleansed and immersed in antiseptic solutions for a week or more, contain no bacteria that can reveal themselves after approved culture methods.

Nevertheless, in order to be absolutely on the safe side, it would appear better, in many respects, to use some cheap absorbent material as a substitute for sponges, which can be used once and thrown away. There are numerous materials which we can thus employ, proper care being given only to see that they are both absorbent and sterile. A final cooking or baking shortly before use will insure at least this latter point.

4. *Suture materials.* These are mainly animal or metal; silk, catgut, horsehair, and silkworm-gut being the best examples of the former, and iron, copper, silver wire, of the latter. Two essentials are requisite in all material for suture, namely, strength and sterility. Power of resorption is a secondary consideration, although very necessary in certain cases. We may at once dismiss metal sutures from consideration, since it is the simplest possible measure to sterilize them. But the proper sterilization of animal suture or ligature material is a problem on which a great deal of time has been spent. (See the researches of Brunner and of others.[1])

Silk may be sterilized by boiling, but this weakens it. The best method is to wind it upon glass spools, to drop these into a large testtube, to plug the tube, and then keep it for an hour in a steam sterilizer, upon two different occasions. Silkworm-gut appears to be much less septic naturally than is catgut, and may be sterilized by immersion in 1 per cent. aqueous sublimate solution for a few hours, and then preservation in alcohol.

But it is with regard to catgut that the greatest study has been excited, and the largest number of preparation methods suggested. It is not necessary here to detain you even with allusion to the work which has been done in this direction, interesting as it may be. Permit me to simply briefly state what I consider the safest and best method by which

[1] Beiträge zur klinischen Chirurgie, vi. 98; Braatz, Ibid., vii. 70; Klemm, Archiv. f. klin. Chir., xli. 4.

to insure the sterilization of catgut. The raw gut, preferably that which
has been prepared in the factories for surgeons' use, should have, first of
all, its fatty material dissolved out by immersion in benzene or ether.
It is then allowed to dry and is soaked for one or two days in a 1 per cent.
watery solution of corrosive sublimate, after which it is dried and transferred to oil of juniper berries, and from this to strong alcohol containing one per mille of sublimate. (In this, if desired, it can be boiled.)
Catgut thus prepared will, so far as we know, resist every attempt to
cultivate bacteria from it. If it be desirable to chromicize it, this may
be done before it is placed in juniper oil.

I have, like many others, tried various experiments to accomplish the
same results by other means, including moist and dry heat, etc., yet
know of nothing which gives such universally satisfactory results as the
above.

5. *The hands.* The hands of all those concerned about the field of
operation should be carefully disinfected. This includes the surgeon,
his assistants, and the nurses or attendants who may handle sponges or
dressings. It has not required such laboratory studies as those of Kümmell and others to show that ordinary methods of cleansing the hands
do not bring about an aseptic condition. The thousands of times that
wound infection has followed contact with the unclean hands of the surgeon or obstetrician bear witness to this fact. It is simply a truism to
state that cemeteries have been filled in time past by the septic hands of
medical attendants.

How then disinfect them? It would seem almost unnecessary to be
obliged to allude here to such measures, yet the use of the penknife and
the nail-brush are not always enough. Is it possible for a surgeon to
go from the post-mortem room or from a case of erysipelas, or for a
surgical teacher to be called from demonstrating on a cadaver to operating in the hospital or in private, without danger of carrying septic
material? I think we are now in a position to say Yes, provided he disinfect his own hands and skin, and change his clothing. I know that I
have, on numerous occasions, gone directly from a class demonstration
on the cadaver to the hospital amphitheatre to operate, and seen patients
recover without a sign of sepsis. But how is this possible? Under such
circumstances, so far as the hands and forearms are concerned, I would
advise to wash them first thoroughly in soap and water, using the nail-
brush freely, then to take a tablespoonful or more of flour of mustard
and wash the hands thoroughly with this, as if it were a powdered soap.
Mustard is certainly an admirable deodorizer, and its essential oil has
been shown to be a most valuable antiseptic agent. (This method will
serve to disinfect the hands and deodorize them after handling any foul-
smelling material or sanious discharge.) Now, before approaching the
patient, no matter what may have been done before, aside from the ordi-

nary scrubbing I would highly recommend the use of the sapo viride (G. P.) to which has been added 5 per cent. of lysol, creolin, or hydronaphthol. Hands and forearms should be thoroughly scrubbed with this, then rinsed and immersed in strongly colored solution of permanganate of potassium. They should then be rinsed again, and now immersed in a solution of oxalic acid, not too strong, and yet sufficiently so to decolorize the skin within two or three minutes. The oxalic solution may be rinsed off, and the hands may now be regarded as thoroughly aseptic. It is expected that occasionally during the course of the operation they will be rinsed in antiseptic solution. This, so far as personal experience goes, is a more reliable method than the use of turpentine or any such material upon the hands.

6. *Drainage materials.* For the most part these comprise horsehair, catgut, soft rubber tubes, hard-rubber tubes, spiral or stiff glass tubes, and gauze strips or wicking. Views and practices concerning drainage have materially changed even since the antiseptic era began. Our predecessors drained to permit escape of pus which they knew would form. Until lately we have drained in order to prevent its formation. We seem now to be on the eve of an era when we need to drain but little or not at all. We resort to drainage now only of necessity, in septic or infected cases. In other cases we drain mainly from habit, or from fear. Indeed, when we start afresh, as it were, without previous infection, the practice of drainage is a confession of fear, or of weakness, both of which are alike unscientific and unfortunate. We have learned that a little blood serum is an advantage rather than a detriment, and we do not need to guard against its presence as we used to. It even seems to me that in many cases, where all other aseptic requirements have been met, we do much more harm than good by the use of drains. Did time permit, it seems to me that it would be justifiable to occupy some moments in a discussion of this single topic. As it is, I will simply justify personal conclusions by mentioning certain classes of operations in which at present I never resort to drainage—never having regretted discontinuing it :

a. Deliberate operations about the brain and calvarium.

b. Amputations when in uninfected tissues.

c. Excisions of joints for conditions other than tubercular.

d. Herniotomy, both for strangulation and radical cure, when the intestine is still viable and no gangrenous condition is met with.

e. Osteotomy, tarsectomy, and other operations for relief of deformity.

f. Most operations for removal of tumors, etc.

This is by no means a complete list, but is simply intended to be suggestive.

7. *Dressing materials.* Two questions come up here : What is the best dressing material ? and what antiseptic is most suitable for the case ?

Naturally wounds need some protection, and, inasmuch as in certain cases there will be at least a slight discharge of serum or blood, this protection must at the same time be absorbent, and the choice of the absorbent material may well be left to circumstances or to fancy of the surgeon. But the selection of an antiseptic is again a confession of distrust of one's self or of what has been previously done; and while such distrust may be in the interest of the patient, it is not in the direction of scientific advance. Consequently we may say that after the ideal aseptic operation we need only a sterilized and protective dressing—protection from the air without, as well as protection from contact contamination and from the restlessness of the patient. Such ideal dressing may be composed of any sterilized material. The majority of operators, however, desire some additional assurance, or an additional safeguard, which they may, perhaps, secure in the impregnation of the wound-dressing with any one of the more or less reliable antiseptic chemicals. These remarks do not pertain so much to a large group of cases where drainage must be resorted to, and where more or less discharge is necessarily expected. If dressings are to be saturated or much moistened with wound discharges, it is well that they should be charged with some soluble antiseptic. In certain cases the conditions of repair necessitate much purulent or puruloid discharge. It is well that this should be taken up by material which may antagonize its decomposition or putrifaction. Whether this material shall be some soluble salt of mercury or zinc, or something like iodoform, salicylic acid, zinc oxide, etc., is scarcely germane to our present subject; so long as the object aimed at is attained the possibility or probability of wound infection is prevented.

8. *Miscellaneous sources of wound infection.* These are almost too numerous to mention, but illustrative examples of sources of danger may be given as follows:

Drops of perspiration are liable to fall into the wound area from the forehead and face of an excited, fatigued, or hard-worked operator. So also may scales of dandruff from his hair or beard. The former will probably be seen, the latter not. Consequently the ideal operator in this respect is he whose hair is worn short, and whose face is devoid of beard. In almost every clinic are certain irrigator tubes and nozzles intended for daily use. It is quite possible for one of these to be used to day for washing out some old abscess cavity and to be then hung up until to-morrow, when it is used in a case about which pus has neither been present nor is expected to be. Infection may thus be carried from one to the other. It is my custom to disinfect these nozzles with strong solutions of permanganate of potassium, as also the hard-rubber atomizing tubes which I frequently use for spraying out wounds or washing off surfaces.

In many severe cases the surgeon is strongly tempted, sometimes imperatively impelled, to place his hand upon the patient's radial pulse. It has been suggested, and it certainly is good practice, to carefully disinfect the area of the patient's wrist before the operation, so that the operator can, if necessary, feel the pulse without the danger of thereby infecting his hands.

In every well-regulated clinic there are regulations with regard to clothing, and a supply of clean linen is furnished for the operator and his assistants. Some even carry this precaution to the extent of allowing no one in the room who is not thus clad in fresh linen, which will dislodge no dust upon contact. And who shall say that this precaution is not a wise one, even if, perhaps, sometimes superfluous?

Another source of danger, which I have not seen elsewhere alluded to, is one to which of late I have given some personal study. It is customary with many, after the wound is ready for its dressing, to anoint the surrounding skin with some unctuous material, which shall prevent such adhesion of wound-dressing as may make change of the same a source of dread to the patient. In my own clinic this is done almost as a matter of custom. It is quite possible for such ointments to come in contact with the wound; often they are deliberately applied over it. It behooves us, then, to know whether such ointments, which are supposed to be antiseptic, are such in effect. In the surgical clinic of the Buffalo General Hospital ointments containing 5 and 10 per cent. of naphthalin, of resorcin, and of hydro-naphthol are constantly kept on hand. These are made up in part with vaseline, to which lanolin is added. For the purpose of ascertaining in the first place whether the ointment material was or was not sterile, in the second place whether these ointments themselves were reliable, and in the third place whether the method of preparation with or without heat made any difference, a series of experiments has recently been made for me by one of my surgical assistants, Dr. E. J. Meyer, who is also well versed in pharmacy. Briefly, the results of these experiments have been as follows:

1. Vaseline and all other bases commonly supplied for ointments, as they come from the shops, are by no means free from bacterial contamination, the majority of culture experiments made with them being successful.

2. Ointments made with resorcin and naphthalin, even of 10 per cent. strength, prepared without heat, give for the most part growths of various bacteria.

3. Similar ointments made up by the aid of heat, where the temperature of the mass has been raised to the boiling-point of water, seem to be absolutely sterile, and when exposed to the air suffer only from air contamination, so far as found, with non-pathogenic bacteria and the common moulds.

I would regard these experiments as not only suggestive, but important, because they show that there is not enough diffusion of the antiseptic itself through the ointment mass to exert any such effect as has been generally supposed. Therefore, I assign this fact as illustrating another of the possible sources of wound infection from well-intentioned but misjudged and overestimated protection.

It is well to recall here the investigations of Liebreich, who claims that a coating of lanolin constitutes an almost impassable barrier for bacteria, keeping them in or keeping them out, as the case may be.

And now, without detaining you further, it is necessary that I should bring to a close a paper in which the endeavor has been made to be suggestive rather than complete. The particular features to which I would especially invite attention may be epitomized in the following conclusions :

1. Study of wound infection and of the septic condition thereby produced is inseparable from a study of what constitutes immunity.

2· By a study of immunity is furnished the best clue to a due appreciation of the principles of asepsis.

3. The surgery of the future must aim to be aseptic, for, so far as fresh cases are concerned, we have passsed the merely antiseptic era.

4. Asepsis is to be achieved, not alone by attention to the wound and the pharaphernalia of operation, but by the closest regard to the condition of the patient's organs and tissues.

5. Sepsis may arise from circumstances and conditions other than those pertaining to the wound itself, although hitherto practitioners have been too prone to scan solely this field when searching for its cause.

6. Sepsis and infection are combated in more than one way by natural agencies and by inherent properties of cells and fluids, totally aside from the measures which the surgeon institutes, and the wisest man is he who studies to take advantage of these vital activities rather than introduce new and conflicting elements from without.

7. A recognition of the power of chemotaxis possessed by organized and unorganized materials, in such varying degree, can be utilized to great advantage so soon as it can be reasonably clearly defined.

8. A study of chemotactic activity appears to impress one with the truth of the phagocyte doctrine, which, if proven, is one having a large bearing upon the principles as well as the practice of the surgery of the future.

9. The proteid material contained within cellular infectious organisms plays such a rôle, both in causing chemotaxis as well as in poisoning the animal infected, that we have reason to eagerly welcome all knowledge concerning it.

10. So fast as such proteid material can be isolated we need, among other things, to study its effects upon the commonly used antiseptic agents.

11. We need to study much further the anti-toxic and bactericidal properties of human blood serum, and the means by which we can avail ourselves of the same.

12. Some such classification as I have attempted to give of the various causes of lowered resistance to infection, or of the causes of *vulnerability* or susceptibility, will certainly assist in a due appreciation thereof, and will often aid in so fortifying the patient that he may resist infection to which he would otherwise succumb.

13. The condition of entero-sepsis, fecal toxæmia, stercoral intoxication, or whatever it may be called, is certainly one which every practitioner has to fear and against which he should assiduously guard. It is not sufficiently generally recognized and combated.

14. A sub-form of this condition might justly be made and be entitled gastro-sepsis, comprising cases where defective stomach digestion, often from .dilatation, brings about a lithæmic or other toxæmic condition which favors infection.

15. Antiseptic agents in the past have worked a revolution in surgical practice and results. We have now reached a time when we know that they all have their disadvantages, and also understand how, if we are strictly aseptic in our work, we can afford to discontinue their application to wound surfaces.

16. But the insurance of the aseptic character of such work necessitates the use of antiseptic agents of some kind upon everything which may directly or indirectly come in contact with these surfaces.

17. When this work is strictly aseptically performed, the use of drains or further employment of antiseptics is either an expression of mental uncertainty or of fear. It may be in the interest of humanity, undoubtedly it often is, but it is not attaining the ideal of scientific work.

TWO CASES OF PREGNANCY WITH BRIGHT'S DISEASE AND ALMOST COMPLETE SUPPRESSION OF URINE.

By G. Ernest Herman, M.B. Lond., F.R.C.P.,

OBSTETRIC PHYSICIAN TO THE LONDON HOSPITAL, AND LECTURER ON MIDWIFERY; EXAMINER IN MIDWIFERY TO THE ROYAL COLLEGE OF SURGEONS OF ENGLAND; TREASURER TO THE OBSTETRICAL SOCIETY OF LONDON, ETC.

An obstetric physician cannot help being interested in the pathology of puerperal eclampsia. The theory of this disease which has the most reason in its favor is that the convulsions of puerperal eclampsia are caused in the same way as uræmia apart from pregnancy.

But the pathology of ordinary uræmic convulsions appears to me to scarcely yet rest on a firm basis. It seems generally accepted that uræmic convulsions are a result of imperfect elimination of certain waste products that ought to have been got rid of by the kidneys. Various views have been put forth as to what these products are, where they are retained, what changes they undergo, and in what form they produce the symptoms of uræmia. But there seems to be agreement as to the fact that in health they appear in the urine, for the most part in the shape of urea.

I have not been able to find in any text-book which treats of kidney diseases any proof, or attempt at proof, or reference to proof, that uræmic convulsions are associated with deficiency either of urine or urea. But in conversation with physicians whose line of practice makes them specially familiar with renal disease, I find that the proposition that in uræmia the elimination of urea is diminished is to them a truism so repeatedly verified by experience that no one thinks that the publication of detailed evidence for its demonstration is needful. Doubtless, then, this view is correct. But I have quite failed to get, either from reading or from verbal inquiry, any information as to what *degree* of defect in the elimination of urea is sufficient to produce uræmia, or how long a great diminution must last before convulsions or other uræmic symptoms are produced. One would, of course, not expect that a very rigid limit could be laid down which should hold good for all cases, but surely some law must be capable of definition.

I have published in the *Transactions of the Obstetrical Society of London* (vols. xxix., xxxii., and xxxiii.) a series of twelve cases of puerperal eclampsia in which the urine was measured and the quantity of urea in it estimated. In every case it was found that while the fits were occurring there was diminution in the excretion of urea. These observations harmonize with what would have been expected if puerperal convulsions are uræmic; and the current conception of the pathology of uræmia is correct.

But there are observations which tend to show that the pathology of uræmia is not quite so simple as this. Carter[1] speaks of "the absence of convulsions so often characterizing the uræmia of absolute suppression in persons healthy up to the time of the suppression, of which probably most physicians have seen examples." Sir W. Roberts[2] says: "Sometimes, however, very great scantiness of urine, or even total suppression (in acute Bright's disease) may exist without evoking any uræmic symptom. In a case of scarlatinal dropsy related by Biermer complete suppression of urine continued for five days without uræmia; then followed a further period of four and a half days in which urine was secreted, but only in the scantiest proportions (a few teaspoonfuls a day), and yet no uræmia.

---

[1] Bradshaw Lecture " On Uræmia," Brit. Med. Journal, 1888, vol. ii. p. 466.
[2] Urinary and Renal Diseases, 2d edition, p. 421.

At the end of this second period the urine began to flow abundantly for a short time, and then again became scanty. Three days later uræmic coma set in, followed by convulsions, which proved fatal."

In the present communication I report a case in which there was almost absolute suppression of urine, lasting a week, and very great diminution in the amount of urine for two weeks; and the excretion of urea was diminished even more than in proportion to the quantity of urine, and yet there were no convulsions.

I report, also, another case in which the diminution in the quantity of urine was not so great as in the first case, and the amount of urea in it was only once estimated; but the flow of urine for more than a fortnight was far below the average of health, and below the quantity passed in some cases of eclampsia.

I refrain from any attempt at generalization, further than to say that Case I. and the case Sir W. Roberts quotes from Biermer seem to me to show that mere diminution of the excretion of urea in the urine cannot be *per se* the cause of uræmic convulsions.

CASE I. *First pregnancy: symptoms of renal disease coming on during the last three months; intra-uterine death of fœtus and premature delivery; almost complete suppression of urine for eight days after delivery; great diminution for two weeks; diminution of urinary solids and urea; albuminuria; vomiting; diarrhœa; œdema; delirium; pericarditis in third week after delivery; parotitis in fourth week; retinal hemorrhages; death eleven months afterward.* (From notes by Dr. Hugh Smith, resident accoucheur, and Mr. A. H. Smith, clinical clerk.)—M. A. McC., aged twenty-five. Admitted to the London Hospital October 29, 1889, under the care of Dr. Herman. Patient was a domestic servant, and remained in her situation until three months before admission. No previous illness, except smallpox when aged about twenty. First menstruated at fourteen. After the first appearance of the catamenia they ceased for six months, then returned, and from that time till her pregnancy she was regular every month, flow lasting two days, and being scanty and painless. Patient was not married, and the pregnancy was her first.

During the first three or four months of pregnancy patient suffered severely from vomiting every morning. At the beginning of the fourth month of pregnancy her legs began to swell. This swelling was as great in the morning as in the evening. About the sixth month she began to suffer from an enlargement of a vein in the right leg, and for this reason, and not because she felt ill in any other respect, she left off work. During the last three months her face was puffy. Three weeks before admission she noticed that her urine was scanty and dark-colored, and at the same time she had a slight aching pain across the loins. These symptoms lasted about six days. From that time until her confinement she had to get up three or four times in the night to pass water. The water was pale in color and she thought more than the usual quantity.

She was delivered of a stillborn child on October 28th. She thought herself about a fortnight short of full term. The labor was easy, only lasting seven hours. Immediately after delivery patient became very restless, could not sleep, and was very thirsty. She passed no urine for fifteen hours after her confinement, when six drachms were drawn off.

Next morning (*October 29th*) she was said to have been feverish, thirsty, and somewhat delirious, and her sight became suddenly indistinct, so that she could only see the outlines of things, but not details. She was brought to the hospital and admitted.

On admission she complained of great pain across the loins and was very thirsty. She was pale and anæmic. Eyelids so œdematous that they could not be separated more than one-quarter of an inch; legs œdematous. Optic discs slightly swollen and outline indistinct, but no retinal hemorrhage in either eye. Sight bad; could count fingers at two feet distance with the right eye; at three feet with the left; could not distinguish faces. Heart's impulse strong and widely diffused. Loud and harsh systolic murmur heard over the whole cardiac area, but especially over the base on the left side. Pulse full, but compressible; 104 per minute. Has not at any time had headache; none now.

30th. At 6 P.M. on the 29th was dry-cupped over loins, and at 7 P.M. had a hot bath, which produced profuse perspiration. At 8 P.M. vomited, and some hemorrhage from the uterus took place. During the night was restless and did not sleep; slight apparent delirium at times.

31st. Patient had a hot-air bath last evening, and sweated freely while in it and for half an hour or more afterward. Loins were again dry-cupped, and this gave great relief, removing a persistent dull pain that had troubled her all day. Eyelids less œdematous than on admission. Is less thirsty. Last night was restless and a little delirious, wanting to get out of bed. No convulsions, nor anything like the premonitory symptoms of one. Is taking milk with lime-water, soda-water, and "Imperial," and tr. ferri perch. $\mathfrak{m}$x ter. die. There is occasional vomiting, which does not appear to be provoked by food or medicine. Bowels open five times in last twenty-four hours; motions loose.

November 1. Hot-air bath last night, which produced free perspiration. A retinal hemorrhage discovered this morning. Bowels open once.

2d. Bowels yesterday open thirteen times; motions loose. Troublesome vomiting of green, bilious stuff. Pulse less full. Murmur not so loud. Milk stopped; patient taking brandy and soda and iced water.

3d. Diarrhœa continues. Vomiting less frequent. No pain. Œdema less. Taking now about eighteen ounces of milk in the twenty-four hours with soda-water or lime-water. Ophthalmoscopic examination by Mr. Warren Tay: discs ill-defined, œdematous; numerous small hemorrhages in both eyes.

5th. Vomited yesterday. Pain in umbilical region complained of. Appetite bad. No headache. Restless. Œdema less.

6th. Some diarrhœa. Still very restless. Chloral last night, which gave some three hours' sleep.

7th. Hot-air bath last night; sweated freely. Also dry-cupped.

8th. Hot-air bath and dry-cupping repeated last night.

9th. Signs of neuro-retinitis more marked. Diarrhœa continues. No vomiting. No headache. Sleeps better. Œdema gone.

12th. A few moist râles at lung bases. Has been dry-cupped every other day, and had hot-air bath, in which she sweats freely. Still restless at night.

14th. Appetite improving; patient less anæmic. Still on milk diet.

15*th.* Vomited once. Complains of a sensation of something swelling in her head. Slight epistaxis.

16*th.* About 4.30 A.M. complained of oppression of breathing, which was relieved by sitting up, and a little brandy. At 10.30 A.M. respirations 38 per minute; complained of weight on the chest. Pericardial friction sound heard over a small area to left of sternum. Fine crepitations at lung bases, but no dulness. Patient looks ill; hands and nose cold.

17*th.* Breathing very distressed. Respirations 40. Pulse 120, small and compressible. Pericardial sound well marked.

20*th.* Breathing now easy. Pulse 104. Now no abnormal cardiac sounds. Patient seems better in every way.

21*st.* Left parotid gland swollen and tender; left side of face so swollen that left eye is completely closed. Temperature 100° last night, normal this morning. Pulse 114.

26*th.* Parotid swelling has disappeared. No pain. Last two days some hemorrhage from rectum, blood being intimately mixed with fecal matter. Pulse 120, very weak. Patient anæmic.

28*th.* Per rectum, some thickening and great tenderness on each side of uterus.

29*th.* Some clots passed per rectum. Last two days patient very drowsy. Still vomits once or twice daily. Is much wasted.

December 3. Patient still very drowsy, sleeping the greater part of the day as well as at night. Appetite bad. Frequent vomiting. Tongue red in patches; lips cracked. Since November 28th taking half a pint of beef tea daily, as well as milk diet. Last night vomited a clot of blood. Pulse small and weak.

7*th.* Vomiting continues. Anæmia marked. The largest of the retinal hemorrhages is nearly absorbed. Outline of discs clearer. Sight better; can read large type.

14*th.* Patient seems improving. Pulse 90; stronger than before. Tongue clean.

19*th.* Can read ordinary print easily. No nausea or vomiting for three days. Appetite good. Sleeps well.

27*th.* Has only vomited twice since last note. Hot-air bath and dry-cupping discontinued. Gets up for an hour every evening. Taking since December 13th ferri-amm. cit. gr. v, t. d. To have now reduced iron gr. iij three times daily.

28*th.* Breathing hurried and shallow; pulse 120. Loud systolic murmur at heart's apex.

30*th.* Dulness and râles at extreme base of each lung. Pericardial friction sound. Morning vomiting.

January 1, 1890. Friction sound still heard.

6*th.* Inflamed swelling over sacrum. Morning vomiting continues.

7*th.* Patient's weight this morning is eighty-eight pounds. She says that a year ago she weighed one hundred and twenty-nine pounds.

15*th.* There has been daily vomiting. Appetite not good; nausea after food. · Anæmia very marked. Sight better; can read small print for a short time, but sight soon becomes misty. Heart distinctly hypertrophied; no murmur. Arteries tortuous and thickened.

29*th.* Vomiting rather less since last note. Weight now ninety pounds.

February 3. Swelling of optic discs has increased again, and there are some recent retinal hemorrhages.

10*th.* Weight now eighty-five and a half pounds. Is sick every morn-ing; appetite bad.

March 5. Retinal changes more marked; fresh hemorrhages; peripheral atrophic patches. Patient cannot sew or read, or distinguish faces clearly at the distance of a few yards. Condition otherwise much the same. During the last week a good deal of sharp and severe headache. Slight puffiness of eyelids. Vomiting on most days. Is less anæmic. Weight eighty-four pounds.

April 8. Weight seventy-eight and a half pounds. Vomiting con-tinues. Very little nourishment taken.

15*th.* Transferred to the care of Dr. Ralfe. She remained under his care until July 18th, when she was sent to a convalescent home at Brighton. She was again admitted under Dr. Ralfe's care on Septem-ber 4th. She suffered much from dyspnœa, sleeplessness and vomiting, and died on September 29th.

Autopsy showed effusion into both pleuræ; pericarditis; hypertrophy of left ventricle; fatty heart; kidneys extremely granular, with lines of calcareous deposit in cortex; weight three ounces each. Liver normal.

Urine. *Quantity:* From the time of the patient's admission until December 23d (*i. e.*, nearly two months) the urine was collected at intervals of two, three, or four hours, but never less than four hours. If the patient did not herself pass water at these intervals, a catheter was passed. Some urine was unavoidably lost with the motions, and, as the patient had a good deal of diarrhœa, these were frequent. In women there is no practicable means of avoiding this source of error. But in the table the number of motions is shown; and it will be seen that the difference in the number of the stools before and after the augmentation of the amount of urine exhibited in the table is not sufficient to account for the difference in the amount of the urine col-lected. Although the diarrhœa prevents the observations from present-ing an entirely accurate account of the renal function, yet it is not enough to explain the difference from the phenomena of health. There is error, but I do not think it material in amount.

During the first week, the amount of urine was so far below the normal standard that the diminution almost amounted to suppression. The average of the first eight days was two and a quarter ounces per diem. During the next five days the quantity increased, the average for these days being eleven and seven-eighths ounces per diem. During the first eight days the average number of motions per diem was seven and a half, and in the succeeding five days seven; so that the difference in the amount lost at stool is no explanation of the deficient quantity of urine at first. By the end of the period just mentioned the urinary secretion may be considered to have been restored to its normal quan-tity. In the second fortnight the daily average was thirty-six ounces;

third, thirty-one ounces; fourth, forty-seven ounces; fifth, fifty-nine ounces; sixth, fifty-four ounces; seventh, fifty ounces; eighth, thirty-eight ounces; ninth, forty-eight ounces. After this date it was not collected with so much care. The number of motions was not, after the first three weeks, recorded so accurately; but it will have been seen from the notes that the patient frequently suffered from diarrhœa, and yet the average amount of urine collected was rather above than below the average of health.

It may be suggested that the deficient quantity of urine was possibly due to deficiency in the amount of fluid ingested. To anticipate this, I have stated in the table the amount of fluid taken each day. It will be seen that this does not explain the scantiness of the urine.

Specific gravity: During the period in which the urine was so scanty the quantities collected were not large enough to allow the specific gravity to be taken with the ordinary urinometer. A specimen of October 30th, mixed with one of October 31st, gave a specific gravity of 1006. The specimens of November 3d mixed together gave a specific gravity of 1011. From November 8th onward, the specific gravity varied between 1010 and 1014. Therefore not only was the urine deficient in quantity, but the little urine that was passed was deficient in solid contents as compared with that of health.

Albumin: The quantity of albumin was measured by the eye when the urine had been allowed to stand after precipitation of the albumin. Throughout the whole of the patient's stay in the hospital the urine was albuminous. The quantity varied from a mere trace to half the bulk of the urine. Toward the end of the first week (the week of scanty urine) the amount of albumin was rather greater than at the beginning. But taking the average of various specimens, there was no great difference between the quantity of albumin at the time when the amount of urine was greatly deficient, and that when the secretion had been reestablished. I am not able to point out any circumstances with which I can connect the minor variations in the quantity of albumin.

The extent to which the albuminous precipitate was composed of *serum-albumin* and of *paraglobulin* respectively, was estimated by separating the paraglobulin with sulphate of magnesia and filtering. There were great variations in the relative amounts in different samples on the same day, from causes which I cannot identify. But comparing broadly the relative quantities during the period of great diminution in the quantity of urine, with those after the reestablishment of the secretion, there is a great difference. During the first week (that of scanty urine) the quantity of paraglobulin was never less than, and usually several times as much as, that of serum-albumin; and on three occasions the albumin was almost all paraglobulin. After the first week the quantities of the two kinds were sometimes equal, sometimes there was more serum-albumin than paraglobulin, and sometimes there was no paraglobulin. Sometimes the paraglobulin was in excess ; but there was never such an excess of paraglobulin as was repeatedly observed in the first week.

Urea : Not only was there, during the period of suppression, the deficiency in the elimination of urea which would have been expected from the scantiness of the urine, but the percentage of urea in the urine was much below the average of health, and below even what would have been expected from the specific gravity of the urine. It was estimated by the hypobromite process.

Day of month.	Day of puerperium.	Urine in ounces.	Urea in grains.	Percentage of urea.	Ounces of fluid taken.	Bowel movements.
Oct. 30	1st	2	5	0.7	110	2
" 31	2d	3	7	0.5	40	5
Nov. 1	3d	2	7	0.6	41	10
" 2	4th	3	8	0.7	36	9
" 3	5th	5½	16	0.7	34	9
" 4	6th	6	18	0.75	25	9
" 5	7th	4	14	0.8	34	5
" 6	8th	2	7	0.85	23	6
" 7	9th	12	50	0.9	35	7
" 8	10th	9	42	1.	37	7
" 9	11th	15	66	1.05	42	6
" 10	12th	14	70	1.05	43	9
" 11	13th	8	36	1.	43	9
" 12	14th	19	90	1.1	42	4
" 13	15th	25	114	1.05	43	6
" 14	16th	29	138	1.05	45	8
" 15	17th	42	212	1.1	58	6
" 16	18th	40	220	1.25	44	3
" 17	19th	39	239	1.4	46	3

On admission the percentage was only 0.7. The next day it fell to 0.5. From this date onward there was a gradual but slow rise till 1 per cent. was reached, on the tenth day. Then the percentage continued from 1 to 1.2 per cent. till the eighteenth day. On the eighteenth and nineteenth days there was a more rapid rise, reaching 1.4 per cent. on the latter day. After this, for the next month it was, on the average, about 1.5. From the combination of a diminished percentage of urea with diminished quantity of urine, the absolute amount of urea eliminated by the kidneys was for a fortnight surprisingly small. For the first ten days it averaged 17.4 grains per diem. The next five days show a slight increase, the average being 53 grains per diem. Then it rapidly rose until an average of 200 to 300 grains per diem was reached. The quantities subsequently were as follows :

Second fortnight, average		.	.	.	231 grains per diem.	
Third	"	"	.	.	. 187	" "
Fourth	"	"	.	.	. 198	" "
Fifth	"	"	.	.	. 215	" "
Sixth	"		.	.	. 265	" "
Seventh	"		.	.	. 163	" "
Eighth	"	"	.	.	. 146	" "
Ninth	"	"	.	.	. 155	" "

It must be admitted that error from the amount of urine lost at stool, unavoidable in women, makes these figures incorrect in the direction of being too low. In relating the quantity of urine passed I have discussed this source of error, and given the reason for thinking that not much urine escaped collection, and that therefore the figures here given are not *much* below the truth.

Deposit: Owing to the very small quantity of the urine, and to this being used for the estimation of urea, the urine was not often examined microscopically. But on the few occasions on which this was done no casts were found.

Briefly: We have here a case in which for eight days the patient passed only about three ounces of urine, and eliminated about ten grains of urea per diem; and yet there were no convulsions.

CASE II. *Eleventh pregnancy: symptoms of renal disease for at least eleven months; œdema; cough; vomiting; labor induced at six months of pregnancy; child living; death two weeks after delivery; no autopsy; urine loaded with albumin and containing casts; almost complete suppression of urine for ten days before admission; for a week after admission urine averaging a little more than three ounces per day; gradual but incomplete reëstablishment of the secretion until three weeks after admission, when labor was induced; after delivery rapid increase in quantity of the urine.* (From notes by Mr. A. F. Peskett, resident accoucheur, and Mr. Cornish, clinical clerk.)—I. R., aged forty-two. Admitted into the London Hospital May 23, 1885. Patient was a street hawker, and had always lived much out of doors. Had taken stimulants freely, mostly rum or gin. Had occasionally suffered from rheumatic pains, but otherwise had had good health until the present illness began. Was married at sixteen, and had had ten children, the last six and a half years ago.

Two years and a half ago she ceased menstruating for two months, then hemorrhage began and lasted ten weeks. She attended for six weeks as an out-patient at the Metropolitan Free Hospital, and got better. Three months after this she found her legs swelling. She went to St. Bartholomew's Hospital, was treated as an out-patient for five weeks, and got better. From this time she continued well until eleven months ago. Then she noticed that her legs were swelling, that her urine looked bloody, and that she had to pass it oftener than she had been accustomed to. She often had shooting pains in the lower abdomen and back. She menstruated the week before Christmas, and she believed herself to be pregnant. For ten days before admission she had passed hardly any water, not more than a teaspoonful at a time.

State on admission: Patient was fairly nourished, and not anæmic. Complained of epigastric pain and flatulence. No enlargement of liver or spleen. Heart's apex-beat in normal position; area of cardiac dulness not increased. Systolic murmur at apex, conducted toward axilla. Arteries rather hard. Breathing rather hurried and labored; bronchial râles over the chest; cough and expectoration. Ophthalmoscopic examination shows nothing abnormal; no retinal hemorrhages or retinitis. Patient complains of severe frontal headache. Abdominal wall and legs œdematous. Uterus reaching to umbilicus.

The catheter was passed on admission, and the night and morning afterward, but only a few drops of urine were obtained each time. All the urine passed or drawn off was collected and measured.

Pulv. jalapæ co., ℨj, was given on the morning following admission, and acted well. Patient was also given pot. acet. ℨss, liq. amm. acet. ℨj, spt. æth. nit. ℳxx, three times a day. In the evening of the day after admission she had a vapor bath, and perspired a little after it. Three times during this day the loins were dry-cupped. The next evening (May 25th) the vapor bath was repeated. On May 26th one-twelfth grain of pilocarpine was administered subcutaneously, and the dry-cupping and vapor bath were repeated. A mustard poultice was applied to the loins, and this was repeated on May 27th. On the evening of May 29th patient had a warm bath, and one-twelfth grain of pilocarpine was given subcutaneously, and these measures were repeated every evening until delivery.

Until June 9th the patient's condition appeared to be steadily improving. The cough and shortness of breath were getting better, and the œdema becoming less. There was throughout occasional vomiting. Pulse was throughout about 76 per minute. The temperature never exceeded 99°.

On June 9th and the following days the patient's breath became shorter, her cough and vomiting more troublesome.

Therefore on June 12th it was decided to induce labor. This was done by the introduction of a bougie between the membranes and the uterus. The patient was delivered on June 14th of a six months' fœtus, which lived about two hours.

The patient died on June 29th; no autopsy was allowed.

The urine was tested on May 24th, June 1st, 8th, and 18th. On the three first occasions it was smoky in color, and loaded with albumin. Its specific gravity on June 8th was 1013, on June 18th 1012. On the two first occasions it contained a deposit of epithelial and blood casts; on the two later, phosphatic crystals. There was no sugar. The urea was estimated on June 8th, by the hypobromite process, and was 0.6 per cent. Its reaction was acid or neutral throughout. The quantities collected are shown in the table which follows. Some was unavoidably lost with the motions, therefore the number of motions each day is also given, so that an idea may be formed of the amount lost.

It will be seen that although the very small quantity of urine may be partly accounted for by assuming that some was lost with the motions, yet that there is no such difference between the number of motions per day in the first week and afterward, before delivery and after, as can account for the great difference in the quantity of the urine at these different periods.

May 24	1 ounce.	2 motions.	⎫	
" 25	3 ounces.	3 "		
" 26	1½ "	3 "		
" 27	1½ "	6 "	⎬	1st week, average per day, 2.9 ounces.
" 28	6½ "	7 "		
" 29	3 "	9		
" 30	4	6	⎭	
" 31	2	5	⎫	
June 1	4	5 "		
" 2	4	2 "		
" 3	10 "	4 "	⎬	2d week, average 5.8 ounces per day.
4	6	3 "		
5	8	3		
6	6½	3	⎭	
7	6	3	⎫	
" 8	10 "	3 "		
" 9	10 "	1 "	⎬	5 days before labor, average 12 ounces per day.
" 10	17 "	6 "		
" 11	18 "	5	⎭	
" 12	2½	4 "	⎫	Bougie introduced. Collection
" 13	6½	3 "	⎬	this and following day im-
" 14	28 "	6 "	⎭	Delivery. [perfect.
" 15	20 "	3 "	⎫	
" 16	10 "	3		
" 17	33 "	4 "		
" 18	30 "	3 "	⎬	Week after delivery, average 25.2 ounces per day.
" 19	40 "	1 "		
" 20	20 "	5		
" 21	28 "	4	⎭	
" 22	30 "	3	⎫	
" 23	30 "	2		
" 24	24 "	4 "		
" 25	30 "	4 "	⎬	2d week, average 29.3 ounces per day.
" 26	35 "	3 "		
" 27	32 "	2		
" 28	24 "	2 "	⎭	

Both in this and in the former case, the diminution in the quantity of urine was far below what has been observed in some cases of eclampsia.

In this case, on the unfortunately few occasions on which the urine was examined, the specific gravity was found (as in Case I.) less than normal, and the percentage of urea even less than would have been expected from the specific gravity of the urine.

Seeing how powerful a diuretic urea is, may not the explanation of the suppression of urine in these and similar cases possibly be a deficient formation of urea? This would account for the small quantity of urine, the deficiency of urea in it, and the absence of so-called uræmic symptoms.

ASEPTIC AND ANTISEPTIC DETAILS IN OPERATIVE SURGERY.

By Arpad G. Gerster, M.D.,
OF NEW YORK.

Though it must be conceded that the process of evolution of the principle which underlies safe operating is a closed chapter in surgery, yet it cannot be denied that means have lately undergone change, and are still undergoing improvement. The main feature of this improvement is the simplification of our procedures. And simplification means an easier comprehension, a more ready acceptance by the general practitioner, and a beneficial spread of the practice of aseptic and antiseptic measures.

One of the most interesting features of the birth and infancy of the Listerian idea was the circumstance that this vast practical revolution in surgical management was based on purely scientific facts, seemingly of mere theoretical interest. I refer to the use made by Lister of Pasteur's researches. To one familiar with the character of these researches, it will be very natural that Lister's first steps in practically establishing the value of Pasteur's results were dominated by the idea of the necessity of chemical sterilization, or, as it was then called, disinfection. How strong and persistent the hold of this thought was upon the minds of men is best illustrated in the remarks made by Lister himself in a lecture or paper delivered not very many years ago. In those days Volkmann taught that in preparing the field for an operation, shaving and scrubbing of the skin ought to precede the application of the carbolic solution. Lister deprecated these measures as over-zealous and unnecessary, and if the printed report can be trusted, the tinge of a sneer was not mistakable in his critical observations. He contended that the great efficiency of carbolic lotion and spray made these plainer methods of disinfection superfluous. Of course, I must add that since then Lister has changed his position.

As a matter of fact there is no doubt now that the powerful action of the razor, of soap, and a stiff brush, goes far beyond anything that can be accomplished in the way of disinfection, even by the strongest permissible antiseptic. We know that, beside the filth adhering to them, epidermis and hair contain not only hosts of harmless and noxious germs, but that epidermis, hair, and clinging filth are all by necessity or accident more or less coated and permeated by various oleaginous substances which form an effective barrier to the penetration of all watery solutions. Hence, to insure the penetration and imbibition of a chemical sterilizer contained in a watery solution it is first necessary to remove this coating of grease. And what agent is better capable of doing this effectually than emollient potash soap, applied with plenty of hot water and the thorough action of a stiff brush made of the bristles of the hog? Grease, filth, and effete epidermis, harmless and pathological germs, are swept away all alike, rapidly and thoroughly, and with admirable impartiality. When the germicidal lotion is finally applied to the cleansed skin, there is very little to kill in the shape of noxious organisms. Lack of time forbids my entering into the scientific demonstration of the facts just related, but I refer those interested in the proofs of the inhibiting effect of oleaginous substances upon the action of aqueous disinfectants to the conclusive article of Schimmelbusch.[1] Far be it from me to depreciate the value of the experiment which demonstrated that a noxious germ finely distributed in a generous quantity of water, to which was added a powerful germicide in a certain minute proportion, would promptly succumb to the deadly influence of this chemical. I only desire to point out the fact that these noxious organisms are not met with in the shape of thin, watery emulsions by the surgeon, but are found imbedded in dense masses of what Lister appropriately called " lumps of dirt," in conglomerations of grease and epidermis, in powerful plugs of sticky slime, pus, and blood-clot. Therefore let us *first* emphasize the paramount antiseptic value of the homely methods employed for cleansing dirty surfaces comprised in the term of *mechanical purification;* and *secondly* point out how infinitely more they accomplish than any form of chemical disinfection by watery germicidal solutions alone.   Both should be combined.

Next in importance to the cleansing of the field of operation stands the question of the sterilization of the hands employed at an operation. Both Kuemmel[2] and Fürbringer[3] have brought abundant experimental proof of what enormous quantities of truly pathogenic germs are habitually lodged under the finger-nails of even the most cleanly persons, and especially of physicians. It matters not how often their hands were washed with soap and brush, the scrapings of the finger-nails always contained an abundance of noxious germs. We know that to facilitate digital examination, the surgeon's finger is lubricated with oil or vaseline. Not inconsiderable quantities of oleaginous matter intermixed with pathogenic bacteria persistently cling to the deepest recesses of the subungual space, and this fatty deposit prevents the effective penetration of germicidal lotions. Fürbringer's investigations have shown that the following process will invariably render the surgeon's hands germ-free: The nails should be kept trimmed short; the hands are to be scrubbed with brush and soap in hot water for one minute, especial attention being paid to the subungual spaces, which then are to be scraped carefully with a nail-cleaner, the hands to be immersed for another minute, first in strong alcohol, then in a 1 : 1000 solution of corrosive sublimate. Even hands that were in prolonged contact with intensely septic matter can be instantly rendered reliably aseptic by this process. This is comforting for the surgeon to know, who during the progress of an operation may be compelled to insert his finger into the rectum or oral cavity for the sake of necessary verification.

When my thoughts revert to the old days of spray and unlimited

[1] Archiv für klinische Chirurgie, 1891, p. 129.
[2] Centralblatt für Chirurgie, 1885, Beilage zu No. 24, p. 26.
[3] Idem, 1888, p. 83.

carbolic acid, the first thing remembered is the habitually shocking condition of our hands. Martyrdom means testimony, and the martyred state
of our hands bore shining testimony of the earnestness of our faith.
We all believed in the necessity of unlimited chemical sterilization,
especially as to our instruments. Fortunately, all this has been changed
for something better, and this we owe to Davidsohn,[1] who taught us to
sterilize instruments by boiling.

But let us first examine whether the usual steps of the mechanical
cleansing to which surgical instruments are subjected are adequate or
not. That they are very important is very evident, inasmuch as by them
is removed the bulk of blood, pus, shreds of animal tissue, and ointments
clinging to their interstices and rough surfaces after an operation. Yet
even the most thoroughgoing scrubbing in hot water with soap and a stiff
brush will not render instruments aseptic. Schimmelbusch[2] has subjected
instruments thus cleansed to bacteriological examination. He found
that especially to artery forceps a considerable quantity of noxious germs
were constantly adherent, and that only the simplest instruments were
irreproachable.

Another factor has to be considered. In the large practice of our
hospitals, where from three to five operations are performed at one
session, the minute cleansing of a large instrumentarium after each
operation is tedious, involving considerable time. We either had to
submit to this, or had to provide a disproportionately large and costly
set of duplicates and triplicates. As a matter of fact, the latter thing
was rarely resorted to, and the cleansing of the bloody instruments being
hurriedly and often inadequately done, main reliance was placed upon
the disinfecting power of our carbolic acid bath. And as consideration
for the assistants' hands had gradually caused the abandonment of the
stronger for weaker solutions, frequent failures in securing primary union
were the result of these evasive attempts.

As mentioned, Davidsohn demonstrated that boiling for five minutes
in a covered vessel charged with water was invariably followed by a
faultless sterilization of instruments thus treated. But the great drawback of this plan was that all steel objects thus treated, unless they were
perfectly protected by nickel-plating, became rusty and were sooner or
later ruined. This objection does not apply to its full extent to sterilization by superheated air ; but the necessity for costly apparatus and the
tardiness of the process[3] make this plan evidently impracticable. Sterilization by steam presents the drawback of rusting in a still greater
degree.

[1] Berliner klinische Wochenschrift, 1888, No. 35.
[2] Loc. cit , p. 147.
[3] Poupinel : " La stérilisation par la chaleur," Revue de chirurgie, 1888, p. 669.

If we then had some reliable means of safely preventing the inroads of rust upon our instruments during sterilization by boiling, we would possess a rapid, simple, and thoroughly practical way of accomplishing our purpose. Common washing-soda, as found in every household, if added in the proportion of one per cent. to water, is endowed with the valuable property of preventing the formation of rust on steel during boiling. And we owe this expedient to the ingenuity of Schimmelbusch.

Let me now practically illustrate in another direction the vast importance of this simple, rapid, and reliable manner of cleansing instruments. It must appeal with peculiar strength to the sensibilities of the general practitioner and country surgeon. Look at the ordinary surgical pocket-case, containing the chief and often only available instrumentarium in a grave case of emergency. Its leather and lining are well worn and more or less soiled, both from long use and the necessity of carrying it about with us in hot and cold weather, rain and shine. Bathed in the vapors of perspiration, freely accessible to dust and dirt, it soon becomes the very negation of what is tidy. Imagine that a fresh case of compound injury to bone or joint, vessel or tendon, has to be dealt with, and that at once. Under these circumstances the instruments drawn from the pocket-case were always employed by me with much reluctance and no little trepidation. Only when the case brooked absolutely no delay and could not be tided over by temporary expedients permitting postponement of the operation to a safer occasion, did I operate. The cleansing that could be bestowed on such instruments on such occasions must needs be inadequate, and one had no choice but to trust to luck.

How different matters are, when we know that to put our instruments in a perfectly aseptic condition we need only a covered pot of boiling water charged with washing-soda, one tablespoonful to the quart. After five minutes of ebullition the contents of the pot, instruments, water and all, are emptied into a clean pan, and the operation may proceed.

In hospitals a sufficient supply of cold sterilized soda solution can be kept on hand, to be poured over the hot instruments as soon as they are placed in the instrument tray. Lately we have used at Mount Sinai Hospital simple boiled water for this purpose, with perfect satisfaction.

In recapitulation, we will say that instruments should be first cleansed with soap, water, and brush, then boiled for five minutes in a covered vessel containing a watery solution of washing-soda 1 : 100 (one heaped tablespoonful to the quart).

We have seen, from the preceding remarks, how important a rôle is played in modern surgery by the humble scrubbing-brush. And yet there is no other implement so generally neglected as this, and none that receives less care in practice. In hospital and the private office we see the brush used indiscriminately on the hands of the surgeon, the skin of the patient, in close contact with vaseline, feces, urine, sputa, blood, pus, ichor, and what not. After use it is deposited on the washstand without any special care as to the removal of filth clinging to thousands of bristles and their interstices. It is no wonder that brushes thus treated become very hotbeds of infection.

Various expedients were employed to overcome this obvious evil, among which shall be mentioned first the exclusive use of new brushes in the preparation for each major operation, especially laparotomies; then the disinfection of brushes by continuous immersion in strong sublimate of mercury solution, and finally, the rejection of all brushes and employment of bundles of excelsior instead, which are thrown away after each single use (Neuber).

On account of its great effectiveness the banishment of the brush could be viewed by the surgeon only with regret. Hence let us examine whether a simple and practical way has not been devised to keep this implement clean.

I have again to refer to Schimmelbusch,[1] who has shown beyond any reasonable doubt, that a single and brief immersion in a strong germicidal solution is inadequate to destroy the noxious forms of bacteria contained in surgical nail-brushes. He found that brushes used in the wards and private rooms of the Berlin clinic, which were simply kept in the stereotyped dish alongside of the wash-basin, literally swarmed with pyogenic organisms. Further, he established that to satisfactorily disinfect a brush containing pathogenic germs, an immersion in strong mercuric solution of at least ten minutes was indispensable. If we consider how often brushes fresh from use on infectious cases and still filled with soapsuds are thrown back into the vessel set aside for their immersion, there to give up their contents of soap, which render the sublimate solution inert, we must conclude that under such circumstances even fifteen or twenty minutes will not accomplish a perfect sterilization. Hence we see with pleasure the demonstration of the fact by Schimmelbusch, that boiling of the most unclean brush for five minutes in a 1 : 100 soda solution will always render it absolutely aseptic. Ordinarily, then, surgical brushes should be always kept immersed in a 1 : 1000 sublimate solution, and should be always boiled before laparotomies, or whenever intensive infection has occurred. Finally, brushes carried about in the open satchel of the surgeon, or those found on the washstands of patients, should also be boiled before use.

Whenever I have watched the process of impregnation of our absorbent dressings, as it is carried on at our large hospitals, I could not avoid the feeling of uncertainty regarding the desired result. The repeated

---

[1] Loc. cit., page 161.

handling of large quantities of material by a certain number of persons required in folding, immersing, wringing, unfolding, drying, refolding, cutting, and final storing, cannot but impress the observer with the suspicion of contamination. Add to this the mistakes made in mixing the solutions used for impregnation, and the resulting over- or under-charging of the dressings with chemicals prone to evaporation or chemical change, and it will be seen that impregnation itself- is apt to be very uncertain as to its absolute value. As to the merits of the processes employed by various manufacturers in preparing disinfected dressings, I will only remark, that as their gauge of success is a purely commercial one directed solely to profit, the work being done by persons to whom the essence of a surgically clean procedure is a matter of utter indifference, their trustworthiness must be a factor not amenable to direct proof and demonstration.

But let us see wherein dwells the antiseptic property of our surgical dressings. Can is be the inconstantly represented chemical agent, which even if present in the prescribed quantity, is nearly inert, or is it some other factor? The answer is that we know that the high antiseptic value of our intensely absorbent dressings depends on their quality of favoring rapid evaporation, rather than on any chemical properties they may possess. The curing of meat and fish by exposure to the sun is one of the most ancient preservative processes, and well known to be highly effective. As to the effect of evaporation upon pathogenic microbes, Schlange[1] has shown that the bacillus of green pus, for instance, inoculated upon moist pads of cotton—was aggressively prolific if kept under a glass cover which prevented evaporation. On the other hand, its proliferation was immediately checked if the pads were freely exposed to air and became dry by the loss of moisture. I cannot but fully indorse the statement made by Schimmelbusch, that the effectiveness of highly absorbent and rapidly drying dressings, even if they contained a moderate amount of schizomycetes, is much greater than that of materials which, however faultlessly impregnated, are lacking the properties just mentioned, as, for instance, Lister's resinous gauze.

Looking aside from the objectionable and unreliable features of impregnation itself, let us not forget the disagreeable influence of the chemicals used in this process upon the skin of surgeon and patients. The intensive eczema so frequently produced underneath our sublimate and carbolic dressings is a serious drawback of not small moment.

All these objections vanish if preference is given to one or another mode of sterilization by dry or moist heat. Of these modes only three need to be considered.

First comes the simple process of boiling. For purposes where a reli-

[1] Archiv für klinische Chirurgie, 1887.

able dressing has to be procured, *extempore* boiling in a soda or potash solution of about 1½ per cent. for ten minutes is incomparably the simplest and most practical manner of getting an absorbent and aseptic material. In this procedure we recognize at once the familiar ways of the laundry, the eminently aseptic results of which have been demonstrated beyond any reasonable doubt by Behring[1] in the Berlin Hygienic Institute. Thus cotton or linen stuff, to be found in every household, can be rapidly rendered serviceable for surgical purposes by a short boiling in soda or potash lye. Well rung out, it can be immediately used, and will dry rapidly *in situ* under the influence of the body-heat and exposure to the air.

Sterilization by hot air has also been shown to be sufficient, and would deserve serious attention but for the necessity of employing costly and complicated apparatus.

FIG. 1.

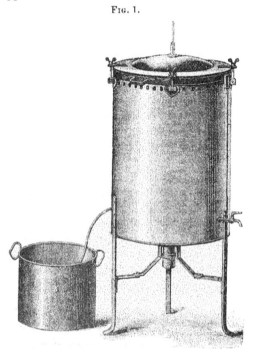

Lautenschläger's apparatus for the sterilization of dressings by steam.

But these objections do not prevail as to a steady current of slightly superheated steam. The apparatus needed for this purpose is simple, cheap, and durable, and as I have ascertained during an extensive tour of investigation, embracing a considerable number of Continental clinics,

---

[1] Zeitschrift für Hygiene. 1890.

has been and is there universally employed with unvarying satisfaction. The apparatus I refer to is made by Lautenschläger, in Berlin, from plans by Schimmelbusch, and has several features to commend it. First, its moderate cost, easily afforded by every hospital, and even a busy surgeon. Secondly, the absence of the danger of explosion, the rapidity with which it is set in motion, and the thoroughness with which every fibre of the articles placed within it is permeated by steam, which enters the receptacle containing the dressings from above, displacing all atmospheric air, finally escaping through a tube at the bottom of the apparatus, whence it is conducted into a pail of cold water to effect its precipitation.

A nother ingenious feature of this apparatus consists in the employment of a number of perforated tin boxes, which can be closed at will, each of

FIG. 2.

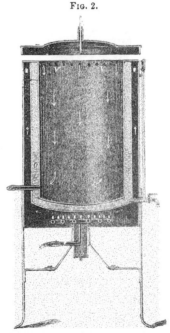

Sectional view of Lautenschläger's steam sterilizer.

these containing everything that is to be used at a given operation. Supposing that three operations are to be done, one after another, three of these boxes are charged each with all the dressings, towels, and surgeons' gowns to be used on that occasion, and are placed within the steam-chamber of the apparatus. The flames are lighted, and counting from the time that the thermometer connected with the apparatus indicates 100° C. the contents are exposed to the action of steam for forty-five minutes. After this the boxes are taken out, their air-holes are closed, and the dressings in them remain clean and undefiled by any contact until the moment when they are taken out and applied to the wound.

Protected from all undesirable contact by the tin case, aseptic dressings can be thus transported anywhere, to be used wherever occasion requires. I need not add that gauze or cotton is not rendered absorbent by steaming alone, and must possess this property before sterilization. This apparatus was recently acquired for Mount Sinai Hospital, New York, where it can be inspected.

Dressings thus prepared possess all the requisites demanded by modern surgery. They are cheap, aseptic, can be kept so indefinitely, and do not irritate the skin.

Fig. 3.

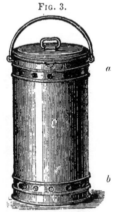

Schimmelbusch's box within which dressings are placed in steam chest of sterilizer. *a* and *b*, air-holes.

The sponge is a surgical requisite so full of excellent qualities that no substitute has as yet succeeded in displacing it. A very good article, known as the Florida sponge, can be bought here for such a trifling sum that we can easily afford to use a sponge but once. Among the many processes recommended for its disinfection, that by boiling is to be absolutely condemned, as it robs the sponge of its most valuable properties—its softness, elasticity, and power to absorb. One of the most effective processes has been abundantly tested by myself in hospital and private practice for seven years, and these are its simple details: The sponge is to be freed of its calcareous impurities by dry beating and a short immersion in standard dilute muriatic acid. Traces of the acid having been washed away, the sponges are left for two days in water to give the spores contained in them a chance to germinate. The reason for this is the fact that proliferating microbes succumb much more

promptly to germicides than their spores. After this process of fermentation the sponges are thoroughly kneaded by hand, each for a
minute, in plenty of hot water and potash or soft-soap, which will thoroughly macerate and mollify hard lumps of dirt that may be imbedded
in the densest and central parts of the sponge, thus rendering them, as
it were, penetrable to the action of germicides. After all traces of soap
are removed, the sponges are thrown into a five per cent. solution of
carbolic acid, which I prefer to corrosive sublimate for this purpose, as
it does not become inert as easily as a metallic compound. An immersion extending over twenty-four hours will render the sponges absolutely
sterile and fit for use. Should it for economic reasons be desired to use
sponges oftener than once, this same process will be just as effective to
purify them.

The large flat sponges so generally used in laparotomy have been
abandoned by me for three years as expensive, and not as handy as
small, well-sterilized compresses of plain absorbent gauze, which, to
prevent unfolding and fraying, are firmly tied with silk at one end.
The surgeon is nowhere so cramped for lack of space as at his operations in the bottom of the pelvis. A sponge used for packing away intestines needs constant pressure to prevent its expansion and encroach-
ment upon available space. A pad of gauze held down for a short
while will become packed, and will retain its shape and position even if
released from digital pressure.

When I approach the vast subject of *operative technique*, indissolubly
connected with the principle of asepticism and antisepticism, I confess
to a feeling of helplessness. Hours would be required to do justice to
the intimate connection and interdependence of these subjects, and I
must content myself with giving you a few glimpses only. The enormous increase in the ratio of safety in operating caused by anti-parasitic
measures has led to curious results. A clumsy and rough operator who
is a thorough antiseptician is often very successful. On the other hand
we see very dexterous men suffer disheartening discomfitures on account
of disregard of the maxims of cleanliness. This is not said to encour-
age clumsy operating. On the contrary, I must declare what all of you
know already, that the most brilliant triumphs of surgery are won in
these days by those who combine technical skill, the cunning of hand
and brains, with the conscientious practice of a thoroughgoing cleanliness. The neglect of cleanliness will meet in no field of human activity with a swifter and more certain retribution than here; hence I
may say that cleanliness is one of the most important and truly ethical
factors in the honorable pursuit of our noble art.

The barbaric elements of the neglect of cleanliness and inattention
to hemorrhage, the rough methods of evulsion, the slashing and tearing,

often made necessary in former days by the absence of anæsthesia, have almost all been eliminated from surgery. Dissection is made safe by adequate incisions and by the control of hemorrhage, which keeps the field of operation comparatively dry. By the skilful use of retractors the track of the knife is laid bare to the scrutiny of the eye; and blunt methods of severing tissues being avoided wherever possible, clean-cut surfaces are left behind, more prone to heal than bruised and torn ones.

The immediate effect of anti-parasitic principles upon the improvement of operative technique is nowhere more evident than in those procedures where internal sources of infection are encountered and set free during an operation, as, for instance, in the excision of tuberculous, suppurating joints and glands, in the removal of the diseased appendix vermiformis, the evacuation of the intra-peritoneal abscesses, and the excision of suppurating abdominal tumors. To prevent accidental contamination of healthy surfaces, or, if unavoidable, to neutralize its bad effects, can be truly said to be a newly developed art. I may also mention the enormous progress in the safety of surgical interference in operating upon organs that can never be called aseptic: as, for instance, the rectum; the oral cavity—in fact, the entire digestive tract; the bladder, and the uterus. Here operative technique in the old sense, and antisepsis or asepsis, are so intimately blended that they cannot be safely separated, and ought to be taught together by book and example.

To illustrate the meaning of these remarks, I may be permitted to mention a few examples. To insure the success of an extensive excision of the rectum for cancer, we perform preliminary colotomy. Thus we divert feces and contamination from the field of operation, rendering it aseptic as far as possible. Likewise we open the membranous portion of the urethra and pass a drainage-tube into the bladder, in order to prevent the infection of a urethroplasty wound by ammoniacal urine. Not long ago, in performing a needful herniotomy upon a boy-child, I have, to prevent the soiling of the wound by urine, performed external urethrotomy with success. All these operations represent improvement of operative technique in a wider sense.

The field we have here touched is one where a clear line of demarcation between aseptic and antiseptic measures cannot be drawn. In many of the cases belonging to this order, *irrigation* is an important element of success; therefore let us devote a few words to the subject of irrigation.

The wholesale condemnation of irrigation as employed in the past is just as sure a sign of superficiality on the part of the critic as the slighting of the important rôle of antiseptic agents in former periods of the antiseptic method. As long as the preparatory measures to an operation were rather perfunctory; as long as the skin, the surgeon's hands, his sponges, instruments, and dressings were indifferently cleansed, the continuous use of disinfectants during and after the operation was necessary to insure success—that is, to ward off virulent suppuration. Similarly, under those conditions, the use of continuous irrigation during operations was justified by the general improvement of results observed after its employment. As we have learned to lay greater stress upon and practice a more exact form of preparatory asepsis, so the necessity for chemical germicides and irrigation has been restricted. But both of these agents have furnished a valuable and necessary link in the chain of development of the discipline. This view is confirmed by the fact that practical experience tells us how indispensable irrigation still is to the safe performance of many operations done in regions which can be rendered and kept aseptic only with great difficulty or not at all. Here, too, the mechanical effect of the stream of irrigating fluid is infinitely more important, in my opinion, than the chemical influence of the weak solutions generally used. It is rather the rush of the fluid washing away impurities than the salicylic or boric acid dissolved in it that is effectual.

Accordingly, we rarely employ irrigation in wounds that are known to be free from infection, and with few exceptions never take strong solutions, the use of which has produced in the past a considerable number of fatal intoxications. By eschewing chemicals we also have seen hæmostasis become easier, and especially have observed that the troublesome oozing of the fresh wound has been almost entirely done away with. Our dressings grew less bulky and cumbrous; they could be left longer undisturbed, and, what is an important item in the amputation of limbs, could be bandaged on with less pressure, whereby the danger of marginal necrosis of the flaps is materially diminished. In short, the dryer the operation, the dryer was the course of healing. How this matter has affected the question of drainage we shall consider presently.

To sum up we shall say, then, that irrigation of an aseptic wound is unnecessary, even harmful; that it should be only employed in wounds which are *per se* not aseptic, such as those in the vicinity of or within the several orifices of the body—as, for instance, the rectum, oral cavity, and vagina; that irrigation is well employed during operations in and about accidentally infected or suppurating areas. *A notable exception to this rule is the abdominal cavity, wherein irrigation is never to be employed.* This statement seems to condemn a widely spread practice, and some courage is needed to express it unreservedly. But both experience and scientific experiment support this view. It will be objected that a vast array of cases is on record wherein irrigation of the abdominal cavity was practised successfully by eminent surgeons. To this we reply, that where harmless substances, as, for instance, blood, non-septic

contents of cysts, or abacteric pus from a ruptured pyosalpinx or
ovarian abscess, have accidentally soiled the peritoneum, the simple
wiping off of the bulk of these substances is sufficient to eliminate
danger; that in these cases irrigation is unnecessary, and that recovery
takes place rather in spite than in consequence of irrigation. How
entirely useless, nay, pernicious, the effects of flushing the peritoneum
are in cases of active septic infection, as, for instance, in the presence of
fetid fecal abscesses due to intestinal perforation, has been abundantly
demonstrated to myself and to other surgeons here and abroad by
numerous unsuccessful attempts. And there is nothing more certain
than that, on account of its complex character, the peritoneal cavity
cannot be completely washed clean; that germicidal solutions cannot
be used in a sufficient strength to be effective, and that finally an inert
or weak solution will only help to spread the elements of infection to
previously unaffected areas. The substance of these assertions was
essentially confirmed by experimental research on animals.[1]

I take this opportunity for a short diversion to a subject still discussed
by surgeons and deserving some notice. Most operations within the
peritoneal cavity afford no very rigid test of the absolute value of the
aseptic measures therein employed. The tolerance of the peritoneum is
almost incredible, and technical sins committed during abdominal
operations against the accepted rules of cleanliness, proper dissection,
hæmostasis, go much oftener unpunished than those incurred at an amputation, resection, osteotomy, or the excision of extra-abdominal tumors
—in fact, at all major operations performed outside of the belly. But let
the limits of peritoneal tolerance once be overstepped and usually the
damage becomes irretrievable; the patient generally dies of septic peritonitis, for which there is no adequate corrective. On the other hand,
if extra-peritoneal regions manifest less tolerance of slipshod methods,
the consequences of surgical shortcomings are here often retrievable by
corrective measures of one or another kind. The tolerance of the peritoneum was only too often the mantle of charity under which were hidden
from view sins of omission and of commission of laparotomists without
surgical training. In laparotomy more than anywhere else the most
rigid asepsis is a conscientious duty.

Intimately connected with the change of views respecting preparatory
asepticism and irrigation is the shifting of our standpoint regarding the
application of *drainage*. Imperfect cleanliness, copious irrigation, and
abundant drainage represent the links of a chain forged by necessity.
A faultless asepsis has often enabled us to do away both with irrigation

[1] P. Delbet: "Recherches expérimentales sur le Lavage du Péritoine." Annales de
Gyn., xxxii. p. 165.

and drainage. Wounds of a moderate extent, for instance, made in herniotomy, if really aseptic, their dissection clean, and hæmostasis perfect, will behave correctly under an hermetic collodion dressing, and exactly like a subcutaneous injury. The oozing will be very moderate, scarcely penetrating the thin coat of gauze soaked in collodion, swelling none, and after the lapse of ten days we shall find the catgut stitches absorbed and the wound perfectly healed. This is a common observation of modern surgeons and does not need specific verification. The same principle finds a different application in certain operations about the joints and bones, when so-called " dead " spaces must needs be left behind. As most of these operations are done with the aid of artificial anæmia considerable oozing of blood follows the removal of Esmarch's bandage. This blood fills up the irregular cavities left by the surgeon, and, coagulating, forms there a solid aseptic plug, which is gradually consumed and replaced by connective-tissue elements of new formation. For seven years I have abandoned the use of drainage-tubes in those excisions of joints and sequestrotomies where it was possible to remove all diseased tissues in an unexceptionable manner. According to Schede's plan, I have only provided an avenue of egress for the first onrush of oozing blood by leaving one or another angle of the wound somewhat patulous. A film of protective over this little gap will prevent the absorption of the blood needed for filling up the irregular cavity of the excision wound, and will maintain sufficient moisture to prevent the exsiccation of the coagulum.

And even in operations where we are not absolutely certain of the aseptic condition of our wound we can often dispense with the use of drainage-tubes, and not incur any serious risk. Bergmann first demonstrated that a wound of doubtful asepticity can yet be made to heal by primary adhesion. He passed his suture points through the edges of the wound, but leaving them untied, and then packed the open wound and all its recesses down to the bottom with iodoform gauze. Over this was placed the usual outer dressing. Through the capillary action of the gauze copious oozing of serum was encouraged, which in about sixty hours lost its sanguinolent character, whereupon the packing being extracted the suture points left *in situ* were closed, and the wound was seen to heal in a manner little differing from primary union. Undoubtedly, much of the success of this plan of packing and secondary suture is to be attributed to the action of iodoform, which has triumphantly withstood various attacks upon its reputation.

Still another modification of this form of drainage is now extensively employed in abdominal surgery, where, on account of much unavoidable denudation or accidental infection, copious oozing is to be expected. Mikulicz was the first one to employ the iodoform-gauze packing successfully in the abdominal cavity, and his plan has met with widespread and deserved acceptance. First, it does away with the use of the drainage-tube, and secondly, its contact* with the peritoneum causes just enough adhesive irritation to insure after its removal rapid agglutination of the raw surfaces. Immediate closure of the wound can be practised after extraction of the packing. But *drainage by tubes* still remains indispensable where acute progressive suppuration has to be dealt with, as an ample way of egress must be provided for sticky and coherent masses of pus, blood-clot and sloughing tissue.

By touching this subject we have entered the realm of *antisepsis* proper. Let us now consider the comparative value of the principal measures employed for combating active, destructive suppuration, the form of infection which the surgeon has to encounter most frequently. I unhesitatingly declare, and lengthening experience tends only to confirm my conviction, that here as elsewhere, purely mechanical measures employed with a view to the removal of excessive tension and the thorough evacuation of noxious matter, such as adequate incision, properly placed drainage, the extraction of sloughs and sequestra, with frequent energetic irrigation, play a much more important part in checking mischief than chemical disinfection. Even in the treatment of destructive ulcers the constant bath and actual cautery are found to be more effective than chemical applications, though the great usefulness of the latter cannot be denied in milder processes of a superficial character.

We have seen that dry absorbent dressings, favoring rapid evaporation, are most useful in the treatment of extensive aseptic wounds, and that smaller aseptic wounds can be advantageously sealed with an hermetically occlusive collodion pad. An entirely different principle obtains in the dressing of septic or suppurating lesions, surgical or accidental.

While capillary attraction, exerted by a dry absorbent dressing, is perfectly adequate to drain an aseptic wound of its serous discharges and while the rapid drying and crusting of these dressings is just the thing we want to seal a sweet wound against the possibility of subsequent infection from without, these very qualities of the dry absorbent and occlusive dressing make it unfit for use in cases where the secretions are purulent. To begin with, pus contains so many corpuscular elements in the shape of leucocytes and shreds of decayed tissue, all suspended in a more or less viscid medium, that capillary absorption alone cannot effect much more than the removal of a portion of its serous components. The remainder, containing the more solid part of the discharges, becomes inspissated and forms a crust. Thus, artificially, retention and an aggravation of the existing mischief is brought about. A moist dressing, protected against evaporation either by remoistening or an outer covering impermeable to moisture, does not possess these disadvantages. Inspissation being prevented, the escaping pus retains at least its original density, and is evenly absorbed and distributed through the interstices of the entire dressing. Crusting and retention will be prevented, especially if the dressings are frequently renewed. An additional and very valuable quality of the moist dressing is the soothing effect it exerts upon the inflamed parts. It soon acquires the temperature of the covered region, and the combination of warmth and moisture presents the most valuable features of the time-honored poultice without its drawbacks.

Is the impregnation by germicides of moist dressings used in cases of suppuration effective and necessary, or not? My answer is unhesitatingly negative. While the microbes contained in dense masses of pus will remain unscathed by the minute quantities of a chemical contained in our dressings, these will be very often sufficient to irritate the skin into florid eczema. Adequate incisions, efficient drainage, frequent change of dressings supplemented by irrigation, contain the essence of the successful treatment of suppuration.

In summing up we will say, finally, that though chemical sterilization is still important, and even indispensable in some fields of modern surgery, main stress belongs to those mechanical measures of purification which comprise the essential part of aseptic preparation.

Having passed in review the present status of anti-parasitic surgery we see that, although incisive changes have befallen the means employed, the principle upon which the discipline was grounded remains unshaken. The living spark of truth has survived the pedantry and over-zeal of the advocates, as well as the sneers and contempt of the opponents of the new departure. Its blessings have soothed and removed untold suffering and misery—have saved, I might say, millions of lives. For all this, humanity is indebted to one man, whose intellect pierced the deadly mists that overhung the practice of surgery. That to the activity of the surgeon, though it still remains surrounded by grave responsibilities, was added a vastly increased element of pleasure, the *gaudium certaminis* against disease and death—for this gift to his fellow-surgeons, we are indebted to Sir Joseph Lister.

THE PATHOLOGY OF OPHTHALMOPLEGIA.

By W. J. Collins, M.S., M.D., B.Sc. Lond., F.R.C.S. Eng.,

SURGEON TO THE LONDON TEMPERANCE HOSPITAL, AND ASSISTANT SURGEON TO THE ROYAL SOUTH LONDON
OPHTHALMIC HOSPITAL,

AND

L. Wilde, M.D. Durham,

LATE RESIDENT MEDICAL OFFICER TO THE LONDON TEMPERANCE HOSPITAL.

Whether we regard the complexity of the structures concerned, or
the rarity of opportunity for post-mortem examination, or the indirect-
ness and consequently secondary character of the evidence on which we
accordingly have to rely, the difficulty of the explanation of the pathology
of ophthalmoplegia is obvious.   Bearing in mind the destination of
the third, fourth and sixth nerves, with the second and parts of the
fifth and seventh, together with the sympathetic, to the eye and orbital
contents, the eyelids and appurtenances; the long and varied course
which several of these pursue from their nuclei to their termination in
the orbit; the more complicated connections of their centres with the
nerve-tracts proceeding from the spinal cord, medulla, and pons, and
those proceeding to the cortex of the brain, the varied and extended
ocular symptoms which may result from even a small intra-cranial
lesion are self-evident.   Probably nowhere has post-mortem examination
been of less service to pathology than here.   We are constrained to
rely upon clinical observations, judicious analogy, and certain experiments upon animals, for a rational explanation of the symptoms with
which we are dealing.   This field of research, common to the physician
and the oculist, it is not surprising to find, was permitted to remain
fallow until within the last twenty-five or thirty years.   The term
ophthalmoplegia had been employed by Brunner as early as 1850, and
was first brought to the notice of Continental oculists by Von Graefe,
who reported a case in 1856, and exhibited a typical example of
this disease to the Berlin Medical Society on January 29, 1868.
The more modern (1878) division into ophthalmoplegia externa and
ophthalmoplegia interna may prove, on further investigation, to be of
as little value pathologically as, according to Mauthner, it is perhaps
incorrect etymologically.

The site and nature of the lesion to which the group of oculo-motor
palsies (for which we employ the term ophthalmoplegia as an equivalent) is due, have been the chief points upon which discussion has taken
place.   It is obvious that disease affecting the nucleus of origin or the
nerve in its continuity or termination, whether such disease be intrinsic
or extrinsic, may be productive of results difficult to separate.   Disease of the second nerve alone of all cranial nerves is recognizable by

other means than those having reference to disturbance of function. The magnified image of the optic disc exhibiting, in the case of optic neuritis, increased vascularity, lymphatic engorgement, intra-neural hemorrhage, proliferation of fibres, gives us an insight into what may be going on in other nerves during life when they are the seats of neuritis, whose evidence is only rendered visible by the less precise method of post-mortem examination, or inferred by reason of disordered function. It is now well recognized that what is called sclerosis, or some other equally precise, more acute, and more truly inflammatory process, is liable to overrun on definite lines, both centripetally and centrifugally, the cerebro-spinal system, and that the same may be scattered sparsely over the brain and cord, or localized in certain parts. It follows that the symptoms may be as diversified as the sites of this degeneration are various, and it is impossible to understand aright the effects resulting from a lesion affecting the deep origin of any one nerve, or group of nerves, without taking a survey sufficiently broad to cover similar lesions affecting neighboring areas. It was at one time argued that a group of oculo-motor paralyses occurred which was sufficiently distinct from the previously recognized single-nerve palsies or single-muscle palsies, on the one hand, and from symptoms indicating invasion of the spinal cord or brain on the other, to warrant their collection into a separate category, and their being dignified with the exclusive application of the term ophthalmoplegia. This appears to have been the view of Hutchinson when he communicated his paper on "Ophthalmoplegia Externa, or Symmetrical Immobility (partial) of the Eyes with Ptosis" to the Medico-Chirurgical Society in 1879.

He therein states that cases of single muscle paralysis, occurring in syphilis and in locomotor ataxia, are to be distinguished from the class for which he "ventured to propose the name of ophthalmoplegia externa" upon the three following grounds:

1. By the fact of non-symmetry of the former.
2. By the early completeness of the paralysis.
3. By the ease with which very frequently they are cured.

He, however, admits that symmetry is not invariable; indeed, one of his fifteen cases was unilateral, and several others exhibited less symmetry than mere bilaterality.

As to the absence of early completeness of the symptoms, it may be true that the affection of the various muscles may be progressive, but the invasion may be sometimes sudden, as in his eighth case; and it is difficult to understand why the cause which he suggests of the unilateral and partial category of cases, viz., a gumma in the nerve-trunk, should manifest itself by suddenness of onset.

As to the comparative facility of cure in the two sets of cases, it is difficult to see why he should regard as more unfavorable those he calls ophthalmoplegiæ, since he says: "The effects of remedies in several cases were very remarkable, the patient having been rescued from a very dangerous condition." And again: "Often it is distinctly influenced for good by treatment."

As showing that the group of palsies which Hutchinson had in view was less capable of sharp separation from the recognized results of similar affections of the neighboring parts, it is important to note that among his fifteen cases, "in six the lower extremities were more or less weak and liable to pain, the condition approaching more or less closely to locomotor ataxia," and several cases exhibited affection of other cranial nerves—e. g., first, fifth, seventh, and eighth—and in two cases there was insanity; and he finally admits that "there can, however, be no doubt that ophthalmoplegia externa is sometimes a part of the general malady known as progressive locomotor ataxia."

The close similarity of these palsies to those spinal palsies common in children, and known as anterior poliomyelitis, has often been remarked, notably by Wernicke, and the term polio-encephalitis superior as opposed to polio-encephalitis inferior, or bulbar paralysis, has been suggested. This would appear to be the view entertained by Ludwig Mauthner in his valuable monograph on the subject, which reviews most of the previous literature and critically investigates the evidence at large.

We have hitherto made no mention specifically of so-called "ophthalmoplegia interna," which has been regarded in this country, in spite of accumulating evidence both physiological and pathological to the contrary, to belong to the category of orbital or peripheral lesions, rather than as of central origin. It is difficult to see à priori why, if a central control be allowed for the muscles of convergence, this should be denied to the muscles of accommodation, and, if allowed to the latter, why the same privilege should not of necessity be extended to the muscle of the iris.

In 1878 Hutchinson communicated to the Medico-Chirurgical Society his paper on "Paralysis of the Internal Muscles of the Eye"—ophthalmoplegia interna—a group of symptoms which probably indicates disease of the lenticular ganglion. He then held that if paralysis of the muscles of the iris and of the ciliary muscle alone coexisted the "seat of the disease can be in no other structure than the ganglion itself."

Curiously enough, out of the eight cases he relates, in five both of the eyes were affected. It will appear at the outset that such symmetry would be more easily explicable by a focal lesion in the neighborhood of the posterior part of the third ventricle where the third nerve takes its origin, than by assuming that the widely separated lenticular ganglia should be similarly and synchronously affected. How such symmetry can be comparable to the symmetry of choroiditis, as Hutchinson suggests, is hard to understand. Indeed, it would appear from a footnote, which he added after the paper was read, that he was not well satisfied with the explanation he had volunteered. He says: " My only hesitation on this point is as to whether in some cases the same symptoms may be due to disease near the nucleus of the third nerve. It is not easy, however, in such cases to see why the vasomotor should be affected. I have, however, seen the pupil motionless and accommodation lost in some cases in which the disease was believed to be in this position; always, however, there were other complications."

This last observation appears to be most important and suggestive, and would seem to us to indicate at once the solidarity of so-called ophthalmoplegia interna, not only with ophthalmoplegia externa but also with bulbar and infantile spinal paralysis, so far as the nuclear nature of such lesions is concerned. Hulke, in the first volume of the *Ophthalmological Transactions* for 1880, traversed Hutchinson's lenticular ganglion theory, and suggested in its place disease of the "intra-ocular ganglionic plexuses in immediate relation with the muscular apparatus," as the approximate cause. Andamuk had demonstrated that after removal of the lenticular ganglion stimulation of the cervical sympathetic produces the usual dilatation of the pupil. This "appeared to be absolutely decisive " that there was a route from the sympathetic to the iris not *via* the lenticular ganglion. Hulke's preference for the ganglionic plexuses may be accounted for by his claim to have discovered these bodies coincidently with Müller and Schweigger in 1858.

Hutchinson, in reply to Hulke, thinks, " so far as the choice lay between a central and a peripheral seat of change, Mr. Hulke and myself are in the same boat." Gowers, who followed, suggested that they might both be in the wrong one, and taking a broader view and following the researches of Hensen and Volkers, he regarded the probable seat of the lesion as being the anterior portion of the nucleus of the third nerve.

The researches here referred to, carried out in 1878, upon dogs, went to show that the most anterior portion of the nucleus of the third nerve at the posterior part of the third ventricle was the centre for accommodation; behind this came the centre for the iris, then that for the internal rectus, and posteriorly the other muscles of the eyeball. Kohler and Picks's clinical researches powerfully support the foregoing observations, while slightly varying the arrangement of the posterior portion of the nucleus, the internal part of which they would devote to the interior and inferior recti, the outer portion comprising the nuclei for the levator palpebræ, the rectus superior, and the obliquus inferior. Both sets of observers agree in regarding the centre for the fourth nerve as practically part and parcel of that of the third, to the posterior extremity of which it is immediately adjacent. The nuclei of the sixth

appear a little further back, close to the median fissure and the olivary fillet. There is reason to believe that a path of connection between the sixth nucleus of one side and the third nucleus on the other is provided by the posterior horizontal fibres, a nexus which appears at once to explain and to be supported by the facts in regard to what is known as conjugate deviation.

It is well to note here that the recent researches of Gaskell led him to regard the lenticular ganglion as the vagrant motor ganglion of the third nerve akin to the sympathetic ganglion connected with the motor root of a spinal or segmental nerve, and composed almost entirely of third-nerve fibres. He does not regard the first division of the fifth nerve as their corresponding sensory nerve, but finds in the third and fourth trunks fibrillar tissue and cells which he considers to be the vestigial remains of long disused sensory roots and sensory (stationary) ganglia of these nerves. If this view be correct, it is doubtful whether reflex central functions can be attributed to the lenticular ganglion with any more assurance than they can be to the submaxillary ganglion. It would appear to be little more than a vestigial incident occurring in the course of distribution of the third nerve, and not to be regarded either as the primary or secondary seat of control of the intra-ocular muscles.

We have hitherto made no allusion to neural as distinguished from nuclear lesion as occasioning ocular palsy. In 1883, in *St. Bartholomew's Hospital Reports*, one of the present author's, in recording thirteen cases of oculo-motor paralysis exhibiting great variety of both unilateral and bilateral palsy, thus recorded his view of the pathology of these cases:

" In those cases where periostitis in the form of nodes or gummata was present, it is probable that the lesion was situated in the orbit or the sphenoidal fissure. In those cases of *bilateral paralysis*, especially when there is implication of the optic nerves, the base of the brain or the central ganglia are presumably the seat of disease."

In apportioning the effects of extrinsic (*e. g.*, tumor or aneurism exciting pressure), or intrinsic (*e. g.*, nucleitis or neuritis) causes it is important to bear in mind, as Mauthner insists, that we may speak of three categories of causation according to the proximity of the cause. Thus syphilis may cause tumor which may cause ophthalmoplegia. Here nerve-pressure is a cause of the first category, the cause of the proximate cause is the tumor, and the remote cause of this is syphilis. The relative irrelevance of the remote cause as compared to the proximate cause is obvious, yet its importance therapeutically is paramount.

In no other situation are there opportunities for a small lesion to affect so many cranial nerves in their continuity as in the cavernous sinus. Putting aside the rather obscure ocular palsies of cortical origin, the floor of the aqueduct of Sylvius and fourth ventricle and the walls of the cavernous sinus would be the most favorable site for small lesions to effect large results; in the former such lesions would be mostly nuclear, in the latter necessarily neural. We would here introduce the following scheme:

OPHTHALMOPLEGIA.

I. *Cerebral.*   (*a*) cortical $\begin{cases} \text{conjugate deviation.} \\ \text{hemi-ptosis (?).} \\ \text{hysterical ophthalmoplegia (?).} \end{cases}$

(*b*) cortico-peduncular.

(*c*) nuclear $\begin{array}{l} \left. \begin{array}{l} \text{1. cycloplegia} \\ \text{2. iridoplegia} \end{array} \right\} \text{"ophthalmoplegia interna."} \\ \text{3d nerve} \quad \text{3. palsy of extra-ocular muscles.} \\ \qquad\qquad\quad \text{ptosis.} \end{array}$

3d nerve 3. palsy of extra-ocular muscles.
        ptosis.
4th nerve 4. palsy of superior oblique.
6th nerve 5. palsy of external rectus.

(*d*) radicular (and ? commissural).

II. *Basal.*   (*a*) region of pons (vi.).
(*b*) " " peduncles (vi. iv. iii.).
(*c*) " " cavernous sinus (vi. iv. iii.).
(*d*) " " sphenoidal fissure.

III. *Orbital* (including peripheral).

Ophthalmoplegia of cortical or cortico-peduncular origin is usually conjugate, not unilateral; this is a corollary to the observation that movements, rather than muscles or nerves, are represented in the cortical colligation. The only exception to this rule apparently is that of ptosis occuring upon the opposite side exclusively to that of the cerebral lesion. (Landouzy.)

In order to complete the cerebral classification of intra-cranial sites of possible lesions resulting in ophthalmoplegia, it is necessary to add the "radicular," to include lesions intermediate between the superficial and deep origins of the various nerves concerned, and perhaps also commisural.

In addition to intra-cranial causes, there are those situate in the orbits, which logically should be made to include the so-called peripheral lesions, which some authors would place in a separate category. It is difficult to deny that in some cases of transient ptosis, symmetrical cycloparesis, convergent asthenopia may not be of peripheral neuro-muscular causation; and it is certain that trauma may be productive of peripheral palsies, whether by extravasation or by more permanent sequelæ.

With a view to elucidate from a clinical standpoint some of the questions we have raised in what has preceded, we have been at some pains to collect and classify such available cases of ophthalmoplegia in English literature as would lend themselves to such treatment. We have kept apart those cases in which paralysis of the intrinsic muscles of the eye only existed—twenty-one in number—and the heads of classification we have adopted have been the following:

1. Sex.
2. Age.
3. Alleged cause.
4. History, personal˙ and family, with duration and cause of symptoms.
5. Seat of lesion as found, or presumed or inferred.
6. Symptoms, including the muscles paralyzed, vision, headache, condition of pupils, reflexes, optic discs, etc.
7, The treatment.
8. The result.
9. The autopsy in the rare instances in which such has been made.

Sex. Of 120 cases of ophthalmoplegia 73 were males, 39 females, 8 unstated, giving 65 per cent. of the stated cases as males, showing a considerable preponderance in the male sex.

Age. Of the 120 cases, in 111 the age was stated. From 0 there were 8 cases; from 10 there were 17; from 20 there were 26; from 30 there were 28; from 40 there were 19; from 50 there were 6; from 60 there were 4; from 70 there were 3; from 80 and upward there were 0; with 9 not stated = 120.

This summary, in the absence of the number of the population living at each decade, of course tells us nothing as to the actual age-incidence of the disease; but, inasmuch as the population living at each ten years' period is less than that at any previous ten-year period, it proves that the increasing number of cases up to between 30 and 40 indicates a greatly increased liability to the disease up to that age. The fall to 19 in the next period—40 to 50, if viewed in relation to population living at such age—would not show any such considerably reduced liability to attack at that age as probably does occur at the ages beyond fifty. ˙

Syphilis as a cause. In 40 cases out of the 120 there was some evidence or other of syphilis apart from the ophthalmoplegia, or in 33 per cent. of the whole. Of the 40 the result in 32 was stated. In 23 there was improvement under treatment, 11 recovered, and in 9 others the improvement was stated to be considerable and substantial; in 7 there was no improvement, 1 was said to be progressive, and 1 was known to terminate fatally. On these facts we would remark that, while quite agreeing with Mr. Hutchinson that a more careful search for evidence of syphilis might most probably have revealed its presence in a larger number of cases, the disease, even in its central form, is probably not exclusively syphilitic; but if syphilitic, and if unaccompanied by other more serious central disease, and especially if treated early, is apt to be very amenable to remedies.

Eye affected. Of 109 cases, 1 eye only was affected in 61 cases, both eyes in 48. In the 61 cases in which only one eye was affected, this was the right in 31, the left in 30; showing that the side affected is a matter of indifference. The above figures, of course, destroy the importance attached to the symmetry of the lesion. Our cases include many in which the affection was in the nerve-trunks, but in some of these the palsy was bilateral; and we think far too great importance has been attached to the question of symmetry as deciding the seat of the lesion.

Distribution of the palsy as regards various portions of third nerve. Of the 120 cases of ophthalmoplegia in which the external ocular muscles were affected, there was evidence of some affection of intra-ocular muscles in 65.

In 29 of the 65 both iris and ciliary muscle were involved.

We would, however, direct especial attention to the mode of linking of extra-ocular palsy with cycloplegia and indoplegia respectively as bearing upon the work of Hensen and Volker and of Kohler and Pick. In the 34 cases in which only one of the two (viz., iris or ciliary) was affected, plus extra-ocular palsy, in no less than 31 it was the iris and not the ciliary, and in only 3 was it the ciliary and not the iris. If it be true that the centres for ciliary, iris, and extra-ocular muscles are arranged in that order—tandem fashion—on the floor of the aqueduct, we can understand why the linking of the palsies should be as above.

Distribution of palsy as regards nerves involved. Of the 116 cases in which the analysis could be made, in 47 the third nerve alone was affected (in 18 complete, in 29 incomplete); in 42 the third, fourth, and sixth were affected in company; in 11 the sixth alone was affected; in 8 the third and fourth failed together; in 4 the third and sixth are presumed to have been associated in palsy; in 2 the fourth and sixth, and in 2 the fourth alone.

The frequent bracketing of the third, fourth, and sixth might suggest the frequency of lesion in the course of the nerve-trunks; but the relative infrequency of attack of the sixth, in spite of its longer and more arduous extra-cerebral, intra-cranial course, would rather suggest an opposite reflection. The direct connections between the sixth nuclei and those of the third and fourth by the posterior horizontal fibres are to be borne in mind.

Result. Of the 92 cases out of the 120 in which the result is noted 53 improved under treatment, 26 completely recovering, and in 14 more the improvement was stated to be considerable; in 15 there was no improvement, in 2 the disease was progressive, and in 22 it was fatal.

Age and fatality. We have previously suggested that ophthalmoplegia of young children was probably more serious and fatal than that of adults. Of 6 cases under ten in which the result is recorded, 3 died, or 50 per cent.; of the 86 over ten in which the result is recorded, 19 died, or 23 per cent.

REVIEWS.

Die Peptone in ihrer Wissenschaftlichen und Praktischen Bedeu-
tung: Studien zur Lehre von der Verdauung der Eiweisskörper
und des Leimes. Von Dr. V. Gerlach. Hamburg und Leipzig:
Leopold Voss, 1891.

The Peptones: Their Scientific and Practical Significance. Studies
toward the Knowledge of the Digestion of the Proteid Bodies
and Gelatin.

This interesting publication of a series of original investigations, made
partly at the physiological laboratory of Professor Kühne in Heidelberg
and continued at the hygienic department of the laboratory of Dr.
Schmitt in Wiesbaden, begins with a historical review of the development of our knowledge of digestion and nutrition, and then dwells on
the present views on this subject. The splitting up of the albumin
molecule into the anti- and hemi-groups of Kühne and Chittenden, and
especially the formation of the albumoses, are freely commented on.
The amounts of nitrogen and anti-albumin and anti-peptone, also hemi-
albumose and hemi-peptone, as found by Kühne and Chittenden, were
gone over by the author, and pure albumoses and pure peptone produced
by him. With these latter he made further studies on their nutritive
value on animals by controlling the nitrogen ingested and that eliminated. In this manner he proves that the albumoses are quite able to
take the place of meat as proteid food ; further, that they are well borne
by the animals and readily taken by them. With the pure peptones he
could not determine any results, as they invariably disagreed with the
experimental animals. He also prepared gelatin absolutely free .from
albumin, and from it gelatin-peptone. He determined the amount of
nitrogen in this also, and made a series of nutrition experiments with it,
both alone and together with meat. He found here that with gelatin-
peptone alone there was a steady loss of body nitrogen, so that it does not
possess nutritive qualities sufficient to take the place of meat; but when
fed with meat together, it increased the body nitrogen over the simple
meat diet. Thus he claims to prove that, though no substitute for meat
by itself, it brings about a saving of the latter when fed with it.
   The practical application of the author's investigations is in connection
with the estimation of the food value of the so-called " meat peptones."
He arrives at the conclusion that, as they are principally composed of
albumoses and of gelatin- (chondrin-) peptones, they are valuable substitutes for albuminous diet, quite able to take their place, and by comparison and comparative experiments with a number of them, claims
the greatest food value for the " Kemmerich's meat peptones."

L. W.

TEXT-BOOK OF MEDICAL JURISPRUDENCE AND TOXICOLOGY. By JOHN J. REESE, M.D., etc. Third (revised and enlarged) edition. Philadelphia: P. Blakiston, Son & Co., 1891.

THE third edition of this well-known work needs scarcely any comment at our hands. It has been so fully and favorably dwelt upon in THE JOURNAL at its former appearances that but little more can be added now. That it is a standard work of American medical literature is not saying too much for it, also that it is a thoroughly reliable guide for the practitioner if called upon to define his position in the judicial forum.

To the student of medical jurisprudence and toxicology it is invaluable, as it is concise, clear, and thorough in every respect. The absence of cumbersome quotations enhances its value.

If any fault were to be found with it, it would be of quantity, rather than quality. Thus, with somnabulism and other conditions of irresponsibility, the question of hypnotism might have been considered in this edition.

The additions especially valuable in the present revision are the chapter on the Ptomaines and Formad's investigation and technique for the restoration and measurement of blood-corpuscles.   L. W.

THE MODERN ANTIPYRETICS: THEIR ACTION IN HEALTH AND DISEASE. By ISAAC OTT, M.D., Ex-Fellow in Biology, Johns Hopkins University; Ex-President of the American Neurological Association; Consulting Physician to the Easton Hospital; Corresponding Member of the German Medical Society of New York, etc. Pp. 52. Easton: E. D. Vogel, 1891.

IN this little volume a preliminary chapter is devoted to an account of original work on the nature of fever. The author's position is that fever, though primarily set up by an increase in heat-production beyond that of heat-dissipation, continues not from excessive production, but from an altered relation between production and dissipation. This is corroborated by experiments on the dog, and by the use of a calorimeter made large enough to hold a man. A detailed record, among others, is given of the study of a malarial paroxysm made with this apparatus, which is described and illustrated. The amount of heat produced by muscular exercise was also investigated.

After a short reference to the chemistry of antipyretics, their general action in health and disease is considered. The conclusion is reached that in fever antipyresis is usually set up by a temporary decrease of heat-production beyond that of dissipation.

Under the head of therapeutics, these drugs are discussed separately as to their physiological action, toxicology, and clinical use. In a few pages much information is condensed which has not been readily accessible.

The value of antipyretics in typhoid fever receives consideration in a separate chapter. The author assigns them a secondary position in the treatment of this disease, particularly because of their depressant heart action. He prefers quinine for occasional use in grave hyperpyrexia, unless there is great cerebral excitation, when antipyrine does better. A description of Brand's method of cold-water treatment is appended.

G. E. S.

————— —

LECTURES ON DIABETES; INCLUDING THE BRADSHAW LECTURE DELIV-
ERED BEFORE THE ROYAL COLLEGE OF PHYSICIANS, AUGUST 18, 1890.
By ROBERT SAUNDBY, M.D., F.R.C.P., Lond., etc. 12mo. pp. 232. New
York: E. B. West & Co., 1891.

THERE can scarcely be a more difficult part in the rôle of medical authorship at the present day than to write a satisfactory book on diabetes. It is a disease that has long been known; an enormous number of clinical facts has therefore been accumulated bearing upon it, while no department of physiology has had added to it so much accurate experimental knowledge as the glycogenic function of the liver; yet we know neither the cause nor pathology of diabetes. As much as is known has been known a long time, and whenever a new book is announced the reader naturally expects more than he receives.

Each carefully collated volume, however, adds to the stock of knowledge whence we must some day extract the kernel of a solution of the vexed problem. Dr. Saundby's book is no exception. The direction in which he has efficiently aided us is in the geographical distribution of the disease and in its morbid anatomy. In the former respect his work is complemental to the equally excellent book of Dr. Purdy, of this country. Dr. Saundby's book is especially complete in this direction so far as Europe and Asia are concerned, while it is signally deficient in the American distribution. On the other hand, Dr. Purdy's account of the distribution of the disease in America is by far the most complete and exhaustive yet published, and he who follows will have the advantage of their joint labors. The most important result of Dr. Purdy's observations is, that the disease is peculiarly prevalent in our northwest and northeast, and hence the conclusion that cold and dampness are important factors in production; and Dr. Saundby's, that the disease is very common among the educated and learned class in India—chiefly non-flesh-eaters. Dr. Saundby has collected many individual cases bearing upon the etiology, but it cannot be said that they add much to what was previously known.

The second feature of Dr. Saundby's book by which it is to be distinguished from others is the exhaustive treatment of the morbid anatomy, no surprise to any one who had the privilege of hearing Dr. Saundby's Bradshaw Lectures, as happened to the writer. The most hopeful organ in this direction at the present day is the pancreas, since not only are there constantly being added to the original cases of Lanceraux others wherein the autopsy after diabetes has disclosed pancreatic disease, but there are now also to be added cases of diabetes consequent on extirpation of the pancreas, not only in animals but also in man. The presence of well-defined cases, however, in which there has been no pancreatic lesion, and of others where the disease followed blows on the stomach or other localities where the semilunar ganglion could be reached, goes to show that it is likely to be the sympathetic system of nerves which is really responsible even in pancreatic cases.

One turns naturally in every new book to the treatment of such an intractable disease as diabetes. It cannot be said that Dr. Saundby helps us greatly, but at the same time the old treatment is well reviewed and the chaff thoroughly sifted from the grain—and it must be said there is a good deal more of the former than the latter. The dietetic treatment remains the best, while opium is the only adjuvant in the shape of a drug which can be relied upon.

Dr. Saundby's book is welcome to our shelves as reflecting the most recent information on the subject, and as a safe guide to the practitioner for the management of any cases which may come under his care.

J. T.

PRACTICAL PATHOLOGY AND MORBID HISTOLOGY. By HENEAGE GIBBES, Professor of Pathology in the University of Michigan, etc. Illustrated with Sixty Photographic Reproductions. 8vo., pp. xvi., 320. Philadelphia: Lea Brothers & Co., 1891.

THE book is divided into four sections: Part I., Practical Pathology; Part II., Practical Bacteriology; Part III., Morbid Histology; Part IV., Photography with the Microscope. The subjects included under the different sections are as well treated as could be the case in the limits allowed. We are unable to agree, however, that "such instructions are given as will enable him (the student) to transfer a specimen of any morbid change directly to his microscope in an unaltered condition, and to recognize it unerringly." Such a result can only be obtained with a much more exhaustive volume than the one here spoken of. It is an omission to have made no mention of the Koch-Ehrlich method of staining the bacillus of tuberculosis—for this method is one that every student should at least be familiar with.

Taken as a whole, the volume will very well carry out its purpose—that of an aid to the student—and the typography and its illustrations are extremely good. H. C. E.

BACTERIA AND THEIR PRODUCTS. By GERMAN SIMS WOODHEAD, M.D. Edin., Director of the Laboratories of the Conjoint Board of the Royal College of Physicians (Lond.) and Surgeons (Eng.), etc. With 20 photomicrographs, and an appendix giving a short account of bacteriological methods, and a diagnostic description of the commoner bacteria. 8vo., pp. xiii., 454. London: Walter Scott, 1891.

THIS book is, in the language of the preface, "an attempt to give some account of the main facts in bacteriology, and of the life-history of the bacteria and closely allied organisms, and also to discuss the more important theories as to the part played by them in Nature's economy; especially in their relation to the commoner fermentative, putrefactive and diseased processes." The result of the author's efforts is a more full work of the sort than any with which we are yet familiar in the English language. The arrangement is very similar to that of Löffler's *Vorlesungen*, and at the end of each section there is placed a series of references to the more important works upon the subject just treated. To one interested in the development of bacteriology, and in its present condition, this book will be of value as containing a fairly extensive epitome of what is known, and especially for the facilities given for further reading upon the subject.   H. C. E.

THE LATIN GRAMMAR OF PHARMACY AND MEDICINE. By D. H. ROBIN-SON, Ph.D., Professor of Latin Language and Literature, University of Kansas. With an Introduction by L. E. SAYRE, Ph.G., Professor of Pharmacy in, and Dean of, Department of Pharmacy, University of Kansas. Pp. 271. Philadelphia: P. Blakiston & Co., 1890.

A CURIOUS outgrowth of the modern tendency to narrow specialism in education is this volume, which is designed for the use of those whose limitations compel a short preparation only for the practice of medicine or pharmacy. Somewhat in the form of a beginner's Latin book, it aims to use words and examples in teaching which will serve to familiarize the student from the start with medical and pharmaceutical terms.

It must be confessed that it is startling at first to find, instead of the traditional and familiar sentences about Balbus or Romulus or the she-wolf, such exercises for translation as these: " Is the syrup of ipecac a good remedy for a bad boy?" " What is on our friend's nose? A capsicum plaster." " Nitric acid bit the boy's third finger." Truly, this is a utilitarian age. While it must be admitted that under ordinary methods a considerable vocabulary is acquired which cannot be directly applied in pharmacy or medicine, there may be an error in the other direction. Large numbers of technical words, as names of drugs, are transferred almost bodily into English. There is little advantage in being familiar with them as words simply, when their meaning is unknown to the beginner, while the use of unwieldy terms would seem to make more embarrassing than ever the Latin construction. After all, a vocabulary can best be acquired by associating a word with an object or its use.

There is much in the exercises here given which can only be of use to students of pharmacy, and it is probable that among these the work will find its chief field. For instance, one of the exercises to be translated into Latin consists of the formula and the method of preparing the compound fluid extract of sarsaparilla. It is doubtful whether there is any practical improvement upon a narrative of the Romulus and Remus type in the translation of the following: " Moisten the powders with twenty ounces of this mixture, and pack it firmly in a cylindrical percolator."

Granted that his whole knowledge is superficial, the question arises whether a man is more likely to write correct prescriptions after learning the declension of *adeps* rather than that of the time-honored *rex*.

The book, which stands alone in its field, is written by a teacher who has been obliged to confront the difficulties caused by poor preparation among students. The general plan is undoubtedly the outgrowth of his experience, and as such deserves respectful consideration. While the method utterly divorces the language from its literature and cuts off the comparative study of other languages, it is conceivable that it should help the short-term student to a working knowledge. Though in the individual case it may serve a purpose, its adoption in a school could not fail to maintain a low standard.

It seems a mistake to advise the so-called Roman method of pronunciation. If ever the English method is justifiable it is here, since all scientific terms are Anglicized. Why, for instance, teach a student of pharmacy to pronounce *gentiana* with "*g*" as in "*give*," or *cinnamomum* with "*c*" as in "*cave*." "*Yalapa*" for *jalapa* strikes one as odd, even in this book of incongruities.

A useful feature is the frequent giving of simple derivations of compound words, including many of Greek origin. The word ὕδωρ, water, looks unnatural when spelled "hudor,". but the end of simplicity is attained. G. E. Š.

A MANUAL OF DISEASES OF THE NOSE AND THROAT, INCLUDING THE NOSE, NASO-PHARYNX, PHARYNX AND LARYNX. By PROCTOR S. HUTCHINSON, M.R.C.S., Assistant Surgeon to the Hospital for Diseases of the Throat. With Illustrations. 12mo. pp. x., 127. London: H. K. Lewis, 1891.

A FAIRLY good primer with a good index. Upon 124 pages no less than 64 subjects noted in the table of contents are summarized, with 38 illustrations, and some of them large ones. Ten pages concerning paralyses of the larynx are by far the best of the batch. The illustrations are excellent. A novel departure is presented in sandwiching the subject-matter between three terminal pages devoted to diseases of the larynx in the lower animals, and two full-page initial display plates illustrating morbid growths of the larynx and trachea in dogs, and atrophied muscles of the larynx of a " roaring " horse. J. S. C.

ATLAS OF CLINICAL MEDICINE. By BYROM BRAMWELL, M.D., F.R.C.P. Edin.; F.R.S. Edin.; Assistant Physician to the Edinburgh Royal Infirmary, etc. Volume I., Part I. Edinburgh: T. & A. Constable, 1891.

THE contents of the first instalment of this work, which will probably soon be widely known as *Bramwell's Atlas*, are: Myxœdema; Clinical Investigation of Cases of Myxœdema; Sporadic Cretinism; The Clinical Investigation of Cases of Sporadic Cretinism; Myxœdema and Exophthalmic Goitre Contrasted; Friedreich's Ataxia; The Clinical Investigation of Friedreich's Ataxia; Notes of Three Additional Cases of Friedreich's Ataxia.

It must not be supposed that the work is, as its name implies, a mere collection of pictorial illustrations of disease. The plates are certainly its most striking feature, both on account of the excellence of their execution and their truth to nature, but they are, after all, but the complements of a verbal description, in every instance admirable, of the subjects they represent. Without the plates the work would take rank as a standard on the subjects of which it treats; with them, it does away with those false conceptions which are sure to arise in the mind of the mere textualist. We cannot recommend this Atlas too strongly, especially to teachers and to those who are deprived by absence from great medical centres of many clinical advantages; but in mentioning these two classes of physicians we do not exclude anyone who has it in his power to obtain the work.   F. P. H.

TEXT-BOOK OF HYGIENE. By GEORGE H. ROHÉ, M.D., Professor of Obstetrics in the College of Physicians and Surgeons, Baltimore, etc. 8vo. Second edition, revised and rewritten. Philadelphia: F. A. Davis, 1890.

A BOOK whose purpose is to teach men how to live long is always welcome. In these days of wonderfully rapid development of the science of hygiene, when only those skilled in bacteriological research can keep pace with its march, it becomes an urgent need to have a book in which the practical results of so much progress are stated in a clear and concise form, intelligible to the ordinary practitioner and student, as well as to the laity. This purpose is certainly filled by the present work. "The author cannot flatter himself that much in the volume is new. He hopes nothing in it is untrue." With this apology, he certainly deserves credit for the clear-cut manner in which he handles the important sanitary problems. In twenty-two chapters the various departments of hygiene are treated in a manner that embodies in practical application all that the later development of bacteriology has taught us. Especially commendable are the chapters giving a concise but pointed description of contagion, infection, and the use of antiseptics, deodorants, and disinfectants. Prophylaxis, *in place*, has been given due importance, and the accurate and comprehensive description of the Quarantine Station, as established and conducted by the Louisiana State Board of Health, is a valuable addition to the merits of the work, giving the student and practitioner the application on a gigantic scale of the principles which he is called upon to use in daily practice, should he wish to be abreast of the times in the fight against infection and contagion. On the whole, we believe that the author's purpose has been fully achieved, and that this volume, though not an exhaustive treatise, is called to furnish much valuable knowledge in a most accessible form.
                    E. L.

PROGRESS

OF

MEDICAL SCIENCE.

THERAPEUTICS.

UNDER THE CHARGE OF

REYNOLD W. WILCOX, A.M., M.D.,

PROFESSOR OF CLINICAL MEDICINE IN THE NEW YORK POST-GRADUATE MEDICAL SCHOOL;
ASSISTANT VISITING PHYSICIAN TO BELLEVUE HOSPITAL.

SALICYLATE OF SODIUM IN THE TREATMENT OF DIABETES.

The treatment of diabetes mellitus by salicylate of sodium is by no means novel. Speaking generally, there are two great classes of diabetics. In the first are those on whom the disease falls while they are quite young, with symptoms of great intensity; as a rule, to which at present there are very few exceptions, this form is quickly fatal. The second class includes those who are attacked when they are elderly and of gouty tendencies. In these it may not be very active; they may even become fat while they are suffering from it; they have not much glycosuria or polyuria, and they often do not die from the diabetes itself.

Dr. Mansel Sympson reports a case where the salicylic treatment was successful in the more fatal class of cases, that is in the younger and more fatal form. The patient was an engineer's apprentice, seventeen years old, who came under Dr. Sympson's care on April 18, 1891. The family history was not good; he had been a fairly healthy lad until about six weeks before. The urine was very pale, greenish-yellow in tint, limpid, also smelling of apples, very acid, of a specific gravity of 1040, free from albumin, but giving a great deal of sugar. He was passing about seven pints in the twenty-four hours. He was at once put on a mixture of ten grains of salicylate of sodium, five drops of tincture of nux vomica, and an ounce of infusion of gentian, to be taken every four hours. He was also cut off absolutely from sugar, pastry, bread (save well-baked toast), and biscuits, and of course from potatoes and starchy vegetables.

In the first week his water became gradually reduced in quantity, from seven to five and a quarter pints in the twenty-four hours, while its specific gravity varied from 1050 to 1040, the amount of sugar remaining about the same, or decreasing a very little. His medicine was only given *sextis horis* at the end of the first week. He suffered a good deal with headache, which was relieved by the salicylate and by citrate of caffeine. By the middle of the second week he was on strict diet, gluten bread, almond cakes, etc., with no starch or sugar in any form. His urine was greatly improved, only three pints being passed in the twenty-four hours, of specific gravity 1024, and containing by Dr. Oliver's test a little over five grains to the ounce. His thirst was lessening, headache had vanished, and his sense of satisfaction with both meat and drink was increasing. About the twelfth day of treatment he was passing about two pints of urine, of specific gravity 1014, with a mere trace of sugar. In six more days there was no sugar at all in his water. On April 10th, having been without medicine for four days, passed about half a pint more water daily, and had suffered from a slight return of the headache. On May 18th had been again off the salicylate mixture for three days, with the result that he passed just twice as much water daily as he had done before. He complained also a little of pains in his back when without the medicine. Since May 19th his water had never been over two and three-quarters pints; it had never contained any trace of sugar; and on June 24th it was acid, specific gravity 1025, no albumin or sugar.

When the patient was on a mixed diet at the very beginning of treatment, salicylate of sodium made a difference of nearly two pints per diem in the amount of water passed; again, when he was on strict diet, the temporary cessation of the medicine on two occasions caused him each time to pass nearly double as much water as he did before or since, and gave him much uneasiness and more desire to micturate.

It may be due to the salicylate that the urine became free from sugar and kept so; it is, however, to be borne in mind that the effect of diet in some cases is marvellous, and the case cannot be considered as cured until the patient has been without the medicine again for some considerable time, and has had a mixed diet without showing evidence of glycosuria.

The action of salicylate of sodium in this case is well worth recording; the more of such cases which are known the more encouraging this method of treatment will be.—*Practitioner*, No. 278, 1891.

The Treatment of Epilepsy by the Combined Use of Bromides and some Agent Capable of Producing Anæmia of the Nervous Centres.

Poulet's conclusions, as given in the *Bulletin général de Thérapeutique*, are as follows:

The bromides constitute the basis of the treatment of epilepsy. Among them the bromide of gold does not possess the advantages ascribed to it by some, and must yield the palm to the bromide of potassium. There are always a number of cases of epilepsy which though benefited by bromide treatment are not as efficiently treated as they admit of being.

In such cases the addition of one of the following drugs—Calabar bean, picrotaine, belladonna, and, in cardiac epilepsy, digitalis—will frequently bring about the desired result, viz., the suppression of the attacks. This will hold in general for epilepsy, pure and simple, as well as for many cases of Jacksonian epilepsy, though in this latter disease the search for the exciting cause, and its removal where possible, must always precede the above palliative treatment. In cardiac epilepsy twenty-four to thirty drops of the tincture of digitalis, or about four grains of the powder may be given along with the bromides.

ANTIPYRINE IN THE TREATMENT OF PLEURAL EFFUSIONS.

CLEMENT, in the *Lyon Médical*, commends the value of antipyrine in the treatment of acute and chronic pleural effusions. The drug to be effective must be given in doses of about fifteen grains every four hours, and continued in somewhat smaller doses for several days after the disappearance of the effusion, a result which he states may be expected in from one to four days. Purulent or bloody effusions are not favorably affected, and when the pleural cavity is completely filled, Clement prefers immediate resort to paracentesis. He is at a loss to explain this singular effect of the drug upon any other ground than its specific action upon inflammatory processes, the kidneys or skin never having shown sufficient over-activity to account for the rapid subsidence of the effusion.

DEATH UNDER METHYLENE.

DR. EDWARD CHAMBERLAYNE recently administered methylene for an operation for the removal of a cancer of the breast. It was slowly given in a Junker's inhaler, and the inhaler was removed from time to time. Besides the supply of air through the valves of the inhaler, there was a space, owing to the falling in of the cheeks, easily admitting the tips of two fingers, on each side of the mouth between the mouth and the inhaler. All went well until about twenty minutes after the administration was begun, when the patient began to heave as if to vomit. The apparatus was at once removed; the heaving lasted a minute and a half, after which she made several deep inspirations of air. A moment later respiration suddenly ceased. Artificial respiration was instantly begun, and kept up for an hour and twenty minutes; it was then decided that the case was hopeless. Six injections of ether and three enemata of brandy had previously been used. About three drachms of methylene were used. There was no post-mortem; her heart had been frequently examined by her medical attendant, and was believed to be healthy. —*Lancet*, 1891, No. 3548.

A NEW ANTISEPTIC.

No sooner is one antiseptic chemical rejected by some disappointed disciple of antisepticism, than he is greeted by a new chemical possessing all the virtues and free from all the vices of its predecessor. DR. BERLIOZ now presents to the Parisian Academy of Medicine a new chemical which already has proved itself worthy, if we accept the statements of its advocates, of general recognition as the best of antiseptics. He names it "Microçidine" —a name to which it is hardly entitled, seeing that its germicidal powers are inferior to those of corrosive sublimate.

According to Professor Polaillon, the new drug is not a definite chemical compound, but rather a mixture of β-naphthol and hydroxylate of sodium. This new product is soluble in three times its weight of cold water, the solution being of a brown color, which disappears on dilution. The chief advantages claimed for this, the latest of antiseptics, was its slight cost and its non-poisonousness. As it is eliminated by the kidneys, it should be found useful in cases of chronic cystitis with fetid urine. The value of the naphthols α and β in the tympany of typhoid is well known, and as microcidine is simply a product of the fusion of β-naphthol with the hydroxylate of sodium, it should prove useful in such cases.—*Medical Press*, September 16, 1891.

The Toxic Dose of Oil of Turpentine.

The daughter of a former Hawaiian missionary states that the natives are so fond of drink that the native house-painters will drink oil of turpentine for its intoxicating effect when they are unable to obtain any other stimulant. They have been known to drink as much as a pint at a time. From this statement it would appear that the toxic dose of this substance is far beyond any dose dreamed of by therapeutists.—*New York Medical Journal*, 1891, No. 25.

A New Mode of Administering the Bromides.

In Paris the pharmacists have been astonished by the increasing number of prescriptions wherein the bromides are combined with naphthol and bismuth. This is simply carrying out suggestions made by Professor Féré, that large doses of the bromides tended, in certain individuals, to beget unpleasant symptoms, chiefly for the reason that the gastro-intestinal tract of such persons was in a condition of sepsis that prevented the proper assimilation of the drugs. He recommended the administration of such intestinal antiseptics as naphthol and salicylate of bismuth as a means of removing drug intolerance from this and from other causes. The following formula is one method found by him to be advantageous, in the treatment of epileptics especially:

R.—Bromide of potassium . . . . . ℥iss.
β-naphthol . . . . . . ℨj.
Salicylate of sodium . . . . . . ℥ss.

Mix, and divide into three doses, one dose to be given three times daily.

It is maintained by Féré that this treatment is curative as well as preventive. He has found that the eczema and psoriasis which sometimes follow in the train of borax will also disappear if the intestinal tract is rendered aseptic.

Peroxide of Hydrogen in Diseases of the Eye.

The following is a summary of the conclusions of Dr. S. S. Golovin regarding the use of peroxide of hydrogen in ophthalmic practice:

In healthy eyes the peroxide causes only trifling smarting and transient congestion of the conjunctiva. In diseased eyes, especially when deep corneal ulcers are present, instillation of the peroxide may give rise to a more or less intense burning sensation, which, however, quickly disappears spontaneously.

A reliable preparation should always be employed. The peroxide solutions are somewhat unstable, but decomposition can easily be prevented by the addition of a small quantity of sulphuric ether, and by keeping the mixture in an opaque glass in a dark place. A 3 per cent. solution may be employed for lotions or irrigations; stronger solutions should be used in the form of eye-drops.

R.—Hydrogenii hyperoxydati (10 to 15 per cent.) ⸱ ℥iss.
Ætheris sulphurici . . . . . . gtt. j.
(Keep in a bottle of dark glass.)
Sig.—A few drops to be instilled into the eye several times a day.

The best results are obtained in corneal affections. Simple ulcers of the membrane rapidly disappear without being complicated with purulent infiltrations. Suppurating ulcers speedily assume a cleaner and healthier appearance, infiltrations undergo absorption, the lesions healing without perforation of the cornea occurring. Even in severe cases the only traces remaining at the site of the ulcers are slight opacities corresponding to the deepest portion of the excavation. The peroxide is also invaluable in cases of hypopyon keratitis. Provided the instillations are made regularly and thoroughly, even cases in which otherwise operative interference would be necessary, yield to the remedy.

Of conjunctival affections, the peroxide is especially of service in cases of phlyctenular conjunctivitis, which is cured by it much more rapidly than by ordinary treatment. It is also useful in the early stages of acute gonorrhœal ophthalmia (in which the instillation should be repeated not less than four or five times daily, or even every two hours), though the effects scarcely go. beyond sterilizing the discharge and preventing or controlling corneal lesions· In simple acute and chronic diffuse catarrhs of the conjunctiva, as well as in trachomatous or follicular conjunctivitis, the peroxide seems to be useless.

[Much of the peroxide sold in this country is acid in reaction, and would be unsuitable to be dropped into the eye unless neutralized, in which case it keeps less well than when its reaction is acid.—ED.]—*British Medical Journal*, 1891, No. 1599.

———

THE METHODICAL EMPLOYMENT OF SULPHONAL IN MENTAL DISEASES.

DR. FORSTER publishes his experience with fifty-six patients of the Königs-mutter Institution. He was much pleased with the result. The drug acted principally as a motor depressant. Noisy, obstreperous patients were quieted down; many who were given to soiling themselves, ceased to do so. This condition of restfulness was induced in excitement stages of acute and chronic insanity, periodical and chronic mania, senile dementia, progressive paralysis, idiocy, and epilepsy. Thirty grains were generally sufficient, but as much as sixty were sometimes given. The single dose was from seven and a half to fifteen grains. In periodical excitement, given continuously, it shortened and ameliorated the period of excitement. It was of special value in acute melancholia and insanity. Epileptic attacks were not so violent; a cure of the epilepsy was not achieved.

He observed two forms of disagreeable by-effects, called by him sulphonalismus. The first was a motor and sensory depressive form, that appeared as paretic weakness, at first of the lower extremities, then of the tongue and upper extremities. The other form was a persistent somnolency, and a diminution of sensation, weakening, or extinction of the cutaneous sensibility. The first stage of this was not dangerous, but the second required careful observation. The symptoms disappeared quickly on reduction of the dose of sulphonal. The pulse was generally regular and powerful. Neither respiration nor the uro-genital system was injuriously affected. Disturbances of the digestive tract were, however, observed twice, with an exanthem. Tolerance of the drug was never observed, so that, unlike morphine, it can be discontinued at any time.—*Medical Press*, 1891, No. 2730.

Oxygen as a Distinct Remedy for Disease, and a Life-saving Agent in Extreme Cases.

On this subject, Dr. A. W. Catlin contributes an article, and cites cases where oxygen has been used with advantage. Primarily, and for a long time exclusively, this agent has been recommended in lung difficulties—more especially to relieve the dyspnœa and cyanotic conditions following in the train of a pneumonia, where a large amount of lung-structure is involved: another way of stating the fact that its use was deferrred until the disease was far advanced, the strength exhausted, and the recuperative powers in abeyance—in other words, a *dernier ressort*, as a palliative, but not as a curative.

Fortunately, however, for our patients, another view is now taken of this life-saving agent, and to-day we recognize the fact that if we can, with a limited lung-capacity in acute disease, pass more or less continuously the same quantum of oxygen into the blood that is normally required when no disease is present, we practically lift our patient to the plane of health, so far as functional activity is concerned, and give him a hundred-fold more strength to battle with than before.

Dr. Catlin desires to show that oxygen is the most sure and satisfactory stimulant we have; that by being exhibited through the lungs, and not by the stomach, its entrance into the circulation is much more certain and immediate; that its effect, felt primarily upon the heart, is almost as quickly seen at the nerve centres and in the digestive organs; that it is preëminently the remedy for profound shock, either from hemorrhage or nervous drain, where vitality is at too low an ebb to take up the intricate history of assimilation and repair.

To get the best results the remedy must be administered at first freely and continuously, especially in those cases of profound shock where the depleted centres of life must have this true stimulation offered unremittingly. The only indications for a suspension of its use is a condition at once recognized by the patient, viz., super-exhilaration and dizziness, and this limitation is rarely reached in these extreme cases where the inhalations are not as deep or prolonged as they are when the strength returns and the demand for the stimulant naturally begins to limit itself. In other words, the patient, once instructed in its use and conscious of its helpfulness, is the best guide in its administration, and can be safely allowed to breathe it *ad libitum*. The fear is they will not get enough, not that they will get too much. This, of course, implies that the pure gas mixed with nitrogen, two parts of the former to one of the latter, is being used.

There are many conditions under which oxygen can be exhibited, always with relief, even if the nature of the case is necessarily fatal. It is no small thing to say that it relieves needless suffering.

The objection so often raised to it as a cumbersome remedy, not easily obtained on short notice, no longer holds, for depots are established all over our large cities.—*Medical Record*, 1891, No. 1086.

DIURETIN.

Von Schröder found that both caffeine and theobromine had a marked diuretic action, and that caffeine had also an undesirable influence upon the brain and vasomotor centres. The fact that theobromine acted only upon the kidneys induced CHR. GRAM (*Therapeutische Monatshefte*, 1890, No. 1) to make clinical trials of its diuretic action. It was, however, soon found to have disadvantages; since it is only slightly soluble, it sometimes caused vomiting. After many attempts, Gram succeeded in finding a compound of theobromine which had not these disadvantages; this was a combination of a sodium salt of theobromine with salicylate of sodium, to which was given the name diuretin. This substance is soluble in water. The dose is fifteen grains, and this amount may be given six times a day. The diuresis after two or three days is marked, and it continues for a time after the withdrawal of the drug. If albumin is present, its amount is unchanged by the drug.

It will act as a diuretic in some cases where digitalis, caffeine, and strophanthus have failed. It has no cumulative action; the system is not readily rendered unresponsive to its action. It may be given with cardiac tonics.

The conclusions of DR. GEISLER are that diuretin unquestionably increases the blood-pressure, as he has found no exception to this in all of the few cases included in his observations, and he feels bound to include the drug among the cardiac stimulants, as well as among diuretics.

In patients with valvular disease its action was most satisfactory; less so in affections of the heart's muscle. In the latter cases its action was that of a diuretic chiefly.

In acute nephritis its action was much greater than in chronic nephritis, as shown by the increase in the urine and the rapid disappearance of the œdema.

In one case of cirrhosis of the liver it caused no diuresis; in a healthy person it increased somewhat the twenty-four hours' urine.

It is probable that the salicylate of sodium also contributes to the diuretic action, and that this is not the result of the theobromine alone.—*Berliner klinische Wochenschrift*, 1891, Nos. 16 and 17.

DR. AUG. HOFFMANN has found diuretin an energetic diuretic, especially in cardiac dropsy; it reaches its maximum effect on the second to the sixth day. As regards its action upon the heart he is not in accord with Schröder or Gram, since he finds the heart's action is made more regular and stronger by it; as a substitute for digitalis it will not answer, though it may well be given with it.

As a substitute for caffeine, as a diuretic, it will be found serviceable.

It is best given in solution, since it will not keep in the form of powder when exposed to the air for some time.

The carbonic acid of the air decomposes diuretin into insoluble theobromine. Fifteen grains in a tablespoonful of water, or—

> R.—Diuretin . . . . ℥jss.
> Aq. menthæ pip. . . . . . . ℥iij.
> Syr. simpl. . . . . ℥j.
> Sig.—One tablespoonful five or six times a day.

All acid solutions and fruit syrups are to be avoided in prescriptions containing diuretin. In all cases it is best to have the solutions freshly made, as they decompose after a few days.—*Therapeutische Monatshefte*, 1891, No. 5.

DEATH AFTER SALOL.

Salol is usually considered a tolerably innocuous drug, but there are not wanting clinical observations which tend to show that, under certain circumstances at least, its use may be followed by dire results. Thus a case was some time ago reported by Aufrecht and Behm, in which death followed its use in acute endocarditis, and more recently DR. CHLAPOWSKI has published in a Bohemian medical journal an account of a case in which a similar fatal result followed a fifteen-grain dose ordered to a patient who was suffering from severe gastric symptoms, and who was being examined by Ewald's method. After taking the salol the patient became restless and unconscious, the pupils dilated, the pulse became irregular, there was constant vomiting, and the urine became dark and contained salicylic acid. Death occurred twelve days later. At the autopsy there were found gastritis and hemorrhagic enteritis, a gastric ulcer cicatrized at the cardiac end, chronic endometritis, and a cyst of the ovary. No doubt was entertained that the salol had caused the symptoms of poisoning.—*Lancet*, May 23, 1891.

[In such cases the early use of the soluble phosphates, such as Glauber's salt, should not be omitted.—ED.]

HYPODERMIC INJECTIONS OF CARBOLIC ACID IN ACUTE ARTICULAR RHEUMATISM.

In 1875 Senator published a paper in which he pointed out that marked alleviation of the local and some amelioration of the general symptoms quickly followed the hypodermic injection of a strong solution of carbolic acid into the neighborhood of the affected joints. This was accomplished without any appreciable ill effects to the patient.

DR. A. L. GILLESPIE has tried this treatment in about twenty-four cases, and publishes notes of five of them.

He injected from four to ten minims of a 10 (?) per cent. solution of carbolic acid. [As carbolic acid is not sufficiently soluble in water to make a

10 per cent. solution, some other solvent must have been added to the water. —Ed.]

A grain of the pure acid may be given at a dose.

In some cases the relief is speedily afforded, and the patients often begged for a repetition of the injection when another joint became painful.

It is said to be of special value in cases of gonorrhœal rheumatism in which no relief has followed the use of salicylates, but does not seem to act so well when many of the joints are affected.

It is best to pass the point of the hypodermic needle through the skin obliquely, and judging where the synovial membrane is, to inject the fluid as close outside the sac as possible.

Injected into the sac itself a 10 per cent. solution of carbolic acid precipitates the albumin present in the serous contents.

The *rationale* of the rapid disappearance of all the symptoms is, first, that it is due to the powerful local anæsthetic action of the acid ; secondly, to some slight specific action against the rheumatic poison exerted by it.— *Medical Press*, 1891, No. 2719.

MEDICINE.

UNDER THE CHARGE OF

W. PASTEUR, M.D. Lond., M.R.C.P.,

ASSISTANT PHYSICIAN TO THE MIDDLESEX HOSPITAL ; PHYSICIAN TO THE NORTHWESTERN HOSPITAL
FOR CHILDREN ;

AND

SOLOMON SOLIS-COHEN, A.M., M.D.,

PROFESSOR OF CLINICAL MEDICINE AND APPLIED THERAPEUTICS IN THE PHILADELPHIA POLYCLINIC ;
PHYSICIAN TO THE PHILADELPHIA HOSPITAL.

MALARIA ON THE GOLD COAST.

Dr. W. T. Prout, in *The Practitioner*, No. 291, 1891, states that the varieties of malaria met with on the Gold Coast of Africa are the same as elsewhere, but there is a tendency toward irregularity and severity in type, especially among Europeans. Well-marked quotidian, tertian, and quartan ague is rare, and met with among natives or in Europeans who have been long resident on the Coast, in whom the type approximates more closely to that observed in the native. In such cases the attack is essentially mild, of sudden onset, with shivering or chilliness, rapid rise of temperature to 104° or 105°, with headache, lumbar pain, etc., followed by a copious sweat and return to health on the next day. In natives, constipation and hepatic torpor are frequently associated, and the attack can be cured by a dose of blue pill. In newly arrived Europeans the attack is usually more severe, and comes under the head of bilious remittent. The cold stage is usually not observed, nausea is invariably present, and frequently vomiting forms a dangerous symptom.

Besides splenic enlargement and tenderness, there is tenderness over the pyloric end of the stomach, and at times along the hepatic margin of the ribs. The stools are dark bottle-green in color and offensive. The attack lasts four to six days, leaving the patient in a very exhausted and anæmic state, from which he slowly recovers.

The third type is the hæmoglobinuric form, which is fortunately the rarest, as it is the most severe and the most dangerous (*Lancet*, 1891, No. 3544). It rarely occurs in Europeans who are in robust health, but in those who have become debilitated and anæmic from repeated attacks of fever, or from mental worry or alcoholic or other excess. Dr. Prout inclined to associate it more particularly with any cause which interferes with the action of the liver, as he has seen it occur several times in beer-drinkers. The onset is sudden, accompanied, it may be, with slight shivering. Vomiting commences early, and is a prominent and intractable symptom throughout. At first it consists of bile, and latterly merely of the liquids imbibed, mixed with dark-green, shreddy particles. The tongue and breath are foul, and there is great thirst The skin, conjunctivæ, and buccal mucous membranes are of a bright canary-yellow color. The temperature need not necessarily rise very high, and may even fall to normal, though the other symptoms persist. If after this there is a constantly rising temperature without remissions, the prognosis is unfavorable. The state of the urine early attracts the patient's attention. In the worst cases it is of a dark porter-like color, is almost syrupy in consistence, froths easily, and stains the sides of the vessel containing it a bright crimson. At this stage boiling and nitric acid show the presence of considerable quantity of albumin. A copious deposit forms on standing, which is seen to consist of pigment granules and pigment casts from the kidneys. A few blood-cells may be present, but they are not common. The quantity of urine is generally diminished. Recovery may take place, and in this case the general symptoms improve, the urine gradually becomes less high colored, increases in quantity, and becomes loaded with urates. Convalescence is naturally slow, and departure from the Coast is indicated. On the other hand, the symptoms may become aggravated; the urine diminishes in quantity, although the color generally improves, and total suppression may take place. Death in these cases results in from three to five days from uræmia and exhaustion.

The blood was examined in ten cases, partly native, partly European. They include two cases of bilious remittent, one of hæmoglobinuria, the rest being of the mild remittent type.

In eight cases distinct changes were observed in the red corpuscles. These were of five kinds:

1. Brightly refracting, rod-like bodies occurred in three cases, and in one of them were very numerous. They varied considerably in number and size, and appeared to possess a certain power of movement, which was possessed also by the other intra-corpuscular forms, which was rather pulsatile than an an amœboid movement, although occasionally a slow alteration of their position in the corpuscle took place.

2. Brightly refracting round spots of various sizes, sometimes combined with the rods in the same corpuscle.

3. Large circular bodies, like vacuoles, lying in the centre or at the side of the corpuscle. Rods may also be seen along with these.

4. Irregular bodies, which may be regarded as transition stages between the above forms.

5. In three cases there were peculiar bodies, which were more like a tadpole or spermatözoön than anything else—possessing, as they did, an oval head with a tapering filament attached to it.

All these forms were characterized by an absence of pigment, which does not agree with other observations. It is possible, however, that the examination of a larger number of cases may result in the discovery of intra-corpuscular pigmented bodies, such as Osler describes.

Pigmented bodies were noticed in five cases :

1. Small corpuscles, about the size of a leucocyte, containing dark-brown pigment granules, distributed evenly throughout the cell.

2. Bodies two or three times the size of a leucocyte, containing similar granules of pigment, but arranged around clear spaces.

3. Pigmented bodies, showing amœboid movement.

4. Amœboid bodies containing large masses of black pigment. These bodies differ from those just described in the character of the pigment, which is in masses instead of fine granules; they are probably the phagocytes on whose scavenging properties Carter lays so much stress. It is possible, however, that all these forms are merely different stages of the same body. The pigmented crescents or spheres described by Laveran were not met with.

With reference to the time of occurrence of these bodies, it may be observed generally that the intra-corpuscular forms were present before the paroxysm and while the temperature was rising, and usually disappeared under treatment; while the pigmented bodies were found at all stages, but persisted for a considerable time after the attack had ceased. In one case the whole of the bodies were found; in one rods, clear spots, and pigmented bodies; in one rods, vacuoles, and pigmented bodies; in two vacuoles and tadpole bodies ; in three vacuoles only ; and in two pigmented bodies only. The effect of quinine in the cases in which examinations were made appeared to be the disappearance of the intra-corpuscular bodies. These observations, then, are of value as corroborating, to some extent at least, the results obtained elsewhere.

As regards the efficacy of quinine in the treatment of malaria, the author considers it the only drug which can be relied upon. Considerable stress is also laid on the influence of the state of the liver on the action of quinine. Thus: "It has been pointed out that quinine forms a salt with the bile which is sparingly soluble, and in practice it is frequently found that it is useless to administer quinine, and, in fact, that it has a distinctly prejudicial action, until the liver has been acted upon by a large dose of calomel or blue pill, which may even have to be repeated before satisfactory results are obtained. I have before me the records of several cases where a cholagogue had to be administered twice or thrice before there was any improvement in the condition. We must remember that we have to deal not only with the malarial organism, but with the results of blood-destruction which themselves are sufficient to cause a rise of temperature, as seen in cases of paroxysmal hæmoglobinuria at home, and in the febrile attacks of pernicious anæmia. The liver, which appears to be the main element in the removal of these morbid products, eventually becomes loaded with them,

538 PROGRESS OF MEDICAL SCIENCE.

which is seen on examination in the altered condition of the liver-cells. These are found to be filled with a fine yellow pigment, which is quite different from the melanæmic pigment, and which has quite different microchemical reactions, blacking with ammonium sulphides, and giving the Prussian-blue reaction on the addition of potassium ferrocyanide and dilute hydrochloric acid. It is evident, therefore, that until we assist the liver in getting rid of these morbid products other treatment will have little effect. Quinine can only be regarded as a poison to the malarial organism, killing it and preventing its further development. There are, no doubt, certain cases in which quinine entirely fails; but they are rare, and I believe are not pure cases of malarial fever, but probably associated with some obscure complication often connected with the state of the intestines."

Quinine in small doses taken over prolonged periods is recommended as a prophylactic. The treatment of the cachectic condition found in tropical climates is another matter. The condition more nearly approaches that of pernicious anæmia, and the most useful drug is arsenic in large doses, or, better than any medicine, removal to a cooler climate. Antipyrine and sulphonal have also been found useful adjuncts.

An Epidemic of Gastro-intestinal Catarrh.

Dr. G. M. Lowe, of Lincoln, refers to an epidemic of this complaint which occurred at the conclusion of the severe frost experienced last winter. According to observations in his own practice the affection occurred only among adults, the symptoms being epigastric pain, vomiting, frequent copious feculent discharges of a successively whitish-green and yellow color; sometimes considerable tenesmus, a dull yellowish color of conjunctivæ; the tongue furred, moist, and viscid; temperature seldom above 102°; anorexia, and great nervous prostration. In no instance any mucous, bloody, or typhoid stools. Complications were: jaundice in 3 cases, severe labial herpes in 7 cases, and bronchitis in 2 elderly persons, who both died; 132 recovered.

Two possible causes are discussed, viz., rapid and great alterations of temperature and pollution of drinking-water, the writer inclining, on the whole, to the former view.

[At the same time cases of an altogether similar type were very prevalent in London.—Ed.]

Influence of Carbohydrates upon Proteid Metabolism.

To determine if the loss of flesh which occurs in cases of diabetes is due to a failure of carbohydrate-metabolism, Graham Lusk, Ph.B. (*Zeitschr. f. Biologie*, Bd. xxvii. p. 459), has endeavored to ascertain if a person in normal health, from the diet of whom the carbohydrates were withdrawn, would present the increase in proteid and fatty metabolism that takes place in diabetic patients. With this end in view, he partook, for three days, of a known amount of albuminoids, fats and carbohydrates; and, for another three days, of the same quantity of albuminoids and fat as in the first experiment, but omitting the carbohydrates; in each instance determining the amount of nitrogen excreted in the urine and feces. As a result, he found that, under the latter conditions, the amount of nitrogen eliminated was 36 per cent.

greater than under the former. Repeating the experiments, using in both, however, less than half the amount of nitrogen used in the first series, he found that the amount of nitrogen eliminated was greater than that ingested, the amount eliminated being increased 32 per cent. when carbohydrates were withheld. The inference is that the omission of carbohydrates from the food brings about a marked increase in proteid metabolism, and, conversely, that the destruction of carbohydrates tends to protect a certain amount of albuminoid matter. The excessive elimination of nitrogen, shown to take place in cases of diabetes, may be explained by the excretion of sugar in the urine, and it is highly probable that the failure of sugar-decomposition in the system is the cause of the loss of flesh. That the amounts of oxygen consumed and carbonic acid given off by diabetics and healthy persons, under conditions otherwise similar, are respectively alike, is indicated by the fact that the number of heat units produced to the cubic metre of body surface is the same in both. The oxygen used in health to burn sugar is in the case of diabetes used in the destruction of fat, of which destruction there is said to be a relative increase.

POTASSIUM CANTHARIDATE IN LUPUS.

SAALFELD (*Deutsche med. Wochenschr.*, March 12, 1891) presented a case of lupus, in which, after five injections of potassium cantharidate, the masses were reduced in size and paler than before.

LANDGRAF did not find the course of acute affections of the larynx shortened by the use of the remedy. From the results of its application in five cases of chronic disease, he concluded that its use, even in small doses, gave rise to an inflammatory œdema of the laryngeal mucous membrane, which disappeared rapidly.

LUBLINSKI had treated sixteen cases of pulmonary and laryngeal tuberculosis of moderate severity, with a varying number of injections. The application of the remedy is painful in most cases, and more painful from the use of the potassium than of the sodium salt. In two cases, strangury occurred after the second injection; in one, after the third. Neither albumin nor blood was found in the urine. In one case the sputum became bloodstreaked for the first time after the third injection; in another after the fourth. Some patients felt a sense of warmth in the throat. The majority stated that the cough was looser and the expectoration freer. After the second, third, or fourth injection, the seat of the disease in the larynx appeared hyperæmic and covered with thin secretion. In one case there was dysphagia. The infiltration, especially of the inter-arytenoid fold, receded in most cases, and the voice improved. In one case, an inter-arytenoid ulcer, and in another, after seven injections, ulceration of the right vocal band healed; in a third case, after two injections, an ulcer at the free margin of the left band became progressively smaller; in a fourth, an arytenoid ulcer had almost entirely disappeared, after four injections had been made. In a case presenting, in addition to pulmonary and laryngeal tuberculosis, lupus of the dorsum of one hand, it was stated that the pains of the latter had disappeared after the fourth injection.

CANTHARIDIN.

Conceiving that the transudation of serum from a healthy capillary caused by cantharidin would be greater from a vessel in an abnormal condition, LIEBREICH (*Deutsche med. Wochenschr.*, March 5, 1891) endeavored to determine the dose which would cause from capillaries of lowered resistance the same degree of exudation as occurs from normal vessels after larger doses. The results he reported at a meeting of the Berlin Medical Society. If the hypothesis is correct, some influence would be exerted upon pathological processes resulting from local irritation, of bacillary or other nature. One-fiftieth of a milligramme of potassium cantharidate was injected into the back of a patient with a tumor of the œsophagus. Expectoration became easy and was increased as the dose was increased. It was determined that 0.0006 was the most that could be given without causing local phenomena, while there was strangury and the urine contained blood. The most suitable dose was 0.0001 or 0.0002. In cases of laryngeal tuberculosis, marked improvement in the voice was perceptible after the second injection. The patients may continue their occupations. The injections are made on alternate days. The bladder and the rectum must be looked after. Diarrhœa or burning micturition indicate a withdrawal of the injections. The remedy is prepared by dissolving 0.2 gramme of pure cantharidin and 0.4 gramme of potassic hydrate in 20 c.cm. of water, and heating in a water-bath until a clear solution results. If sufficient water is added to make a litre, every cubic centimeter contains 0.0002.

HEYMAN reported that he had observed striking improvement in the voice and in the general condition in severe cases of laryngeal tuberculosis, usually after the third or fourth injection, given daily. No influence upon the number and appearance of the bacilli was observed. In three cases the râles had diminished or disappeared. In one case the area of dulness had diminished, expectoration became easier and less frequent, the sputum thinner, and the cough moderated in frequency and intensity—in four cases it almost entirely disappeared. Night-sweats occurred less frequently or ceased. Redness and infiltration of the larynx diminished. The granulations became pale and flat; the ulcers cleared up and became smaller from the periphery. A number of well-defined ulcers had healed; others were in process of cicatrization. In some of the worst cases acute exacerbations occurred. Rapid improvement was also observed in a number of cases of catarrhal affections.

B. FRÄNKEL has treated fifteen cases, mostly severe. He found the injection painful, though submitted to by the patient, the pain disappearing in a day or two. The usual symptoms following the internal administration of cantharidin were observed—strangury and tenesmus. The general condition improved, the voice returned, infiltration receded, and ulcers cleared up and healed.

A METHOD OF ACCELERATING DESQUAMATION AND THEREFORE OF SHORTENING THE INFECTIVE PERIOD IN SCARLATINA.

DR. W. ALLAN JAMIESON, of Edinburgh, advocates the use of resorcin on account of its well-known action of causing the outer layers of the epidermis to separate without injury to the deeper ones. A 3 per cent. resorcin-salicylic-superfatted soap was employed, and when used, with warm water, from the commencement to the close of desquamation a notable diminution in the period of "peeling" was observed.

From the consideration of a large number of unselected cases the conclusion has been arrived at that, while the commencement of desquamation may be as early as the fourth day of the disease, or may, in exceptional instances, be delayed as late even as the sixteenth, the average day on which it is first visible is the ninth. Again, from the onset of the disease till the completion of desquamation in sixty-two unselected cases the average was 55.5 days, no treatment having been employed to interfere with the natural process. But when washing with the resorcin-salicylic soap was begun as soon as signs of desquamation could be noticed, or shortly before, the desquamation was entirely completed in 40.26 days. There is thus a gain, on the average, of more than a fortnight. In two cases washing with the soap was practised on only one side of the body, a commencement being made in one three, in the other four, days prior to the appearance of any trace of scaling. In the case in which the right side was washed, peeling began on the right palm, and then subsequently on the right side of the trunk and limbs; in that in which the left side was so treated, the left palm, then the left side of the trunk and limbs, showed the earliest indications of desquamation. In all cases it was found advantageous, after washing with the soap and drying the body, to smear on a small quantity of some bland oil, such as olive, almond, or purified whale oil. The nurses, too, found it necessary to protect their hands with India-rubber gloves, or to use a sponge carefully in washing the patients, else their palms became tender from a thinning of the epidermis. Such of the patients, also, who were old enough or far enough advanced in convalescence to wash themselves, noticed that the hand used in washing desquamated earlier than the other.—*Lancet*, 1891, No. 3550.

Convulsions as a Cause of Cerebral Hemorrhage in Early Life.

DR. HENRY ASHBY, of Manchester, reports a case which, in his opinion, strongly supports the view that a series of convulsions may give rise to a multiple hemorrhage.

A boy, aged twelve years, was admitted to hospital suffering from tuberculosis and old hemiplegia. He was well and strong until two years old, and free from hereditary taint. At this time he had a fit, followed by unconsciousness for ten minutes, attributed to eating pie-crust. Two weeks later he had another more severe fit, lasting half an hour, affecting especially the right arm and leg. After this the right arm hung useless, and he dragged the right leg in walking. Both limbs have recovered to some extent, but have remained more or less stiff and rigid. From this time until ten years of age he had two fits a week on an average. There was no evidence of mental weakness. He died of tuberculosis in February, 1891. The brain was examined on the following day. The outer surface was normal everywhere.

A section made exposing the lateral ventricles, without slicing the corpus striatum, showed an old cyst with brownish contents, $\frac{5}{8}$ inch in length, situated on the left side in the white substance between the fissure of Rolando and the corpus striatum; and four small cysts, situated on the right side in the white substance. One cyst was apparently about $\frac{1}{2}$ inch in depth. There was no sclerosis or induration in the neighborhood of the cysts. A third section, made lower than the above and on a level with the upper surface of the cerebellum, and slicing the optic thalamus, caudate nucleus, and internal capsule, showed the lower limit of the cyst just described, a second old blood-cyst, and another small one. Another similar cyst was found in the white substance of the frontal region at a lower level.

Sections of the cord made in the cervical, dorsal, and lumbar regions did not show any sclerosis or wasting of the descending tracts, neither was there any wasting of the internal capsule or crura.

In reviewing the history of the case in the light of the morbid anatomy, there seems to be little room for doubt that the initial convulsions were the cause and not the consequence of the multiple hemorrhages. It is hardly conceivable that these should be caused by any thrombosis, embolism, or arteritis; they must presumably have been due to a sudden engorgement of the veins due to asphyxia, in consequence of spasm of the respiratory muscles.

Cases of this kind are by no means uncommon, and the view put forward in this communication has been expressed by several recent writers, among others by Goodhart, Osler, and Angell Money.—*Practitioner*, 1891, No. 276.

THE INFLUENCE OF DISEASES UPON THE RESPIRATORY INTERCHANGE
OF GASES.

To determine if disturbances involving the exchange of gases between the air and the blood, and if anomalies of tissue metamorphosis in conjunction with which the need of oxygen or the capability of the tissues to unite with oxygen may be altered, do in reality materially influence the respiratory interchange of gases, KRAUS and CHVOSTEK (*Wiener klin. Wochenschr.*, Bd. iv. 1891, p. 33) made forty observations in twelve persons with various forms of anæmia (pernicious and secondary anæmia and chlorosis), leukæmia, and the carcinomatous cachexia. Under ordinary conditions no aberration from the normal was observed in the gaseous interchange. The taking of nourishment invariably augmented the interchange, as happens also in healthy persons during digestion. In a small number of cases muscular activity increased the combustion of oxygen and the production of carbonic acid, but not in the same degree as in health; in the anæmic patients, the respiratory coefficient (which normally arises) was lowered.

To determine the activity of the bodily oxidation, benzole was administered to six patients with diabetes, anæmia, carcinoma of the stomach, and leukæmia, and the quantity of phenol excreted was measured. The proportion of phenol was found small in conditions of impaired nutrition, but no special change was observed for any single affection.

In investigating the influence exerted upon the respiratory process by an increased volume of oxygen in the inspired air, an admixture of ten volumes of nitrogen and ninety volumes of oxygen was used. The subjective condition of healthy and ill persons was not materially influenced by the continuous breathing of such a mixture; nor did objective manifestations appear. During the first ten minutes of easy breathing a considerable increase in the comparative quantity of oxygen absorbed was noted; subsequently the absorption of oxygen fell to the normal or lower. That this primary increase took place in anæmic patients with a decided deficiency of hæmoglobin makes it evident that the excess of oxygen taken up combines with the tissues. For a short time at the beginning of the experiment the exhalation of carbonic acid was increased, though not in the same degree as the absorption of oxygen. These observations indicate that there is no more substantial basis for the employment of oxygen in disease than has hitherto existed. Clinically, inhalations of oxygen were inefficacious. The most important indication for such a measure would be the sudden occurrence of respiratory insufficiency.

SURGERY.

UNDER THE CHARGE OF

J. WILLIAM WHITE, M.D.,

PROFESSOR OF CLINICAL SURGERY IN THE UNIVERSITY OF PENNSYLVANIA; SURGEON TO THE
UNIVERSITY AND GERMAN HOSPITALS;

ASSISTED BY

EDWARD MARTIN, M.D.,

CLINICAL PROFESSOR OF GENITO-URINARY SURGERY IN THE UNIVERSITY OF PENNSYLVANIA; SURGEON
TO THE HOWARD HOSPITAL AND ASSISTANT SURGEON TO THE UNIVERSITY HOSPITAL.

SURGICAL TREATMENT OF PILES.

On the basis of 200 cases of operation on hemorrhoids, ALLINGHAM (*Medical Press and Circular*, 1891, No. 2724) discusses the surgical treatment of this disease.

He divides hemorrhoids into two groups: the first including those which come down at stool, and those which are almost always in a state of prolapse and bleed profusely at each act of the bowel. In this class of cases the quickest operation is the best, since as a result of long-continued hemorrhage there is always considerable anæmia, and therefore it is of prime importance that as little blood as possible should be lost from the operation, and that there should be a minimum of risk of secondary hemorrhage. These requirements are fulfilled by the ligature, which can be applied in a very few minutes and is practically free from any danger of after-hemorrhage.

The second group comprises those piles which are chiefly troublesome because of the inconvenience they occasion, since they are prone to come down and prevent the patient taking any active exercise. These piles rarely bleed and do not otherwise interfere with the enjoyment of good health. Here the great point is to select the least painful operation. The best modes are crushing or simply cutting off the piles and picking up any vessels that may bleed.

In the operation of ligation with incision the pile is drawn down by a vulsellum and separated from the muscular and submucous tissues upon which it rests. The incision is made upon the skin at the junction of the

mucous membrane, and is carried up the bowel, so that the pile is left connected by vessels and mucous membrane only. A strong silk ligature is
then tied as tightly as possible, and the ligatured pile is returned within the
sphincter.

This method is very well suited to piles which are large and vascular and
are inclined to be sessile rather than pedunculated. It should be applied to
patients who have any tendency to cardiac or kidney disease, or where there
is a thrombosed condition of the vessels. It is the best to use when patients
are feeble. Ligature is, in fact, the safest operation. Its drawbacks are that
the wound takes some time to heal, there is more pain after operation and
on the first motion of the bowels, than after crushing or simple excision.
There is more sloughing and suppuration until the ligatures have separated,
and hence there is greater liability to some contraction.

The crushing operation consists in drawing the pile by means of a hook into
a powerful screw-crusher, which is tightly screwed up, and distal end of pile
cut off. The crusher should be applied on the longitudinal aspect of the
bowel and should be left on the pile for about two minutes. This operation
should be used when the piles are medium-sized and rather pedunculated,
and the patients are in good health; but in bad cases it is not so safe as the
ligature. In ordinary eases its advantages are that there is freedom from
pain after operation; retention of urine is of rare occurrence; suppuration is
not likely; there is little or no pain on the first action of the bowels, and
recovery is usually rapid; after-contraction is not common. The clamp and
cautery are not favored by Allingham. He states that statistics show that it is
quite six times as fatal as ligature or crushing; and burning gives more pain
after operation, as is the case with all burns. Hemorrhage is more likely to
occur, there is greater sloughing of the rectal tissue. More time is required for
healing and greater contraction is common, as is also the case with all burns.
The excision of piles is best applied to one prolapsed pile, to the single
perineal pile, so common in women, or to one pile which is complicated with
fistula, ulcer, fissure, etc. As a rule, one or two vessels require clipping. It
is, therefore, inexpedient to excise many piles, for there may be trouble in
picking up the divided arteries.

Allingham believes that Whitehead's excision method—that is, removal of
the entire pile area and stitching of the healthy bowel above to the sphincter
—is rarely necessary. It is a slow and bloody operation, and is at times followed by contraction. Few cases are really well under three weeks after
operation, and premature resumption of the ordinary ways of life may cause
a greater tendency to contraction, or, what is worse, troublesome and tedious
ulceration may supervene and take months to heal.

———

FIXATION IN THE TRACTION TREATMENT OF HIP DISEASE.

Attention is called by LOVETT (*New York Medical Journal*, vol. liv., No. 6)
to the important place which fixation should occupy in the traction treatment
of hip-joint disease. The ordinary traction splint now commonly used is a
device which gives passive motion without friction. Fixation was not considered one of its attributes. The author has many times shown that this
splint allows of very wide motion in mild cases of hip disease. Where joint

motion is not painful in a fairly wide arc, motion within the limits of that arc is not wholly harmful. In cases where the disease is severe, and where the patient is constantly and harmfully active, the ordinary traction splint is not followed by good results. With the idea of combining traction and fixation, Lovett has devised a splint which should be bent to fit the curve of the back; practically it is a combination of the Taylor and Thomas splints, and has the hip-band of the Taylor splint with two perineal bands, and the leg-piece is in a measure like the Thomas splint, excepting that it is-prolonged beyond the foot to end in a traction apparatus. The splint does not attempt to force the leg into position by using the lever principle; it simply aims to make a traction, and while doing this it fixes the hip as much as can be done by any portative appliance. By means of the pelvic band this splint firmly holds the leg, pelvis, and thorax.

The author uses this appliance where sensitiveness of the hip is present to any extent, where the temperature is high, or where there is much induration of the soft parts—in short, in all bad cases. In addition, he applies it to unruly children, and to those whose parents are ignorant or shiftless.

Fixation in bed is desirable when sensitiveness occurs in the joint or malposition in the limb begins to appear. Statistical study seems to show that fixation in bed, when malformation occurs, not only is an important means of cure of this malposition, but serves to prevent the occurrence of abscesses in a very large proportion of cases.

LAPAROTOMY FOR WOUNDS OF THE LIVER.

BROCA (*Le Mercredi Medical*, 1891, No. 29) reports two cases of wound of the liver, each treated by surgical intervention, and each terminating fatally.

The first patient was seen six hours after the infliction of the stab wound. He exhibited the symptoms of large hemorrhage. The wound was enlarged; the source of bleeding was found to be the liver; blood was flowing freely from the incision upon the anterior surface of this organ. An attempt to suture this wound proved futile, the threads tearing through. Thermo-cautery also failed to check the bleeding; an iodoform tampon was, however, entirely successful. An hour was consumed in the operation.

The patient perished two days later of abdominal septicæmia.

At the autopsy several other wounds were found, in some of which there had been bleeding after operation.

The second case was also a stab wound. The patient was seen four hours after the injury, and presented all the symptoms of intra-peritoneal hemorrhage. The abdomen was opened and a non-penetrating and penetrating wound of the stomach were found. A wound three inches long was observed on the lower surface of the liver. By means of a silk suture this wound was closed and the bleeding ceased. The patient died in a few hours with symptoms of continued hemorrhage.

At the autopsy it was found that the knife had passed completely through the liver, the wound of exit being located on the upper surface of this organ one-fifth of an inch behind the suspensory ligament. From this source sufficient blood flowed to entirely fill the pelvis.

CONTRIBUTION TO THE KNOWLEDGE OF SARCOMA.

COLEY (*Annals of Surgery*, vol. xiv., No. 3) reports a case of round-celled sarcoma of the metacarpal bone, which he treated by amputation of the forearm about four months after the observation of the first tumor. In a little more than a month there was general dissemination of the disease, and death followed six weeks after the operation.

Coley has made a careful analysis of 90 unpublished cases of sarcoma, embracing nearly all those treated in the New York hospitals for the last fifteen years. He succeeding in obtaining the subsequent histories of 44. Of these 9 were living at periods ranging from three to ten years after operation, and 4 were living free from recurrence twelve to eighteen months after operation.

The chief characteristics of subperiosteal sarcoma are: there is usually a history of traumatism ; the pain precedes the tumor and remains throughout the disease; the tumor is usually fusiform and seldom encapsulated, there being rapid infiltration of the surrounding tissue; it increases rapidly in size; the skin is discolored in the later stages ; there is a slight elevation of temperature and an abnormally rapid pulse, and that there is very little tendency to ulceration.

After citing Brune's famous paper upon the curative influence of erysipelas upon sarcoma and carcinoma, Coley reports 3 cases of sarcoma in which inoculations of pure cultures of erysipelas streptococcus were employed. These inoculations were made repeatedly and were followed by local reaction; the tumor seemed to be distinctly lessened in size. No cures are mentioned. To the 5 cases collected by Brune, Coley has added 6 others in addition to the 3 he inoculated : 6 were cured and 2 were greatly improved.

CRANIECTOMY FOR MICROCEPHALUS.

VICTOR HORSLEY (*Internat. klin. Rund.*, v. Jahrg., No. 38), after a careful review of the subject of craniectomy for microcephalus, and after a report of 2 cases, concludes that operative treatment in cases of microcephalus and synostosis is fully justifiable, since the condition is in itself absolutely hopeless, and since surgical intervention has been followed by decided improvement. There are, of course, in these cases special dangers, but these may be limited by restricting the operation both in time and extent.

THE RESULTS OF RADICAL OPERATION FOR NON-STRANGULATED HERNIA.

LUCAS CHAMPIONNIÈRE (*L'Abeille Médicale*, 48 an., No. 43) states that he has performed 254 operations for the radical cure of non-strangulated hernia, beginning this series of cases ten years ago. Of this number but two perished —one because he was in very bad condition, the other because of internal strangulation. In spite of this excellent result, in so far as life is concerned, the operation is found useless and fatal unless it is undertaken under certain definite conditions and carried out under a well-considered system.

The results of operation have been excellent. The greater number of patients have not been compelled to wear trusses or supports ; or, in less favorable cases, this has been found necessary for not longer than two months.

The indications which have been fulfilled in the radical operation are: 1. As extensive an ablation of the peritoneum as possible. 2. Removal of as much omentum as can be reached, or can be drawn into the sac. 3. Formation of a strong and extensive cicatrix in the hernia region.

Of the 254 cases 222 were inguinal, 14 were crural, 17 were umbilical, 1 was traumatic. The most satisfactory results in the operations upon inguinal hernia were obtained in cases of the congenital form of this rupture.

The results of radical cure of umbilical hernia are said to be particularly satisfactory.

The author believes that the radical cure of reducible hernia should be the rule and not the exception. In very young infants, however, he does not counsel operation, not because such cases can be cured by other means, but because the tissues are not sufficiently firm to make a reliable cicatrix. After the sixth and seventh year, however, the operation is strongly advised. In old persons operation should be avoided unless there are pressing reasons for resorting to the knife. Finally, even those of the proper age—that is, between seven and forty, should not be operated upon when the abdominal walls are weak, or there is a tendency to giving way in several regions. Congenital inguinal hernia invariably should be operated upon. This admits of no exception. The same rule applies to all hernias in young women.

[Since the operator began this series of cases ten years ago, he might furnish valuable figures in regard to the ultimate effect of hernial operation. This, unfortunately, he neglects to do.—ED.]

OPHTHALMOLOGY.

UNDER THE CHARGE OF

GEORGE A. BERRY, M.B., F.R.C.S. ED.,

OPHTHALMIC SURGEON, EDINBURGH ROYAL INFIRMARY;

AND

EDWARD JACKSON, A.M., M.D.,

PROFESSOR OF DISEASES OF THE EYE IN THE PHILADELPHIA POLYCLINIC; SURGEON TO WILLS EYE HOSPITAL, ETC.

SYMPATHETIC OPHTHALMIA NOTWITHSTANDING RESECTION OF THE OPTIC NERVE.

DR. A. TROUSSEAU reports a case of this kind in the *Revue Générale d'Ophthalmologie*, Tome x., No. 3. The exciting eye had been wounded by the blow of a stone six years before, and after remaining quiet three and a half or four years became again troublesome, and he applied to have it removed. It was shrunken, red, the seat of violent cyclitis. The other eye, except for the excessive secretion of tears from time to time, was absolutely healthy, with full acuteness of vision.

On account of the slight deformity, and the previous long period during which it had remained entirely quiet, it was judged an especially appropriate case for resection of the nerve, rather than enucleation. Accordingly, the nerve was resected, the piece removed measuring four or five millimetres in length, and the parts bathed with a sublimate solution 1 : 2000. The operation was followed by protrusion of the globe, which lasted but three or four days ; at the end of ten days the eyes were in very satisfactory condition, the sound one relieved of its attacks of lachrymation, and on the twentieth day he was discharged and the case reported as a cure in the *Bulletin des Quinze-vingts* for 1890.

Within two months after his discharge the patient returned with redness of the better eye. He was put upon mercurial inunctions, which he used regularly for three weeks, when he returned with vision reduced to counting fingers at two metres, iris inflamed, and vitreous opacities. The exciting eye was then enucleated, and after four or five days the other began to improve. When the case was reported at the end of three weeks after the enucleation, vision had risen to one-half the normal.

————

TRANSPLANTATION OF THE CORNEA.

VON HIPPEL reports in the *Berliner klin. Wochenschrift*, xxviii. Jahrg., No. 19, his seventh case subjected to this operation. The patient had a dark-brown opacity which covered the pupil, and which had been produced by repeated cauterizations of the cornea with nitrate of silver. He also had cataract. After extraction of the opaque lens, with iridectomy, he had vision equal one-fifth, but he insisted on the removal of the spot on the cornea. The corneal tissue, down to Descemet's membrane, was removed from a circle four millimetres in diameter, and replaced by the full thickness of the cornea from a young rabbit. The eye was afterward dressed with iodoform and both eyes bandaged. Although there was temporary clouding of the thin layer of original tissue behind it, the transplanted flap remained clear. In two weeks the epithelium was continuous from the cornea to the flap. After discission for a secondary cataract, the patient obtained vision equal one-third. It does not appear from the report that the transplantation caused any improvement in vision. But the operation deserves to be called successful in that it secured the continued life and health of the graft, and removed an unsightly scar.

————

MERCURY IN SYPHILITIC DISEASE OF THE EYES.

GALEZOWSKI, in the *Recueil d'Ophthalmologie*, An. xiii., No. 3, points out that mercury administered by the digestive tract acts very rapidly on iritis, either plastic or gummatous, not that a radical cure is effected, but the ocular inflammation disappears. Not so with syphilitic choroiditis, which yields to no mercurial administered by the mouth, but is cured almost without exception by mercurial inunction.

It is still otherwise with the ataxic atrophies of the optic papilla, which are without doubt usually syphilitic. Here, unfortunately, any anti-syphilitic treatment gives unsatisfactory results. This Galezowski explains on the hypothesis that the action of such medicaments is slow in the case of certain affections occurring in closed cavities, as in choroiditis and affections of the spinal cord.

While iritis can be cured in two or three months, choroiditis requires two years; and in the case of optic atrophy the disease outruns the treatment, and produces permanent injury before the cure can be effected. Probably by a course of daily mercurial inunctions, carried out for two consecutive years on the occurrence of the earlier lesions of syphilis, optic atrophy, cerebral syphilis, and such later lesions could always be prevented.

HERPES OF THE CORNEA FROM INFLUENZA TREATED WITH PYOKTANIN.

GALEZOWSKI (*Recueil d'Ophthalmologie*, An. xiii., No. 4) regards this affection as essentially one of the fifth nerve. It has been met with very frequently during the last two years in Paris, more particularly during the epidemic of influenza. The form of eye disease most commonly connected with the influenza was a phlyctenular conjunctivitis, or a superficial herpetic keratitis, with loss of epithelium, anæsthesia of the cornea, and which did not yield to the ordinary treatment for that affection. The two measures found to hasten the cure were the internal administration of large doses of quinine and the applications of apyonine or pyoktanin. The solution of pyoktanin, one part to one hundred parts of distilled water, was brushed on the cornea five or six times a day, and produced excellent and rapid improvement.

THE LIGHT-STREAK ON THE RETINAL VESSELS.

VAN TRIGT put forth the hypothesis that this streak was due to reflection from the anterior wall of the vessel or the anterior surface of the blood-column in the vessel, and this explanation was adopted by Jäger, Donders, and others. Loring ascribed it to refraction of the light passing through the blood-column and reflection from the tissues behind the vessel, and using a watery solution of carmine in a glass tube, he showed that under the conditions that exist in examining a retinal vessel the light-streak was seen when the tube was placed in front of a reflecting surface, and not seen when placed in front of a non-reflecting surface. Donders, however, claimed that the blood of warm-blooded animals was not transparent like the carmine solution, and therefore the conditions were essentially different in Loring's experiment from those the experiment was intended to elucidate. DR. A. E. DAVIS (*Archives of Ophthalmology*, vol. xx., No. 1), repeating the experiment, but using the blood flowing from the carotid of a cat, obtained precisely the results reported by Loring with the carmine solution. This seems to prove conclusively that the light-streak does depend on the refraction of the blood-column and reflection by the tissues back of the vessel.

PLATINUM INSTRUMENTS IN OPHTHALMIC SURGERY.

DR. E. GRUENING urges (*Archives of Ophthalmology*, vol. xx., No. 2) the use of such instruments on account of the ease with which they are sterilized. He has had cystotome, iris repositor, wire loop, spoon, iris and fixation forceps, and speculum made with the working parts consisting of an alloy of platinum and iridium. This alloy by hammering becomes very firm, can be polished, and is not blackened in the flame of a spirit-lamp. By heating to a white heat, such an instrument can be certainly sterilized by the operator at the time of operation, without his having to depend on the skill and care of an assistant.

ANIRIDIA AND GLAUCOMA.

E. T. COLLINS, F.R.C.S., reports in the *Ophthalmic Review*, vol. x., No. 114, three cases in which these conditions coexisted. It might be that in such cases at least glaucoma could not be due to closure of the filtration angle of the anterior chamber, and that some other explanation would have to be found for its occurrence. But in two of these cases of congenital aniridia, although no iris was visible, the ciliary body was found at the microscopical examination to end anteriorly in a rounded nodule that had become applied and adherent to the filtration space of the cornea in such a way as to block it entirely. In the third case, although the iris had been entirely torn away by traumatism and the ciliary muscle was atrophied, the most anterior of the ciliary processes was intimately adherent to the region of the cornea in question. Exceptions of this kind may truly be said to prove the rule that glaucoma is due to blocking of the filtration area by the iris.

GUMMA OF THE CONJUNCTIVA.

Gumma of the conjunctiva is of rare occurrence, and partly on that account is very apt not to be recognized. DR. CAUDRON (*Revue générale d'Ophthalmologie*, Tome x., No. 4) reports a case, and quotes a few others previously reported. In his patient, a man of forty years, giving no history, it appeared external to the cornea, the tumor measuring about ten millimetres in the horizontal, four millimetres in the vertical direction, and three millimetres in thickness. Its color was reddish-yellow, and it was surrounded by an area of vascularization. Its consistence was firm, being almost cartilaginous at the periphery. Thorough examination revealed numerous other evidences of syphilis. Placed on anti-syphilitic treatment, improvement was rapid. A complete cure was effected in two months, and there had been no subsequent manifestations. A study of the reported cases shows that the cure of such lesions is usually rapid and easy under appropriate treatment.

OBSTETRICS.

UNDER THE CHARGE OF

EDWARD P. DAVIS, A.M., M.D.,

PROFESSOR OF OBSTETRICS AND DISEASES OF CHILDREN IN THE PHILADELPHIA POLYCLINIC; CLINICAL LECTURER ON OBSTETRICS IN THE JEFFERSON MEDICAL COLLEGE; VISITING OBSTETRICIAN TO THE PHILADELPHIA HOSPITAL, ETC.

THE PATHOLOGY AND TREATMENT OF PUERPERAL ECLAMPSIA.

In connection with the interesting paper of HERMAN (page 485 of the present issue of THE JOURNAL) the recent literature of eclampsia offers much of interest.

In a discussion on the subject at the British Medical Association during the summer, GALABIN inclined to the uræmic theory of the causation of eclampsia. He quoted the statistics of Guy's Hospital, which showed an improvement in the mortality following the substitution of chloroform for bleeding. Mortality at present was reduced to 20 per cent. Moderate venesection, to relieve extreme vascular congestion, he thought advisable in some cases; bleeding to stop convulsions is inadmissible. BYERS had found the chloroform and chloral treatment, with the speedy termination of labor, most advantageous. AUVARD, of Paris, regarded eclampsia as caused by toxæmia, from failure of the emunctories. Treatment consisted in causing prompt and free elimination, in narcotizing the nervous system until the uterus can be emptied. SWAYNE had seen 36 cases of eclampsia in private consultations. In 24 bleeding was used, in 1 thirty ounces of blood were taken. The convulsions ceased, although other agents had failed. GODSON induced labor when albumin was abundant and urea deficient in the urine.

In general, the opinion was adverse to bleeding, except where marked engorgement was present; labor is to be induced when albuminuria and deficient urea are present.

PATHOLOGY OF ECLAMPSIA AND ALBUMINURIA, WITH REPORT OF A CASE.

VAN SANTVOORD (*Medical Record*, vol. xl., No. 8, 1891) describes the case of a patient whom he observed during two pregnancies, who had albuminuria and diminished excretion of urea. Symptoms of toxæmia were present during both pregnancies, and one eclamptic seizure occurred two months before labor, without apparent reflex cause. The patient bore two healthy children and recovered. The theory of toxæmia from deficient liver action, attended by diminished formation of urea, seems most rational to Van Santvoord. In the treatment of his case, nitroglycerin, digitalis, and citrate of potassium were efficient.

THE TREATMENT OF ALBUMINURIA AND NEPHRITIS IN PREGNANCY.

MIJULIEFF (*Geneesk. Cour.*, 1891, No. 18) has derived the following indications for treatment from three cases of nephritis in pregnancy in which the fœtus perished in the uterus: when a woman previously healthy shows symptoms of nephritis during the first months of pregnancy, abortion should be induced; in the second half of pregnancy it is rarely necessary to interrupt pregnancy, except for urgent symptoms. In chronic nephritis during pregnancy, labor should be induced in the interest of mother and child as soon as viability is possible.

THE TREATMENT OF ECLAMPSIA DURING PREGNANCY BY RAPID DELIVERY.

HAULTAIN (*Edinburgh Medical Journal*, 1891) treated four cases of eclampsia during pregnancy by ½ grain pilocarpine subcutaneously, with the external application of heat; croton oil; and 30 grains of chloral, followed by 10 grains every hour for four hours; milk diet; 5 minims of tincture of digitalis thrice daily, and saline purges were also continued. Haultain performed delivery as soon as possible, in the following way: after the patient has perspired freely and been purged and has taken 30 grains of chloral the previous evening, she is deeply chloroformed and the cervix is dilated by the fingers; the membranes are ruptured, and the child is delivered by forceps. From sixty-five to ninety minutes were required to dilate the cervix; the entire delivery consumed between two and three hours.

THE OPERATIVE TREATMENT OF ECLAMPSIA: CÆSAREAN OPERATION.

SWIECICKI (*Der Frauenarzt*, 1891, Heft 9) performed Cæsarean section on a patient comatose in eclampsia, in whom the os and cervix were undilated and the child lived. The child was asphyxiated at delivery, and could not be resuscitated. The mother perished of pulmonary œdema. This is the tenth Cæsarean operation for eclampsia, six having been done in Holland, one by Von Herff at Halle, one by Rosthorn, and one by Müller at Berne. The operation is only justifiable when the child lives and the genital canal is entirely undilated.

A SUCCESSFUL CÆSAREAN SECTION FOR ECLAMPSIA.

VON HERFF (*Berliner klin. Sammlung klin. Vorträge*, Heft 32) advises the induction of labor when the upper portion of the cervix is dilated, and only the vaginal portion remains closed. When no dilatation is present Cæsarean section is indicated. In a case of severe eclampsia he operated by Cæsarean section; mother and child survived.

A PARASITIC MONSTER.

NORRIS describes a parasitic monster, recently exhibited in Philadelphia, as follows:

The boy Laloo, a monster of the dipygus parasiticus variety, is nineteen years of age, and apparently enjoys good health. The parasite consists of the two upper extremities and a rudimentary pelvis with the two lower extremities closely joined together. It is attached to the boy firmly at the lower right side of the sternum near the ensiform cartilage by a bony pedicle surrounded by soft tissues and covered with integument, and hangs over the lower portion of the chest, the epigastric and right hypochondriac regions, the anterior surface of the parasite looking toward the abdomen of the boy. The skin contains venous capillaries, and is sensitive to touch, the degree of sensibility decreasing as the hands and feet are approached. The hands and feet are contorted, the feet being better developed than the hands. The fingers of the left hand are diminutive and webbed, those of the right hand are more developed, the phalanges being distinct. The glutei are separate and distinct, having between them a natal fold, in which can be found a trace of an anal aperture. The legs are flexed upon the thighs. Careful examination failed to discover respiratory murmur or cardiac pulsations. Coils of intestines could be felt. Discharge of feces from the parasite does not occur, and urination takes place without the boy's knowledge until after the urine has been voided. Perspiration and elevation of the temperature occur simultaneously with these phenomena in the boy. The sex of the parasite is undetermined, it being most probably a pseudo-hermaphrodite.

To pander to the morbid propensities of the curious, the managers of the museum have shrewdly clad the parasite in female attire. The boy, whose intelligence is quite remarkable, states that the surgeons who had examined him had generally decided that the removal of the parasite by surgical means would be directly dangerous to his life.

GYNECOLOGY.

UNDER THE CHARGE OF

HENRY C. COE, M.D., M.R.C.S.,
OF NEW YORK.

The Early Diagnosis of Cancer of the Uterus.

WINTER (*Berliner klin. Wochenschrift*, 1891, No. 33) reviews the recent results of extirpation of the cancerous uterus in Germany, showing that the total mortality of the five principal operators is only 8.4 per cent., the lowest being Kaltenbach's (3.3 per cent.). Although a certain number of fatal cases is inevitable on account of the difficulty of absolutely eliminating sepsis, other dangers ought to be avoided by improved technique, so that the mortality can be reduced to 5 per cent. The statistics of high amputation are still better, the Berlin Klinik showing a mortality of 6.5 per cent. (in 155 cases) previous to 1884, since which time no deaths have followed the operation in 64 additional cases.

Unfortunately, the remote results of both operations have not been as favorable as could be desired. A local recurrence (in the cicatrix) can usually be expected within two years at the utmost, while recurrence in the lymph-glands and pelvic connective tissue occurs later. This difference has not been clearly defined in the statistics. According to the writer's observations, after high amputation 38 per cent. of the patients were well at the end of two years, and 26.5 per cent. had no recurrence five years after operation, after which time a return of the disease is exceptional. Fritsch has noted 36 per cent. of cures after vaginal hysterectomy at the end of five years, and Hofmeier 33 per cent. at the end of four.

Only a small proportion of the patients with cancer of the uterus are suitable cases for a radical operation (about 25 per cent.), and if one-fourth of these are cured, it follows that only 7 per cent. of the entire number of cancerous patients are cured. In other words, the diagnosis of malignant disease is not made at a sufficiently early stage, and this neglect is traceable to the general practitioner. "The physician to whom the patient first applies decides her fate in the majority of the cases." Hence it is extremely important that he should be familiar with the initial symptoms. Of these a watery vaginal discharge is the most constant, especially in carcinoma of the portio. Menorrhagia, in a patient whose flow has formerly been normal should always awaken suspicion and lead to an examination. Hemorrhage after coitus is an initial symptom of great importance, and when occurring some time after the establishment of the menopause it is almost pathognomonic of malignant disease.

Pelvic pain is usually a late symptom, due to secondary parametritis; but intractable sciatica, developing after the menopause, is significant. When a patient with these symptoms applies to her physician she ought certainly to be examined, and if the portio does not present a suspicious appearance, search should be made for cancer higher up in the cervix or corpus uteri. Fragments should be removed for microscopical examination. Patients themselves are often to blame since they defer seeking professional advice until too late, because they have no severe pain, the irregular hemorrhages being attributed to the approaching change of life. It is a peculiar fact that women who have cancer are less likely to fear it than those who have not. In conclusion, the writer urges that both physicians and patients should be trained to recognize the initial symptoms of cancer of the uterus, and to have the diagnosis settled at once.

Pseudo-intraligamentous Ovarian Tumors.

Pawlik (*Centralblatt für Gynäkologie*, 1891, No. 38) reports seven cases which he thus characterizes. They are usually small ovarian tumors associated with diseased tubes, the disease being of puerperal or gonorrhœal origin. They develop posterior to the broad ligament, to which and to the mesovarium they contract firm, broad adhesions; they are also prone to adhere to the sigmoid flexure and to the bottom of Douglas's pouch. They become covered with pseudo-membranes which closely resemble peritoneum, so that they present the appearance of being actually intra-ligamentous. When the broad ligament is split for the purpose of enucleating the tumor, it will be seen that the latter lies behind the posterior fold. In removing these growths it is advisable to tie off the uterine end of the tube first, then to separate the adhesions from behind and below. By drawing the mass upward the adherent peritoneum forming Douglas's pouch will be elongated in such a way as to form a pedicle. Pressure may be advantageously exerted through the rectum by means of a colpeurynter. The writer prefers the latter method to operation in Trendelenburg's posture, since there is less danger of pus escaping among the intestines.

Localized Meteorism in Intestinal Obstruction.

Kader (Inaugural Dissertation: abstract in *Centralblatt für Gynäkologie*, 1891, No. 38) has conducted elaborate experiments on animals, his deductions being as follows: In every case of intestinal obstruction the portion of gut immediately above the point of obstruction becomes distended, but there is no marked increase in the distention in the course of twenty-four hours. When the obstruction is so complete that venous stasis is marked, serious tissue-changes occur in a few hours, which threaten the life of the subject; complete paralysis of the muscle is present and the meteorism is then strictly localized at the affected area, so that it may be readily recognized before the abdomen is opened.

Primary Cancer of the Vagina.

Hecht (Inaugural Dissertation: abstract in *Centralblatt für Gynäkologie*, 1891, No. 38) has made an exhaustive study of the literature of this subject. Among 4507 cases of cancer in females who were examined at the Vienna clinics in ten years he found only 50 cases of primary cancer of the vagina, or 1.1 per cent. It was most frequent between the ages of thirty and forty. Among the probable etiological factors were excessive childbearing and mechanical irritation, such as long-standing prolapsus and the wearing of pessaries. The disease appears under two forms—the cancroid and the diffuse scirrhous—and is usually located on the posterior wall. The initial symptoms are profuse leucorrhœa, which later becomes a foul watery discharge, and irregular hemorrhages during coitus and defecation. Later, pain and vesical symptoms appear. The portio and external genitals are involved late, if at all, but the lymph-glands are usually affected. Metastases are rare; among the whole number of cases analyzed there were only two of general carcinosis. Death is due to exhaustion. It is sometimes difficult to distinguish primary cancer of the vagina from disease originating in the portio; condyloma, sloughing fibrous polypus and sarcoma are distinguishable microscopically. The only treatment is radical removal with knife, scissors, or sharp spoon, followed by thorough cauterization. Cæsarean section has been performed on account of obstruction due to cancer of the vagina, but with bad results, only two patients having been saved out of twelve.

The Diagnosis of Non-Puerperal Abscess of the Ovary.

Rheinstein (*Archiv für Gynäkologie*, Band xxxix., Heft 2) thinks that acute inflammation of the ovary is rarely observed outside of the puerperal state. The follicular form described by Slavjansky, which occurs in acute exanthemata, possesses rather an anatomical than a clinical interest. The interstitial form is very seldom encountered, except in the puerpera, when it is practically impossible to distinguish it from localized peritonitis.

Olshausen admits that a probable diagnosis can be made only when the enlarged ovary can be felt and the pain localized in it. The writer believes that it is only possible when the gradual enlargement of the affected gland has been traced from the outset by the finger of the observer, all other inflammatory conditions in the same region having been excluded. It is doubtful if a positive diagnosis can ever be made before the abdomen is opened.

The following illustrative case is cited: An unmarried woman, æt. twenty-three years, had aborted in June, 1888, and recovered without sequelæ. In November, 1889, she was sick with acute rheumatism for a month and had leucorrhœa, but no other local trouble. In February of the same year she had a chill and fever at the beginning of a menstrual period, accompanied with pain in the left side. The fever persisted, and the pain became so severe that she was often unable to go about. When admitted to the hospital she had an evening temperature of 101.6°; her abdomen was tense but not sensitive on pressure, with the exception of slight tenderness in the left iliac region. To the left of the uterus could be felt an intra-pelvic tumor, as large as an apple, perfectly movable, its consistence being generally hard, but with soft spots. The diagnosis of suppurative disease of the right adnexa was made, laparotomy was performed, and a pus sac was found so firmly adherent to the intestines that a considerable portion of it was left behind. The patient made a good recovery. On microscopical examination of the specimen remains of ovarian stroma were found, but no traces of ovisacs. This fact, together with the location of the abscess behind the broad ligament, indicated its origin.

The history of the case seemed to point to pyosalpinx, but the latter condition does not, as a rule, develop so rapidly; moreover, the tumor was unilateral, which is seldom the case with pyosalpinx. On vaginal examination the mass was felt to be circumscribed, and could not be traced outward from the cornu uteri. The pain and fluctuation in the mass were not characteristic. As regards the etiology, it might be referred to gonorrhœal infection, the virus having perhaps entered a ruptured ovisac during or just after menstruation and caused an abscess of the ovary before there was time for the development of a corresponding pyosalpinx.

[The writer's review of the literature of the subject has been superficial, else he would not have overlooked a number of cases of non-puerperal ovarian abscess that have been reported at the New York Obstetrical Society, especially at a recent meeting. The condition is certainly not so rare as he states. We are surprised that he makes no reference to the differential diagnosis of abscess of the ovary and perityphlitic abscess—which is frequently impossible, especially when the suppurating ovary is buried in coils of intestine high up in the pelvis, so that it cannot be felt *per vaginam*, and when the sac ruptures into the gut. We have had two cases in which, after careful observation, laparotomy was performed for appendicitis and revealed the presence of ovarian abscess.—ED.]

PÆDIATRICS.

UNDER THE CHARGE OF

JOHN M. KEATING, M.D.,
OF PHILADELPHIA ;

A. F. CURRIER, M.D.,   AND   W. A. EDWARDS, M D.,
OF NEW YORK,   OF SAN DIEGO, CAL.

THE USE OF STROPHANTHUS IN CHILDREN.

DEMME reports (*Jahrbuch f. Kinderheilk.*, xxxi., Nos. 1 and 2) that a 1 : 20 preparation of tincture of strophanthus produces a strengthening of the systolic contraction of the frog's heart somewhat less decided than is produced by digitalis. This effect can be sustained a long time by careful dosage, but as the dosage is increased the contractile force diminishes and gradually a cessation in systole results. The toxic effect of strophanthus on the heart-muscle may occur unexpectedly and more suddenly than with digitalis, hence the necessity of great caution in administering the drug to

children. Strophanthus also causes a prolongation of the diastole and a
diminution in the frequency of the pulse as long as the energy of the systole
increases. The author used the drug in seven cases of uncomplicated mitral
disease, in five of scarlatinal nephritis, in three of exudative pleuritis, and
in two each of bronchial asthma, pulmonary tuberculosis, and whooping-
cough in children between five and fifteen years of age. Dyspepsia was
produced in the younger children, so that the treatment could not be continned. The initial dose for children from five to ten years of age was one
drop, three times daily; for older children, one drop, four times daily. After
four to seven days the dose was increased to three drops four or five times
daily. Nausea and cold-sweating indicated a suspension of the treatment
and the administration of wine, cognac, or coffee. In heart-failure diuresis
was increased after three or four days, the pulse becoming slower and stronger
and the breathing easier. The dropsical phenomena became less marked.
The diuretic effect ceased after three or four days in five of the cases of
mitral disease, and compensation could be effected only by the combined
action of strophanthus with digitalis. A prompt diuretic effect was produced
by strophanthus in two of the cases of chronic scarlatinal nephritis, while
in the acute cases no benefit was experienced. The effect in exudative
pleuritis was satisfactory, and also in the two cases of bronchial asthma, in
which strophanthus was given in connection with iodide of potassium. In
pulmonary phthisis no positive result was observed, but in the two cases of
whooping-cough, in which there was persistent dyspnœa and œdema of the
lower extremities in consequence of dilatation of the heart, the results were
satisfactory. The action of strophanthus consists in elevation of the blood-
pressure and favorable influence upon the respiratory centre. It can complete the action of digitalis when both drugs are given, and neither
cumulative effect nor diminished activity were observed in cases in which it
was used during a long period.

BRONCHIECTASIS IN YOUNG CHILDREN.

The subject of bronchiectasis receives but scanty notice in the ordinary
works on children's diseases.

In the new Cyclopædia by Keating it is not even mentioned. In the recent
text-book by Ashby and Wright it is dismissed in a few sentences as a complication of broncho-pneumonia. Henoch only briefly refers to it as an
occasional result of chronic pneumonia. In Dr. Charles West's lectures it
is merely incidentally mentioned under bronchitis. Goodheart says that it
occurs mostly between five and nine years of age, and that bad pertussis frequently precedes it. Eustace Smith describes it under the head of "fibroid
induration of the lung," but says that cirrhosis of the lung rarely attacks
infants, and is usually found in children of five years old and upward; but
J. WALTER CARR (*The Practitioner*, London, 1891) records four cases whose
ages are as follows: Five and three-quarters years, sixteen months, two years,
eleven months.

Yet it is probable that bronchiectasis is by no means uncommon in childhood, though during life it is undoubtedly very apt to be overlooked, the
case being regarded merely as one of bronchitis—with which it is usually
coexistent—or, perhaps, in the later stages as one of phthisis. Moreover, the

supervention of bronchiectasis, though it seriously increases the gravity of the prognosis, does not, so far as we know, call for any important modification in treatment.

As regards etiology and pathology, the cases given illustrate fairly well the chief ways in which the disease may arise. . It is, of course, always secondary to some antecedent lung trouble—bronchitis, pneumonia, or pleurisy. It is true that the acute specifics, especially measles and whooping-cough, are frequently its precursors.

We must remember that, whilst for convenience of description and of teaching we classify and describe bronchitis, collapse, broncho-pneumonia, lobar pneumonia, pleurisy, etc., in reality these conditions are generally intermixed—more so in children than in adults, and most of all in young children.

Some recorded cases, in which the bronchiectasis seems to have been congenital, were probably due to congenital atelectasis, the unexpanded pulmonary parenchyma having been gradually converted into fibrous tissue, which, subsequently contracting, caused a purely secondary bronchial dilatation.

The physical signs alone suggest, as a rule, a very rapid destruction of lung tissue. The most important points were the gradual supervention upon the ordinary evidences of bronchitis or broncho-pneumonia of distinct cavernous signs, with moderately loud gurgling and bubbling râles, and the variations from day to day in the number and character of these moist sounds. In some of the cases the variability in the physical signs, of course, pointed strongly to bronchial dilatation.

Bronchiectasis limited to part of one lung may be almost indistinguishable from a localized empyema; both are often preceded by a broncho-pneumonia. The loud, gurgling râles in the former condition may help in the diagnosis, but in many instances only the aspirating-needle will decide; and in such cases it may be well to remember the possible danger of penetrating a dilated bronchus, as was done in the second case of Carr.

The prognosis must necessarily be bad if the disease be at all extensive; but the cases show that it must be founded on the results of repeated physical examinations of the chest rather than on delusive hopes which may for a time be afforded by an improvement in the child's general condition. At the same time it is necessary to remember that the physical signs alone would seem to justify a far more immediately serious prognosis than experience shows to be correct.

A New Method of Dressing the Chest in Pneumonia, Pleurisy, Pleurodynia, etc.

William Hunt (*Annals of Gynecology and Pædiatry*, 1891) advises the following method to dress the chest in a case of pneumonia, pleurisy, pleurodynia, etc.:

Do it on a large scale, in the same way that we now dress abrasions, bruises, etc.

If there is to be any cupping or other preliminary operation, have that attended to; then all the ingredients wanting are pure collodion and absorbent cotton, in smooth layers, and a good broad brush, like a mucilage-brush.

Apply a very thin layer over the side affected, from spinal column to sternum, and secure it with collodion smeared thoroughly over it. Then go on with thicker layers, securing them with collodion until a good padding is obtained, paying particular attention to the edges. In double cases you can act accordingly. The advantages are:

1. The one dressing, if well applied, will last throughout the case; thus
2. The fatigue and discomfort of frequent poulticing are avoided.
3. The side, in single cases, is held as in a splint, while the free side does the breathing. A first-class non-conductor is covering the chest. It is possible that the contracting collodion may have some influence in controlling the blood-supply.
4. There is no particular interference, in one who has a good ear, with physical examination. May be it would be a good thing if there was; for having once made the diagnosis, what is the use of exhausting the patient every day by trying to find out whether one-eighth of an inch, more or less, is involved? The general symptoms will tell that.

PLEURITIC EFFUSION IN CHILDREN.

HERBERT B. WHITNEY, in the *Denver Medical Times*, in reporting ten cases of latent serous effusion into the pleuræ of children aged respectively two and four years, remarks that there is little value in Smith's remarkable statement as to the variation in the line of flatness on change of posture. No such variation in the level of the fluid ever takes place in a pleuritic effusion at any age. It does occur in pneumo-hydrothorax, and possibly, also, in simple hydrothorax; but that books should still mention this as a sign of pleuritic effusion can only be explained by the well-known frequency with which errors of this sort are handed down from author to author. The laws which govern the shape and position assumed by a lung under pressure are difficult to determine, but one thing is certain: the lung does not simply float about on the surface of the fluid, nor do either lung or fluid readily alter their relative position. Whitney considers the curve of the upper line of flatness to be pathognomonic. This line has two varieties, according to the amount of effusion, the one being a simple curved line with upward convexity, and the other, more characteristic, the so-called "letter S" curve. This second variety of curve, which appears abruptly as soon as the effusion gets beyond a certain size, was first described by Garland, of Boston, as the "letter S" curve. The curve is found only in effusions of moderate extent; in a very large effusion the line becomes again a simple curve, but this time with upward concavity. This "letter S" curve, beginning at the sixth, seventh, or eighth dorsal vertebra, according to the amount of fluid, passes first outward, then upward, and is lost for a while in the upper axilla, or shoulder-joint; appearing again anteriorly, it either passes downward with a gradual slant to the base of the lung, or, in larger effusions, it passes more horizontally inward along one of the ribs to the sternum.

PUBLIC HEALTH.

UNDER THE CHARGE OF

EDWARD F. WILLOUGHBY, M.D.,

OF LONDON.

THE BACILLUS OF DIPHTHERIA.

Although the multiplicity of bacteria present in the "false membrane" of most cases of diphtheria has induced persons of a sceptical disposition, and not practically familiar with bacteriological manipulation, to question the existence of a specific pathogenic microbe in this disease, there can be no reasonable doubt as to the claims of that known as Klebs-Löffler's to this character, and such being the case its detection affords a ready and positive means of diagnosis in difficult cases. We have long insisted that diphtheria is a disease of far more frequent occurrence than many medical men are inclined to admit, and that not only should all, or nearly all, cases of so-called "membranous croup" and of deaths referred to croup be returned as laryngeal diphtheria, but that the great majority of tonsillites, pharyngites, and post-nasal catarrhs plainly originating in insanitary conditions are really diphtheritic, as is occasionally shown by the occurrence of numistakable cases of diphtheria in families where such suspicious "sore-throats" have already been observed. We do not, however, deny that there are or may be sore-throats of septic origin which are not specific, or that a foul tonsillitis or pharyngitis of the simply catarrhal kind may, at times, assume a more alarming character than many cases of mild diphtheria; but considering the insidious course that the latter often exhibit, arousing no suspicion of danger until the fatal termination is imminent, and the fact that those which pass off favorably may be the means of communicating the infection in a virulent form to other and more susceptible subjects, a ready means of diagnosis—some pathognomonic symptom or characteristic phenomenon, if such could be found—would be of inestimable value to the physician.

Such, we are convinced, is to be obtained in the detection of the Klebs-Löffler bacillus, and we commend a careful perusal of the "Contributions to the Study of Diphtheria," by MM. E. ROUX and A. YERSIN in recent numbers of the Annales de l'Institut Pasteur. The method followed by these experimenters is to remove a fragment of the "false membrane" or exudation from the throat by a piece of cotton-wool held in a long forceps. This is then dried on blotting-paper and rubbed between microscopic glass covers, care being taken that the smear be produced by particles of the membrane itself and not by the salivary mucus and epithelium. The glasses, previously dried and passed through the flame of a spirit lamp, are stained, one by Löffler's blue, the other by gentian-violet after the method of Gram. The preparation, washed in water, is examined with a homogeneous immersion objective. The diphtheritic bacilli appear, among other microbes, in the form of unequally stained slender rods, often grouped in masses, and with ends rounded, slightly curved, and pear- or club-shaped.

Instead of Löffler's blue, another composed of dahlia-violet and methyl-green may be used with advantage. One part of a one per cent. watery solution of the violet is to be mixed with three parts of a similar solution of the green, and enough distilled water then added to give a fine but not too dark a blue tint. This solution is very stable and does not deposit on standing. One drop is placed on a clean cover, which is to be immediately applied to another on which is the object to be stained. With either solution the specific bacilli take up the color sooner and more deeply than do the other microbes, and a little practice makes their recognition an easy matter.

In some typical cases the exudation is almost a pure culture of Löffler's bacillus, and it is always more abundant in portions of membrane taken from the pharynx than in those removed from the larynx after tracheotomy. In fœtid putrefying membranes the proportion of other microbes is greatest. The like predominance of saprophytes is observed as the case progresses toward recovery; and even at the commencement of the attack such a disparity between the numbers of specific and indifferent bacteria may justify a favorable prognosis.

Should any difficulty be experienced in discovering the bacilli, portions of the membrane may be hardened in alcohol and sections stained by Gram's method, when beneath the superficial layer, rich in common microbes, the specific bacilli will be seen in well-defined groups.

If the membrane be rapidly dried on linen or blotting-paper, its subsequent desiccation scarcely interferes with the staining process, so that the examination may be made by an expert on specimens sent through the post by medical men who have not the means of doing it themselves. But with a proper microscope and a little practice a few minutes is generally sufficient to obtain satisfactory evidence as to the nature of any given case.

For pure cultures, coagulated serum is by far the best medium, and in it sowings of the false membrane give rise to colonies of the specific bacillus within twenty-four hours, before saprophytes, or the streptococci always present in the exudation, have begun to grow.

This cultivation in gelatin-serum is, indeed, essential to an absolute diagnosis, for, as Dr. Klein has shown,[1] there are two forms of the Klebs-Löffler bacilli, which he calls Nos. 1 and 2, but which would be better described as two species of bacillus morphólogically alike, though distinguishable by their behavior in gelatin cultures. No. 1 is not constantly present in diphtheria, and does not act pathogenetically on animals; in fact, is not the specific bacillus or cause of the disease, which the so-called No. 2 is. The pseudo-diphtheritic bacillus, or No. 1, grows freely enough in pure serum, but not on serum rendered solid by gelatin at temperatures of 70–72° F., which the true bacillus of diphtheria does. Hitherto no one seems to have been aware of the existence of the two forms, for Löffler himself and Flügge state that the bacillus does not grow in gelatin at temperatures below 76° F., while Zarniko and Escherich assert positively that it does so even below 72° F., clearly

---

[1] Report of Medical Officer of Local Government Board.

showing that while the latter experimented with the true one, the former made these observations on the false, though in his inoculations Löffler must have used the pathogenetic form.

According to Dr. Klein, the surest way to obtain pure cultures of the specific bacillus of diphtheria is to wash the pieces of membrane by shaking them up in three successive portions of sterilized solution of common salt, and from the particles in the last to sow plate cultivations on solid serum-gelatin.

The bacilli in diphtheria, as it occurs in the human subject, are confined to the false membrane and perhaps the subjacent tissue; at any rate, they are never found in the blood—a fact which suggests irresistibly that the phenomena, febrile, neurotic, etc., of the disease are caused by the absorption of ptomaines, toxines, or other matters produced by the bacilli, which themselves remain in the original site. This supposition is confirmed by the fact that when guinea-pigs or other animals are inoculated subcutaneously with pure cultures of the bacillus, sections of the tumor produced exhibit under the microscope appearances closely resembling those of the diphtheritic tissue from the human pharynx, but that, though the general phenomena of the disease, nephritis, etc., are induced, the bacilli cannot be found in the blood.

Klein has, however, detected them in the neighboring lymphatic vessels and glands, and has obtained pure cultures from these; but this very limited extension, which we do not doubt would be found to apply to the inflamed submaxillary glands in man, and would indeed seem inevitable, does not detract from the local character of the primary process, and though the usual mode of infection by inhalation or imbibition would, at first sight, seem to offer a ready explanation of this localization in the pharynx, larynx, or nares in man, Dr. Klein's remarkable observations on the cow point to some more occult causes varying with the peculiar constitution of the animal.

The occasional appearance of a similar false membrane on the vaginal or other mucous membranes, and on parts of the skin denuded by blisters, by abrasions, or eczema, and on the surface of wounds, would seem to be comparable to the experimental inoculations in animals.

The theory which attributes the general phenomena to toxines, is fully confirmed by further experiments of Roux and Yersin, who separated the bacilli and their chemical products from artificial cultivations, and by injection of the latter alone produced in guinea-pigs all the general effects of the disease without any local manifestations whatever.

Dr. Thursfield, Dr. Downes, and Mr. Shirley Murphy have recently reported cases in which cats had been ill, and in some instances died, from a disease of the respiratory organs, and children who had played with and nursed them had sickened soon after with diphtheria, and others in which cats had been affected in like manner after association with children suffering from diphtheria. In two instances, post-mortem examinations of the cats revealed, besides evidence of broncho-pneumonia, renal lesions identical with those observed in diphtheria.

Doubts have been expressed as to the identity of the natural diphtheria of cats with that of man, from the fact that, though artificial inoculation of the pharynx or nares may lead to local manifestations resembling those of diphtheria in man, the natural disease in the cat is distinctly pulmonary. But no one now questions the identity of human and bovine tuberculosis, though the peculiar lesions presented by the pleura in Perlsucht were formerly urged as evidence to the contrary. This, however, is by no means the only instance of a specific and communicable disease producing different phenomena, "accidents" in the logical sense of the word, in different animals, and the experiments of Klein at the Brown Institute in the production of diphtheria in cats by the use of infected milk, have confirmed the suggestion that in that animal the lung is the chief seat of the morbid phenomena, while the same tendency to pulmonary localization was observed in other cats that were subsequently infected by association with these.

A far more important question from a standpoint of practical hygiene is the communicability of diphtheria by means of milk. That such a mode of propagating the disease is possible, has been amply proved by the history of numerous epidemics. The evidence, however, had hitherto been wholly circumstantial, though none the less conclusive. We mean that the questions had not been solved, whether the milk served merely as a vehicle, perhaps a cultivation fluid also, but merely as a vehicle for the conveyance of the poison from man to man, as from the milker or dealer to the consumer, or whether the cow herself were capable of contracting the disease and thus becoming an active intermediary. We are not aware of any observations on the effects of the milk of nursing mothers suffering from diphtheria, but it is quite conceivable that such milk, whether of woman or cow, would, by being impregnated with the toxines present in the blood, acquire highly poisonous properties. At the same time, the experiments of Roux and Yersin with the pure chemical products of artificial cultures, suggest by analogy that the disease induced by the use of such milk would, though resembling diphtheria in its general phenomena, be marked by the absence of the bacilli and of the local manifestations of their action on the pharyngeal mucous membrane. This would not be the case were the cow to be inoculated on her udders by the hands of an infected milker, and such a contingency is not improbable.

But Dr. Klein, having learnt that in one undoubted instance of the spread of diphtheria by means of milk, the cows at the inculpated dairy, though apparently in good health, had suffered from " chaps " on their udders, determined to investigate the whole question experimentally. He inoculated two cows with pure cultures from a case of human diphtheria, using a Pravaz syringe and selecting the subcutaneous tissue of the shoulder as a neutral or indifferent spot. A swelling appeared, attended by some febrile disturbance and loss of appetite, but it, as well as the general symptoms, subsided after the third day. Between the eighth and tenth days, they began to suffer from a slight cough, and they left off feeding on the twelfth and twenty-third days respectively. The former died on the fifteenth and the latter was killed on the twenty-fifth. In both, from the fifth to the eleventh days, in fact, during the interval of freedom from any evidence of general disease, a succession of papules appeared on the teats. These papules were followed by vesicles, changing into pustules and ultimately forming brown or black crusts, which fell off in the course of five to seven days, leaving dry healing sores. Some of the vesicles and pustules were one-half or three-fourths of an inch in diameter, but the majority were not more than one-fourth or even one-eighth of an inch across.

The milk drawn from these cows on the fifth day, before even a single papule had made its appearance, was found to be so charged with the bacillus of diphtheria that thirty-two colonies free from any admixture of other bacteria were obtained in pure cultures from one cubic centimetre of milk. When the vesicles first appeared, their serous contents were examined and found to be swarming with the bacilli, as were those of the succeeding pustules up to the last.

These experiments, conducted with every antiseptic and other precaution, demonstrate unequivocally the fact that in the cow the localization of the bacterial phenomena of the disease tends to the udder, and that the milk contains the bacilli in enormous numbers, though the means by which they are conveyed from a distant inoculation are extremely difficult to conceive, and can only be explained by further observations. It may be that the bacilli are not restricted as in man and the rodents to the site or proximity of their entry. It was by some of this milk, taken before the formation of the papules and while the teats were to all appearances perfectly sound and healthy, having been unintentionally given to a couple of cats that the epidemic among those animals in the Institute was set up.

For the post-mortem appearances presented by the cows, as well as the cats, and other details, we must refer our readers to the report of the Medical Officer to the Local Government Board, 1888–89 ; we have here only space for so much of Dr. Klein's discoveries as directly bears on and proves the fact that the cow is susceptible of diphtheria, and that, while in seeming health, her milk may be charged with the specific bacillus and be an active medium for the communication of the disease to mankind.

Corrigendum.—The order of figures 3 and 4, pp. 381 and 383 of the October issue, has been erroneously reversed ; the description of each figure applies to the other.

Note to Contributors.—All contributions intended for insertion in the Original Department of this Journal are only received *with the distinct understanding that they are contributed exclusively to this Journal.*

Contributions from the Continent of Europe and written in the French, German or Italian language, if on examination they are found desirable for this Journal, will be translated at its expense.

Liberal compensation is made for articles used. A limited number of extra copies in pamphlet form, if desired, will be furnished to authors in lieu of compensation, *provided the request for them be written on the manuscript.*

All communications should be addressed to

Dr. EDWARD P. DAVIS,
250 South 21st Street, Philadelphia.

THE

AMERICAN JOURNAL

OF THE MEDICAL SCIENCES.

DECEMBER, 1891.

INTRA-THORACIC SURGERY; BRONCHOTOMY THROUGH THE CHEST-WALL FOR FOREIGN BODIES IMPACTED IN THE BRONCHI.[1]

By De Forest Willard, M.D., Ph.D.,

SURGEON TO THE PRESBYTERIAN HOSPITAL, CLINICAL PROFESSOR OF ORTHOPÆDIC SURGERY,
UNIVERSITY OF PENNSYLVANIA.

The extraction of foreign bodies that have become impacted low down in the air-passages has always been a subject of great surgical interest, since such impactions are necessarily of serious import. This paper is only intended to deal with those cases where the body has become lodged in the bronchi, as those arrested in the larynx or trachea are much more easily reached by surgical measures.

In order to determine the possibility of successfully reaching the bronchus through the chest-wall, the following experiments were instituted upon dogs, since so serious an operation demands thorough experimental work before it is attempted upon the human subject; and as this question may be brought to any of us at a moment's warning, it cannot be too speedily settled.

I approached the subject free from bias as to its possibility, desiring only to prove or disprove its feasibility. The experiments are, of course, too few in number to settle the question, but they are placed on record as additional testimony, and to show the extreme inherent difficulties and dangers which must be met in our attempts to invade the thorax.

We have so successfully advanced both in cranial and abdominal

---

[1] Read before the American Surgical Association, at the Congress, Washington, September 22–25, 1891.

surgery that we are warranted in reviewing anew all the conclusions of the past in an honest effort to secure substantial and life-giving progress in the surgery of the future.[1]

My experiments thus far tend to prove :

1. That the collapse of the lung on opening the thorax, when a lung has not been crippled by disease, is an exceedingly serious and dangerous element, adding greatly to the previous shock, and threatening at once to overpower the patient.

2. The difficulties of reaching the bronchus, especially upon the left side, are exceedingly great and the risks of hemorrhage enormous.

3. Incision into the bronchus necessarily leads, after closure of the chest wound, to increasing pneumothorax, with its subsequent dangers.

4. The delays in the operation from the collapse of the patient must necessarily be great. Rapid work is impossible when the root of the lung is being dragged backward and forward at least half an inch in the efforts occasioned by air-hunger, and precision is almost impossible.

5. To reach the bronchus is sometimes feasible, but to successfully extract a foreign body from it and secure recovery is as yet highly problematical and will require many advances in technique. The anatomical surroundings are those most essential to life.

EXPERIMENT I.[2] *Death from ether; subsequent tracheotomy and bronchotomy.*—Large white and liver-colored blind setter, weighing seventy-five pounds. On account of his size this dog was selected, with a view of performing tracheotomy and of introducing a foreign body into the right bronchus, which, by reason of the large diameter of the trachea, could readily be done.

Before the dog was thoroughly etherized, however, he suddenly ceased to breathe, and all efforts to resuscitate him by artificial respiration were unavailing. He was accordingly utilized by opening his trachea and introducing a pebble the size of a chestnut. An opening was then made in the chest-wall about midway between the sternum and the spine in the fourth interspace. The trachea was easily found, and the stone

1 Interest in this subject has recently been reawakened by a case in a neighboring city, where a cork half an inch in diameter became lodged at the bottom of the left primary bronchus. The case is reported by Dr. Rushmore in the New York Medical Journal of July 25, 1891.

Dr. Rushmore, after two unsuccessful attempts to extract the body through the trachea, attempted an operation for reaching the bronchus through the thoracic wall, but he was obliged to suspend his procedures by the collapse of the patient before the chest was actually opened.

2 These experiments have been made possible by the helpful assistance of Drs. Sailer and Hinkle, and Mr. Nicholson, whose efficient aid and suggestions saved much loss of time. I have also made a number of experiments in pneumonectomy and pneumonotomy in continuation of those made by Dr. Sailer and Messrs. Patek and Bolgiano (Univ. Med. Mag., May, 1891, p. 473), which I shall endeavor soon to publish.

passed down into the bronchus on the left side. Search was made for the stone, but it could not be discovered. The bronchus was opened, the aorta being displaced to reach it, and the pulmonary vein pushed forward. No stone could be found.

The sternum was then removed, as in ordinary post-mortems, but search was still unavailing. The left bronchus lay covered by the pulmonary vein, with the aorta a little behind and to the left. The bronchial arteries and veins were of large size and were wounded at the right bronchus in the search. The vena azygos minor crossed so close to the root of the lung that it would have been wounded during any operation. This bronchus was opened, but it contained no stone. After deliberate search through the substance of the lung, and also in the trachea, the stone was at last found in the larynx, although the dog had been held in a sitting position during its introduction. The same thing happened on another dog while being experimented upon, showing the remarkable power of reverse action in the trachea and bronchi, if such it was.

Favier and Sabatier, in experimenting for the removal of foreign bodies from the air-passages in dogs, also found that the objects were always expelled voluntarily after tracheotomy, even when pushed well down into the bronchus and buried with the forceps. They were rejected whether the dog was lying down or upright.

EXPERIMENT II. *Pebble in bronchus; bronchotomy; death; stone found in larynx.*—White cur dog, male. Etherized, shaved, and antiseptically cleansed. Incision was made far back toward the spine in an endeavor to reach the bronchus from behind at the root of the lung. Division of the skin and pectoral muscles gave but little hemorrhage. The incision was carried back into the erector spinæ group, from which free hemorrhage occurred, requiring the use of hemostatic forceps, ligatures, etc. The periosteum of the fourth rib was split longitudinally, and the bone enucleated with a blunt knife and curved hook. The fifth rib was treated in the same manner, and an inch and one-half removed from each with bone-forceps. When the pleural cavity was reached the lung immediately collapsed. Stripping the ribs from the periosteum permitted later opening of the chest cavity.

Before the pleura was opened tracheotomy was performed, and a stone carried well down into the bronchus with a pair of forceps before it was dropped. Search was then instituted, but from the time the lung collapsed the dog was in an extremely bad condition, and died before the bronchus could be opened, although the stone could be easily felt in the right tube. Artificial respiration was of no avail.

After death the bronchus was opened, and although the stone had been carried well down into place, and had been felt in that position, yet the result was the same as reported in the previous case, the stone being ultimately found in the larynx. By what means it had worked its way there could not be ascertained, as the dog was upon a level table and was not inverted.

The difficulties in securing and maintaining perfect antisepsis in dogs are very great. Their distaste to dressings of all kinds is so persistent that the only method of enforcing continuous cleanly applications seems to be by an enveloping outside bandage of gypsum.

EXPERIMENT III. *Bronchotomy through the thoracic walls; death in two days.*—Large, white, male bull-dog, strong and vigorous. Etherized, shaved, and made antiseptic. A large incision was made on the right side, commencing two inches from the spine, in order to avoid the erector spinæ group and to have less hemorrhage. One rib was resected subperiosteally, as in Experiment II. As soon as the pleural cavity was opened the lung collapsed, and the dog became deeply cyanosed. Respiration was shallow, and soon ceased—the heart's action, however, continuing. The wound was closed with a sponge and artificial respiration instituted. After a few minutes the color returned in his tongue, and he was placed upon his back. This process had to be repeated every few minutes during the entire operation. As soon as he was turned upon his left side the weight of the lung and the air-pressure were so great that he immediately ceased to breathe. As the operation could not be proceeded with when he was turned with his right side uppermost, the opening was closed, artificial respiration performed, and he resumed breathing. When on his back respiration could be maintained but two minutes, and it was not deemed safe to do tracheotomy or actually to introduce the foreign body. The upper lobe of the lung was, therefore, turned forward, the bronchus cleared from the surrounding vessels and incised for one-half inch. Very free hemorrhage occurred from wound of the pulmonary vein. This was controlled by hæmostatic forceps, and afterward by chromicized catgut ligatures above and below the wound. The opening in the bronchus was then stitched with chromicized catgut, the gut being threaded upon a small, sharply curved needle. Three interrupted sutures were thus inserted and tied. The chest cavity was cleared of blood. The incision in the chest was then thoroughly sponged and rendered as clean as possible. The deep muscles were drawn together by deep sutures and superficial stitches added.

The dog rallied well, and on the following day ate and drank. Two days later, however, he died. Cause unknown, as through an error I was not notified until after he had been buried, consequently the postmortem was lost.

EXPERIMENT IV. *Thoracotomy; excision of ribs; bronchotomy; puncture of pulmonary vein.*—Liver and white colored male dog; weight, forty pounds. Etherized, shaved, etc. Incision on the left side in the mid-lateral region between the third and fourth ribs. Four inches of the fourth rib resected periosteally without opening the chest. The pleura was then incised and the upper lobe drawn out. As the dyspnœa in the former case was greatly relieved when the wound in the chest was closed or rendered smaller, an attempt was made to prevent the great inrush of air by drawing out the lobe of the lung and passing it through a slit in a sheet of rubber-dam, thus making an impervious veil and assisting in the relief of air-pressure. The dam was pushed back until the bronchus of this lobe was exposed outside of the slit. The bronchus was bare of pulmonary vessels, and was quickly and easily incised without injury to them. The amount of collapse was less than in the former case, possibly because the left side was being operated upon, and the weight of the heart did not press so heavily upon the left lung, as the heart was in the reverse position. The dog suffered but little from air-hunger. One stitch was easily placed with a curved staphylorrhaphy needle, and matters looked favorable for a speedy and safe completion of the operation, as the dog was doing well. In placing the second stitch, however, a sudden movement of the root of the lung caused the point of the needle to enter the pulmonary vein, and a gush of blood ensued. This was conducted from the chest by the rubber-dam trough, and the punctured vessel was seized with a hæmostatic forceps and thoroughly tied by passing a catgut ligature beneath the vein with a blunt-pointed aneurism needle. The vein was tied above and below the wound. The placing of the second suture was followed with like result, the lung being dragged out of the hands of the operator during the strong inspiratory movement. More hemorrhage ensued, but was controlled in the same way. Other ligatures were placed, but the blood ran into the opening of the bronchus, and the dog was finally killed, since there was no prospect of his more than rallying from the operation. After death it was found that one stitch had been nicely placed in the bronchus, and that the pulmonary vein had been torn by the point of the needle, but had been secured by ligature. The bronchus was not thoroughly cleared from the surrounding structures before incision was made, hence the accident.

EXPERIMENT V. *Thoracotomy; death from ether and collapse of lung.*— Incision on the left side opposite the seventh rib, which was resected periosteally. Anterior part of the bronchus of the left upper lobe exposed and cleared, when the dog suddenly collapsed from heart failure, or perhaps from pressure upon the pericardium, with probable rupture of the septum between the lungs. Artificial respiration proved of no avail.

In this case the posterior part of the bronchus of the middle lobe was easily reached and seen. The aorta lay to the left, with the pneumogastric a little posteriorly, so that it would have been easy to have reached the bronchus. The upper bronchus anteriorly was also easily exposed. Incision at the seventh rib is a little too low. The bronchus had been thoroughly isolated when the collapse occurred, and could have been easily incised. Rubber-dam was used as a valve.

EXPERIMENT VI. *Thoracotomy; bronchotomy; suturing of wound; death fifteen minutes after completion of operation.*—Large black and white mongrel; weight, thirty pounds. Incision on right side. Fifth rib excised subperiosteally, but a serious hemorrhage occurred from the intercostal artery, which was finally controlled by ligature. The bronchus of the first lobe proved to be inaccessible, both anteriorly and posteriorly, being deeply concealed and covered with the pulmonary vessels. The bronchus of the second lobe was reached anteriorly and incised for one-third of an inch.

Three chromicized catgut sutures were introduced into the side of the bronchus wound and tied, a staphylorrhaphy needle being employed. The difficulties and delays in the operation were found to be the same as in the previous cases from the fact that resuscitation had to be performed many times after apparent death. The dog, however, was kept alive and the wound closed. He did not rally, and died in fifteen minutes.

The post-mortem revealed no hemorrhage; bronchus cleanly cut, without injury to surrounding structures, and sutures well placed.

EXPERIMENT VII. *Excision of ribs; bronchotomy; large pulmonary veins; death.*—Skye terrier, male. Etherized. Incision laterally from the point of the scapula. Fourth rib resected. A three-inch incision on the left side. Immediate collapse of lung on admission of air. Shock so great on collapse of lung that but little ether was subsequently required. The bronchus of the upper lobe found concealed by enormous pulmonary arteries and two huge pulmonary veins which lay in front, completely covering it. These were carefully isolated, but the great depth of the bronchus rendered it entirely impossible to incise it, as the vessels could not be held out of the way. The bronchus of the middle lobe was exposed posteriorly. The aorta and pneumogastric lay absolutely upon it, so that operation seemed hopeless, but it was at last incised without injury to the vessels. One stitch was safely inserted with a staphylorrhaphy needle, but the bronchus being very brittle the second stitch tore out, and the dog, having been resuscitated eight times during the operation, finally died.

The relation of the bronchus to the pulmonary vessels was found entirely different from the previous cases, being much larger and the bronchus deeper. The root of the lung, also, was situated low down in the thorax, so that the incision was too high. The fifth rib would have been better.

EXPERIMENT VIII. *Simple incision of bronchus without stitching; death from increasing pressure of pneumothorax.*—Black and white mongrel, male; weight, twelve pounds. Etherized, shaved, and rendered antiseptic. Incision on the right side. Excision of the fifth rib one inch and a half. The bronchus leading to the right upper lobe was exposed. The bronchial and pulmonary veins were pushed aside. Very large azygos vein. The bronchus was incised for one-third of an inch without wounding any other structure. No hemorrhage took place. The pleural cavity was cleaned of a few drops of blood issuing from the divided intercostals. The intercostal muscles were stitched with continuous suture of catgut; pectoral muscles ditto, securely closing the chest. The skin was also closed in the same manner. The line of suture of the muscles showed a constant tendency to bulge, and the air soon burst through it at each inspiration. The dog breathed with comparative ease, and was rallying, while the wound was partially closed. So soon, however, as complete closure was accomplished, the dyspnœa became more marked, the tissues being pushed out more and more at each inspiration. The pneumothorax steadily increased, pushing the heart to the left and with it the septum, thus interfering with the left lung. Death speedily ensued.

The opening in the bronchus evidently permitted the air at each inspiration to escape through the incision into the pleural cavity, but from the cylindrical shape of the tube return was prevented by closure of the slit. The action was that of a force-pump driving more air into the pleural cavity, which is probably the explanation of the increasing pneumothorax.

An examination of the parts after death showed that the incision had been cleanly made in the bronchus, and that no injury had been done to any vessel or nerve-structure in the line of the wound. There was no hemorrhage, and death was apparently from the cause mentioned.

This experiment was made to observe the effect of a wound left open in the bronchus without stitching. The increasing pneumothorax seemed to be caused by the valve action of the bronchial slit.

It has been demonstrated that the air of the bronchi is septic, and that it only becomes aseptic by the time that it reaches the bronchioles and air-vessels.

My experiments show that upon the left side the bronchus of dogs is enveloped by the pulmonary veins and arteries and bronchial vessels, and although the aorta and pneumogastric can be speedily recognized, yet the cardiac and pleural branches of the pneumogastric run so closely to the root of the lung that the dangers upon the living animal are simply enormous, and in a human patient I cannot imagine a more appalling array of difficulties than would meet the surgeon in such an attempt, with these enormous vessels on either side and the heart in close proximity. Combined with the labored movement of the lung, the operation is one beset with extreme difficulties.

On the right side, while the array of obstacles is not quite so serious, yet the danger is increased by the close proximity of the azygos vein, and in dogs the pressure of air upon the septum, together with gravity, pushes the heart so far to the left, and interferes so greatly with the action of the only lung which is capable of rendering service at this time, that it occasions greatly increased risks from apnœa.

Dr. Rushmore states that in the cadaver, however, the operation is not difficult, but expresses doubt as to the condition of a living subject. I can say that in a dog the aspects of the parts during life and after death are as absolutely different as they can possibly be. A bronchus which after death is easily exposed, and which is reached with the greatest ease, I have seen five minutes previously absolutely enclosed with huge pulsating vessels of twice the size, any one of which if punctured would seriously complicate if not render the operation absolutely fatal. The alteration of the parts in life and in death can only be appreciated when seen.

I attempted a posterior entrance in a number of experiments, but found a much more serious delay from hemorrhage of the great veins which supply the erector spinæ group of muscles.

The plan of Nesiloff consists in opening the thoracic cavity in the posterior mediastinum from behind by the resection of the ribs without touching the pleuræ. As the relation of the parts is different in dogs, this cannot be so readily accomplished in experiments.

The patient should be laid upon his abdomen and a vertical incision made parallel to the vertebræ, three inches to the left; two horizontal incisions are carried toward the vertebræ from either extremity of the first, and the flap raised. A sub-periosteal incision of the third, fourth, fifth, and sixth ribs is then performed either by removing them or by bending them by fracture, so as to replace them after the operation. The pleura is then pushed forward and the bronchus searched for.

This operation has been employed to reach the œsophagus, and it is possible that it may yet be used in searching for the bronchus.[1]

The operation which was attempted by Dr. Rushmore, but which was not completed, was the making of a flap three inches long and three inches wide, with its detached edge along the left clavicle. He had cut through and pushed back the pectoral muscles, and was about making the section of the ribs with a saw, when he was compelled to desist his efforts in order to revive the patient.

The difficulty in extraction through the trachea in this case was that the round body, half an inch in diameter, accurately fitted the cylindrical bronchus, and gave no opportunity for the forceps to grasp it unless the bronchus could be first dilated sufficiently to allow the jaws to pass between the walls of the tube and the cork. He employed various devices for securing the object after tracheotomy with division of the second, third, and fourth rings. Air-pump suction worked perfectly well in experimenting upon rubber tubing and cork, yet it could not dislodge the object when held by the swollen mucous membrane of the bronchus. Instruments with concealed hooks he discarded as useless on account of the impossibility of accurately distinguishing between the cork and the mucous membrane. This I have found an exceedingly difficult thing even with rougher bodies than cork, as the cartilaginous rings give a firm sensation to the probe, greatly resembling a foreign body. Piano-wire loops were also tested by experiment on tubing, but the loop would not pass beyond the body. Adhesive substances were found to be useless on a moist surface. With Tiemann's œsophageal forceps he was able to distend the rubber tubing and grasp the cork. These seemed the most hopeful methods of relief offered, and they were used at the first operation. At the second operation he thought his instrument touched the cork. This, however, was only conjecture.

At the first operation the patient was etherized forty minutes, when, as the object was not found, he was allowed to recover. His temperature varied subsequently from 100° to 103°.

The second operation was attempted five days later. The patient labored under increasing difficulty of respiration. There was dulness over the left thorax, and he was evidently sinking. A corkscrew, concealed in a hollow tube, 30 French calibre, twelve inches long, slit from end to end for the purpose of respiration, was employed. This apparatus consisted of three portions, an outer envelope, an inner tube with two concealed spikes, and within this a long-handled corkscrew, which could be easily rotated. He was able to reach the cork and was satisfied that the spikes were not fixed in the wall of the bronchus by rotating

---

[1] In the Journal of the American Medical Association, June 25, 1891, it is stated that Figuiera was experimenting upon this subject by the posterior incision, but I have seen nothing published by him.

the whole instrument on its long axis. The screw having been presumably driven into the cork, traction was made. The coil, as was proven
later, pulled from the cork. The patient coughed up a moderate amount
of bloody mucus, and, breathing with markedly increased difficulty,
became deeply cyanosed, which cyanosis continued until the end of the
operation.

The difficulty of respiration was increased, and it was believed that
the cork had passed over to the right bronchus. After ten or fifteen
minutes' further search the anterior operation, as described, was attemped
but abandoned. Death occurred five days later, the condition never
again warranting operative procedures.

At the post-mortem the cork was found at the bifurcation of the left
bronchus. The lower end of the cork was broken off, probably before
it was swallowed. The mucous lining was sloughing and congested. Pus
oozed from the small bronchi. The lung was hepatized. The right lung
was slightly congested and œdematous. Two punctures were found upon
the upper surface of the cork, and a small piece was missing.

When a foreign body becomes impacted in the bronchus, the gravity
of the injury becomes more and more serious. According to the statistics
of Weist and others, a large percentage of these are fatal ultimately
either from pneumonia, gangrene, abscess, or other complications.

On a careful physical examination to determine the site of the impaction the quality of the sounds elicited on percussion will vary from
slight dulness to flatness according to the amount of blockade, and also
with the nature of the body itself. The primary percussion note will
not be altered except where there is complete obstruction. Later, if
pleurisy or pneumonia supervene, of course the ordinary physical signs
will be present. If there is entire obstruction, or if complete collapse
occurs, there will be but little, if any, movement of the ribs.[1]

A metallic substance will, of course, give forth a more whistling
sound, and peculiar-shaped bodies may occasion strange notes. The
respiratory murmur may be altered in tone—may be extinguished or
altogether lost, while upon the opposite side respiration will usually be
puerile.

The primary symptoms of bronchial impaction are usually dyspnœa,
livid face, spasmodic cough, pain in the chest, and less interference with
the voice than in laryngeal impaction. Thoracic pain is usually present and very constant. Expiration is ordinarily more difficult than
inspiration.

---

[1] Stengel (Univ. Med. Mag., August, 1891, p. 729; Brit. Med. Journ., April 25, 1891)
says that we can determine definitely by auscultation which bronchus is filled. If the
air does not pass in, then it is entirely occluded ; if the sounds are sibilant on inspiration, the obstruction is incomplete and the opposite side will be normal. The sound
will, of course, vary as the object is tubular or solid. In partial obstruction of the
bronchus a portion of the lung may be resonant.

The prognosis of these cases is much more serious than in tracheal and laryngeal obstruction, and the chances of securing the body either by operation or by voluntary expulsion are greatly diminished.

It must be remembered that foreign bodies sometimes shift from one bronchus to the other. The right bronchus, being almost in line with the trachea and occupying as it does nearly three-fifths of the area of the tube (from the fact that the spine of division lies to the left of the median line), is most likely to receive the foreign body. Cheadle found that in thirty cases, sixteen were on the left side. Kocher gives Sander's tables of twenty-one deaths without operative interference or expulsion, of which ten were in the right bronchus, none in the left. In thirty-four cases operated upon, thirteen were on the right, five on the left.

Beleg gives thirty cases, in which nineteen were in the left bronchus.

The right bronchus is three-quarters the size of the trachea ; the left, one-half. The right is about one inch in length ; the left, two inches.

VOLUNTARY EXPULSION.—This is so common an occurrence that this end should not be despaired of even when the body is within the bronchus. Of course, much will depend somewhat upon the character of the body. Seeds of all kinds will naturally swell under the action of heat and moisture, and may, at first, occasion increasing obstruction, but as softening occurs, expulsion may be accomplished by a voluntary effort of the patient. Hence the policy of non-interference in seed impaction is usually the wise course. Expulsion usually occurs in the first few hours, but it may be delayed for weeks ; one case is on record where a bone remained for sixty years. Secondary expulsion may occur after ulceration and abscess, and, although these cases even end in recovery, yet such degeneration of the lung frequently results in death. A body occasionally becomes encysted ; night-sweats and emaciation often follow, and the tubercular process may be engrafted upon the inflammatory lesion.

INVERSION.—Many authors advise against inversion of the body, but in my judgment this procedure is advisable in bronchial impaction, especially when the substance is metallic, and particularly after tracheotomy, when the risk of its lodgement in the larynx has been greatly diminished. Campbell reports a death from hemorrhage during inversion, but this is exceptional.

Statistics of foreign bodies impacted in the bronchi show a slight increased percentage in favor of non-interference. When, however, the obstruction can be located, a low tracheotomy is justifiable with cautious attempts at extraction. These should not be prolonged, nor should imprudent force be used.

Considerable difference of opinion exists upon the propriety of operation in bronchial impaction. Kocher says that operation for the removal of foreign bodies is but an experiment. Weist proves almost conclusively that nearly 90 per cent. will recover without operation. Westmoreland favors operation when the foreign body is in the upper air-passage, but when in the bronchi it is not advisable. When a foreign body becomes impacted in the bronchus, extraction is an impossibility in 78 per cent. of cases even after tracheotomy.

Weist considers that the mortality is increased by tracheotomy in bronchial impaction, since the risks of the operation are added to the primary danger together with the perils arising from the temptation in the hands of a rash surgeon to prolong operative efforts. Ulceration and perforation may result. Small, hard bodies are the ones most liable to drop into the bronchus, but they seldom pass beyond the binary bifurcation.

Gross advises that not more than three attempts of one minute each should be employed with forceps to remove a foreign body.

The danger of the operation is largely increased by injurious instrumentation. Thirty per cent. of the deaths following operation are from pneumonia, while this disease causes death only in 18 per cent. of non-operative cases. Still, as Rushmore wisely remarks, when the deaths from broncho-pneumonia are added, the results are practically similar. The failure to extract a foreign body even after operation in 78 per cent. of cases is certainly an unfavorable showing, but, from my experiments upon dogs, I certainly am not inclined to believe that the chances of recovery would be increased by approaching the bronchus through the chest-wall.

For the purpose of extraction, forceps of various curves are required. Gross's, Cohen's, Mackenzie's, or Cusco's lever-bladed ones are the best. D'Etiolle's spoon, or a bent wire, or a blunt hook, may sometimes be required, varying with the nature of the body to be extracted.

The forceps, though slender, should be exceedingly strong and should have simple serrated edges, so as not to wound the mucous lining of the tube. After the body has been fixed by inflammatory action, however, extraction is often impossible with these forceps. In the case of round bodies, as peas, beans, and peculiar-shaped substances, forceps with sharp teeth are permissible in order to prevent slipping. The manipulations must be performed with extreme caution, and the withdrawal must be slow. Instruments acting upon the plan of a corkscrew are occasionally employed, but a soft substance capable of being penetrated by such a device would render the diagnosis of its having been grasped an obscure one.

Suction by a Bigelow litholapaxy pump through a tube with an open end would be useful for the removal of small articles. Such a tube could be made much larger than the ordinary urethral one, or rubber tubing can be employed. I am experimenting with a rubber tube that can be expanded so as to occupy the entire calibre of the bronchus, and thus give strong suction-power.

After tracheotomy the wound should be kept open by blunt hooks or by stitches: never by a canula, which would block the exit and prevent the voluntary expulsion which is so common even after failure with instruments. The dressing should be simply loose gauze, to exclude the dust without interfering with the exit. The air should be heated after the operation to 80° or 85°, as I am satisfied from experience that all tracheotomies do better in a high temperature.

When the opening in the trachea gives entire relief from dyspnœa, it is very improbable that any object is fastened in the bronchus. Tracheal mirrors with electrical illumination, as well as laryngeal ones, should be employed in the diagnosis after tracheotomy. The greater the extent and duration of the dyspnœa the greater will be the danger from pneumonia after tracheotomy.

The work of Avonssohn, Gross, Durham (Holmes' *Surgery*), Weist, and others have made possible many successful results.[1] It is certainly impossible for any surgeon to diagnosticate beforehand whether his individual case is one of those in which the obstruction will be loosened and coughed up, or whether it will remain, producing gangrene, pneumonia, or subsequent abscess, consequently each case should be most thoroughly considered:

Bronchus originally meant the windpipe, while the two primary divisions were named bronchia, hence the term bronchotomy was used to designate any opening in the air-passages of either larynx, trachea, or bronchus; and Gross and other writers, even as late as Weist, still use the term to designate the high operation. It should be confined to operation upon the bronchus, as laryngotomy and tracheotomy properly designate these higher operations.

Weist (*Trans. Amer. Surg. Assoc.*, vol. i.) gives an accurate and careful analysis of 1000 cases of foreign bodies in the larynx, trachea, and bronchus, as will be remembered by all the members of this Association. In it he shows conclusively that the simple presence of a foreign body is not an absolute indication for operation, as had been previously held by most surgical teachers. While operation is the rule, yet there are modifying circumstances. His conclusions were that 76 per cent. of non-operative cases recovered, and 72 per cent. of those operated upon, but, of course, the latter were the worst class, as the former included many in which early expulsion took place. Weist does not advise opening simply because a foreign body is present; there must be some other indications. He advises non-interference when a foreign body

---

[1] Bourdillat gives a large collection of cases (Poulson, On Foreign Bodies, p. 33). Also Maurice Perrin gives statistics.

remains quiet and the symptoms are not serious, but favors operation when the body is movable and when there are frequent attacks of suffocation.

Smith gives 1600 cases, with 70 per cent. of recoveries of non-operative cases and 76 per cent. of operative ones, the proportion being one death to every three and a half cases not operated upon, and one death to every four of those operated upon.

Durham gives 50 per cent. of recoveries in non-operative cases and 77 per cent. of operative ones; also, he gives 74 per cent. of tracheotomy recoveries. Guyon and Durham, in 1674 cases, give 70 per cent. of recoveries in non-operative cases and 75 per cent. in operative ones.

Medico-legal cases arise in connection with impacted objects in the bronchi, as death is sometimes sudden. Only a few days since a mother was arrested for killing her child. Post-mortem revealed the fact that during the operation of spanking the child had swallowed a button, which had caused almost immediate death.

Conclusions.

1. The bronchus in dogs can be reached either anteriorly or posteriorly through the chest-walls, but the anatomical position is in such close proximity to large and important structures that safe incision is a matter of extreme difficulty and danger.

2. Bronchotomy through the walls of the thorax is an operation attended with great shock from collapse of the lungs, and until technique is further advanced is liable to result in immediate death.

3. Collapse of the lung is more serious in a healthy organ than in one previously crippled by disease.

4. The serious inherent difficulties are shock, suffocation from lung collapse, enormous risks of hemorrhage from pulmonary vessels, injury of or interference with the pneumogastric, great and fatal delays owing to the exaggerated movement of the root of the lung caused by the excessive dyspnœa.

5. Closure of the bronchial slit is slow and dangerous. To leave it open causes increasing pneumothorax by its valve action, and also permits the entrance of septic air into the pleural cavity.

6. Although a foreign body can be reached by this route, yet removal is hazardous. To secure a subsequent complete cure seems in the present state of knowledge very problematical.

7. When the presence of a foreign body in the bronchus is definitely determined, and primary voluntary expulsion has not been accomplished, there is great danger in permitting it to remain, even though it may but partially obstruct the tube. The risks both of immediate and of subsequent inflammation are serious.

8. Low tracheotomy is, then, advisable when the presence of a foreign body is certain ; it adds but little to the risks and affords easier escape for the object even when extraction is not feasible.

9. *Subsequent dangers arise from severe and prolonged instrumentation, not from tracheotomy.*

10. Voluntary expulsion is more probable after than before tracheotomy.

11. Tracheotomy is permissible even after an object has been long in position, unless serious lung changes have resulted.

12. The question of tracheotomy will depend largely upon the form, size, and character of the foreign body.

13. The term bronchotomy should be limited to an opening of the bronchus, and should not be employed to designate higher operations.

14. The risks from thoracotomy and bronchotomy following unsuccessful tracheotomy are much greater than the dangers incurred by permitting the foreign body to remain.

1818 CHESTNUT STREET

THE KINDRED OF CHOREA.

By OCTAVIUS STURGES, M.D., F.R.C.P.,

PHYSICIAN AND LECTURER ON MEDICINE AT THE WESTMINSTER HOSPITAL; PHYSICIAN TO THE HOSPITAL FOR SICK CHILDREN, GREAT ORMOND STREET.

THE help which statistics can bring to the pathology of chorea is of doubtful value. As regards its rheumatic relations in particular, figures are appealed to year by year to support conflicting views, and while it can hardly be said that opinion is less sharply divided to-day than a generation ago, it has certainly lost in vigor of expression. Thus the statements of Sir Dyce Duckworth,[1] that "chorea is a manifestation of the rheumatic habit," and that "rheumatism holds the first place in its etiology," though not wanting in boldness, are less daring and less direct than the simple words of Henri Roger thirty years back, declaring rheumatism and chorea to be one and the same affection under two forms. On the other hand, writers of repute, especially in Germany, deny altogether the kindred of the two disorders. Between these extremes there is much variety. Osler reckons the association of rheumatism with chorea, near and remote, to be 15 per cent., the Collective Investigation Committee makes it 26 per cent., Romberg and Steiner almost nothing per cent. The nearest approach to agreement may, perhaps, be stated thus: Cases of chorea occurring in immediate connection with rheumatism are very few, certainly under 10 per cent.

[1] International Clinic, April, 1891.

Cases of connection, either near or remote, are very differently stated by different observers, but according to most they fall below 30 per cent.

It is easy to account for this discrepancy. Rheumatism in children is apt to be so evanescent that we cannot assert positively of any child whatever that it has not been the subject of it. It can be invoked at pleasure. Of the many pains attributed to children, no one can separate for certain the rheumatic from the non-rheumatic. Apart from the parent's report, which is worthless in such a matter, even our immediate judgment as to the rheumatic nature of joint pain in young children is often open to question. There are growing pains and there is the fever of growth.[1] In the case of those choreic children who best resist an imputation of this sort, which can never be wholly disproved, there still remains the family to fall back upon, including, it is probable, some old persons who so name the pains of senility. But even so, the resources of the rheumatic advocate are not exhausted. Rheumatism—that is, in Sir Dyce Duckworth's phrase, "overt" rheumatism—may be before or after. The child has its life to live and its morbid manifestations to develop, rheumatic and other.[2]

Better than the expenditure of time and ingenuity in exercises like these is a frank admission that the precise admixture of chorea and rheumatism in the same subject is not ascertainable. Attention may then be directed to some unquestioned facts, clinical and anatomical, which not only render the kindred of these two affections a matter of certainty, but may also suggest something of the nature and method of the association.

The points I refer to are two, and they concern respectively (1) the cardinal anatomical feature of chorea, namely, endocarditis, and (2) the well-ascertained clinical fact that in the case of children exceptionally young—at that age, I mean, when both chorea and articular rheumatism are rare—there is a frequent and an intimate connection between the two affections which disappears in later life.

Of the first of these points, the morbid anatomy of chorea, it behooves us to speak with caution, inasmuch as death is its very rare event, so rare, indeed, that there are many with large experience of the disorder who have never seen it fatal. Partly on that account, and partly because post-mortem records of chorea are concerned mainly with the nervous system, the most striking feature in these fatal examples—I do not say the only striking feature—namely, the frequent presence of recent endocarditis (meaning by that term a fringe of soft, fibrinous beads at the edge of the mitral valve), has been too little regarded.

---

[1] Bouilly: Journal de Médecine, December, 1879.

[2] According to the Collective Investigation Committee's Report on Rheumatism (Brit. Med. Journ., September 29, 1888), this unknown quantity—the rheumatic yet to be—would not amount to much. In 655 rheumatic people 13 only, or about 2 per cent., had had chorea.

Some years ago I collected from various sources 80 cases of death
in connection with chorea,[1] or at least with symptoms so accounted.
Only half that number are reported with sufficient detail to be of much
value. Of the 40 that may be so described there are not more than 6
(one of them an elderly woman, who probably ought not to count) who
are free from " vegetations " on the mitral valve. Yet, as will be seen
presently, only a small proportion of the 40 have a rheumatic history.
Taking the 25 cases most completely reported, 22 by Dr. Dickinson and
3 by Dr. Peacock,[2] it appears that of the 22 as many as 17 have vegetations and 5 have none; of the 3 (all dying of the exhaustion of
chorea, and on that account the most apt examples) 2 have vegetations and only 1 has none. But this one, as we shall see, is among the
most striking examples of death by chorea anywhere recorded.

Notwithstanding this very common presence of endocarditis (using
the term here and elsewhere in the sense just given), only a few of these
fatal cases, I say, have a rheumatic history. Out of 32, 7 only could
be so accounted. Eighteen of these 32 may be said to have died not
only *with* but *of* chorea. Only 3 of them, so far as is known, are of
rheumatic origin. In other words the fatal cases, though mostly exhibiting endocarditis post-mortem, are not rheumatic, so far as their history
shows, in much larger proportion than other subjects of the disease.

It may be observed, by the way, of the majority of these fatal cases,
that they are not children, but growing-up boys and girls. In 35 examples of patients dying of or with chorea—an obvious distinction—20
are over thirteen and only 15 under that age. It would be easy to
show, further, that while fatal chorea happens mostly at the emotional
age, and to the emotional sex, its exciting cause is commonly some
obvious mental disturbance,[3] a fact which, taken in conjunction with
familiar experience of nervous children frightened into chorea, makes

---

[1] Chorea, p. 72.

[2] See Med. Chir. Trans., vol. lix. p. 27, and St. Thomas's Hospital Reports, vol. viii.
p. 27.

[3] See Chorea, p. 79, etc. A case of fatal chorea occurring lately in the practice of my
friend and colleague, Dr. Donkin (and which I have his permission to mention), is the
latest of many illustrations of this that have come under my notice. It illustrates also
certain points in connection with non-rheumatic endocarditis in chorea, presently to be
noticed. Thomas D., aged fifteen, has never had rheumatism, nor is there rheumatism
in the family. He was much alarmed by seeing a man killed by a tram-car. Three
weeks after, twitching movements were noticed. These were much aggravated three
days later, when the patient, being already in a highly nervous state, was startled by a
cat. Shortly after admission the chorea became very violent. The heart-sounds were
normal throughout. A week before death bedsores appeared. Admitted April 24.
Died May 23, 1891.

Post-mortem: Heart weighed five and three-quarters ounces; on the edge of the
mitral valve a complete ring of coarseish, small, but recent vegetations; endocardium
elsewhere normal.—Westminster Hospital, P. M. and Case-book, vol. vi. 292.

amazing the statement of Sir Dyce Duckworth that "rheumatism holds the first place in the etiology of chorea."

If it be considered how much larger is the total number of children suffering from chorea under thirteen than above that age, the fact that fatal cases (extremely rare at whatever age) are most frequent with the elder children, becomes the more significant. Fatal chorea in a young child becomes conspicuous by its rarity. In all my search I can discover but two examples of it—a boy aged eleven and a girl aged twelve—to be presently mentioned more particularly. And it so happens that these children aptly illustrate the fact already noticed, that endocarditis, although so common, is not a constant feature in the morbid anatomy of chorea. One of the children had it, the other had it not.

Now, the position brought to view by the foregoing facts is this: Endocarditis (in the sense just described) is to be found in the hearts of the great majority of patients dying with chorea, whether with or without rheumatic history. Is this condition of the endocardium to be regarded as of itself a proof of the "rheumatic habit," as Sir Dyce Duckworth puts it? If so, then it must follow upon post-mortem evidence, which is amply sufficient, that choreic patients are almost always rheumatic, and this notwithstanding that in the past history of most of them (as I have shown) no "overt" rheumatism appears.

Accepting the premises, all that could be urged against the conclusion, and this with no great force, would have reference to the extreme rarity of fatal chorea and the danger of basing pathology upon the showing of exceptional cases. But there is a word to be said before making the admission in question. It is this: While the frequency of endocarditis in fatal chorea is beyond all possible cavil, a broad distinction is to be drawn between those subjects who exhibit it post-mortem, and only so, and those who both in life and death are veritable examples of rheumatic chorea. In the one case endocarditis is only recognizable after death. It has no living signs, no progressive history of heart failure, and often no known rheumatism; in the other, endocarditis (anatomically similar, but not the same) is one of a series of well-marked cardiac changes, having their origin in rheumatism, and ending sooner or later in death, to which the chorea contributes nothing. In other words, the endocarditis attending chorea is of two forms. In one, the non-rheumatic, it is a post-mortem phenomenon, affecting the mitral valve, but not affecting the heart either clinically or anatomically—a liability of chorea as such; in the other, the rheumatic, it early becomes manifest, produces obvious physical changes, which, from their character and from the history of the patient, no one doubts to be rheumatic, and in its usual course, whether the chorea persist or not, is at last fatal by heart failure.

That the occurrence of endocarditis, both in chorea and rheumatism, supplies evidence of affinity between the two affections I shall not deny. It is no evidence at all that the subject of the former is personally rheumatic or of "rheumatic habit." It happens in chorea in one way and in rheumatism in another way.

In witness to the fact that the endocarditis of chorea is *sui generis*, that it has no objective signs, and that the manner of dying is precisely the same with it as without it, let me return to the two cases already referred to as among the most striking examples of their kind—one reported by Dr. Peacock, the other by myself—the patient being the late Dr. Fuller's, at St. George's Hospital. Both died of the exhaustion of violent and persistent chorea. Dr. Peacock's patient[1] was a girl of twelve, who had never had rheumatism, scarlatina, or any other serious illness. The attack was attributed, as it so often is in these fatal cases, to a nervous cause, the teasing of a mistress where she served as a nurse to a baby. She died thirty-four days after admission and forty-four from the commencement of the symptoms, exhausted by the constant movements. And in her case the heart and pericardium were found "quite healthy, and there were no vegetations on any of the valves," nor any other abnormal appearance. The St. George's patient, a boy of eleven,[2] showed precisely similar symptoms, and died like the other, worn out after two months' residence in the hospital and more than five months' endurance of the most violent chorea of unknown cause. No cardiac symptoms had been discovered in his case any more than with the girl. Post-mortem, however, the inner edge of the mitral showed a line of soft beads easily detached. Here, as in other instances that might be quoted (including Dr. Donkin's, just referred to), the endocarditis makes really no difference or distinction. But for post-mortem inspection its presence in the boy would never have been known. It was without objective sign, and the mode of death was exactly the same with it as without it.

It is not so that rheumatic endocarditis behaves. In those striking yet not common cases where acute rheumatism and chorea occur in close proximity, or alternating the one with the other, valve disease, the product not of the chorea, but of the rheumatism, tends early, as everyone knows, to mitral stenosis and consecutive changes in the heart's size and shape. In such children[3] it is in the intervals of the

---

[1] Loc. cit.   [2] Chorea, p. 174.

[3] In illustration of the class of cases here contemplated, and not for any special interest of its own, let me mention that of Mary E. H., under my care for a while at the Convalescent Branch of the Hospital for Sick Children (December, 1874), eventually dying in the London Hospital of heart disease. This child, aged eleven, had five or six attacks of chorea, the first preceded by rheumatism, but caused immediately by fright. She was admitted to the hospital for chorea, and had then well-marked mitral disease. When convalescent from the chorea, and at the Convalescent Hospital, peri-

rheumatic attacks, a little before or a little after, that chorea is apt to appear ; but its advent, unlike the rheumatic visitations, each of which brings new mischief, is of pathological interest rather than practical importance. The heart disease progresses the same, with the chorea or without it, and, as a common rule, death comes eventually through heart failure long after the child has outgrown the nervous disorder. Contrast such a case with any of those wherein recent endocarditis—a fringe of beads, that is to say, surrounding the mitral valve, but no other heart change—is found post-mortem in a choreic child who has never had rheumatism or shown any symptoms whatever of cardiac disturbance. Recent endocarditis, I say, taken alone without articular rheumatism, without pyrexia, and without physical signs, cannot be identified as rheumatic. If it be so found in chorea, as we know it is, it must be accepted as choreic ; there is no other place for it.

It would be possible to pursue the same line of argument further by reference to clinical facts indicating the essential difference between rheumatic and choreic endocarditis. For example, it is highly improbable that the latent endocarditis of chorea, such as I have described, is confined to fatal cases. What, then, becomes of it in those cases who recover ? If it follow the rheumatic pattern (as some, no doubt, will assert that it does), then chorea should be as fruitful a source of valve lesion as rheumatism, and a previous history of chorea would serve as well as a previous history of rheumatism to account for organic heart disease. It is not the habit of clinical observers so to regard it, nor are there many, I will venture to assert, who will deny that the common rule is for the abnormal cardiac sounds developed in chorea— and which, in the course of it, sometimes acquire a character closely resembling structural murmurs—to disappear altogether on the patient's recovery.

To what conclusions do such arguments tend ? Anatomically, endocarditis is the chief, if it be not the sole distinguishing feature of chorea, and in it rheumatism and chorea have a common factor. That is all. In its birth, its progress, and its consequences, rheumatic endocarditis is pathologically distinct from choreic endocarditis. Its occurrence in both affections does not show chorea to be rheumatic any more than it shows rheumatism to be choreic. Keeping in mind the specific character of endocarditis in the two cases respectively, there is no more

carditis set in; this was followed by lobar pneumonia, and the girl died two months after admission, the chorea entirely disappearing on the advent of the pericarditis.

Post-mortem the pericardium was universally adherent, but the adhesions were easily broken down. Recent endocarditis involved all the valves, and both auricles and ventricles were dilated. Middle lobe of right lung was hepatized. The left lung was œdematous and solid in patches. Both pleuræ were extensively adherent.—Hospital for Sick Children, vol. iii. 182.

ground for saying, as Sir Dyce Duckworth would have us say, that chorea is a manifestation of rheumatism than that rheumatism is a manifestation of chorea. The truth is that both are manifestations, and probably not the only ones, of some underlying condition yet to be defined.

From this point of view, indeed, if I may stay a moment to observe it, considering the indefinite and equivocal nature of symptoms often described as rheumatic, it seems remarkable that rheumatism, or "the rheumatic habit," should be put forward as the chief member and representative of a supposed pathological group, and especially that it should be regarded as the source of chorea. When mental disturbance is so described, there is no want of direct evidence to support the assertion. But it wants some physical basis, and offers no distinct image to the mind as to the mode of causation. When embolism is invoked to the same end, the physical changes suggested are definite and plausible enough, and the hypothesis only wants the sanction of fact. But to attribute chorea to the "rheumatic habit' may mean anything. It is, as we have seen, a statement beyond the reach of contradiction. It asserts nothing and suggests nothing, and no theory of causation has ever been proposed that has long held its ground.

Facts are accumulating which render it probable that the common symptom uniting a group of morbid phenomena we have been long seeking to reconcile and adjust, is arthritis. To narrow that word by any such epithet as rheumatic is misleading, especially in early life. It is time to abandon this easy method of lumping together the joint pains of chill, of fatigue, of growth, of certain ill-defined neurotic states, and, it may be added, of chorea itself. A certain disposition of body, so to speak, may show itself in chorea at one time of life, in rheumatism at another, in subcutaneous nodules or nervous arthritis at another. "Any form of nerve lesion," says Dr. Weir Mitchell, "the brain included, may develop in the joints conditions so precisely resembling rheumatic arthritis that no clinical skill can distinguish them." To set up one of these conditions above the others, to make one the parent of all the rest, is not only gratuitous, it is proved to be incorrect by the separate behavior of each. So it is, indeed, elsewhere. Evidence of kindred is not wanting in other morbid groups besides that which includes rheumatism and chorea, and over which rheumatism is assumed to preside, yet we do not, after the same arbitrary fashion, select one out of the group and subordinate the rest as its manifestations. Thus, when labial herpes occurs, as it often does, without lung signs, no one would say that it is a manifestation of pneumonia. But it is most reasonable to say, in virtue of their frequent concurrence and parallel symptoms, that these two affections are allied in their pathogenesis.

But apart from the argument supplied by endocarditis in its relation to chorea and to rheumatism respectively, there is, I think, a further reason for supposing that chorea and rheumatism are two members of one family. It is afforded by the fact of their close alliance in early childhood. They separate more and more widely as life goes on, the differing circumstances of the two serving to draw them apart until, at length, the signs of kinship are hardly discernible.

Some three years ago I had the good fortune to encounter chorea at an unusually early time of life[1] in a girl a month under three years of age. A year before her birth the mother, aged thirty-seven, had acute rheumatism. The father, aged forty-three, was said to be " rheumatic." The child had been very " nervous " since an accident, starting and screaming in sleep and tossing the arms and legs about. During the last month she had been weak and uncertain on her legs, and on admission she was unable to feed herself. The patient was extremely emotional, and choreic movement was pretty generally distributed over face, hands, and feet; the right arm was partially paretic. Now this child, though with no open sign of rheumatism, had at the heart's apex in the fourth space, half an inch within the left nipple line, a loud and (on admission) musical systolic murmur conducted into the axilla and heard distinctly behind; evidence, that is to say—congenital heart disease being excluded—of endocarditis, not choreic, but rheumatic.

In the previous year I published the case of a girl,[2] three years and six months old, and with no family history of rheumatism, who became my patient for slight choreic movement of the right hand and arm, with imperfect control of the right leg and difficult speech. She, too, had a loud and conducted systolic murmur, with feeble thrill. Three weeks before admission the child had been noticed to be " feverish," and the night before the movements began she had been frightened by a quarrel between her parents. In the second week of the child's admission a pericardial friction rub was detected, and the chorea ceased. Presently the back of the right hand was found to be swollen and painful ; the left wrist followed, two subcutaneous nodules appeared, while at the same time the heart became uneven and the area of its dulness increased upward. The patient ultimately died, and no post-mortem examination was permitted. We had ample evidence, however, not only of rheumatism and endocarditis, but of pericarditis also. The case was, in fact, an example of rheumatism, with its usual cardiac accompaniments. It was, at the same time, intimately connected with chorea, and the subject was exceptionally young.

I need not repeat here the figures quoted in the paper referred to,

1 Lancet, January 21, 1888.
2 " The Rheumatic Element in Chorea," Archives of Pædiatrics, May, 1887.

showing (1) the rarity both of rheumatism and chorea under four years of age, and (2) the frequent and intimate association of these two affections at this exceptionally early period of life for the occurrence of either. A mere numerical statement, indeed, does not disclose the full strength of the case, unless the intimacy of the connection is considered as well. My own personal testimony[1] is to this effect: In 177 cases of chorea there are eight under six years old; *all but one are girls.* One of these must be omitted owing to defective information. Of the seven only three were certainly exempt from rheumatism. Three certainly, and a fourth probably, were rheumatic. Add to this the only examples procurable, so far as I know, below the age of four, the two I have just quoted, both showing chorea and rheumatism intimately associated, and the conclusion is not to be resisted that the rheumatic element is conspicuous in the chorea of very young children, almost all of them being girls.[2]

Now, if chorea be considered without reference to age, this close connection with rheumatism is less apparent. It is seen chiefly, as I have said, at that early period of existence when the two affections are first discernible. As the time of life approaches when chorea becomes rare, while rheumatism—the acute polyarthritis rheumatica of young men and young women—attains its fullest development, this near connection is rarely seen. That the interval which separates these two affections should thus go on widening with growth, so that in the end sometimes rheumatism, sometimes chorea, emerges (not to speak of forms of neurotic arthritis, of which we know little), is not wonderful when we consider that each of these affections has its own separate exciting cause, and that each, once excited, is very apt to recur. The accidents of life will favor one rather than the other—exposure tending to rheumatic arthritis in one case, mental strain to chorea in another. In early life, when the affinity is the strongest, and before these separating causes have come into operation, rheumatism and chorea may alternate. But chorea tends to die out with puberty, while rheumatism waits for puberty for its fullest development. Every repetition of the latter affection strengthens its hold and enlarges its clinical features—the rheumatism of seventeen being more express and distinct than that of seven. Meanwhile the natural disposition to chorea is weakening, and the time of life approaches when it ceases altogether.

The several points I desire to affirm are these:

1. Recent endocarditis, with no further heart change, is the cardinal anatomical feature in those dying with chorea without reference to

---

[1] Chorea, p. 180.

[2] The single case quoted by Dr. Dickinson (loc. cit.) under five was in immediate connection with rheumatism, " general articular rheumatism just before chorea."

rheumatism.   Yet it is not constantly found, and some of the most striking examples of deaths by chorea are without it.

2. Choreic endocarditis is distinguishable from rheumatic endocarditis both clinically and anatomically.   Clinically it is without physical or general signs, often without rheumatism, and only disclosed post-mortem. Anatomically the inflammation is recent, its chief, often its only seat, is the mitral valve, and there are no consecutive changes in the heart. The contrast to this condition is seen in rheumatic children with valve disease who are or who have been choreic.   In them the physical signs observed during life correspond with well-recognized changes in the valves and heart chambers found after death and due to the rheumatism and not to the chorea.

3. Choreic endocarditis, therefore, is not accurately described as a manifestation of rheumatism.   Both chorea and rheumatism are liable to this inflammation, each after its own manner.   The common feature may be taken as evidence that the two affections are pathologically allied, not that either of them is a form or expression of the other.

4. The fact of this alliance is best seen by the observation of chorea in very early life, at which period it is often intimately associated with rheumatic polyarthritis in the same subject and at the same time.   But with growth, in obedience to the natural history of the two affections respectively, and influenced by the several accidents of life, this association is relaxed, and at puberty it has ceased to be intimate.

5. Both chorea and rheumatism are, it is probable, members of a pathological group which has arthritis for a common factor, and of whose underlying source we are yet in search.

JACKSONIAN EPILEPSY; TREPHINING; REMOVAL OF SMALL TUMOR, AND EXCISION OF CORTEX.

By CHARLES K. MILLS, M.D.,
NEUROLOGIST TO THE PHILADELPHIA HOSPITAL, ETC.,

AND

W. W. KEEN, M.D.,
PROFFSSOR OF SURGERY IN THE JEFFERSON MEDICAL COLLEGE.

MEDICAL HISTORY BY DR. MILLS.

S. W., female, twenty-seven years old ; height, five feet; weight, ninety-eight pounds.   Until the first symptoms of the spasmodic affection for which she applied for treatment she had been in excellent health, with the exception of an attack of chronic otitis when a child, which had left her with a perforated membrana tympani and the occasional recurrence of a slight discharge.   Ten years before coming under observation, while in a cold room in the northwest, she had for the first time a slight attack of left hemiparæsthesia; her left hand, arm, and foot became numb and heavy. The sensation passed off in a few moments and was not accompanied by spasm or vertigo; but from this time, at intervals of weeks or months, she had attacks, usually slight, of the same character. Handling or unusual movements of the left arm would sometimes bring them on; at other times they would come on without any apparent exciting cause. Between four and five years after the first of these sensory seizures, she had for the first time, as an accompaniment, a spasm involving both the left upper and lower extremity, but more marked in the former. From this time on she had at irregular, but more frequent intervals, these sensory and motor attacks, the spasm beginning on the left side, but after a time markedly attacking the right arm as well. The seizures increased in frequency, until after a few months she had them almost every day, and often six or seven during the twenty-four hours. The only time when she was free from them for a long period was in the spring of 1890, when, while suffering with a fever, she had no attacks for about three weeks. Although the attacks increased in severity and frequency, they had for many months remained much the same as they were when she first came under observation. She had been treated by various physicians, and on several occasions bromide treatment had been pushed, but always without any improvement, and usually she thought she grew worse under the use of drugs. She was sent to me for diagnosis and treatment by Dr. H. C. Yarrow, of Washington, D. C. Her general health, mental and physical, was good, and she had no evidence of paralysis.

Soon after coming under observation I had several opportunities of witnessing her seizures, and one description would answer for all, with the exception that sometimes her consciousness was more deeply affected than at others. She would feel a prickling sensation in her left arm, and would utter a plaintive cry. The left arm would immediately extend at the shoulder and elbow, and almost coincidently the left leg would become spastic in extension, and the head would be twisted to the right. The right upper extremity would then be strongly flexed at the elbow, and the whole limb carried over the chest, as if the hand was grasping at the precordial region. The spasm continued for a few seconds, passing off with a laughing sound and facial expression. In the shortest attacks she did not appear to lose consciousness at all, and during the early weeks that she remained under observation she never seemed to be completely unconscious during the seizures, and could detail most of what was said and done by others during them. She sometimes complained of having pain in the precordial region. She repelled any touching or handling during the spells, and explained afterward that it hurt her and made her worse.

At first the case was regarded as probably one of hystero-epilepsy, and the patient was treated with tonics and gymnastics to improve her general and nervous health, but in spite of such treatment and the best of care her attacks grew more frequent and severe. About three months after coming under observation, an attack, which began in the usual manner, became extremely violent, and was attended with total unconsciousness. In November the patient began to have day and night as many as ten to fifteen serious attacks. After several consultations with Drs. Mitchell, Keen, Sinkler and Lloyd, it was finally decided that an operation should be performed.

In deciding on a site for operation the history and character of the sensory and spasmodic attacks were carefully considered. The case had begun with sensory disturbance in the limbs of the left side, particularly in the upper extremity. The spasm had first affected this side, and usually, as nearly as could be determined, was initiated with a shoulder movement on this side, although the spasm diffused and extended so rapidly to all parts of the left arm and leg, and to the right upper extremity, that it was sometimes difficult to determine how it began. Sometimes, however, the right side escaped. On the left side the patient showed slight drooping and apparent weakness of the muscles about the mouth, although this was so little marked as to be scarcely more than is not infrequently present normally.

Operation was performed December 10, 1890, by Dr. W. W. Keen. The following were present at the operation : Dr. Roswell Park, of Buffalo ; Dr. Raphael Lorini, of Washington ; Drs. W. J. Taylor, Wharton Sinkler, J. H. Lloyd, F. X. Dercum, J. B. Deaver, De F. Willard, M. I. Bassette, and J. W. McConnell.

On the day preceding the operation Dr. Bassette examined the patient and made the following report of her condition : Pupils normal; slight drooping of the left upper lip, but otherwise the face normal ; no paralysis of the limbs ; no impairment of touch, sight, taste, or smell. Hearing much impaired on the left side. Dr. C. S. Turnbull had previously examined her ears, and had reported a chronic otitis media with perforation, which required but little treatment, and which he thought had nothing to do with her brain symptoms. Knee-jerk was present ; no ankle clonus. Heart and lungs were normal.

SURGICAL HISTORY AND REMARKS BY DR. KEEN.

On the day before the operation the carpet was taken up, the walls wiped down, and the floor, woodwork, etc., were washed with a solution of carbolic acid, 1 to 40. The patient's head was shaved and carefully disinfected. The position of the fissure of Rolando was outlined first by means of Hare's method, and then by that of Horsley, the cranial index being determined from measurements made as follows :

Antero-posterior diameter 19.1 cm.; biparietal diameter 14.3 cm. $14.3 \div 19.1 = 0.748 +$. Practically the cranial index was therefore 0.75 ; and this corresponded to an angle of 69° for the Rolandic fissure. From glabella to inion was 13.25.

The position for the trephine centre was fixed 1.75 inch to the right of the median line, in the line of the fissure of Rolando and was marked on the scalp by a small puncture in the bone. The fissure of Rolando was also marked at its two extremities by two similar punctures in the bone, so as to identify it after its surface marking was lost by the lifting of the flap.

A large horseshoe flap was made, and on turning this back no abnormal appearances of the skull were found. The centre pin of a 1½ inch trephine was now inserted 1.75 inch from the median line as before determined, the upper edge of the trephine reaching to a point 1 inch from the median line.

Dr. Roswell Park kindly did the trephining for me, so that my hands should not be unsteadied by the muscular fatigue involved in this part of the operation. It was very fortunate that I asked him to do so, for the skull was very thick and the trephining required time and a good deal of muscular effort. The thickness of the button removed varied from $\frac{5}{16}$ inch to $\frac{7}{16}$ inch, and the diploë was almost entirely obliterated. The under surface of the button of bone was eroded in a number of connected small pits corresponding to the small growth described below. The little pits resembled a miniature bunch of grapes, the stem of the

FIG. 1.

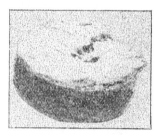

The button of bone removed, showing its thickness and the erosion caused by the tumor of the dura and the vessel supplying it.

bunch consisting of a vessel of considerable size which had also eroded the bone. On the removal of the button of bone, free hemorrhage took place from the dura at the margin of the trephine opening where this vessel ran, but the bleeding was soon controlled by a ligature. The tip of the growth was $\frac{1}{16}$ inch in front of, and the same distance internal to the centre of the trephine opening. The growth was elevated $\frac{1}{4}$ inch above the surface of the dura, and after cutting the dura and lifting the flap, it was found that the granulation or growth had its origin apparently from the pia, and had bored through the dura and formed a nest for itself in the skull. The dura and the pia were adherent at the point where the growth lay.

A triangular bit of the dura, including the growth, was removed by the scissors and placed in Müller's fluid. The exposed pia-arachnoid was œdematous with enlarged veins and capillaries. Nothing else abnormal was found. A fissure corresponding to the line of the fissure of Rolando was seen, and five convolutions were exposed, all of which appeared to be normal. (See Fig. 2.) From the moment that the brain was exposed no antiseptics were applied to it, but only warm, boiled water.

Careful investigations were then made with the faradic current with a view of determining the cortical centres exposed. A small bipolar antiseptic electrode was used. A secondary current was applied; the electrode was connected with the terminal of a Flemming faradic battery, and the current was obtained by passing the switch to the first button of the instrument, and withdrawing the regulating cylinder to a distance of $2\frac{1}{4}$ inches.

Several spots were selected, marked 1, 2, 3, and 4 (see Fig. 2). The first electric tests were made at the spots 1 and 2. From the measurements that had been made, the fissure of Rolando was in the direction indicated by the line seen in the illustration.

Electricity was first applied to the spot marked 1 for a moment only.

Movement at once resulted, beginning in the upper extremity on the left side, the first movement being protraction and moderate adduction of the shoulder and upper arm. This was followed by a series of jerks, involving the upper, and to a more moderate degree, the lower arm. No differentiated movements of the hand and arm, and no face or upper leg contractions, were observed. The left toes and foot, however, slightly flexed coincidently with the shoulder movement.

Fig. 2.

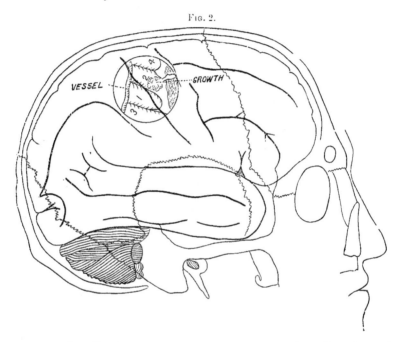

A second application was made at the point marked 2. The effect of this excitation was again to produce decided shoulder and arm movements, with greater adduction and some protraction of the entire arm. The thigh was flexed upon the pelvis at an angle of about 130°, and the leg upon the thigh to about the same, with abduction of the thigh and extension of the toes and foot. At the same time, active, coarse, clonic movements diffused through both extremities. This series of movements of the left upper and lower extremities strongly resembled the spasms which occurred in the patient's ordinary attacks, with the exception that the head was not turned to the right, and no face movements were noted. The application was repeated at 2, with similar results, with the addition that the face and head turned to the left, and the head was drawn downward and to the left, chiefly by platysmic action.

The electrical tests clearly indicated that the centres for the shoulder, upper arm, thigh and knee had been determined, or probably the region which represents the merging of the movements of the upper and lower extremities. A consultation was held with reference to the propriety of excising this region, and it was determined to do this, first, in order to make a sub-cortical exploration for any further lesion, and secondly, to prevent the recurrence of the spasms by removing what seemed to be their primary seat.

With a pair of scissors and sharp bistoury a portion of the cortex. three-quarters of an inch in diameter, was removed. It included all the cortical gray matter under the tumor and corresponding to the centre for the shoulder as ascertained by the battery. The arm, leg and face were carefully observed during excision, but this mechanical excitation was absolutely without effect in producing movements.

After excision the electrodes were now applied to the points 3 and 4 on the border of the excision.

Excitation at the point marked 3 flexed the elbow, hand and wrist with slight shoulder abduction, protraction closely following.

Excitation at 4 caused primary movements of abduction and flexion of the thigh upon the pelvis, and the leg upon the thigh at an angle of 135° or 140°. No foot movements or movements of the upper extremities occurred. In all the trials after the excision of the cortex the movements were confined to the left half of the body.

After the excision had been performed considerable trouble arose in checking the hemorrhage from a large vessel, but this was controlled by two ligatures passed into the brain, and by temporary packing with iodoform gauze. During the operation small bits of iodoform gauze were packed between the dura and the skull to check some hemorrhage. The pulse fluctuated markedly, becoming for a short time weak and rapid. The extremities also became cold. The hemorrhage having been checked by pressure and hot water, after the ligature referred to had been applied, a small rubber drainage-tube was inserted through the defect in the dura. A small bundle of horsehairs was also passed through and through under the flap, which was then sutured into place and dressed as usual. The bone was not replaced, as this was not deemed wise in consequence of its thickness and its sclerosed condition.

On December 11th, the first day after the operation, the drainage-tube was removed. On the 13th, the third day, the horsehair was removed, and a slight escape of cerebro-spinal fluid occurred. On the 15th, the fifth day, nine stitches were taken out and five were left. On the 21st, the eleventh day, the last stitches were removed from the wound, which was entirely healed except at one or two of the stitch-holes and where the flap was at a slightly different level.

Temperature record for ten days after operation.—*December* 10. 4.40 P.M., 96.6°; 8 P.M., 100.6°.

11th (first day after operation)	8 A.M., 99.8°;		4 P.M., 99.4°;		8 P.M., 100.2°.
12th (second day)	"	100.2°	"	100.4°	"	100.2°.
13th (third day)	"	99.2°	"	99.4°	"	99.4°.
14th (fourth day)	"	100.6°	"	99.2°	"	99.2°.
15th (fifth day)	"	98.4°	"	99.2°	"	99.4°.
16th (sixth day)	"	98.4°	"	98.8°	"	98.6°.
17th (seventh day)	"	98°	"	98.8°	"	99.2°.
18th (eighth day)	"	98°	"	98.8°	"	98.6°.
19th (ninth day)	"	97.6°	"	99°	"	98.6°.
20th (tenth day)	"	97°	"	98.6°	"	98.8°.

REMARKS.—The bone was so much thickened and sclerosed as to raise the question whether there was not possibly an element of hereditary syphilis in the case, but this it was learned could be positively excluded. In the absence of such an explanation it was, of course, possible that the thickening of the bone was due to the irritation caused by the pressure of the little growth. Whether it was only a local thickening could not be accurately ascertained at the operation. In either case it seemed unwise to replace the bone.

Accuracy of localization. The accuracy of the localization of the shoulder centre and also of the centres in its neighborhood is worthy of remark. The tip of the growth was found within one-sixteenth of an inch of the point selected as the location of the shoulder centre and the probable seat of the irritation.

The nature of the growth. Its appearance suggested that it was a hypertrophied pacchyonian body, but the microscopical examination showed that it was sarcomatous, with some hemorrhagic pachymeningitis. That it was the probable cause of the epileptic attacks seems very reasonable. Unfortunately, the irritation had possibly continued long enough to establish the epileptic habit, and to this may be due the fact that the attacks have continued since the operation, though with lessened frequency and severity ; or, as suggested by Dr. Mills, sarcomatous growths or infiltration may be present elsewhere in the brain. Whether the attacks will ultimately disappear or not is a question which we are not yet in a position to decide.

Excision of the cortex. The operation might have been limited to the removal of the growth and the dura which contained it, and then later, had the attacks not disappeared, a second operation might have been done and the shoulder centre removed. Against this, however, is the argument that a second operation involves a second peril to life, and also that the convolutions might be so adherent to the flap and the new tissue which would fill the opening, that it might be difficult at the second operation to recognize them, and to delimit the centres to be removed with the same accuracy that we could at the primary operation. All the questions which present themselves on reflection upon such cases should be stated with a view to their consideration, and the determination of what is the wisest course.

Drainage. Since this operation was done I have operated on a number of cerebral cases, with absolute closure of the wound without drainage. In two cases there has been considerable accumulation of bloody serum which has been evacuated by gentle separation of the flap between the sutures. In one case this had to be done four times, and in the other but once ; so that I am now quite convinced that, as a rule, drainage can be dispensed with in cerebral operations. Had it been dispensed with in this case the apparent risk of a fungus cerebri would have been avoided. In fact, I think this one of the strongest reasons why drainage should not be employed in cerebral cases. Possibly a few strands of horsehair might be used to advantage for twenty-four hours, but a drainage-tube should not be used.

After removal of the dura, cannot the loss of substance be made good by the transplantation of a piece of the pericranium? In the after-history of the case one point was purposely not mentioned, but reserved for consideration here. A few days after the operation the flap bulged to such an extent that I was afraid that the union of the flap to the rest of the scalp would give way, and that a fungus cerebri would appear, especially at the site of the drainage-tube. Fortunately, this did not occur, but the bulging gradually subsided and the wound healed without incident. In reflecting upon this case, it occurred to me that the conditions were most favorable for the formation, almost inevitably, of a fungus cerebri, which I believe actually took place subcutaneously, but fortunately subsided without appearing on the surface. Under the flap was a deep well, corresponding to the thickened bone, the dura, and the excised portion of the brain; in depth perhaps an inch or more.

When the dura is opened and closed by suture there is little danger of a fungus cerebri, but where there is a loss of substance of the dura, and especially where the cortex is excised, there is a marked tendency to the formation of a fungus cerebri, especially where the distance between the scalp and the surface of the excised portion of the brain is as deep as in this case. To avoid this it occurred to me that we had ready means at hand in the transplantation of a piece of the pericranium similar to the transplantation of skin by Thiersch's method.

On the 10th of May, 1891, in another case operated upon at the Jefferson College Hospital, an opportunity occurred to me to test this. A piece of the pericranium was separated from the scalp, cut loose, and attached by a few interrupted sutures at its margin to the dura, thus filling the gap produced by the excision of a piece of the dura. The transplanted bit was turned upside down, so that the osteogenetic surface lay upward, in order that if bone should form from it, it should grow upward into the gap in the skull, rather than downward, and so possibly press upon the brain. The result was all that I could wish. No fungus cerebri formed, and up to September 1st he had not only been entirely free from his epileptic attacks, but no mischief had arisen from the transplanted pericranium, which presumably therefore has retained its vitality.

Can we differentiate normal from apparently normal, yet, in fact, diseased cortex, by means of the battery? This question I cannot yet answer positively, but I am inclined to think that it may be answered possibly in the affirmative. If we faradize a normal cortical centre (motor) by a single application, for a moment we get response in a single motor expression of its function, and the muscles cease to respond the moment the electrodes are removed. In several cases of visibly diseased cortex, by a similar single and short application of the electrodes, I have evoked not a single motor response, but have started an epileptic fit, resembling in the part in which it started and in its march the fits from which the patient had suffered. After excision of the diseased cortex similar brief stimulation has produced only the normal single motor response. It may be that this is explained by the fact that the first stimulation was of gray matter, and the last of white matter after the excision of the former. In some cases in which I have operated on the brain after injury and loss of brain-substance, presumably cortical (chiefly so, at least), faradization of the diseased and disintegrated brain-substance, presumably chiefly white matter, has started the characteristic fit, and, after excision, faradization of the underlying apparently normal matter has again given me a single normal response. If, then, faradization of apparently normal cortex induces a typical epileptic fit, instead of a single motor response, can we conclude that, though normal to the eye and finger, it is really diseased and should be excised? If so, this will be a most important and valuable aid to us.

My observations on this point are yet too few to warrant a definite conclusion.

MEDICAL HISTORY AFTER THE OPERATION, AND CERTAIN SPECIAL FEATURES OF THE CASE, BY DR. MILLS.

History of loss and recovery of power in the left limbs after the operation; sensory investigation. When the patient came to from the effects of the ether, she had a feeling of numbness and heaviness in the left arm and hand, and also at times in the back of the left shoulder—what she described as a " battery sensation," or a feeling of prickling. Five hours after the completion of the operation she was cautiously tested for motion and sensation. The tests were not elaborate, for fear of disturbing her too much. The left shoulder movements were paralyzed, but all the forearm, hand, and finger movements were retained, but weak. The power of flexion at the elbow was very feeble, probably abolished; extension was present, but much diminished. So far as could be determined, sensations of touch, pain, and temperature were preserved.

December 11 (first day after operation). The loss of power in the left arm and leg were about the same as noted the day before. Dynamometer: Right hand, 50; left hand, 26. Sensation was carefully tested for and found to be normal.

12th (second day after operation). The paralysis of the shoulder persisted, that of the upper arm was increased, and the loss below the elbow and in the hand and fingers was more marked. The left leg was growing much weaker; the loss of power was most decided below the knee.

13th (third day after operation). The foot movements were almost entirely abolished, but some power of flexion and extension of the thigh remained. The left upper extremity was completely paralyzed. No loss of sensation could be made out in the shoulder or anywhere in the upper or lower extremities.

From December 13th to 20th (third to tenth day after operation) the paralyzed left extremities remained the same—paralysis was total in the arm and almost so in the leg, the only power retained in the latter being that of pushing the leg downward after it had been thrust upward and held by the examiner. On December 20th (the tenth day after operation) the patient had slight power of extension and flexion of the thigh, and marked increase of power of extending or thrusting the limb downward against resistance. Gradually power returned in the lower extremity, as nearly as could be made out in the following order: Thigh extension, thigh flexion, abduction, adduction. Until January 3d (the twenty-fourth day after operation) no foot movements below the knee returned. At this date signs of flexion and extension at the ankle appeared. January 2d, she could flex the leg over the thigh, and cross the left leg over the right, and could perform, but in a feeble manner, all movements of the foot and leg.

No change was observed in the paralysis of the arm until December 29th (nineteenth day after operation) when, if the forearm was slightly flexed, she could extend it; at this time, as above noticed, she had regained considerable power in the lower extremity. January 1, 1891 (twenty-second day after operation) she began to flex the distal and second phalanges, but had no power of phalangeal extension, and no wrist movements. On January 3d (twenty-fourth day after operation) she could flex, extend and separate the fingers and hand, but had no elbow or shoulder movements. On January 6th (the twenty-seventh day after operation) she gained decided power in flexing and extending the elbow, and on January 7th the (twenty-eighth day after operation) she could elevate the arm nearly in a horizontal line. On January 12th (the thirty-third day after operation) she had regained all movements of both upper and lower extremities, and had been able to walk for several days. The limbs remained weak, and this weakness continued most decided for shoulder movements. All true paralysis, however, had practically disappeared.

The order in which paralysis of different muscular groups appeared and disappeared is of considerable physiological interest.

Knee-jerk was found to be increased on the left side, and ankle clonus was present on the day after operation. Gradually the exaggerated knee-jerk diminished, and on December 23d (thirteen days after operation), when the power of flexing and extending the thigh had greatly improved, ankle clonus disappeared.

History of spasms after operation. At 4.30 P.M, on the day of the operation, the patient had a slight attack without unconsciousness, in which the right arm at the elbow and wrist was flexed, but the arm was not carried over the chest as in the old attacks; the head was drawn to the right. The left extremities and face and the right leg were not involved.

December 11 (first day after operation). She had light seizures at 5, 6 and 8.30 P.M. The spasm affected both arms and the left leg.

12th (second day after operation). Attacks at 4, 7.30, 8.30 and 10.30 A.M., and 12.50 P.M. Both arms and left leg were involved in the spasm; the head was drawn to the left. At 7.30 P.M. she had an attack, the spasm affecting both arms and left leg; the head was drawn to the right.

13th (third day after operation). Attacks at 1.35, 5.40 A.M. Both arms and right leg were affected; the head was drawn to the right. She had other attacks in the afternoon and evening.

14th (fourth day after operation). Attacks at 6.45, 8.30, 9.30 A.M.; none P.M. Both arms and right leg were involved; the toes were flexed; the head was drawn to the right.

15th (fifth day after operation). Attacks at 12.15, 1.15, 7.45 A.M., affecting the arms and right leg; the head was drawn to the right.

16th (sixth day after operation). No attacks.

17th (seventh day after operation). Attacks at 4.30, 6.45, 7.45 A.M., spasm invading both arms and left leg; the head was drawn to the right.

A careful daily record was kept of the spasmodic seizures until February 1, 1891—that is, for a period of nearly eight weeks after the operation. She averaged four or five attacks daily, occasionally only one, two, or three. The majority of these seizures were in the early morning hours, between 1 and 2 A.M. They were commonly of moderate severity, none of them as severe as the frequent attacks which she had had several weeks just preceding the operation. The character of the attacks was usually as already described, but they varied somewhat at different times. As a rule, both arms took part, the right upper extremity becoming spastic in flexion, the left either in extension or extended and affected with some clonic spasm; the left leg was usually extended, but was sometimes flexed. The right leg, when included in the spasm, was usually semi-flexed at the hip and knee. During the week from January 26th to February 1st, the average number of seizures was somewhat smaller, on the 26th being only three, on the 31st two, and on the other days three, four, and five. So far as the distribution of the spasm in different parts of the body was concerned, their severity was somewhat influenced by the varying degrees of loss and recovery of power on the side paralyzed after the operation. About three days after the operation, as will be recalled, the paralysis of the upper and lower extremity was almost complete, and for several days the left leg took little part, or no part, in the spasm, taking, however, an increasing part as power was recovered. The same was true of the left arm. During most of the time that these notes were taken the spasms preponderated on the right side, the morbid ascendancy of the left side, however, reasserting itself as power was more and more recovered.

This patient has been seen at longer or shorter intervals from the time of operation—December 10, 1890—to July 7, 1891. Her history has been a monotonous one, and can be condensed into a few sentences. Usually she has had about three attacks of spasm in twenty-four hours, these, as a rule, occurring during the night, most commonly in the early morning hours. Sometimes she has had an attack after daylight, between 6 and 8 o'clock in the morning. Occasionally she has had two attacks in succession. The spasms have never attained the severity or frequency which they had for a short time prior to the operation. She had then as many as twelve to fifteen in twenty-four hours, often with total unconsciousness, involuntary urination, and subsequent great dazing and confusion of mind. At the time of the last examination and report, and for some time previous, the attacks usually began with a feeling of numbness in the left shoulder and a lifting and jerking movement of the entire left arm. The spasm spread, involving the left side and sometimes also the right side. Sometimes she was unconscious in the attack, but as often not. She now has good use of both the left arm and the left leg, all movements being preserved. The left arm, however, shows some general weakness, is easily fatigued, and the patient thinks that over-use of it brings on the spells. Her general health is good—better than for a long time—and she has gained from five to ten pounds since the operation.

The small growth of granulation, with the attached piece of dura mater, and also the excised segment of cortical and subcortical tissue, were placed in the hands of Dr. Allen J. Smith for microscopical examination. Dr. Smith has prepared six slides showing the appearance of the membrane, growth, or granulation, and of the excised cortex. He reports that connected with the growth or granulation are spots of hemorrhagic pachymeningitis, and several points in its interior which are decidedly sarcomatous. He also reports that beyond the engorgement of the vessels and the presence of hemorrhage at the surface, and at one point at the margin, that the excised cortex was apparently normal.

At the time of the operation the general impression of those present was that the small growth was a large, isolated, pacchyonian granulation, which had perforated the dura and eroded the inner wall of the skull. The microscopical examination throws a doubt upon that view, and makes it more likely that after all we had a real neoplasm of very small size; but perhaps, without further investigation, the question may not be regarded as absolutely decided. If the growth was sarcomatous, other sarcomatous foci may be present in the brain; and it was in part because of the suspicion that a subcortical mass might be present that the cortex was excised. It is not improbable that the other hemisphere may contain a growth, as the localizing symptoms were at times confusing. The patient had clonic spasms of the right arm, although, as has been stated in the clinical history, the symptoms began on the left side and the attacks were initiated by both sensory and motor disturbances on this side. Since the operation right-sided spasms have often been a striking feature.

Supposing that the small tumor was a pacchyonian formation, it would be by no means certain that this had not to do with the causation of the spasmodic phenomena; and still another view that might be taken is that such a formation had resulted from the frequent and long-continued localized cortical discharges with their accompanying hyperæmia. The question of pacchyonian formations in general, and particularly of those which we sometimes see either isolated or in small groups, may have some importance in connection with the subject of cortical epilepsy and paresis.

The nature of these granulations is probably still an unsettled matter. Little, at least in late years, has been written about them; but an interesting article is that by W. Browning,[1] from which I may cull a few

[1] THE AMERICAN JOURNAL OF THE MEDICAL SCIENCES (N. S.), vol lxxxiv., October, 1882, p. 370.

facts and views applicable to the present case. These formations grow from the pia-arachnoid, both over the sulci and over the crests of the convolutions. It seems to be universally admitted that these formations are limited to certain parts of the pia-arachnoid, showing a decided preference for the sides of the longitudinal sinus and the vicinity. Some, but not all, of these granulations are connected with the veins and sinuses.

Other structures connected with them are the parāsinoidal spaces, which occur along the sides of the longitudinal sinus, and are of the largest size at the crown of the head. Browning suggests that these are important accessories to the veins and sinuses as regulators of the cerebral pressure. Sometimes the pacchyonian granulations and para-sinoidal venous spaces are combined and connected. When venous spaces are present the granulations are not likely to cause depressions in the skull. It would seem from these facts that whether a pacchyonian granulation would or would not cause greater or less cortical irritation might depend upon its peculiar location, and the presence or absence of venous spaces into which it could grow. A growth such as was found at this trephining may have caused considerable irritation.

On the other hand, as already intimated, such a formation may have been the result of repeated discharges of the adjacent cortical area. As Browning states, and as I can verify from abundant experience at the Philadelphia Hospital, many morbid conditions may favor the development of these bodies, one of which of great importance is chronic alcoholism. This writer also states that in cases of brain tumor an excessive development of these pacchyonian bodies has often been found. They have often been found in adults and children suffering from meningitis, and probably some granulations, particularly those associated with meningitis, may be inflammatory in origin, and in reality somewhat different from the usual pacchyonian growths. Formerly they were all regarded as inflammatory. Browning shows that, while much evidence may be had in support of hyperæmia as their cause, some facts do not harmonize with this hypothesis. He holds rather to a mechanical cause, depending in some way upon the ebb and flow of the blood of the veins just above the sinuses. It is not hyperæmia of the venous blood as such, but the blood acting as any other fluid of its consistence would do.

Some clinical symptoms have been attributed to pacchyonian granulations, but only a few can with any positiveness be regarded as due to these formations. Browning refers to cases where such granulations were present near the Gasserian ganglion and the motor nerves of the eye, causing ocular neuralgic and paretic symptoms. Meyer refers various neuralgias to them. Headaches have been attributed to them in some instances, but with doubtful propriety. Possibly they may cause sinus thrombosis. They sometimes produce little flat elevations of bone along the median line of the crown of the head. I do not know of any record of cases of spasm, local or general, which could be clearly attributed to pacchyonian bodies. Browning refers to a varix of the sinus longitudinalis which he believed developed from the parasinoidal spaces, and quotes a case of Meschede in which a patient had suffered from epilepsy for thirty years, and after death a varix the size of a bean, which had reduced the bone to paper thickness, was found.

THE BILATERAL PARESES AND PSEUDO-PLEGIAS OF CHILDHOOD, WITH SPECIAL REFERENCE TO A TYPE OF MALARIAL ORIGIN.

By WILLIAM BROWNING, M.D.,

LECTURER ON ANATOMY AND PHYSIOLOGY OF THE NERVOUS SYSTEM AT THE LONG ISLAND COLLEGE HOSPITAL, MEMBER OF THE BROOKLYN SOCIETY FOR NEUROLOGY, AND OF THE ASSOCIATION OF AMERICAN ANATOMISTS.

THE occurrence of partial paralysis in childhood is not very infrequent, though its interpretation is still a subject of dispute. As the lower extremities are principally and most often affected, only the various incomplete and pseudo-plegias (parapareses) will here be considered. If those known to be dependent on marked organic changes (neuritis, myelitis, bone-disease, etc.) be excluded, the remaining types that claim recognition may be grouped into two general classes :

A. Reflex. It is this class of assumed reflex origin that has so many times offered a field for discussion. Some of the best authenticated types of this are briefly recapitulated under the first four sub-heads below. The cases on which they were originally founded were many of them observed in the adult; still it is reasonable to suppose that like causes might produce quite as severe results in children.

B. Resulting from systemic conditions (toxic ?). Whether such a distinct class is wholly warranted, it has a sufficient clinical-etiological basis for present convenience.

A. REFLEX PARAPARESES.

1. *From Injury to Peripheral Nerves.*

Such acceptance as this form has received must be attributed to the great weight of Weir Mitchell's authority. But the cases that he relates (*N. Y. Med. Journ.*, February and March, 1866) do not, so far as the present subject is concerned, bear any close scrutiny. He says on p. 402: "Among some two hundred or more of carefully studied instances of wounds of nerves, we have met with only seven cases of reflex paralysis of remote organs, in which the influence was prolonged or severe."

The phenomena occurred, not in cases where some large nerve was injured, but from wounds of other soft parts, or from slight and indirect injury to nerve-trunks. There does not appear to have been any authoritative observation of these cases at the most important period, viz., directly after the injury, and as (p. 423) " in almost every instance some relic of the paralysis existed even after eighteen months or more from the date of the wound," it is quite as reasonable to suppose that the assumed reflex was the result of some organic lesion. - One of his cases was wholly sensory, and in most the reflex was to an upper extremity. In but one were both lower extremities reflexly affected (Case IV., Injury of Testicle), and as this was in an adult its interest here is but theoretical.

2. From Genital Irritation.

Sayre's writings on this subject are well known : (a) " Partial Paralysis from Reflex Irritation caused by Congenital Phimosis and Adherent Prepuce," Trans. Am. Med. Assn., 1870 ; (b) "Spinal Anæmia with Partial Paralysis and Want of Coördination from·Irritation of the Genital Organs," Ibid., 1875; (c) " On the Deleterious Results of a Narrow Prepuce and Preputial Adhesions," Trans. Ninth Internat. Med. Congress, 1887.

These titles indicate briefly his views.   They have been variously corroborated (as recently, 1888, by Reverdin and by Pinto Portello), but also justly criticised (e. g., by Gray in Annals of Anat. and Surg., January and February, 1882).   The evidence so far offered is not very convincing as to the reality of such paralyses or their dependence on the cause assigned, and still less of the proposed explanation (spinal anæmia).   There is not much uniformity of type in the reflexes described ; nor, strange to say, have such observations often been made in nerve clinics. In the profession, however, there is a widespread belief that cases like those given by Sayre do occur, and it is possible that peculiarities in the published descriptions have prejudiced many authorities against the whole matter.   Considerable inquiry amongst the most careful observers in Brooklyn has failed to discover any case showing paraplegic phenomena, although a couple are noted in which other troubles seemed to have been favorably influenced by circumcision.

3. In Certain Cases of Spina Bifida.

It is well known that a variety of paralytic and spastic troubles, including foot deformities, perforating ulcer (Kirmisson, 1887), etc., frequently accompany this defect in spinal development.

In a case published by Dollinger in the Wien. med. Wochenschr., 1886, No. 46, there was urinary and fecal incontinence, with contractures in the lower extremities, etc.   Puncture and withdrawal of fluid produced each time temporary relief, and osteoplastic closure of the spinal opening was followed by lasting improvement. Apparently quite independent of this, Zenenko, of St. Petersburg (*vide* abstract in *Annals of Surgery*, September, 1889, p. 223, 224), relates a case of sacral meningocele in a boy of fifteen years, with incontinence of urine and feces, "extreme wasting of the muscles of his lower limbs, and flexory contractures in the knee-joints." Here also an osteo-plastic operation on the vertebral cleft—after extirpation of the tumor, some integument, and loops of the cauda—led to a fairly complete recovery.

Cockburn (AMERICAN JOURNAL OF THE MEDICAL SCIENCES, August, 1890) gives the case of a vigorous boy of nine weeks. "This tumor was but slightly reducible, and pressure on it elicited none of the nervous symptoms which are produced by pressure." It was found on operating to connect by a pedicle through an opening in the first sacral vertebra. "The hips were then raised and the tumor compressed, in order to return as much of the spinal fluid within the membranes of the spinal cord as possible, and a stout catgut ligature was now tied around the pedicle. At the moment the ligature was tightened a sudden and rigid extension of the lower limbs took place, and also a marked change in the respiration." On removing the ligature these symptoms soon abated. "The cauda equina was found included in the ligature. . . . About three-fourths of an inch of the extremity of the cauda with the adherent dura was excised." Recovery without further nervous symptoms.

The fact that various cases of spina bifida have been cured as to the tumor, yet without relief of coexisting paralytic conditions, in no wise detracts from the significance of the cases quoted. In those of Dollinger and of Zenenko it was observed that the sheaf of nerves constituting the cauda was stretched out over the tumor-sac, and it was to the irritation produced by this tension on the nerves that these writers attributed the symptoms from the side of the lower extremities and pelvic organs.

A close relationship might be inferred between these cases and those of genital reflex. The sensory path from the prepuce and adjacent parts passes up through the cauda (third sacral nerve according to Thorburn, 1888). The symptoms noted by Sayre in some of his cases are not unlike those seen at times in spina bifida—only less severe. Hence, the morbid phenomena in the apparently quite separate classes of cases *may* be due to irritation of the selfsame set of nerve-fibres. But such symptoms are not the rule, even in apparently like cases of spina bifida ; and where they do occur it is more rational to conclude that not the tension on certain nerves as such, but the dragging at the nerve-roots, and hence direct irritation of centres in the cord, is the real cause.

It might seem that the correct explanation could be decided by anatomical considerations. For, whilst a reflex impulse would at the cord choose functionally rather than physically related parts, direct pulling would probably exert its maximal effects on the nearest centres. But in these few cases the morbid conditions are so complicated that little light is thus obtainable.

4. *From Visceral Irritation.*

Brown-Séquard, in his *Lectures on Paralysis of the Lower Extremities* (Phila., 1861 and 1873), as is well known, divided all cases of paraplegia into those of central and those of reflex origin. Since the time of his writing our knowledge of this subject has greatly increased, especially as to the important part played by neuritis of various kinds. Moreover, the irrelevancy of his cases of reflex—from enteric, intrapelvic, pleuritic, and other troubles—was long since shown by various writers. To discuss this matter by later published reports would require a special paper.

The following case well illustrates the easy possibility of error. A girl of four years was brought to the dispensary in May, 1889, with the history that for two and a half years she had been subject once or twice a month to attacks of loss of power in the lower extremities, accompanied by fever (101°–102° F.) and a tendency to lie on the side or abdomen with feet drawn back toward head. Treatment was refused without previous observation of the girl at such a time. From the physician, Dr. De Castro, who saw one of these attacks and relieved her by the removal of a large mass of pin-worms, I learn that there was no paralysis at all, but "prolonged epileptoid spasms with considerable opisthotonos" leaving her perhaps a little weak.

Hence, although much has been written on this subject, there is as yet no convincing proof that paraplegia, partial or complete, is ever of reflex origin. Certain it is that such cases are exceptional, and that recourse to this explanation is less necessary the more carefully cases are studied. The theory of an hysterical neurosis may in this connection be a real advance—or only a shifting of terms.

B. PARAPARESES RESULTING FROM SYSTEMIC CONDITIONS.

The cases of the other class, to which we now come, though not as widely studied, have a more uniform cause and course. The three types described below are known only in children. To these there may be others that can suitably be added.

5. *From Rickets.*

Attention has recently been called to this form of weakness in the lower extremities by Berg (" Rhachitic Pseudo-paraplegia," *N. Y. Med. Record*, November 16, 1889). He says it has received but little notice from writers on rhachitis. A few quotations will show that it has been fully recognized by American, English, and German observers.

Seitz's *Niemeyer* (edition of 1879, p. 600) says: "Stiebel, most true
to nature, tells how the children, who otherwise took the greatest pleasure in moving their limbs or perhaps putting their toes in the mouth,
now lie down with their legs stretched out straight and stiff. Apparently, they do not dare to move, they cry out on being turned, and begin
to cry when they fear being taken from the bed and carried about."
This, of course, refers more to the hyperæsthetic conditions so common
in this trouble than to any real paralysis.

Samuel Gee, in *St. Barth. Hosp. Rep.* for 1868 (vol iv. p. 72):
" Pseudo-paraplegia—'*Veluti inferiorum artuum paralysis*,' as Stoll says
—the rickets falling, as it were, upon the muscles; the bones being left,
in some cases, comparatively unaffected. An exaggeration, this, of the
inability to stand or walk, which is so commonly met with in rickets.
That the muscles are at fault more than the bones is shown by those
cases in which, notwithstanding great softening of the bones, the children
are able to walk at twelve months of age, and become bandylegged in
consequence." This is given by Gee as the first evidence of latent,
masked, incomplete, or larvated rickets.

Parry (AMERICAN JOURNAL OF THE MEDICAL SCIENCES, January,
1872, p. 30) treats of this trouble very fully : "In these cases it is not
uncommon to find children who had been walking cease making any
effort of this kind, and even to become the subjects of ' pseudo-paraplegia.' In no other disease excepting paralysis, it has been said, is the
muscular power more interfered with than in this. In scrofula, tuberculosis, and the other cachectic disorders, children may continue to walk
with considerable energy even until near the close of life, and when the
emaciation and atrophy are far greater." "*Pseudo-paraplegia* (p. 51).
There is one form of rickets to which we wish to call especial attention.
This is the more important since it is repeatedly mistaken for paralysis,
and the helpless infant subjected to a course of medication for disease of
the brain or spinal cord. . . . Indeed, it seems as if the disease had
expended itself upon the muscles. The common form of this variety is
loss of power in the lower extremities. . . . The condition is often
unassociated with any serious or even with any visible deformity." In
a footnote he tells of an autopsy on a girl of four years: "A typical
example of pseudo-paraplegia. The brain, spinal cord, and nerves
coming from them were found perfectly healthy, while the muscles of
the thigh and leg were wasted and very pale." Berg's article, already
mentioned, is so excellent and complete, and fortunately so accessible to
all, that further quotation or description is unnecessary. That this affection runs a slow course if untreated was shown by a colored girl of six
years, referred to me in August, 1889. The lower extremities showed
extreme general weakness—inability to stand alone—though not complete paralysis. Musculature of arms as well as legs very scant, with-

out any localized atrophy. The general evidence of rickets was ample, and a prescription therefor was given. But on looking up the case in April, 1890, it was found that this had been lost, and the child had remained untreated. She was in practically the same condition as eight months previously.

6. *Of Malarial Origin.*

CASE I.—In June, 1886, a boy, Frankie B., was brought to the dispensary for loss of power in the lower extremities and peculiar associated symptoms. He was six years old, and came from the malarious Red Hook. The father, a chronic alcoholic, showed old bilateral wrist-drop, the result of some metallic poisoning. Frankie's trouble was already of three months' duration, though worse "by spells." He likes to lie around, especially on his stomach. Complains of pain in feet and finger-tips. Has a way of pulling off shoes and stockings and holding his feet in his hands; this he would do, if undisturbed, even when brought for examination. Is not inclined to say much even when questioned. Sleeps well. Has lost flesh greatly, though no special atrophy is discoverable. Cervical glands large. Eyelids red. Later he lay down all the time, cried more at night, and then had his worst attacks about 3 A. M., crying and doubling up as his mother said. At the time no cause was discovered (no genital trouble nor helminthiasis), and it was simply called a neuritis. Various lines of treatment proved futile. Many features of the case were so striking and peculiar, however, that the matter was kept in mind with a view to its eventual solution.

In January, 1887, the mother applied for treatment of what was evidently a brow-ague—and this in part suggested the treatment in the subsequent cases.

In March, 1890, it was learned that for a couple of years Frankie had ceased complaining, is well, and uses all his extremities perfectly. He took no medicine; hence recovery was spontaneous, unless influenced by moving to another neighborhood.

Seen again in December, 1890, when he was suffering from a keratitis. Some two years previously he had had a similar trouble of the same right eye. Dr. Lennox, in whose care he has recently been, kindly informs me that it was the ordinary form of keratitis and not in itself characteristic of malaria. Still, as it did not improve, he was then put on quinine and soon relieved. Dr. Lennox considers that the keratitis was without doubt of malarial origin.

CASE II.—German-Irish boy of five years, brought to the dispensary September 17, 1889. Sick all summer. Was at the Seaside Home for a while with asserted malaria. For three weeks now he has been losing the use of his legs; this has become much worse the last two days. He can still walk a little, but soon gets so tired that he has to be carried. He has a slow swinging gait, not simply an excessive waddling but also a laborious dragging. This resembled that sometimes seen during recovery from spinal injuries, where there is simply weakness in the lower extremities with a slight tendency to toe-drop. He likes to sit or drop on his knees. The hands are not stretched out fully, the left one being worse than the right, and appearing like an ulnar paresis (of the type so well shown by Bowlby, *Injuries and Diseases of Nerves*, 1890, Figs.

15 and 16). There was also some undetermined difficulty in speech. He is cross, peevish, and losing flesh. Of late has a bowel movement after each meal, though the evacuation is described as quite natural. Nuchal glands rather large, splenic dulness ditto. Reflexes all normal. A trial was first made with anti-rhachitic treatment, but as this did not affect his condition, and it was found that he lived on the first floor in a very malarial neighborhood—Sackett St., adjacent to Gowanns Canal— quinine with a little arsenic and iron was substituted. In five days he was reported a little better, and in nine more as decidedly improved.

Seen again two months later, when he was almost and perhaps quite free from any motor disturbance, and wholly recovered as to other symptoms. The mother was very enthusiastic over his rapid and full cure, and as later reports are all that he is well, it is certain that he has had no relapse. The anti-malarial treatment had probably lasted about three weeks altogether.

It seems that this boy had been seen also in May, 1888, when the following note was made : "Healthy fellow up to just a week ago, though nervous and old in manner. On that day he came in complaining of pains in his legs, and wanted to be put to bed. Varying since, sometimes he wanted to go about on his knees, again he walks fairly. Comes to the dispensary, walking with knees half bent; can be straightened out without much pain, and in fact the condition seems to be functional (spasmodic) contracture. No knee-jerk. Moans in sleep. Does not eat very well this week. No preputial adhesions. Urinates well. Bladder not full." As both he and his sister had passed intestinal worms, medicine therefore was given. His history up to the next attack given above is not known to me.

CASE III.—Samuel W., six years old. Dispensary December 26, 1889. Brothers and sisters said to be weakly ; mother dead. Sammy's legs first became weak about a fortnight since. He walks clumsily, with an uncertain waddling gait, much after the manner of the preceding boy, though not quite as badly. Stands with legs apart. He is uneasy ; does not sleep well, though he is sleepy mornings and looks sleepy. Eats well, though he cannot swallow solids as well as liquids. A slight disturbance in speech has already improved. Tongue a trifle coated. Face pale and said to show that he is not well. Spleen large. Knee-jerks normal ; faradic reactions good. He had lived for three years in one of the most malarious parts of the city. Last October moved to a much healthier neighborhood.

To test treatment he was first put on iron and arsenic. For a week he seemed to improve a little, but then no further. Finally, he was put on quinine with Donovan's solution. He then mended rapidly, and in three weeks was able to walk on the street alone. His gait had become natural. He was no longer inclined to lie down all the time; is lively, active, and does not look sleepy.

March 11, 1890, reported to have kept perfectly well. He has his strong voice again. Goes to school, runs, and plays.

CASE IV.—Vigorous boy of three and two-thirds years (mother epileptic). Seen August 7, 1890. Thought not to have been as active in running and playing this summer. For a week especially some loss of appetite, grinding of teeth at night, etc. Since yesterday high fever (over 104°). Constipation. This fever was soon relieved. Next day he went on an excursion, and in the following night awoke complaining of pain in

the legs. This continued on the 9th, with a disinclination to walk. Brought
to the office August 10, P.M., in his father's arms. This morning the pain
was in the left ankle but now it has shifted to the right, the outer anterior
surface in each case. No certain swelling at this spot, but pain on pressing, twisting, or standing; some tenderness of left ankle also. Gentle
squeezing of either calf is well borne, but of lower thighs makes him
cry. Arms not tender. Will only walk by leaning on something, and
even then has to be compelled and at first cries. Now toes-in when
walking, though when well walks toes-out. No speech-impediment observed. Very peevish. Sighs now and then deeply. No longer feverish. Spleen a trifle large. Put on quinine and Warburg. For two
days more he continued to complain of his legs. On the third morning
he came down himself, shouting, " Papa, I can walk!" Since then in
good health.

A younger brother (of two years) had a febrile attack believed to be
intermittent, and yielding only to anti-malarials some three months later.
The mother thought that he also had some difficulty in walking, until
the fever was broken, but it might not have been noticed had she not
recalled the brother's trouble.

Amongst the asserted nervous complications and sequelæ of malaria
are: Neuralgias, including sciatica and cruralgia; limited contractures
(Holt, *N. Y. Med. Journ.*, 1883); intra-cranial inflammations of a meningitic type; pigmentary deposits in the brain; epilepsy (Hammond, *Trans.
Am. Neurol. Soc.*, 1875, 1 case; Hamilton, *Pepper's System*, vol. v., p.
472, 3 cases);[1] hysteria (Regnault, *Gaz. des Hôp.*, 1890, No. 3, 1 case);
mental disorders (Lemoine et Chaumier, *Annales Médico-psychologiques*,
1887, i., pp. 177–209; their fourth conclusion is that " There very probably exists a form of paludal general pseudo-paralysis "); multiple
neuritis; and, according to Morton Prince (*Journ. Nerv. and Ment. Dis.*,
October, 1889), even tabes and desseminated sclerosis. Vought, in Starr's
" Familiar Forms of Nervous Disease," attributes 3 out of 124 cases of
chorea to malaria.

Neuritic malarial paraplegia is specially considered by Strachan, of
Jamaica (article in *Sajous' Annual*, 1888, vol. i., p. 139); by Singer (one
case reported in *Wien. med. Wochenschr.*, 1887, No. 22, pp. 730-1), and by
Cardoso Fonte (" Impaludismo larvado; paraplegia complete," *Brazil
Med.*, 1888-9). An intermittent form of malarial paraplegia has also
been variously observed (*v.* Birdsall, in *Sajous' Annual*, 1889, ii., 110).

Motor disturbance of malarial origin and of the type illustrated by
the preceding cases (paraplegic, non-intermittent, though sometimes

---

[1] Ferreira (*Archivio Italiano di Pediat.*, 1889; *v. Arch. f. Kinderheilk.*, Bd. xii.) "dis-
tinguishes four different varieties of the cerebral form (of malaria), which are especially
seen in children during the heated seasons, and which are very frequent and very
dangerous. These varieties are: 1. The eclamptic form. 2. The comatose form. 3. The
delirious form. 4. The meningitic form. The last two are observed more in older
children." Earlier cases of malarial epilepsy are quoted in Hanfield Jones's work, 1868.

varying in extent and severity, not severe and protracted but yielding
readily to treatment, occurring only in the young) has been fairly recognized by at least one observer (Holt, " The Symptoms and Diagnosis of
Malaria in Children," *Am. Journ. Obstet.*, 1883). His remarks on this
subject are worth quoting in full:

" Neuralgic pains in the back, the extremities, the neck, and general soreness have all been noted occasionally. The general cutaneous hyperæsthesia is often acute, and, when accompanied by fever, may
lead to the diagnosis of some affection of the central nervous system.
In the subjoined case the febrile symptoms were slight. It, however,
illustrates well the point under consideration."—p. 213.

" CASE I.—Robert M., aged eleven years, was brought to the dispensary May 19, 1882. His mother stated that he had been complaining
for several weeks of headache, and of late seemed to be growing stupid.
She thought that he was losing his memory. For two days he had been
having severe pains in the calves of both legs, of a neuralgic character,
and had also complained of the parts being sore to the touch. His
limbs were so weak he could scarcely walk a block and a half. A slight
fever had been noticed to come on toward evening, but there had been
no chill, no sweating, and no vomiting. His axillary temperature was
found 101° ; he was pale and anæmic ; pulse regular ; pupils normal.
He walked unsteadily, not clearing the floor well with his feet, and
seemed inclined to drag the left limb slightly.

" On testing the different muscular groups separately no real paralysis
could be discovered, but all the muscles seemed weaker than normal.
Over the whole of both lower extremities there was great hyperæsthesia,
so that even moderate handling caused him to cry out with pain. This
was much more acute in the thighs than in the legs. None was present
in the upper extremities. Cinchonidia was ordered, and two days later
he reported. There was no hyperæsthesia to be found, and he said the
pains were much less severe. He could walk much better than before.
Slight fever continued for a few days, and the pains steadily improved,
the medicine being kept up. He was not seen after a week from his first
visit until November 8th, when he was found walking perfectly well, and
said he had no return of the symptoms since I last saw him."

" Motor disturbances are less frequent than the sensory. I have.
met with three cases in which paresis of the lower extremities was
present. In two cases it was associated with severe pain, and improved
rapidly under anti-periodics until a perfect cure took place. The third
case was not traced ; when last seen there was some improvement ; some
lameness existed."—p. 433.

Two similar cases in children were described by Gibney (*Am. Journ.
Neurol. and Psychol.*, 1882, No. 1). They were not intermittent in the
same sense as malarial fever, but rather recurred after further exposure
to the paludal poison.

It is remarkable that all these patients have been boys, and generally
of vigorous rather than puny appearance.

In each of my cases genital irritation. helminthiasis, and vertebral
disease were excluded. The possibility of latent rhachitis was considered

but no further evidence of it discovered, and though the symptoms resemble somewhat those at times seen in that trouble, it is fair to conclude that malaria was the prime and predominant if not exclusive cause. Microscopical evidence from examination of the blood is wanting—though in one case, kindly sought for by Dr. Van Cott, of the Hoagland Laboratory—and in such atypical forms of malaria may well prove negative. As to the malarious districts of Brooklyn the Thayer-Baker committee report (*N. Y. Med. Journ.*, May 8, 1886) is not very explicit; but E. D. Page (*Ibid.*, 1887, ii., p. 566) briefly says that, "Usually, these cases (of malaria in children) can be traced to those districts skirting the bay or in the vicinity of Gowanus Canal, regions known to abound in malaria." The first three of the above cases came from the worst parts of this neighborhood.

The symptoms are few. Apparently there is a general motor weakness of both lower extremities, without special atrophy or change in reactions, reflexes, or local circulation. The main complaint for which they are brought is that their legs have become very weak or paralyzed. The children have been too young and uncommunicative to say whether it was tenderness and pain that interfered with their walking. They object to making any attempts, and when stood up remain where placed with feet somewhat apart, or make clumsy attempts at progress and drop down helpless. In one of these and in one of Holt's cases the thighs were found to be more tender than the calves, though some general oversensitiveness to touch and pressure may exist.

The children are ill-humored and fretful. They are not, however, as timid and inclined to cry as choreics, though a slight early speech trouble —more a disinclination to speak than any distinct defect—might lead one to think of chorea. This, as also Morini's recent case, corroborates Singer's observation that aphasic affections are common in disorders of the nervous system due to malaria. This, with the arm trouble in one case and slight impediment to swallowing in another, indicates a more than local implication of the nervous system. The variable pains in the extremities are also frequent in children suffering from other forms of malaria.

Little value attaches to any enlargement of the spleen, since this occurs also in rickets. There is a marked difference between the favorite attitude of these patients—as also of those from rickets—and that attributed to paraplegia from genital reflex or spina bifida. In the latter there is frequent mention of a tendency to adduction of the thighs, whilst in the former quite the opposite prevails.

The distinction of malarial from rhachitic paraplegia may not be as easy, and, in the absence on the one hand of febrile attacks, past or present, on the other of distinctive rhachitic marks, one has to depend partly on determining which etiological factor is more probably present, or on therapeutic experiment.

7. *In Chorea* (*Rheumatic?*).

In this disorder there are two distinct forms of paralysis that do not appear, however, to have been very carefully distinguished. Only one of these, the first below, belongs to the clinical forms under discussion.

(*a*) True choreic paralysis usually incomplete. This commonly appears either very early in chorea or else at the beginning of convalescence, A paralysis varying from partial to very pronounced may usher in the more characteristic phases of chorea. The child is brought by the anxious parent with this complaint alone. Inquiry shows that though it may have developed rapidly its onset was not strictly sudden. Such cases are far more misleading than where the trouble follows a typical chorea. Though this form is usually unilateral (monoplegic or hemiplegic), in rare cases a paraplegic or paraparetic type, or a condition like general motor exhaustion occurs. However, the mono- and hemi-pareses in the prejactatory stage of chorea, not infrequent in any large nerve clinic, sufficiently attest the fact that motor impairment may be due to the choreic process alone; and they further indicate that the general paralytic condition, seen in or following many cases of chorea, is not wholly due to the tiring of the nerve motor apparatus.

Souza-Leite and E. Cherbuliez (*Progrès Med.*, 1889, No. 19) have published two observations on girls—or really young women—with neuropathic family history, in whom for a time there was paresis of both lower extremities (arsenic as a factor excluded). They also quote a corresponding case from Ollive's thesis. The choreic paralyses, including paraplegia without marked jactation, are also fully considered by Cadet de Gassicourt (*Rev. mens. d. Mal. de l'Enf.*, 1889 ; seen only in abstract).

Paralysis during or after the characteristic period of chorea will rarely be misconstrued. In early and doubtful cases something in the mental condition of the child, a greater impairment of one side, an occasional choreic twitch, or a history of past chorea, usually gives a clue to their real nature.

(*b*) Neuritis (arsenical or rheumatic) following chorea. This is a far more frequent cause of paraplegia than chorea alone.

Sherwell (*Brooklyn Med. Journ.*, April, 1890, p. 273) has added a recent case to others by Brouardel and Fouchet. Railton's case of paralysis following chorea is attributed by others (*v. Sajous' Annual*, 1888) to arsenic; and the same possibility is suggested in Fry's case ("Chorea with Multiple Neuritis," *Journ. Nerv. and Ment. Dis.*, June, 1890). Several other cases have been published. In fact there has been some question whether the cases attributed to chorea were not in reality all due to arsenic. But such is certainly not the case. In Ashby's case (*Manchester Med. Chron.*, 1890), occuring in the course of a choreic attack, both arms and legs were affected; the sensitive contractures, atrophy, etc., indicate that it was a neuritis, evidently rheumatic.

Do these cases of the second class (B) represent the initial or slightly developed stage of severer trouble, or, are they always self-limited? As to the malarial group, one of the above cases, as well as one of different character given by Holt, indicates that spontaneous recovery may be expected; and the same holds for the rhachitic and choreic forms. There is evidently no gross pathological basis, as these cases do not in themselves present any proof thereof, and under suitable management recover so rapidly. The paresis may be the immediate effect of toxic matters in the circulation; or it may be a pseudo form, the consequence of muscular and fascial tenderness; according to prevailing views, however, some mild form of neuritis seems most probable, though, as is the case in common pressure paralysis, the change may be too slight to be demonstrable.

However, it is quite possible that the seat and nature of the trouble may be very different in the different forms. That the condition in each seems to favor the development of poly-neuritis is indicated by various cases, some of which are mentioned in this paper.

8. *Other Forms of Paralysis to be Distinguished from the Preceding.*

(*a*) The possibility of confounding any of these cases with infantile spinal paralysis or that following meningitis, especially cerebro-spinal, is slight; but certain other motor disturbances in childhood are at times confusing.

(*b*) The nearest analogy is furnished by certain forms of neuritis. That malaria in children, usually after a more typical course, may induce undoubted neuritis with resulting atrophies in both upper and lower extremities was made probable by two cases observed late in their course. Both were in boys, one of five, the other of seven and two-third years. The trouble followed intermittent febrile attacks without the intervention of any such condition as that in the previous cases.

(*c*) Another form of neuritis occurring in children is that, now so well recognized, from arsenic. Various recent writers note that at least in adults diabetic neuritis preferably attacks the lower extremities, and is more often bilateral. Alcohol, lead, and the rest of the category of neurotoxics might doubtless be included as possible analogous causes of paraplegic phenomena in the young.

(*d*) The post-infectious paralyses (after diphtheria, scarlatina, measles, etc.) are sufficiently common. At present they are largely classed as cases of neuritis. That following diphtheria is familiar to all, and probably that after scarlet fever is essentially similar. A form of extensive and for a time severe (complete) paralysis after measles has been described (principally by French writers within the last decade), and "a certain tendency to simple paraplegia" noted. According to the two cases seen by the writer—one, a girl of six years, at the dispensary in the spring of 1885; the other, a boy of two years, in the practice of Dr. McNaughton—this form is somewhat distinctive in character. At first all the voluntary muscles below the head, except the respiratory, were involved. Improvement began in a few weeks, and went on to entire recovery in from one to two years.

(e) Hysterical cases of this type must be very rare in American children at least. S. P. Denhope (*Cincinnati Med. Journ*, Nov., 1890, p. 366-9) gives a case of hysterical paraplegia in a German girl of twelve years.

(f) Incipient paraplegia from Pott's disease should be carefully excluded.

(g) Syphilitic or osteo-chondritic pseudo-paralysis, often called Parrot's disease, is apt to attack but one extremity, whether a lower or an upper, at a time. It has been described in this country by Van Harlingen and others.

(h) Infantile spastic paraplegia (of Osler, Fergusson, and others) cerebral in origin.

It is certainly of the greatest moment, for practitioner and patient, to recognize the difference between the essentially functional and the tedious organic paralyses of childhood. Though relatively rare, these lighter forms are nevertheless worthy of further study and fuller recognition. Treatment follows from the diagnosis; and the prognosis also, usually excellent, depends on the primary trouble.

THE DIAGNOSIS OF POTT'S DISEASE.[1]

By ROBERT W. LOVETT, M.D.,
OF BOSTON.

IN considering the question of the diagnosis of Pott's disease, one must start with the assumption that the *history* is of little or no value in establishing the presence of the disease. It may be significant enough to make one suspect very strongly the existence of vertebral disease; but without definite physical signs, it can never be positive enough to justify the diagnosis of Pott's disease. With this understanding, it may be asserted that particularly significant symptoms are paroxysmal pain in the chest or abdomen, which is aggravated by jarring or movement; and pain coming on at night when the child is first falling to sleep (sig-

---

[1] Read by title before the American Orthopædic Association at Washington, September 23, 1891.

nificant as the well-known night-cries, simulating very closely those of hip disease). Other symptoms which should excite suspicion are: tiring easily, leaning on tables and chairs, carrying the chin in the hand, and supporting the weight of the trunk by placing the hands upon the knees. These symptoms should all be considered significant and suggestive, but it may be said once more that they cannot be considered, in the absence of physical signs, as establishing the diagnosis of Pott's disease. Such a history should be allowed especial significance when it occurs in the children of tuberculous parents, or when it follows some months after the exanthemata, or comes on as the remote result of a fall which has injured the spine. It should be mentioned that the absence of pain can in no way be assumed to show the absence of Pott's disease.

The diagnosis, then, must be made wholly from the *physical examination*, and the chief physical signs upon which one must rely can be divided into two classes: (*a*) those occurring from bony destruction, and (*b*) those dependent upon muscular spasm.

(*a*) *Signs Due to Bony Destruction.*

Since these are made evident by the presence of angular deformity of the spine, which is the result of bony destruction, they are so conspicuous that they can scarcely be overlooked. And the prominence of one or more of the vertebral bodies, associated with muscular spasm, is a positive sign of the presence of the disease, unless it is the result of a fracture of the spine, or in adults the outcome of malignant disease. In the larger number of cases, as they come to the surgeon, this bony deformity has occurred, and the diagnosis can be made at a glance; but the most important class of cases, so far as the diagnosis is concerned, are those where bony destruction has not yet begun, and where the need of an early diagnosis is evident, in the hope that it may lead to treatment which may be sufficient to prevent the occurrence of deformity.

(*b*) *Signs Arising from Muscular Spasm.*

These are:

1. Stiffness of the spine in walking and in passive manipulation.

2. Peculiarity of gait and attitudes assumed, according to the location of the disease.

3. Lateral deviation of the spine.

4. High temperature.

Of the two latter it may be said that they do not receive general recognition as diagnostic symptoms, hence the writer feels inclined particularly to call attention to their importance.

Lateral[1] deviation of the spine he believes to be practically a universal

---

[1] R. W. Lovett: Boston Med. and Surg. Journal, October 9, 1890.

sign in Pott's disease,[1] and high temperature as a constant accompaniment of active tuberculous joint disease has been already discussed at length. Further experience has only served to confirm, in his opinion, the value of these two signs.

1. MUSCULAR STIFFNESS.—On examining for muscular stiffness of the spine, the child is most conveniently laid face downward on a table or bed, and lifted by the feet. In a normal back the lumbar spine can be markedly flexed, and a general mobility is seen of the whole column. In patients where Pott's disease is present the region affected is held rigidly by muscular contraction when manipulation is attempted. In certain instances the erector spinæ muscles stand out like cords when the child is lifted, and it is questionable how much importance should be attributed to this sign. After having depended much upon it, the writer has come to the belief that it is not a sign of Pott's disease, and that it occurs in cases of hip disease, and in certain instances in excitable children where no joint disease is present. Lifting the patient by the feet in this way is practically sure to show the existence of lumbar or lower dorsal rigidity; but it does not detect high dorsal Pott's disease. In lumbar Pott's disease lateral mobility of the spine, as well as anteroposterior flexibility, is lost.

2. PECULIAR GAIT AND ATTITUDES.—In considering the gait as a diagnostic symptom of Pott's disease, one must be prepared to find any or all the characteristic features absent. In general the walk is careful, steady, and military, and the steps taken with such care that jars to the spine are avoided; in other instances, however, the child walks with comparative freedom, even when the presence of the disease is manifest, and the well-known test of having the child pick up objects from the floor may fail to detect anything. It is only necessary to allude to the fact that these symptoms, usually assumed as characteristic, may be practically absent in clearly marked cases of Pott's disease.

Assuming, then, the extreme importance of the early diagnosis of the disease where practicable, it becomes necessary to consider in detail the general and local physical signs, according to the region of the spine affected.

Cervical Pott's Disease.—The most common symptom of the disease in this region, due to muscular rigidity, is the occurrence of wry-neck with stiffness of the muscles of the back and neck. This is often accompanied by distressed breathing at night, and intense occipital neuralgia. The head is held sometimes in a very much distorted position, and the most characteristic attitude is when the chin is supported in the hand; and when the patient turns sideways to look at objects, the whole body is turned. In severe cases one notices flattening of the back of the neck,

---

[1] Ibid., April 17, 1890.

with sometimes bony deformity. When spinal caries occurs in this region the early symptoms are most often confused with sprains, muscular torticollis, and inflammation of the cervical lymphatic glands.

From sprains the diagnosis is almost impossible. In the early stages of sprains of the neck the head is often held stiffly and to one side ; motion is resisted and is painful, muscular spasm is present, and in the case of children of unintelligent parents the history cannot be accepted as valid. The writer has in mind a case which presented every symptom of Pott's disease in this region, where two weeks in bed cured all the symptoms, and the recovery has been permanent.

From true muscular wry-neck the diagnosis is often extremely difficult. In true torticollis manipulation is generally not painful, and one muscle is firmly contracted while the rest are relaxed. In congenital cases the head and face are distorted, and the eyes often are not upon the same plane. In Pott's disease, on the other hand, the muscular fixation involves all the muscles, and movement in any direction is resisted. It is more apt to be painful, and in most cases comes on with considerable rapidity. This applies fairly well to cases of anterior wry-neck ; but in cases where the true muscular torticollis is of the posterior variety, and is due to a contraction of the deeper muscles, the diagnosis is much more difficult, for no one muscle is contracted, and movement is limited by a general muscular resistance. The writer has in mind certain cases where the diagnosis has been impossible, and some in which an operation of tenotomy has been performed in cases of Pott's disease where a most careful examination had seemed to establish the diagnosis of true muscular wry-neck.

In these obscure cases the differential diagnosis is extremely difficult, and can be most easily made by putting the patient to bed and seeing if the application of the extension is sufficient to overcome the distortion, as it will do in the course of a few days if due to Pott's disease. It is in this class of cases that the writer would particularly insist upon the value of high temperature as pointing to the presence of Pott's disease.

Inflammation of the lymphatic glands of the neck is likely to give rise to a position of the head simulating wry-neck, associated with muscular spasm. These cases simulate Pott's disease very closely, and in two cases under the writer's observation recently the diagnosis has been impossible until the inflammation of the glands was subdued, and it was found that the head again became perfectly movable. In these cases it was impossible to determine whether the inflammation of the glands was secondary to the Pott's disease, or the muscular spasm was the result of the adenitis.

Upper Dorsal Pott's Disease.—In this region detection is the most easy because any bony destruction at once results in angular deformity, on account of the posterior curve of the spine in this part, and it is on this deformity that one must depend rather than on symptoms due to muscular stiffness.

The shoulders are, however, held high and squarely, the gait is military and careful, and lateral deviation is almost certainly present. In dorsal Pott's disease, paralysis may exceptionally be the first perceptible symptom.

The two affections with which dorsal Pott's disease is most likely to be confused are scoliosis and round shoulders. From rotary lateral curvature the distinction may be difficult in cases where the kyphosis is rounded and involves several vertebræ. The fact that lateral deviation of the spine is so constantly associated with Pott's disease is another factor in making the distinction more difficult.

In a case recently under the care of Dr. Bradford and the writer, for some weeks it was impossible to make a diagnosis between scoliosis and vertebral disease, in the case of a girl twelve years of age, and it must come to the mind of everyone under whose observation these cases come that there are certain cases where a distinction between the two is extremely difficult. As a rule, this is in very early cases, but in the case just alluded to the disease had been in progress for many years.

Here, again, the writer would call attention to the importance of high temperature as pointing to the presence of Pott's disease.

From round shoulders, Pott's disease is generally to be distinguished by the fact that in the former the spine is flexible, and the deformity rounded and not angular. In some cases of round shoulders, however, where the affection is of long standing, the curvature is more or less fixed, and pain may also be present, so that the resemblance to Pott's disease is marked; but these cases are uncommon, and the distinction is generally easily made.

Lumbar Pott's Disease.—Vertebral caries in this region of the spine is difficult of detection on account of the anterior curve of the spine in the lumbar region, so that in any moderate amount of destruction of the lumbar vertebral bodies no posterior angular curvature is developed, and it is only in the later stages of the disease that any angularity becomes prominent. The occurrence of deformity is preceded by a flattening of the lumbar curve, which is characteristic and very significant. The attitude is that of lordosis, which in some cases becomes very marked; the gait is military and careful, and lateral deviation is always present, sometimes to a very marked degree. It is in this region of the spine that it is most conspicuous.

In using the ordinary tests to detect the disease in this region one is liable to be deceived by the readiness with which some children can bend the spine in picking up objects from the ground when lumbar Pott's disease is markedly present. This is due to an increased flexibility of the upper part of the spine. In many instances of lumbar Pott's disease the first noticeable symptom is a limp which is due to unilateral psoas contraction, the result perhaps of abscess, or perhaps only of psoas irritability, and psoas contraction must be set down as one of the common symptoms of lumbar Pott's disease. If the child is laid on its face and an attempt is made to flex the lumbar spine, it is found to be entirely rigid, and any attempt to hyperextend the leg in this position leads to the detection of the slightest psoas irritability.

Lumbar Pott's disease is most liable to be confused with single or double hip disease, with rhachitic curvature of the spine, and with primary inflammation of the psoas muscle.

The differential diagnosis between lumbar Pott's disease and hip disease is one which the writer often finds extremely difficult, although it is not generally considered so; but a long series of mistakes made by other surgeons, as well as by himself, have led him to consider the diagnosis as one which should be made with very great care. In general, when the hip symptoms are due to Pott's disease, and the joint symptoms are caused by psoas irritability, the restriction of motion in the hip is simply in the loss of hyperextension; while abduction and internal rotation are free and not affected. This limitation of motion in only one direction is generally sufficient, in connection with the other symptoms, to establish the presence of Pott's disease. On the other hand, in some cases the limitation of the hip's motion is in all directions, and simulates very closely the limitation of true hip disease.

In a case of lumbar Pott's disease, which had been for some years under the writer's observation, suddenly a complete limitation of all the motions of the right hip occurred, and it seemed as if hip disease must be present. The child was kept quiet, and in the course of a few weeks the symptoms entirely disappeared, leaving the hip perfectly well, and in the whole time there never was any evidence of psoas abscess. The child in the last two years has been free from all hip symptoms. This case simply serves as a type of several which have occurred under the writer's observation where psoas irritability very closely simulated true hip disease.

Another element which leads to the confusion of the two affections is the rigidity of the lumbar spine which often occurs as an accompaniment of acute hip disease. If a child with hip disease is laid upon its face, and an attempt made to flex the lumbar spine by lifting the feet from the table, the irritability of all the muscles is so great that often the lumbar spine will appear to be completely rigid, and only a very careful examination will show that this is secondary to the hip disease.

Rhachitic deformity of the spine is a posterior curvature often so sharp as to be angular. It occurs at the junction of the dorsal and the lumbar regions. This junction is also the most frequent site of Pott's disease.

Rhachitic curvature of the spine is characterized not so much by muscular spasm as by persistent stiffness in most cases, so that if the child is laid upon its face, and an attempt is made to flex the spine, the curve is not obliterated. The symptoms, therefore, are the same that would be presented by Pott's disease occurring under the same conditions, and much dependence must be placed upon the coexistence of rickets.

In general, a posterior curvature of the spine in young children is much more apt to be rhachitic, but it may simulate Pott's disease so closely that a diagnosis is impossible. It has been the writer's custom to treat all such cases by rest in bed or on a frame, with the experience that in nearly every instance where the general signs of rickets were present, complete mobility was restored to the back within the course of a few months.

Primary inflammation of the psoas muscle would simulate lumbar Pott's disease, accompanied by psoas abscess, so closely that a distinction between the two might be difficult. There would, however, be no symptoms of flattening of the lumbar curve of the spine. There would probably be, however, some stiffness of the lumbar spine in making the ordinary tests, and lordosis would be present to a certain extent. Primary inflammation of the muscle, however, is very rare, and its existence should lead to the suspicion of Pott's disease, and the only distinction that could be made would be the absence of bony change, and a greater flexibility of the lumbar spine where only the muscle was involved. In most cases, however, it would be safer to assume that lumbar Pott's disease was present, and fortunately the treatment of the two affections would be identical.

Pain. A word should be said with regard to the significance of pain as a diagnostic symptom in Pott's disease. In most cases it is referred to the terminal part of the spinal nerves, and the pain is most often complained of in the front of the chest, and in the abdomen, where it often passes for stomach-ache. In other instances severe pain is felt in the legs where the disease is low down, and in cervical disease it takes the form often of a severe occipital neuralgia; but the absence of pain, as has been said, is not to be taken as evidence of the absence of the disease. Pott's disease is in general more often accompanied by pain than hip disease, for example; but, on the other hand, certain cases pass from the earliest to the latest stages with little or no pain, and the former diagnostic tests of lifting the child suddenly, making pressure upon the head and the like, can be set down as not only harmful, but entirely useless.

The same may be said with regard to tenderness over the spine, which is often assumed to be a diagnostic symptom. It is in most cases absent, and if it is present it shows nothing, and is of no diagnostic importance whatever. On the other hand, the occurrence of persistent abdominal or chest pain in a child is a symptom which should be allowed more weight than it ordinarily receives in the hands of the family physician, and although it is in no way a diagnostic symptom of Pott's disease, yet it is so often due to that affection that its presence should lead to a very careful examination to detect, if possible, the early stages of the disease.

3. LATERAL DEVIATION OF THE SPINE.—The writer believes that a noticeable amount of lateral deviation of the spine is an early symptom of the existence of Pott's disease, and occurs in practically all cases of dorsal or lumbar disease. It is a symptom due to muscular spasm, and is early rectified by treatment. In cervical disease it is often present, although it cannot be set down as a uniform accompaniment of the disease in this situation.

4. HIGH TEMPERATURE.—In a large series of observations relating to Pott's disease in the acute stages it has been the writer's experience that a high evening temperature is almost uniformly present, and that it occurs independently of abscess formation, and is no higher in cases of abscess than in cases without abscess. The rise of temperature is from one to three degrees, and in general it can be accepted as indicating roughly the degree of severity of the disease.

The Diagnosis of Abscess.—The diagnosis of abscess in Pott's disease rarely presents any difficulty, but in certain instances their occurrence is attended with peculiar symptoms which may give rise to some obscurity. In the cervical region the most common seat of abscess formation is in the back wall of the pharynx, where it often persists for some time unrecognized, giving rise to a peculiar series of respiratory symptoms. The pharyngeal wall is pushed forward, and the child breathes at night with a peculiar snoring respiration, which is to a certain extent characteristic. There is some difficulty in swallowing food; the pain is apt to be severe; and occasionally a swelling extends so much to the side as to be noticeable at the sides of the neck. The finger introduced into the mouth comes upon a projecting swelling of the back of the pharynx, which is characteristic and not to be mistaken.

In the dorsal and lumbar region the abscesses point for the most part in the loin, or follow down the course of the psoas muscle to appear in the upper part of the thigh or groin. Appearing in the back the abscess is not likely to be mistaken for anything unless for a cellular abscess of the back muscles, which is not an uncommon occurrence in young children.

Appearing in the groin the abscess may be mistaken for hernia which it sometimes resembles rather closely, and gives a certain obscure impulse on coughing; but it is irreducible and the part of the psoas muscle within the abdomen can be felt to be enlarged and resistant. Psoas contraction is present, which causes flexion of the leg. Psoas abscess due to Pott's disease cannot be distinguished from psoas abscess due to other causes except by the presence or absence of the diagnostic signs of Pott's disease.

The Diagnosis of Paralysis.—Paralysis in Pott's disease, although ordinarily one of the later symptoms, may occasionally precede the deformity, and be the first sign of the presence of vertebral disease. Such cases are not so rare that they should be overlooked. The occurrence of myelitis in a young child should be considered as extremely suspicious, and as being more likely to be due to Pott's disease than to any other cause, even if the signs of vertebral disease are obscure or apparently absent. In general the paralysis is preceded by a stage of the disease in which this pain is much increased, and this pain may be paroxysmal or steady.

The first thing noted generally in the paralysis is a tendency to tire easily, and to hit the toes in walking. A disability to use the legs much and a staggering gait follow this very closely, and along with it is often a jerking and twitching of the legs at night, with an occasional cramp of the muscles. When such paralysis occurs in connection with disease of the cervical and dorsal regions, the patella reflexes are much increased and ankle clonus is present to a marked degree. In disease of the lumbar region, however, the pressure may be upon the cord below the reflex centres of the cord, and the patella reflex may be absent as well as the ankle clonus. The paralysis is generally one of motion only, but in severer cases sensation is impaired or lost. The paralysis may be either a slight disability or a complete loss of power, and its general diagnostic symptoms are those of myelitis.

A CASE OF PEMPHIGUS FOLIACEUS ENDING FATALLY WITHIN EIGHT MONTHS.

By HERMANN G. KLOTZ, M.D.,

OF NEW YORK.

THE history of the following case of pemphigus chronicus vulgaris, turning into pemphigus foliaceus and ending fatally within about eight months, has been taken from my notes, principally at the suggestion of my friend, Dr. J. W. Gleitsmann, Professor of Laryngology in the New York Polyclinic, on account of its bearing on the incidental affections of the oral cavity and the larynx. Dr. Gleitsmann having abandoned the idea of writing a paper on the subject, the case, I believe, is of interest enough in itself to justify its publication, since only very few cases of pemphigus foliaceus have been recorded in this country, those of Dr. Sherwell, of Brooklyn, and of Dr. Graham, of Toronto, Canada, mentioned by Duhring, being the only ones I could find after a careful search of the *Index Medicus*. Besides, interest in the case will be somewhat increased by the fact that recently the pathology of pemphigus was brought into greater prominence by the discussion of the subject before the late meeting at Vienna of the German Congress for Internal Medicine, in connection with a report by Mosler, of Greifswald, in which the participation of the mucous membranes formed an important part. The present case has been briefly mentioned by Dr. L. D. Bulkley in a paper published recently.[1]

Mr. F. T., cigar manufacturer; a native of Germany; forty-nine years of age, with a good family record; married, and father of six healthy children. Was first seen by me at my office on May 7, 1887. A man of strong physique, he had generally enjoyed good health; he at one time was a member of the police force of this city; he never had syphilis;. in 1876 he had pneumonia, and, somewhat later, trouble with the left tonsil, which he subsequently had removed. In December, 1886, he contracted a severe cold at the inauguration of the Montefiore Home, and on another occasion soon afterward had his feet thoroughly chilled. Within a short time he began to suffer with bronchitis. In January, 1887, he noticed a blister on the left breast, and soon after blisters in the mouth, particularly on the gums, which caused a great deal of annoyance, especially during eating and otherwise. He consulted several specialists for mouth and throat diseases, without relief. It appears that the lesions in the oral cavity were considered as specific, and were treated accordingly. I saw the patient first in consultation with his family physician, Dr. J. Scheider, and with Dr. Gleitsmann, because the latter had some doubt as to the nature of the lesions of the skin as well as of the mouth.

On inspection of the oral cavity the gums, from the edge about halfway to their base, appeared devoid of epithelium, leaving a dark-red, nearly cherry-colored surface, with intervening yellow spots here and there. The mucous membrane of the cheeks, of the uvula, and of the soft palate showed the same loss of the epithelial cover, forming irregular and variously outlined dark-red patches, partly covered with yellowish membranes resembling mild diphtheritic exudations. Between the upper and lower maxillæ this condition was particularly severe, shallow fissures of a deep-red color appearing on the generally yellowish surface. On the upper surface of the tongue, as well as on the lower one, numerous dark-red raw spots were likewise noticed.

On the scalp, which, particularly in the front parts, was but thinly covered with dark-brown hair, a number of bullæ of different sizes, more or less tensely distended with a clear, watery fluid, were observed; the largest one, about the size of a fifty-cent piece and rather flat, was located just within the hair, several smaller ones over the vertex, and some on the forehead. Beside these blebs a number of pale reddish spots could be noticed on the face and scalp, some of them quite smooth, some covered with thin scales resembling gold-beater's skin. On the right aspect of the neck a number of similar bullæ were found, one behind the left

ear covered with a blackish crust owing to the application of nitrate of
silver, and further down on the same side a larger cluster of smaller
bullæ or vesicles containing a perfectly clear fluid.

Quite a number of similar bullæ and scaly or smooth spots were scattered over nearly the entire front and back of the thorax without forming distinct groups, while on the abdomen only a few blisters could be
observed, besides numerous reddish spots, which, according to the patient's
observation, mark the first stage in the development of blisters.   The
bullæ vary in size from a hemp-seed to a small filbert; the more recent
ones are all hemispherical and tensely distended, while some of the older
ones are flaccid and overlap their bases like a bag.   The contents of
the blebs were in almost all cases perfectly clear, only in the dependent
portions of some of the older ones a somewhat opaque or even pus-colored
fluid could be observed.   Close to the frenulum glandis penis two small
excoriated depressions of a remarkably dark-red color, resembling that
of raw smoked beef, were found; on no other part of the body, particularly not on the extremities, could blisters or scars or other pathological
changes be detected; the lymphatic ganglia were nowhere enlarged or
otherwise affected.

On the strength of these symptoms, in connection with the condition
of the mouth, and with the history of their development, the diagnosis
of pemphigus chronicus vulgaris was made.   The patient was ordered
to take arsenic and iron (Fowler's solution with the tinctura ferri
pomati, 1 part to 12; 20 to 30 drops three times a day); locally, baths
and a dusting powder composed of bismuth, zinc, and starch were given.
Considering the comparatively small extent of the disease after a duration of over three months, it could be regarded as of a mild type.   Up
to May 11th very few new blebs had made their appearance, except in
both axillæ, where clusters of smaller bullæ were visible, some containing a transparent fluid of a light-yellow color; others were dried up
into a yellowish crust.   The maculæ on the abdomen had entirely disappeared.

May 17*th.* No new blebs were found; almost all the former ones had
dried up, leaving brownish spots, some of them scaly.   Even the axillary
eruption showed great improvement, but the excoriations on the penis
had not undergone any change.   The dose of the medicine had been
increased to 40 drops without any trouble, except slight costiveness.

25*th.* While only a few new bullæ have broken out on the body,
numerous clusters of smaller ones have developed between the toes and
on the soles of both feet, while the large one on the scalp, as well as
another quite conspicuous one over the right clavicle, have entirely dried
up.   The nail of the right thumb shows a brownish color, suggesting the
formation of a blister beneath that had rapidly dried up again.   The
patient's general health is fair; he has retained the weight of one hundred and seventy-two pounds to which he had previously fallen.

June 1*st.* A few new bullæ on the right arm and the thorax have
appeared, but quite numerous ones beneath and between the toes which
are very annoying on account of itching and of the offensive smell of
the easily decomposing contents.   After removing the cuticula as far as
possible with a pair of curved scissors, the parts were cleansed with a
solution of boric acid, dusted with bismuth, and covered with borated
cotton.

In this way the disease continued, taking a still comparatively mild course, up to June 20th; although constantly new blisters formed, some of them in groups, still they had the tendency of drying up rapidly and to leave the skin but little impaired, except as to its color, which was changed into a reddish-brown. From that date on, however, it assumed a different character. Not only did the isolated bullæ all over the trunk become more numerous, but also, first on the right forearm and very soon afterward on the left one, more flaccid bullæ appeared in great numbers; they extended within a few days from the shoulders to the wrists and to the backs of the hands, and soon began to run together, detaching the epidermis over a considerable space in the centre and leaving a denuded, bright-red, shining or glazed surface, as in eczema rubrum, or that beneath the blisters of a burn of the second degree. Although in the central portions of such patches new epidermis was formed, it never became solid and firm again, but remained brittle, divided by superficial fissures, or slightly scaling. In the peripheral portions, particularly around the wrists, the bullæ lost their sharply defined form and the epidermis was raised in a continuous outline, clearly exhibiting the character of pemphigus foliaceus.

After June 20th the patient was unable to dress, and had to stay at home. Arsenic, the dose of which had heretofore been gradually increased, was now omitted, owing to loss of appetite and dyspeptic symptoms, and 5 grains of the muriate of quinine were given every three hours. Local baths were applied to the arms; but on the 22d the eruption of bullæ became so general all over the trunk that the patient was ordered to stay in the bath-tub as continually as possible at a temperature of 80° to 85°. This he did from that date with little interruption up to August 1st, generally repairing into the bath-tub at 5 or 6 o'clock A.M., and remaining there as late as 9 P.M., taking all his meals while there. The warm weather prevailing throughout July, 1887, favored the use of a bath as continuously as circumstances would permit. During the night lotions or powders were applied, and the compound salicylated soap plaster which I have devised[1] was used on the larger raw patches with good effect.

A slight remission followed this first stormy eruption, lasting, however, but a few days. The bullæ now numbered by hundreds, and new ones were constantly added, while the old ones rapidly dried up and even the denuded surfaces showed considerable improvement. Except a feeling of weakness the general condition of the patient was fair, appetite good, bowels regular; sleep at night was not very quiet, but the patient had a number of naps during the day. The urine at this time and through the entire course of the disease never showed any irregularities; it was voided, without any trouble, in normal quantities, was generally of a light-yellow color, and never showed the presence of albumin or sugar.

A new feature manifested itself after June 27th. Heretofore all the new blebs appeared on skin of normal condition (except on the arms, where it was considerably swollen and red during the intense eruption), and had caused but slight burning or itching preceding the eruption. On the above date it was noticed that some of the bullæ on the trunk rose on top of a wheal-like, reddish elevation, accompanied by considerable itching. On the next day numerous slightly elevated patches of a

---

[1] New York Med. Journal, Sept. 17, 1887.

dusky-red color were observed on the lower part of the trunk, extending nearly symmetrically to the thighs, varying in size from a silver half-dollar to a dollar. Over these patches numerous small blisters with perfectly clear contents could be observed, principally studding the borders of the patches, most of them yet half-hidden in the skin, causing intense itching before and after eruption. This condition answered very well to the description of pemphigus pruriginosus given by Kaposi.

While the general condition of the patient remained satisfactory, on June 30th it was noticed that for the first time bullæ appeared on parts previously unaffected; on the back and abdomen several blisters attained the size of a walnut, raised more than half an inch above the surface of the skin. On July 1st the patient was seen in consultation by Dr. George H. Fox, who proposed mainly a change of diet to a more vegetable and less stimulating one.

It is no longer necessary to follow so closely the course of the disease. During the first part of the month of July there followed a general improvement. Still, new blisters were forming constantly and on some localities large areas denuded of epidermis could always be found, while in certain portions, particularly around the joints—above all, about the wrists—the foliaceous character never entirely disappeared. The patches, resembling urticaria, gradually flattened down and coalesced, forming extensive areas of a dark, bluish-red color, which, at first beginning only around the borders, soon changed into a brighter, almost scarlet, tint, and presented its former deep hue only after the patient had assumed an upright position for some time. The groups of smaller vesicles, often half-hidden in the skin, with their intense itching, continued to appear beside the isolated larger bullæ arising from the uninfiltrated skin. After July 6th the quinine was omitted and 10 grains of salicylate of soda were given every three hours. This drug seemed to have a beneficial effect on the itching and on the formation of the smaller blisters, but the general condition was not much altered; therefore, on the 17th Fowler's solution was again resorted to, increasing from 2 to 5 drops three times a day.

About July 19th an extensive eruption over the buttocks obliged the patient to relinquish the bath-tub for several days, as the pressure on these parts became unbearable; but he soon returned to the bath, as apparently he found more comfort in the water than in the bed. About the same time the affection of the mouth and lips, which so far had continned in a moderate degree, began to cause intense suffering, and obliged the patient to avoid solid food almost entirely. Dr. D. L. Bulkley, who saw the patient for the first time on July 26th, recommended a more effective administration of arsenic, which now was tried in the form of the solution of sodium arsenatis, 2 to 10 drops every two hours.

A short period of improvement set in again about August 1, although the formation of new blisters did not cease entirely, and several portions remained at all times severely affected; in general the tendency to form a new epidermis decidedly prevailed over that of destruction. The affection of the mucous membrane of the mouth and its adnexa, however, remained exacerbated, and considerably annoyed the patient by the discharge of a copious serous secretion, which originated either in the pharynx or the œsophagus or the trachea or the larger bronchi.

Heretofore the temperature had always remained normal and the pulse seldom exceeded 72. On the evening of August 5th Dr. Scheider, who continuously attended Mr. T., found the temperature at 101°, pulse 120, with frequent respiration, and the patient in a state of great weakness. The next day at noon, with a temperature of 102°, pulse 112, respiration 30, he was very low and weak, continuously expectorating large quantities of a sero-purulent fluid from the throat. The symptoms suggested congestion of the lungs or beginning pneumonia, of which, however, no physical signs could be detected by careful examination. Under the administration of valerian with the carbonate of ammonia and stimulants, the temperature remained between 101° and 100.5°, the pulse about 96, the respiration somewhat more frequent than normally for the next three days. After August 10th the temperature again became normal, the pulse less frequent, the secretion gradually less, and the general condition of the patient improved considerably, leaving him, however, a great deal weaker physically and psychically much more depressed. He repaired to the bath-tub only occasionally and for short periods on account of increasing weakness, although he longed for the relief afforded by the bath.

Throughout the remainder of August the disease continued its course with little change; the temperature showed occasional elevations to 100.8° and 101.4°; the pulse retained a frequency of 90 beats and over. While the patient was able to take sufficient quantities of nourishment, as the mouth and throat were in much better condition again, and the secretion therefrom had almost entirely ceased, the bowels exhibited a tendency to looseness, three to five passages a day being the rule. The local process on the skin showed occasional remissions, but short and slight. From the time the bath was given up the scaling became much more conspicuous, and on some parts considerable accumulation of the brittle, grayish or yellowish scales took place, often hiding from view the real condition of the denuded corium underneath and exhibiting more distinctly that condition to which the name of pemphigus foliaceus owes its origin. At the same time a peculiar smell, mentioned by several authors, became noticeable, to gradually give way to the more decided offensive odor of decomposing epidermis. Altogether the patient presented a most pitiable sight: new blisters were constantly appearing all over the body, repeated eruptions taking place on the same localities, and hardly a square inch of normal skin could be found. Now the inguinal, now the popliteal region, now penis and scrotum, now neck and back, were the parts principally affected, generally showing the corium exposed over a large area, with bleeding and oozing fissures wherever the skin is exposed to flexion and extension ; even the face became affected extensively, particularly the chin, lips, and eyelids, which at different times were entirely devoid of epidermis or covered with black crusts. The conjunctiva of the lids and of the bulbs blistered in their turn, and sores remained on the swollen mucous surface for some time. Around the heels the blistering process became extremely painful, owing in part to the thickness of the epidermis, which could not be detached so easily, and with its sharp, hard edges cut deep, extremely sensitive fissures. To relieve the local lesions, lotions, powders, ointments, plasters, and cotton padding were employed wherever it was found possible to do so, but scarcely had the last spot been attended to when the first ones again required attention, so that there was not a moment of real rest or comfort. Arsenic was continued as regularly as possible, together with opiates to check the diarrhœa.

About the 1st of September the mouth, throat, and larynx again became worse, while externally several places began to dry up. Owing to my absence from New York, I did not see the patient again after that date. From personal communications from the attending physician, Dr. Jul. Scheider, and from notes taken by the nurse, I shall briefly report the final course of the disease: The rise of temperature was more constant and more pronounced, reaching 102.4° on the 2d and again on the 5th of September, after a slight remission; it attained 103° on the 6th, to fall again to 102.6° on the following days. The pulse became much more frequent: after rising to 108 on September 4th, it increased to 128 on the 5th, 130 on the 6th, 136 on the 7th, and continued about 120 to the end. Diarrhœa became much more profuse from day to day, six passages occurring on the 1st of September, eight on the 2d, nine on the 3d, ten on the 4th and 5th, twelve on the 6th, twenty-one on the 7th, 8th, and 9th. The patient gradually lost strength, without ever losing consciousness, and died on the morning of September 10th. During the last few days, with the rapid increase of diarrhœa, no more new blisters appeared.

There is a certain temptation to range this case among the cases of dermatitis herpetiformis on account of the intercurrent appearance of the clusters of small, very itchy vesicles on hyperæmic patches, which, indeed, were more or less herpetiform, but otherwise the disease did not exhibit the characteristic features of dermatitis herpetiformis. In the later stages the disease had much in common with impetigo herpetiformis, the contents of the bullæ being purulent from the start, in many instances; but for a long period there existed only bullæ with clear, serous contents and no pustules at all, thus distinctly differing from impetigo. Unfortunately, no autopsy could be obtained, which certainly would have elucidated one point in which I was particularly interested—the origin of the diarrhœa. I have little doubt that it was due to the extension of the pemphigoid process (of forming bullæ and destroying the epithelial cover) to the intestinal tract. There is certainly some probability of such an occurrence in view of the participation of the mucous membranes of the oral cavity, the larynx, and the œsophagus; and this supposition finds a valuable support in the observation in Dr. Graham's case, where the report on the autopsy says:[1] "Mucous membrane along the lesser curvature of the stomach was congested, and about twenty spots were discovered which nearly resembled some of the patches of eruption on the skin. The spots varied in size from that of a pea to a ten-cent piece, and on close inspection were found to consist of superficial ulcerations, some extending partly and some altogether through the mucous membrane. The mucous surface of the large intestine was very much congested and thickened in some places. Death seems to have been hastened by the eruption, so to speak, on the mucous surface of the stomach."

Concerning the effects of treatment, I must candidly confess that I do

---

[1] Canadian Journal of the Medical Sciences, 1879, p. 172 et seq.

not believe the course of the disease was at all influenced by the same. There were, indeed, several periods of improvement, but I consider them rather as spontaneous fluctuations—exacerbations and remissions being more or less the rule in all cases of chronic pemphigus. I therefore cannot agree with Dr. Bulkley as to the effectiveness of arsenic, certainly not in the case of Mr. T., although I am well aware that in a number of cases it has undoubtedly been given with great benefit and is considered almost the only remedy worthy of a trial. It was given early and later on certainly in abundant doses, but, as the final result proved, without real effect. I cannot suppress a suspicion that arsenic had something to do with the profuse passages, although I cannot bring forth any positive evidence in favor of this opinion. Generally, arsenic shows its best results in skin diseases accompanied by dryness and scaling, rather where an excessive formation of the corneal layer of the epidermis takes place. Why it should have the same effect in a disease where the formation of epidermis is defective, rather, and a constant loss of the same takes place, as in pemphigus, is not easily understood. Although we have lately heard less of the advantages of the internal use of ichthyol as proclaimed by Unna, I should feel inclined to try it whenever I may meet with a similar case again.

The external applications were made with the purpose rather of relieving the suffering of the patient than of effecting a cure. There is no doubt in my mind that the use of the protracted bath gave the greatest relief, and that it ought to be resorted to wherever practicable.

42 E. TWENTY-SECOND ST., NEW YORK.

DR. FINLAY'S MOSQUITO INOCULATIONS.

BY GEORGE M. STERNBERG, M.D.,

LIEUT.-COL. AND SURGEON, U. S. ARMY.

MY friend Dr. Finlay, of Havana, has recently published in THE AMERICAN JOURNAL OF THE MEDICAL SCIENCES (September, 1891) the statistics of his " preventive inoculations" against yellow fever by means of mosquitoes. As the editor of a prominent medical journal[1] has devoted an editorial article to the subject in which he says " the results would seem to show that this insect is a good attenuator of yellow-fever virus," I think it proper to make a few remarks with reference to these so-called " mosquito inoculations," especially as I did not consider it necessary to refer to them in my published reports upon the etiology and prevention of yellow fever. I have not considered the subject as demanding serious attention, for the reason that *the mosquito does not inject the blood drawn from a yellow fever patient into the inoculated individual, but it*

1 The Medical Record, New York, September 19, 1891.

enters the insect's stomach, and whatever remains after its meal has been digested is passed per anum.

When the mosquito introduces its proboscis into the individual who is to be inoculated it is for the purpose of withdrawing blood, and it is difficult to see how any inoculation can occur, unless some virus has adhered to the exterior of the delicate instrument during the considerable interval which elapses after one full meal before the insect can be induced to fill itself again.

This supposition, viz., that a minute quantity of virus adhering to the surface of the proboscis of the insect is sufficient to produce a mild attack of the disease in an unprotected person, does not appear very probable, and very positive experimental evidence will be required before it can be accepted, especially as we have some experimental evidence which indicates that the blood of an individual sick with yellow fever may be injected beneath the skin of an unacclimated person without producing any noticeable effect.

In my official report, published in 1889,[1] I gave the following account of experiments made in my presence by Dr. Daniel Ruiz, of Vera Cruz:

" If the infectious agent in yellow fever is present in the blood, we would expect that the disease may be transmitted by inoculating a susceptible person with blood drawn from one sick with the disease. Dr. Finlay, of Havana, believes that the disease is commonly transmitted by mosquitoes, which, after filling themselves from a yellow fever patient, transmit the germ by inoculation into susceptible persons. Evidently the most satisfactory and direct way of determining whether the infectious agent is present in the blood would be to make inoculation experiments in susceptible persons. Before going to Brazil I had considered the possibility of making this crucial experiment, and had determined to make it if opportunity offered. When in Vera Cruz I learned that the experiment had already been made in 1885 by Dr. Daniel Ruiz, director of the civil hospital in that city. Dr. Ruiz is an entire unbeliever in the infectious nature of yellow fever, and had no confidence in the alleged discovery of a yellow fever germ by Dr. Carmona, of the City of Mexico. In order to test in a practical manner the truth of his views, he made, in 1885, injections of blood and of urine from typical cases of yellow fever into the subcutaneous connective tissue of an ' unacclimated ' person. The result of these inoculations was negative. At the time of my visit to Vera Cruz he expressed his entire willingness to repeat these experiments in my presence. This was exactly what I desired, and accordingly Dr. Ruiz made three inoculation experiments upon three unacclimated persons in the hospital. Unfortunately, the blood used for two of these individuals was obtained from a case in which the pathological appearances did not fully sustain the diagnosis of yellow fever made during life. This case is one of great interest with reference to the question of diagnosis, and I shall give a tolerably full account of it. The third inoculation was made from a non-fatal case in the eighth day of sickness; urine still albuminous; skin yellow. Fifty cubic centimetres of blood were drawn from the median vein of this patient by means of a hypodermic syringe, which had been carefully sterilized. This was immediately after injected, subcutaneously, in the deltoid region, into the arm of a man aged forty years, from the interior of Mexico, who had been in Vera Cruz only twenty days. The man from whom the blood was taken was apyretic, and the experiment is open to the criticism that it was perhaps too long after the inception of the malady. I was, there-

[1] Annual Rep. Sup. Surgeon-Gen. Marine-Hospital Service, 1889, p. 166.

fore, anxious to make other experiments before leaving Vera Cruz, but the tim fixed by my orders expired without my having had an opportunity to do so."

I do not consider the experiments made as entirely conclusive; but, on the other hand, I know of no experimental evidence which goes to show that the blood of yellow fever patients contains the virus of the disease, and that yellow fever can be transmitted by inoculations with such blood. Before admitting that the virus can be attenuated by passing through the body of the mosquito, I think we should have some satisfactory experimental evidence that the infectious agent is present in the blood. But, as stated, if it were present it would be passed with the excrement of the insect, and not injected into the inoculated individual.

In Dr. Finlay's last paper he says:

" I infer that the insect has some way of rendering its outer surface aseptic, and probably does so through a very peculiar operation, which I have often seen it perform. This consists in collecting with its hind or middle legs a secretion expelled from the posterior part of its body, and besmearing very persistently with it every part of its body—legs, wings, head, and proboscis."

If the exterior of the proboscis is rendered aseptic by this operation, it is difficult to see how any inoculation can occur even if the blood of the yellow fever patient constituted the true virus of the disease.

The transmission of the filaria sanguinis hominis by the mosquito is a very different matter from the mode of transmission imagined by Dr. Finlay in the case of yellow fever. The embryo filariæ are taken into the body of the insect with blood drawn at night from the infected individual, and, according to Manson, undergo certain developmental changes in the intermediary host, and are subsequently discharged into water with the larvæ of the insect. Other individuals are presumably infected by drinking this water.

But the à priori objections raised against Dr. Finlay's so-called " inoculations " must give way if it can be shown that decided and constant results follow the application of a mosquito, which has filled itself with blood from a yellow fever patient, to an " unacclimated" person. We fail to find satisfactory evidence that this is the case. In Dr. Finlay's published reports of his experiments we find that of 52 persons inoculated, only 12 (Group II.) " experienced, within a period of days varying between three and twenty-five after the inoculation, an attack of fever with or without albuminuria." Now that 12 out of 52 unacclimated persons arriving in Havana should suffer mild attacks of fever, " with or without albuminuria," is not surprising; and inasmuch as 40 other persons inoculated did not suffer similar attacks within twenty-five days after the supposed inoculation, we see no reason for ascribing the slight attacks of fever suffered by these 12 to the application of a mosquito by Dr. Finlay. If these 12 had all suffered characteristic attacks of yellow fever within a few days after the so-called inoculation, the experimental evidence might have some weight; but the attacks recorded occurred at intervals of from three to twenty-five days, whereas the period of incubation in yellow fever is generally admitted to be comparatively short, and probably does not exceed three to five days. Moreover, the slight febrile attacks experienced without albuminuria cannot be identified with yellow fever, and if they could, would be more rationally accounted for by ascribing them to the recent arrival of these individuals in a yellow-fever-infected city.

As to Dr. Finlay's Group IV., "twenty-four who did not experience pathogenic effects within the twenty-five days, but subsequently had fevers of a mild type, either non-albuminuric or with slight or transient albuminuria," we do not see any reason for supposing that the mosquito inoculation was in any way concerned in the development of these attacks. Such attacks are common in Havana and in tropical or semitropical countries generally. Whether such attacks in newcomers in yellow-fever-infected ports are to be considered "fevers of acclimation," and to what extent they afford protection against subsequent attacks of yellow fever, has not been fully determined. But that such attacks frequently occur, and that strangers arriving in Havana or in Rio de Janeiro frequently remain in these infected cities for several years without suffering any more pronounced attack of yellow fever than this so-called "acclimating fever," is a matter of common observation among physicians in the cities mentioned.

Finally, we call attention to the fact that four of the individuals inoculated by Dr. Finlay subsequently suffered genuine attacks of yellow fever; that one of the four died, and two of the remaining cases are said to have been severe.

As to Dr. Finlay's comparative statistics we shall say nothing at present, except that such comparisons call for a very careful analysis of the facts relating to surroundings, exposure, etc.; and that medical literature abounds in similar comparisons, in which the value of a certain treatment appears to have been established by statistics, but in which, unfortunately, a more extended trial by other members of the profession has failed to confirm the sanguine expectations of the author of the method. So far as I am aware, there has been no confirmatory evidence by other members of the profession in Cuba, and no one has felt sufficiently impressed with its value to repeat the experiments of Dr. Finlay and his associate, Dr. Delgado. I esteem both of these gentlemen very highly, and I would welcome most gladly a demonstration of the value of the method which they faithfully endeavored to test. But a justifiable scientific scepticism makes it necessary to demand more direct and satisfactory proof that the so-called inoculations produce any pathogenic effect before any great importance can be attached to the results of Dr. Finlay's laudable efforts to discover a method of prophylaxis in yellow fever.

REVIEWS.

LEÇONS DE THÉRAPEUTIQUE. Par GEORGES HAYEM, Professeur de Thérapeutique et de Matière Médicale à la Faculté de Médecine de Paris; Membre de l'Académie de Médecine. Troisième série. Pp. 450. Paris: G. Masson, 1891.

LECTURES ON THERAPEUTICS. By GEORGES HAYEM, Professor of Therapeutics and Materia Medica of the Faculty of Medicine of Paris; Member of the Academy of Medicine. Third series.

THIS work on Therapeutics, coming from a country of which the medical literature has been, each year, enriched by contributions from the clinics of Germain Sée and Dujardin-Beaumetz, justly claims our attention. The name of the author, well known for nearly two decades, is a sufficient guarantee for sound laboratory work, extensive reading, and wide experience. It is, then, with more than ordinary interest that we take up this volume discussing the action of remedies.

The first twenty-two pages are devoted to a general introduction, closing with a brief statement of the results of intra-venous transfusion of blood, considered as a prophylactic measure, in which the observations of Wooldridge, Richet, Héricourt, Büchner, Behring, Kitsato, and the author are recorded. The fact that we are apparently about to enter upon a scarcely explored territory, the resources of which we can only surmise, gives great value to the clear statement of the results thus far recorded. The completion of a study of the drugs for the relief of pain, commenced in the preceding volume, occupies one hundred and sixteen pages. Although the older drugs have been less studied during the past few years because of the great interest that the synthetic compounds of organic chemistry have excited, yet the clearness with which the presentation of the useful and harmful effects of opium and its derivatives is set forth, calls for commendation. The subject of mixed anæsthesia, at one time a theme so fruitful for discussion, has received full justice, and the advantages as well as the dangers are fully recorded. Although the standpoint taken is that of the use of chloroform, yet the views there expressed will find acceptance amongst American practitioners.

Taking up the Solanaceæ, one is reminded of the interesting work of Harley, *The Old Vegetable Neurotics*, so thoroughly is the task performed, while in this section the more recently discovered alkaloids receive full attention. The treatment by aconite, the products of conium and of gelsemium suggest many uses known to the last generation, when pharmaceutical resources were not so abundant.

When we reach the chapter on sedatives of the aromatic series, we find a carefully considered *résumé* of the effects upon man, of quinine, salicylic acid, antipyrine, acetanilide, the phenacetines and exalgine. The poisonous effects of acetanilide are shown to be due, citing Lépine, Weill and Herczel, to the transformation of hæmoglobin into met-hæmoglobin, while the harmlessness of phenacetine, which does not give rise to aniline by decomposition in the blood, is clearly stated. The reviewer would submit that a daily dosage of fifteen grains of exalgine is considerably larger than is warranted by American practice. With-out undue enthusiasm, yet with full consciousness of the value of these drugs, we consider this section to be excellent. Its careful perusal will lift many a physician from the rut in which he is unconsciously moving. Electricity for the relief of pain, revulsive and surgical measures, with a very complete *exposé* of the plan of therapeutic action, brings this part of the work to a fitting conclusion.

Three lectures are devoted to a discussion of the hypnotic drugs. Dividing insomnia into two classes—that of (1) nervous and of (2) dys-crasic origin—he presents for consideration, paraldehyde, amylene hy-drate, urethan, sulphonal, and hypnone. The more recently discovered derivatives of chloral, as chloralamide, ural, and somnal, are timely acquisitions to our pharmacopœia in view of the great demand for remedies that shall be as efficient as chloral but without its harm-ful effects. Hypnal, a combination of chloral and antipyrine, receives praise as a hypnotic even if the insomnia be due to painful symptoms. Methylal, cannabis Indica, piscidia and its active principle, piscidine, receive perhaps more attention than their importance would seem to justify. The subject is concluded by a review of the physical means of producing sleep.

About sixty pages are occupied by a presentation of remedies known as anti-spasmodics. The author gives an excellent review of the numer-ous and interesting researches concerning the phenomena of convulsions, taking into consideration both central and peripheral causes. In the treatment by the bromides, and especially by the bromide of potash, we find evidence of a careful study; while the drugs more properly anæs-thetic and hypnotic, as Calabar bean, picrotoxine, nicotine, curare, hydrocyanic acid, the derivatives of valerian, pilocarpine, camphor, asa-fœtida, the nitrites, and the salts of zinc, are fully discussed in this con-nection. We notice that even simulo is not passed without comment, although no opinion is expressed as to its value. Physical measures, such as the various methods of hydro-therapy and electricity, conclude the presentation of the subject.

Under the head of remedies for the relief of anæsthesia we find a most interesting discussion of results from the application of electricity, metallo-therapy and metalloscopy, including that of magnets. In the forty pages concerning excito-motor remedies, we find much for our con-sideration. The careful physiological investigation of nux vomica and its alkaloids, and the therapeutical indications deduced therefrom, have prominent place. The action of arnica, ergot, phosphorus, and arsenic receive due mention. The electrical treatment and methods of diag-nosis by electricity are so fully and accurately set forth that one can readily believe that he is reading more than the usual information con-tained in text-hooks on general therapeutics.

Ten lectures are occupied with the study of drugs especially directed toward the relief of cardiac diseases. The author believes that the subject can best be considered by dividing the morbid elements, so far

as the symptoms are concerned, into three classes, each calling for a
particular medication. For the description of the first class he has
coined the word "kinesitaraxia" (from κίνησις, movement, and τάραξις,
trouble). This class includes the mechanical disturbances, the heart-
muscle and nerves being healthy; for the second class, "asystolia,"
an enfeeblement of the heart of nutritive origin or cardiac weakness;
for the third class, "ataxia," the nervous troubles of the heart, primary
or secondary, the cardiac neurasthenia. He presents a clear view of the
subject because he accepts, with the physiologists, the statement that
cardiac tonics are really cardiac poisons. Taking this view, then, we
follow his argument with great interest. Digitalis, and its derivatives,
the drug above all others whose physiology gives accurate indications
for its therapeutic use, are fully treated; even the physiological experiments of Williams, the importance of which is too little recognized in
his own country, have by no means escaped the observation of the
author, nor have they failed of proper appreciation. Squill, convallaria,
adonidine, and strophanthus have received the same careful attention as
digitalis. If we accept, with Schmiedeberg, the hypothesis that digitalis
increases blood-pressure by modifying the cardiac energy, and that this
action has as a consequence a greater filling of the arteries, we have a
good basis for the accurate therapeutical indications unfolded by the
author. These indications are equally well marked out for squill,
sparteine, caffeine, adonidine and strophanthus. In the treatment of
cardiac weakness the author believes in the use of such stimulants as
alcohol, ether, ammonia and caffeine in acute cases. In the chronic
form, sparteine, strophanthus, opium in small doses, the nitrites, iodide
of potash (Sée), iron and arsenic. Further it is insisted that great care
shall be exercised to ascertain the exact physical competency of the
heart. In the treatment of the disturbances of cardiac innervation are
considered the bromides, chloral, quinine and the valerianates. In
general the treatment of cardiac diseases, following the plan described
by the author, is based on sound physiology, confirmed by careful clinical observation.

One cannot lay aside this book without feeling that he has placed
himself abreast of the times as regards therapeutics, and that he has
a more just conception of the value of the newer drugs than those
interested in their commercial possibilities have given him; that he has
received from a master's hand the latest authoritative statement concerning many remedies not ordinarily found in the text-books; and that
(and it is by no means of little value) in the form of lectures this volume
has imparted to him the enthusiasm born of the speaker's personality.
The work has the thoroughness of that of Fonssagrives, with which, as
a student, the reviewer was familiar, together with the vigor of the
modern French school, tempered by the results of a careful review of
the opinions of eminent clinicians. In an English translation it would
be a welcome addition to the library of every practical physician.

R. W. W.

LEAD-POISONING IN ITS ACUTE AND CHRONIC FORMS. (The Gulstonian
Lectures, delivered in the Royal College of Physicians, March, 1891.) By
THOMAS OLIVER, M.A., M.D., F.R.C.P., Professor of Physiology, Uni-
versity of Durham ; Physician to the Royal Infirmary, Newcastle-upon-
Tyne. Pp. 121. Edinburgh and London : Young J. Pentland, 1891.

THE profession is indebted to Dr. Oliver for an interesting and instructive essay on lead-poisoning, a condition the manifestations of
which are unfortunately so protean and often so insidiously developed
that not rarely we fail to trace them to their origin. As stated by Dr.
Oliver, the subject of plumbism is not only of local but of national
importance. This applies to other nations than Great Britain, but
especially to our own, than which none is more heedless of the physical
well-being of its denizens. Adulteration of food here runs riot, uncon-
trolled by statutes which, if they exist, have actuality only in name,
and ill-health thus generated is too frequently perpetuated through the
ignorance of our *medici*, who are permitted by the flimsiness of our laws
to juggle with human life without other than a primer-like knowledge
of the rudiments of medicine.

How frequently lead-poisoning arises, not only in other trades than
lead-making, and through other channels than occupation, none save
those having this fact constantly in mind are well aware. The occurrence of lead-poisoning through drinking-water, food, the use of
cosmetics, hair-dyes, and the like, is sufficiently common, and its manifestations sufficiently insidious and unexpected, to permit the unwary
practitioner to be often misled.

Dr. Oliver's brochure is not an extended treatise on lead-poisoning,
the limit of three lectures not permitting the subject to be considered in
some directions more than in outline. This is the more to be regretted
because of his ample experience. As it stands, however, the book contains numerous original pathological and clinical facts of value. Some
of the former are based on experimental work which reflects great credit
on Dr. Oliver.

We note that Dr. Oliver is inclined to regard the gingival blue-line as
of local origin, due to absorption of the metal from the mucous membrane of the gum rather than to its precipitation from the blood by the
action of sulphur, originating from decomposing food elements in contact
with the teeth forming an insoluble lead sulphide from the soluble salts of
lead circulating in the loops of vessels in the gingival margin and in the
plasma of the perivascular spaces. The former view, which is that of
Grisolle, Bouillard, Gubler, and others (Dechambre's *Dictionnaire
Encyclopédique des Sci. Méd.*) who do not regard the blue-line as a sign
of lead-intoxication, appears to the reviewer to be negatived by the fact
that a very marked line occurs in cases of plumbism arising solely
through drinking-water containing too small an amount of the metal
sufficient to be absorbed from the gum margin to originate a decided
blue-line. The reviewer has seen a number of cases of plumbism due
to drinking-water slightly impregnated with lead, in which a marked
blue-line was present, and Dr. Oliver records on page 13 two cases of
lead-poisoning with a blue-line occurring similarly, in which the water
contained but 0.0028 grains per gallon.

Dr. Oliver holds, with Erb, Oeller and Romberg, that the primary
seat of the lesion in lead-palsy is, in all probability, usually in the spinal

cord, a view that has much in its favor, though it is at present far from being generally accepted. If the lesion is primary in the intra-muscular motor nerves, Dr. Oliver justly inquires, why should motor fibres, which are efferent, suffer from an ascending lesion, while the sensory (afferent) nerves nearly always escape? Pathological changes are probably not detected in the cord, because but a limited cornual area is allotted to functionally related groups of muscles, which may be readily overlooked in the examination. Erb (*Electro-therapeutics*), who reasons similarly, states: "*Gross* lesions cannot be looked for in a toxic process which usually recovers in a short time, and the *function* of the anterior gray columns and their ganglion cells may be very markedly disturbed, although no change can be demonstrated microscopically. And this disturbed function may produce degenerative atrophy of the peripheral nerves as readily as a primary affection of these tracts." In addition to citing other cases in which central lesions were found, Oliver also quotes Monakow and Oeller, each of whom have reported a case of lead-palsy in which decided changes were detected post-mortem in the anterior cornu. In the latter's case alterations were also found in the peripheral nerves, but far less advanced than those in the cord. The character of the cord lesion in this case—hemorrhages and softening in addition to advanced atrophy of the ganglion cells—indicated beyond doubt its primary character. To the reviewer's mind the fact that the palsy affects functionally related muscle groups, and is usually unaccompanied by sensory alterations, is the strongest argument against the peripheral origin.

Dr. Oliver's view regarding the probable cause of lead-eclampsia and other symptoms of encephalopathy is interesting. He looks upon the cerebral manifestations of plumbism as due rather to the retention in the body of animal poisons (leucomaïnes?) through deranged metabolism, and imperfect action of the excretory organs, especially the liver and kidneys, than to the deposition of lead in the brain, however intimately it may be combined with the protoplasm of nerve-cells. In his opinion it is usually found in too small an amount to account for the symptoms.

Blythe (*Journal of Mental Science*, January, 1888), it may be recalled, has shown that the greater portion of lead found in the brain in cases of encephalopathy ending fatally, exists in chemical union with the complicated nitrogenous and phosphorized fats, as lead-kephalin, forming a definite substitution compound, in which a molecule of hydrogen is replaced by one of lead. It appears to the reviewer that but a grain of lead so disposed (the amount found in the brain in one of Oliver's cases) would be sufficient to originate the various phases of encephalopathy. As suggested by Blythe, so important a modification as the replacement of hydrogen in its molecule by lead, which is not a structural change, but one of composition, must profoundly modify, if not annihilate, whatever function kephalin may possess. Hughlings-Jackson's view of the origin of epileptiform seizures (*Lumleian Lectures on Convulsive Seizures*, 1890) is very suggestive in this connection. He regards them as due to an unstable condition of a few nerve-cells, owing to an unduly free interchange occurring between the contents of the cell and the surrounding fluid which bathes it, leading to an alteration in composition while its constitution remains unchanged. He instances stable glycerin being transformed into explosive nitro-glycerin without alteration in its constitution, by a substitution of a molecule of hydrogen by one of nitrogen peroxide. Is it not likely that a cell thus lead-saturated would be not only incapable of proper function, but highly unstable, constantly tending toward discharge?

Curiously, Dr. Oliver nowhere speaks of lead-arthralgia, a form of joint pain unattended with redness or swelling, and probably due to a neuralgia or neuritis of the intra-muscular and articular sensory nerve filaments. In this country it is a very common and early symptom of lead-intoxication. He deals very briefly with the therapeutics of plumbism, and here offers us nothing new. For the convulsive phase of encephalopathy he advises amyl nitrite, mentioning no other remedy save pilocarpine, which he resorts to when the seizures are accompanied by suppression of urine. The reviewer has used amyl nitrite and nitroglycerin alternately, the former by inhalation, the latter subcutaneously, successfully as regards breaking the spasm, but he has found both of scant avail in preventing a return. He prefers to rely on a very full dose (a half-grain or more in an adult) of morphine hypodermically, and chloral and potassium bromide by the mouth or rectum to prevent recurrence where the convulsions show a tendency to rapid repetition. Acute seizures of this sort, if not early controlled, terminate very early fatally.   D. D. S.

A CLINICAL TEXT-BOOK OF MEDICAL DIAGNOSIS FOR PHYSICIANS AND STUDENTS, BASED ON THE MOST RECENT METHODS OF EXAMINATION. By OSWALD VIERORDT, M.D., Professor of Medicine at the University of Heidelberg; formerly Privat-docent at the University of Leipzig; later, Professor of Medicine and Director of the Medical Polyclinic at the University of Jena. Authorized Translation from the second improved and enlarged German edition, with Additions. By FRANCIS H. STUART, A.M., M.D., Member of the Medical Society of the County of Kings, New York; Fellow of the New York Academy of Medicine; Member of the British Medical Association, etc. With 178 illustrations, many of which are in colors. Philadelphia: W. B. Saunders, 1891.

THIS is an octavo volume of 700 pages, of which the last 93 are devoted to the index.

The work is divided into three parts, the first being introductory, and, therefore, largely concerned with the explanation of terms of frequent recurrence, and with the proper mode of recording cases; the second, dealing with the general examination of the patient, such as—1, his physical condition; 2, his decubitus; 3, his general structure and state of nutrition; 4, his skin and subcutaneous cellular tissue; 5, his temperature and pulse; while the third is devoted to special diagnosis.

The various diagnostic methods in diseases of the respiratory and circulatory systems, the digestive and urinary apparatus, and the nervous system, are detailed with great clearness, and are evidently described by one who is himself an expert in them all. In addition, there is a short appendix containing directions as to laryngoscopical and ophthalmoscopical examinations and the staining of bacilli. The translator has performed his arduous work in an excellent manner, and has interpolated some practical additions.

Allusion has been made to the apparently disproportionate size of the index to this book, but not with the object of unfavorable criticism, for it is in a work of this class that one wishes to turn as rapidly as possible to the facts concerning a symptom which may be common to many diseases, and which are, therefore, widely scattered through its pages. An elaborate index is, therefore, a necessity.

Both the typography of the book and its illustrations are good, and we heartily wish it the success it has met with in Germany.

F. P. H.

HANDBOOK OF DISEASES OF THE EAR, FOR THE USE OF STUDENTS AND PRACTITIONERS. By URBAN PRITCHARD, M.D. Edin., F.R.C.S. Eng., Professor of Aural Surgery, King's College, London, etc. Second edition, with illustrations. Pp. 238. Philadelphia: P. Blakiston, Son & Co., 1891.

IN preparing a second edition of this book the author has revised the whole, rewritten a large portion of it, and added much new matter. The increasing attention which is being paid to the effects of naso-pharyngeal disease upon hearing has led the author to give a special chapter to these subjects. Another chapter is devoted entirely to the consideration of the important complications and sequelæ of middle-ear suppuration, including mastoiditis and cerebral abscess. Otomycosis and exostosis in the external ear receive fair consideration. We are surprised that when chronic suppuration in the attic is under consideration the author offers no method of treatment which he considers efficient in curing the disease, but condemns, evidently without ever having tried it, as he considers it "obviously a serious operation," the only means of a radical cure in these cases, viz., excision of the diseased membrana, malleus, and incus. This operation has never, so far as the reviewer knows, been followed by any reaction; on the contrary, it has invariably been followed by a cure of suppuration in the antro-tympanic space. It is no more "obviously a serious operation" than perforation of the mastoid. It is amazing that so useful an operation should be condemned, apparently purely on à priori grounds, without any evidence that the author of the book has either tried it or seen it performed. We regret that in a work offering so little that is new, there should be found a rejection of the only rational modern means of curing chronic suppuration in the attic space, while pages are devoted to discussing artificial drum-membranes, though no aurist of experience often resorts to their use. No one should wear such a thing in his diseased ear, excepting perhaps for a very short period in some special cases, under the constant supervision of an aurist. Patients should never be allowed to apply any form of artificial membrana tympani to their ears by themselves. To say the least it is a septic proceeding, unless carefully carried out and watched by a competent surgeon. The chapter on mastoiditis is a succinct account of the best methods of combating this very important malady.

C. H. B.

COLLECTED CONTRIBUTIONS ON DIGESTION AND DIET.   By SIR WILLIAM
ROBERTS, M.D., F.R.S., formerly Physician to the Manchester Royal Infirmary, and Professor of Medicine in the Victoria University. Small 8vo,
pp. xi., 261.   Philadelphia: Lea Brothers & Co., 1891.

IN this volume Sir William Roberts has collected all his contributions on subjects relating to Digestion, Dietetics and Dyspepsia, beginning with the Lumleian Lectures of 1880, "On the Digestive Ferments
and Artificially Digested Foods," and including an address "On Some
Practical Points in Dietetics," delivered before the Manchester Medical
Society in 1890.   A certain degree of order and coherence has been
given by some re-arrangement of materials and grouping of subjects,
but no attempt has been made to produce a systematic treatise.   All the
articles have been carefully revised.

To Sir William Roberts, above all others, we owe that great advance
in the feeding of the sick represented by the employment of predigested
foods ; and the number of lives he has thus been directly instrumental
in saving is simply incalculable.

The four sections in which the subject-matter is now grouped are—
I. Digestion and the Digestive Ferments ; II. Dietetics ; III. Preparation
of Food for Invalids ; IV. Dyspepsia.

Upon questions in the physiology of digestion that are still unsettled
the author expresses himself with proper reserve ; upon all others with
the authoritative clearness we expect from a teacher.   In practical
applications of the principles derived from the study of physiology he
is fertile.   His directions are clear, full, precise.   S. S. C.

A TREATISE ON THE DISEASES OF INFANCY AND CHILDHOOD.   By J.
LEWIS SMITH, M.D.   Seventh edition, thoroughly revised, with fifty-one
illustrations.   Philadelphia: Lea Brothers & Co., 1891.

A BOOK which has reached its seventh edition surely demands no critical review.   We have always considered Dr. Smith's book on Children
one of the very best on the subject, and as each edition appears, the
weeding that it has undergone, the planting that has taken place, the
cultivation of untouched soil, shows the careful gardener, the successful
cultivator, the fruits of whose toil are evident throughout this continent.

Dr. Smith's book has always been a practical book—a field book ;
theoretical, where theory has been deduced from practical experience—
he takes his theory from the bedside, and from the pathological laboratory.   He does not conceive his theory first and practice afterwards.

The very practical character of this text-book has always appealed to
our fancy.   It is characteristic of Dr. Smith in all his writings to collect
whatever recommendations are found in medical literature, and his
search has been wide, comprising the medical journals of the day.
Indeed, in many instances, after reading pages of what others think, one
sometimes says: But what does Dr. Smith say, and what are his recommendations ?

Possibly, he carries this too far.   Nevertheless, one seldom fails to find
a practical suggestion, after search in other works has been in vain.   We
cannot agree with several of the best authorities of the day that pædi-

atrios is not a specialty in itself. It may not be to-day, but it will be to-morrow. The symptoms, course, ultimate result, and treatment of diseases of children—indeed, many of the diseases themselves—are entirely different from those of adults, and, in our opinion, the sooner the profession recognize this, the sooner will infant mortality diminish.

In the seventh edition we note a variety of changes in accordance with the progress of the times. Obsolete material has been excluded, and the text condensed, and such matters added as conjunctivitis, icterus, sepsis, umbilical diseases, hæmatemesis, sclerema, œdema, pemphigus of the newborn, epilepsy, tetany, appendicitis, typhlitis, perityphlitis, and intubation.

But, to show how thorough has been the revision, one need only turn to the article on diphtheria. In the sixth edition this occupied thirty pages; in the present one we find a most exhaustive article of eighty-four pages, giving us the pathology up to date, and a most exhaustive section on treatment, in which the author for the first time in this text-book recommends the use of corrosive sublimate. We expect soon to see the seventh edition exhausted, and that when the eighth edition is called for we shall see the article on scrofula rewritten, and a section devoted to the diseases of the heart—a subject of great importance—the diseases of the liver, the diseases of the kidney, the diseases of the nervous system, the diseases of the blood, malaria in its various types, and such matters, that are of equal importance to any mentioned in the book before us, but which need discussion under special sections, that they may be referred to by the busy practitioner. The article on malaria, (at present, on intermittent and remittent fever), we think will scarcely satisfy the practitioner outside of New York. Indeed, the whole subject of fevers is one of the most unsatisfactory in Dr. Smith's book. The article on cerebro-spinal fever is a most exhaustive one. We should say far too much space has been given to it; whereas no mention whatever is made of the subject of ephemeral fevers which are so common during child-life, so annoying to the physician, so great a cause of anxiety to the parent, so difficult to differentiate, and so unsatisfactory to treat.

Dr. Smith's work still stands foremost as the American text-book. The literary style could not be excelled; its advice is always conservative and thorough; the evidence of research has long since placed its author in the front rank of medical teachers. For many years he has led the advance as the able and conservative teacher of pædiatrics, and we surely voice the feelings of his vast array of students and admirers throughout the continent when we wish that he may live long to give us the results of his great experience. J. M. K.

DIE KRANKHEITEN DER ATHEMORGANE, MIT SPECIELLER RÜCKSICHT AUF JAPAN. Bearbeitet von DR. E. BAELZ, Professor der klinischer Medicin an der Kais.-Universität zu Tokio. Mit 1 Titelbild in Farbendruck und zahlreichen Holzschnitten. Tokio, 1890.

DISEASES OF THE RESPIRATORY ORGANS, WITH SPECIAL REFERENCE TO JAPAN. By DR. E. BAELZ, Professor of Clinical Medicine in the Imperial University, Tokio.

THE rapid progress made by the Japanese in the appropriation and assimilation of Western science is nowhere more marked than in the domain of medicine. The domination of Germany in scientific medicine is perhaps shown by the fact that Berlin and Vienna, rather than London and Paris, furnish teachers to the Japanese schools. The present volume is the first one in which an attempt has been made to set forth concisely and authoritatively, for the principal benefit of Japanese students and practitioners, the present status of medical knowledge in a special field ; and the work has been apparently very well done. The nose, the larynx, the trachea, the bronchi, the lungs, and the pleura are studied. Each section begins with a brief elucidation of the anatomy and physiology of the parts, and is appropriately illustrated. The colored frontispiece, for example, gives a fairly accurate representation of the gross topographical anatomy of the contents of the chest and abdomen. The first woodcut shows a side view of the nasal chambers in relation with the pharynx, tongue, etc. Next follow methods of examination, and illustrations of the instruments necessary. We notice, in passing, that the author employs Zaufal's long nasal specula, and that the illustration of a laryngoscopic examination has a peculiarly Japanese appearance. Then general diagnosis is taken up, first giving local symptoms, then distant symptoms. There is next a section upon general therapy. After this the individual diseases are taken up in order ; their etiology, pathology, symptoms, and therapy being treated briefly or at length, in accordance with the importance of the affection under discussion, and always with special reference to the disease as manifested in Japan. Thus there is a careful study of " parasitic hæmoptoë " or " distomatosis pulmonum," with an excellent illustration of the parasite and of the sputum in this disease, which, of course, we do not ordinarily find elaborated in text-books for the use of European and American practitioners. Of the development of the parasite and the manner of its introduction into the human body, very little is positively known. Japan, Corea, and Formosa are the principal regions in which the disease occurs. In Kumoto it is estimated that no less than 39 per cent. of the school children suffer from it, small children and older persons being less frequently affected. In Nagamo the author saw one family in which five out of six members were affected. Women are very seldom attacked, but one having been found among 102 patients. The only diagnostic point is the expectoration of bloody sputum in which the ova are found.

                                                                    S. S. C.

PROGRESS

MEDICAL SCIENCE.

THERAPEUTICS.

UNDER THE CHARGE OF

REYNOLD W. WILCOX, M.A., M.D.,

PROFESSOR OF CLINICAL MEDICINE IN THE NEW YORK POST-GRADUATE MEDICAL SCHOOL AND
HOSPITAL; ASSISTANT VISITING PHYSICIAN TO BELLEVUE HOSPITAL.

The Treatment of Typhoid Fever.

DR. SICARD, after discussing the inconveniences and dangers in the use of salicylate of bismuth, charcoal, iodoform, naphthalin, and β-naphthol as intestinal antiseptics, in the *Revue de Thérapeutique Médico-chirurgicale* for 1891, No. 17, p. 458, recommends salol in daily doses, from fifteen to forty-five grains. Calomel, given in fractional doses, following the method of Bouchard, although diminishing the mortality, yet gives rise to a long convalescence. He believes chloroform in small doses to be one of the most useful and least dangerous of all. Used by Desprez in 1867 in cholera, and by Stepp in 1888 in gastric ulcer and in typhoid fever, the author administers it in five-drop doses, thrice daily. This dose is dissolved in one thousand parts of water. He further insists that large quantities of fluids shall be prescribed in small doses, frequently repeated, up to six or seven quarts per day; two quarts of milk, one quart of bouillon, in addition to water in which sugar-of-milk is dissolved. The amount of urine passed is frequently five or six quarts daily. This treatment not only favors the elimination of toxic matters, but restores to the organism the water lost through the lungs and skin.

Ergot for Hypodermatic Use.

In the *Therapeutische Monatshefte* for 1891, Heft 7, S. 369, DR. BIEDERT gives us a method for using ergotin subcutaneously without danger of producing either indurations or abscesses. He dissolves the extract of ergot in a 2 per cent. watery solution of carbolic acid. In the intervals between the injections the syringe remains filled with a 3 to 5 per cent. solution of carbolic acid, the needles being kept in a similar solution. At the time of the injection the site selected is cleansed with cotton moistened with the carbolic solution,˙ and the point of puncture covered by a second pledget of cotton dipped in the same solution.

———

EUROPHEN.

In the same number of the *Therapeutische Monatshefte*, S. 373, we find a bacteriological study of europhen by DR. W. SIEBEL. This product is the result of the action of iodine on isobutylorthocresol in the presence of an alkali, and its name, following its chemical composition, is isobutylorthocresoliodide. It is a fine yellow powder, soluble in alcohol, ether, chloroform and oils, but insoluble in water. In view of the widespread use of other derivatives of iodine, as iodoform, iodol, and aristol, this study is timely. On p. 379 DR. EICHHOFF presents the results of a very carefully conducted clinical research, from which he arrives at the following conclusions : It is of value in all cases of venereal disease, gonorrhœa excepted. In two cases of chancroids, simple dusting of the europhen was followed by rapid healing. Constitutional syphilis was favorably influenced by the remedy in all stages, whether applied externally or used by subcutaneous injection. In doses of a quarter of a grain there was no pain, neither general nor local reaction, but large doses (one and a half grains) gave rise to pains in the head and in the abdomen, especially in women. The advantage of the internal administration of this drug lies in the fact that in the organism the decomposition, with the setting free of iodine in the nascent condition, is a slow process. Among dermatological patients cases of parasitic eczema, psoriasis, and favus were not influenced by the application of europhen, but, on the other hand, favorable results followed in crural ulcer, scrofuloderma, exulcerating lupus and burns, the explanation apparently being that the separation of free iodine takes place only in the presence of moisture and not upon a dry surface, like that of the unbroken skin. Iodoform will be of more limited usefulness, because europhen has all of its advantages with none of its disadvantages, while aristol will not be displaced by europhen, but rather be complementary to it. For external use, a 5 or 10 per cent. salve, with 10 per cent. of olive oil in lanolin, or as europhen-traumaticin, one to twenty, is prescribed.

———

ELECTRIC CATAPHORESIS.

In the *Revue Internationale d'Electro-thérapie*, 1891, No. 12, p. 397, DR. IMBERT DE LA TOUCHE gives the results of this treatment of gout and rheumatism, using bryonia and iodide of lithia. The immediate results are greater mobility of the joints, lessened local pain ; the subsequent results are, tophi and swellings diminish, the patients gain in strength, can more readily bear fatigue, the appetite improves, digestion becomes easy, sleep becomes calm, and the general health markedly improves. Although the author's experience has been limited and of recent date, yet he believes that this treatment protects against relapses, and also against future attacks.

In the same number DR. GAUTIER relates his interesting experiences with electro-chemical punctures in local tubercular manifestations. This method

combines the chemical injections of Lannelongue with the electrolytic punctures of Le Fort, and promises to combine the valuable features of each.
The author has chosen patients suffering from diseases notoriously rebellious
to treatment, and although yet too early to announce the final results, yet he
believes that its field is one where a practice of this method will yield brilliant results.

METHYL-BROMIDE.

In the *Asclepiad*, No. 31, vol. viii. p. 239, in commenting upon the dangers
from the administration of the methyl- and ethyl-bromides, DR. B. W. RICH-
ARDSON calls attention to the fact that they decompose readily, and free bro-
mine may be liberated during inhalation, causing rapid spasmodic contraction of both the pulmonary and coronary arteries, with death by syncope.
The reasons for this warning are—1st, that these compounds are unstable,
being influenced by light, temperature, and exposure to the air; 2d, even
when the compounds are unchanged they are irritants; and 3d, they are
insoluble. They act quickly, and upon the minute pulmonary circulation,
but this very speediness of action is of great disadvantage.

THE IODIDES OF ANTIPYRINE.

In the *Bulletin général de Thérapeutique* for 1891, p. 158, M. DUROY gives a
most interesting account of his researches concerning two new organic iodides,
the iodides of antipyrine. Dating his investigations upon the antiseptic properties of the iodides from 1853 he believes he has now found a combination
superior to those previously known. The proto- and biniodides of antipyrine
are pleasant to the taste, and yet in solution prevent the putrefaction of meat,
which the iodides of potash and soda do not. Doses of six to nine grains *per
diem* are borne without any inconvenience. The proto-iodide appears suited
to such conditions as tuberculosis, and glandular enlargements, while the
more powerful biniodide should be used in typhoid fever, diphtheria, organic
diseases of the alimentary canal, and epidemic diseases. These iodides can
be administered in wafers, or rubbed up with sugar, or even placed dry upon
the tongue.

MORPHINE *vice* CODEINE AND NARCEINE.

In the *Dietetic Gazette*, 1891, No. 9, p. 177, DR. J. B. MATTISON makes an
eloquent plea for the use of less morphine, and in place thereof to prescribe
codeine and narceine. No one should be more conversant with the terrible
conditions brought about by the use of morphine, since his experience has
been extensive in his own special field, and probably no one more appreciates
the ease with which the habit is acquired than one whose particular work
consists in the care of *habitués*. Referring to a paper by Lauder Brunton, in
the *British Medical Journal* for June 9, 1888, in which the analgesic properties
of codeine are insisted upon, he believes that with pure codeine we can
obtain relief from pain in precisely those cases in which morphine seemed our
only resource. He believes, also, that it has distinct and decided hypnotic
properties. The gastric symptoms, the dulness and headaches, so often com-

plained of from the administration of morphine, do not follow codeine. The dose need not be increased, nor does it give rise to the indescribable craving of morphine. In following Fischer, with whose valuable contributions he is evidently familiar, he states that the dose is three times larger than that of morphine; the sulphate for administration by mouth, the phosphate for hypodermatic use. Narceine is not an anodyne, and it will not succeed as a soporific, if pain be present. In double the dose of morphine it is efficient in producing sleep. The hydrochlorate (of Merck) can be used for subcutaneous administration.

THE TREATMENT OF SYPHILIS.

Hefte 8 u. 9, 1891, of the *Wiener Klinik* contain the valuable work of DR. ELSENBERG on the treatment of syphilis. After discussing the curability of this disease, the question of re-infection, the results of the excision of the primary lesion, he comes to a consideration of the means at our disposal for the successful treatment. For the primary lesion, if phagedenic, the ordinary antiseptics are recommended: corrosive sublimate, carbolic acid, iodoform, derivatives of iodine. He recommends the method of inunction as the best of all for external use of mercury. He insists that a full warm bath which contains a pound of soda, the patient being well rubbed with soap, shall be taken for two or three days before treatment; that the teeth shall be put in order, and any inflammation of the mucous membrane of the mouth shall be treated by washes of 5 per cent. solution of salol dissolved in alcohol and well diluted with water. For inunction he advises the ordinary blue ointment popularized by Lebeuf, in doses from one-half to one and a half drachms. The time required for thorough inunction of the minimum quantity is upward of half an hour. This treatment is to be continued until all symptoms have disappeared, or eight or ten more treatments have been made, or there intervenes swelling of the oral mucous membrane. For six or eight weeks succeeding this treatment the iodide of soda or potash is to be employed. Although placing his reliance upon the inunction method, yet the author gives a very complete history of the various mercurials used for internal medication, as well as those used hypodermatically, both the soluble and insoluble salts.

In the administration of the iodides he prefers the iodide of potash, in doses sufficient to accomplish his purpose, even to one hundred and fifty grains *per diem*. The iodide of soda is to be substituted when potash is contra-indicated, because of the condition of the heart. In rare cases iodoform or odol (thirty to forty-five grains *per diem*) may be substituted.

[Although but little that is new is to be found in this monograph, yet the literature has been so thoroughly studied, the opinions of the clinicians discussed with so much fairness, the indications for treatment so clearly given, the methods to be employed so accurately described, that the careful perusal of this work will amply repay one who wishes to keep himself fully informed on the subject.—ED.]

CREASOTE.

In the *Revue de Thérapeutique Médico-chirurgicale* for 1891, No. 18, p. 497, we find described the method of DR. LEGROUX, who believes that creasote is of great value in preventing the broncho-pneumonia which so frequently follows the operation of tracheotomy. He recommends a formula as follows:

Beechwood creasote, pure .	. . . . . .	ʒss.
Glycerin .	. . . .	ʒiij.
Rum .	. . . .	ʒv.

To be administered in doses of from two to four teaspoonfuls, according to the age of the child. The treatment is to be commenced as soon as it is suspected that the diphtheria has extended to the larynx, and it is of advan_tage to impregnate the broncho-pulmonary mucous membranes before the operation is performed, so that their resistance to infection may be increased, As soon as the operation is completed it is well to place over the external opening of the canula a thin layer of cotton moistened in a mixture of which the following is the formula:

Creasote .	. . . .	♏xv.
Alcohol .	. . . .	ʒijss.
Glycerin .	. . . .	ʒv.

The internal medication, using the creasote mixture, is to be continued. This treatment does not appear to be as successful if the broncho-pneumonia has set in before the operation.

LAVAGE.

In the same number, page 498, we find the method of DR. LIENEVITCH, who proposes to relieve the vomiting which follows the administration of chloroform, by lavage. He believes that not only the chloroform, but as well the irritation of the peritoneum produced by the antiseptics, is accountable for this symptom. He employs the tube of Faucher and washes out the stomach with warm water in which ½ to 1 per cent. of bicarbonate of soda has been dissolved, until the water returns clear. The abdominal walls are compressed (after an operation of laparotomy has been performed) during the washing. The results are excellent, in that, if necessary, water sufficient for the needs of the patient can be left in the stomach. The general condition improves, because there is freedom from nausea, gaseous accumulations, vertigo, and epigastric distress.

METHYL-BLUE.

In the *Berliner klinische Wochenschrift*, No. 39, 1891, S. 953, DRS. PAUL GUTTMAN and P. EHRLICH give a valuable report of their investigations at the Moabit Hospital in Berlin. Taking the statement of Celli and Guarnieri, that the *plasmodium malariæ* was dyed by methyl-blue in fresh blood as well as in dry specimens, the authors set themselves at work to ascertain if this substance was of value in the treatment of malaria. Owing to the rarity of intermittent fever at Berlin but two cases are reported. The first patient suffered from the tertian variety and the diagnosis was undoubted, the temperature chart, condition of the spleen, and the presence of the plasmodium being confirmatory. On the evening of the day preceding the expected chill seven and one-half grains of methyl-blue were administered

Two hours after the dose there was slight strangury. During the night there were chilly sensations, a rise of temperature of about one and one-half degrees, with subsidence under gentle perspiration. Twelve hours after the administration of this dose the plasmodium was not dyed, nor indeed was there any change in the blood corpuscles. The same amount of methyl-blue was continued, but divided into five doses administered between noon and midnight. The chill did not again recur, and after the third day it was impossible to find plasmodia in the blood, and the spleen rapidly diminished to its normal size. In the second patient, suffering from the quotidian variety, an equally good result was obtained. This treatment must be continued for eight or ten days after the cessation of the fever. For the prevention of bladder irritation it is well to administer this medicament in powdered nutmeg (preferable to the ethereal oil, which is uncertain). Although the urine is increased in amount and deeply dyed, no albumin has been detected.

In Prof. Brieger's clinic methyl-blue has been used as a remedy for neuralgia (DR. ROBERT IMMERWAHR, *Deutsche medicinische Wochenschrift*, 1891, No. 41, S. 1147.) Here the drug has been used in somewhat smaller doses, to one and one-half grains daily. Eight cases of unilateral sciatica were treated without benefit. Two patients suffering from facial neuralgia, three from angio-spastic migraine were speedily relieved. Several cases of purely nervous headache, of alcoholic depression (*vulgo*, "Katzenjammer"), were cured within an hour. Muscular rheumatism and the neuralgia of herpes zoster were greatly benefited.

IODISM.

MR. F. W. ELSNER, in the *Australian Medical Journal*, 1891, No. 8, p. 377, reports a fatal case of iodism. A woman, forty-nine years old, for four days had taken less than four grains of iodide of potash every six hours. She suffered from a severe coryza; vesicles, blebs, and bullæ appeared on her face, backs of hands and forearms; hemorrhages were found in the scalp. Vomiting of blood, bloody stools, œdema of the feet, hemorrhages confined to face, hands and scalp, were the marked symptoms before her death. "This case illustrates, what has often been urged, viz., that the small doses of iodide produce iodism most rapidly; but most authorities differ as to the dose, etc., which ought to be administered."

THE CUTANEOUS ABSORPTION OF DRUGS INCORPORATED IN FATTY SUBSTANCES.

M. L. GUINARD has been carrying out some interesting experiments to ascertain—1st, if fatty substances, lard, vaselin, or lanolin, are absorbed by the unbroken skin; 2d, if cutaneous absorption is established, whether there exists any difference in the facts as regards absorption; 3d, if fatty absorption is not demonstrated, what excipient would yield more of the active drug incorporated in it. (*Lyon Médical*, 1891, No. 36, p. 6, and No. 37, p. 37.) The results are: Iodide of potash in lard, vaselin or lanolin, well rubbed in, is not absorbed. The same result was obtained with mercury, morphine, strychnine, and atropine. The conclusions are, that with man the absorption of drugs that are not irritant fails to take place through an unbroken skin, and that lanolin is not of more value than vaselin or lard.

OXYGEN INHALATION IN CARDIAC ASTHMA.

In the *Centralblatt für die gesammte Therapie*, 1891, Heft 10, S. 578, DR. M. HEITLER relates his success in the inhalation of oxygen in a case of cardiac asthma dependent upon atheroma of the aorta. Treatment by morphine and ether injections not being satisfactory, with likewise a failure after administration of large quantities of alcohol, it was found that oxygen afforded relief. If there is, however, pulmonary œdema, ether injections are necessary.

DANGERS OF CREASOTE AND IODOFORM INJECTIONS.

In the *Journ. de Méd. de Paris*, 1891, No. 38, p. 429, M. MOREL-LAVALLÉE warns the profession that the subcutaneous administration of creasote and iodoform may be ₁ dangerous in tubercular patients. Practising injections of iodoform dissolved in olive oil, to which eucalyptol is added (method of Besnier), the author found in a case of cutaneous tuberculosis that there was a marked amelioration of the symptoms, but as the dose was steadily increased there was a dull-red halo about the site of the disease, and points of suppuration with excavation appeared. According to the observations of Besnier, precisely the same result may occur with creasote. This congestion could readily become dangerous in cases of pulmonary tuberculosis, so that, on account of the popularity of the treatment, this warning is timely.

BITES OF VIPERS.

PROFESSOR KAUFMANN, of the Veterinary School of Alfort (*Lo Sperimentale*, 1891, No. 16, p. 352), has found permanganate of potash and chromic acid to be the best remedies against the bites of vipers. As soon as possible he places a ligature above the lesion, and then with a hypodermatic syringe injects deeply into the point of penetration two or three drops of a 1 per cent. solution. Three or four similar injections are made around this point. If there is swelling, injections are made into it, and the remedy diffused into the tissues by gentle pressure of the hand. Scarification, with compression, is the next procedure, then a protective dressing, dipped in the solution, after the surface has been thoroughly cleansed with it. Small and frequently repeated doses of ammonia and alcohol should be administered to keep up persistent stimulation.

THE TREATMENT OF ERYSIPELAS.

DR. STANISLAUS KLEIN, in the *Berliner klinische Wochenschrift*, 1891, No. 39, S. 958, presents a very valuable contribution from the clinic of Professor Stolnikow, in Warsaw. Quoting Fessler's observation that ammonia ichthyol in bouillon, one to four thousand, prevented the growth of streptococci, and that soda ichthyol in weaker solution hindered the growth of streptococci, and, to a less degree, that of the staplylococcus aureus, he presents his conclusions based upon the experience of two years.

The method which is employed is as follows: The diseased surface is cleansed by washing with soap and water (or with concentrated aqueous solution of carbolic acid, Fessler), and an ointment of equal parts of vaselin and ichthyol, or of equal parts of ichthyol, water, and lanolin, thoroughly rubbed in with the hand over the area of disease, and for a distance of a hand-breadth around it. Over the anointed surface a thin layer of salicylic acid cotton dressing, covered by a thick layer of absorbent cotton, is applied. This is reapplied two or three times daily until the temperature has been normal for three or four days. He concludes that ichthyol is beneficial by its reducing action on the tissues, or by its influence upon the microörganisms, or by both together; that it shortens the duration of the disease one-half; that the duration of treatment is three or four days, and that the course of the disease is much milder.

The following articles are worthy of note :

"Salol," by M. ED. ÉGASSE, in the *Bulletin Gén. de Thérapeutique*, 1891, No. 36, p. 241, is an excellent study of salol, dealing with its chemistry, physiology, and therapeutics. Its value in the diagnosis of diseases of the stomach and pancreas is clearly stated, and its very great usefulness as an intestinal antiseptic duly set forth.

DOTT-DOMENICO MARINUCCI, in *La Riforma Medica*, 1891, No. 218, p. 803, presents the results of his investigations in "Sterilization of Drugs for Hypodermatic Use." The problems were—1st. Do these solutions contain living germs? 2d. In sterilization is their therapeutic value changed or lost? Conclusions: All solutions studied can develop organisms, although probably not all harmful ; in sterilization by heat, strychnine, curarine, bichloride of quinine and borate of eserine are unchanged; with morphine and atropine the dose after sterilization must be increased ; sulphate of eserine markedly changed. Since heat changes atropine and sulphate of eserine these drugs are best sterilized by a sublimate solution, 1 : 10,000, renewed every two weeks.

DR. R. DUBOIS presents an interesting theory, to account for the "Action of Anæsthetics" (*Revue Générale des Sciences*, 1891, No. 17, p. 563). Recounting the effects of anæsthetics on vegetation, quoting the experiments of Bernard and Javal and the curious studies of Graham, he believes the mechanism of the action of anæsthetics is really a dehydration of the protoplasm, which does not, however, produce any change of structure recognizable by our ordinary methods of investigation.

COCAINE.

In *La Médecine Moderne*, 1891, No. 37, p. 653, PROF. G. SÉE furnishes us with a short and practical statement concerning the cocainization of internal organs. As a remedy for pain, it is inferior to injections of morphine or antipyrine, and presents many more inconveniences. In diseases of the stomach it fails, although less dangerous when administered by the mouth than hypodermatically. It is not prophylactic against fatigue. As an antidote to the morphine habit "it is not a triumph but a martyrization of the human race." Acute cocaine poisoning is difficult to foresee, the poisonous dose being so variable and the conditions not easily determined. The vaso-constriction produced by cocaine may be combated by nitrite of amyl, which is often without effect, while chloral is still more uncertain.

MEDICINE.

UNDER THE CHARGE OF

W. PASTEUR, M.D. Lond., F.R.C.P.,

ASSISTANT PHYSICIAN TO THE MIDDLESEX HOSPITAL; PHYSICIAN TO THE NORTHEASTERN HOSPITAL FOR CHILDREN;

AND

SOLOMON SOLIS-COHEN, A.M., M.D.,

PROFESSOR OF CLINICAL MEDICINE AND APPLIED THERAPEUTICS IN THE PHILADELPHIA POLYCLINIC;
PHYSICIAN TO THE PHILADELPHIA HOSPITAL.

THE DIURETIC ACTION OF FRESH THYROID JUICE.

A year ago, E. HURRY FENWICK (London) found that on rubbing the glairy juice from the cut surface of a fresh sheep's thyroid into the subcutaneous tissue of a myxœdema patient, at the request of Dr. Sansom, the quantity of urine passed by the patient rose from twenty to fifty ounces on the following day. Since then he has made hypodermic injections of the fresh juice mixed with an equal quantity of distilled water, with striking results. About twenty drops of the mixture are injected into the subentaneous tissue of the arm, or over the shoulder-blade, with a Koch's syringe. Some pain and slight swelling are sometimes complained of, but toxic symptoms such as have been described by Ewald have not been encountered. The urine increases in amount during the next day or the day after, and the effect in the myxœdema case continued for fourteen to twenty-one days.—*British Medical Journal*, 1891, No. 1606.

SALICYLATE OF SODIUM IN THE TREATMENT OF DIABETES.

DR. E. MANSEL SYMPSON (Lincoln) records a case of acute saccharine diabetes in a youth, aged seventeen years, in which marked improvement took place under sodium salicylate. When first seen, on April 18th, he presented the usual symptoms in a marked degree, and was passing seven pints of sugary urine (specific gravity 1050) in the twenty-four hours. On a mixed (though partly restricted) diet and ten grains of salicylate every four hours, at the end of a week the daily quantity of urine had diminished by two pints. During the second week he was put on strict diet, and had salicylate every six hours. On the twelfth day of treatment he was passing two pints of urine daily, of specific gravity 1014, with a trace of sugar (less than one grain to the ounce). On the eighteenth day sugar had disappeared from the urine. Meanwhile the symptoms gradually subsided, and he gained weight rapidly. On two occasions, when the drug was temporarily suspended, the amount of urine passed was doubled in quantity. The blood presented no abnormalities, and the motions did not contain fatty matter. In July the patient was well and healthy-looking, and able to take plenty of exercise. The author discusses at some length the action of sodium salicylate, and indorses the view of Haig that it may do good in the neurogenic form—that due to vascular eccentricities of the liver—by promoting the excretion of uric acid, so as to lessen irritation of the vascular system of the liver and consequent abnormal transformation of glycogen into glucose. He further draws attention to the large number of cases of diabetes in which post-mortem evidence of disease of the pancreas is met with, and quotes recent experiments which would tend to show that the pancreas secretes a ferment capable of transforming the glucose in the blood. In view of the many reports given of obstructed ducts and of atrophy and degeneration of the gland itself in fatal diabetes, these experiments, if confirmed, would clear up the pathological difficulty.

"There is one rather weak link at present in the chain of argument—namely, that this glycogenic ferment has not yet been isolated.[1] It probably is poured out into the portal vein (if it went into the duct it would be neutralized by the glucose-forming ferment already present there), and carried thereby to the liver. As long as there is a normal supply there, it keeps carbohydrate material in hand as glycogen. When, either from too great blood-supply to the liver (which will expose the glycogen to the action of the glucose-forming ferment in the blood) or from failure of the pancreatic secretion, the sugar formed by digestion passes into the blood—and, moreover, as there is no restraining influence—the glycogen already formed in the liver is converted into sugar, and diabetes mellitus is the result. Then it becomes a very interesting question as to whether many of the more acute cases, occurring in youthful patients, may not be really due to pancreatic disease ; the severity and the issue will depend on the cause of that pancreatic disease. This suggests at once the treatment, which has been carried out with some success, of giving these patients liquor pancreaticus, calves' sweetbreads, etc. Finally, if salicylate of sodium does any good in these cases, I would suggest that it stimulates the pancreatic gland, just as it certainly does good to nursing mothers by stimulating the mammary gland. Again, as it makes the bile more watery and less likely to form gall-stones, so with much probability it does the pancreatic juice."—*Practitioner*, No. 278, 1891.

PULSATING EMPYEMA.

DR. E. M. LIGHT (Leeds) records three cases of this affection.

In the first case, a boy, aged four years, the whole left chest was absolutely dull. There were two localized swellings—an anterior one over the fifth, sixth, and seventh ribs, in which pulsation was most marked, and a posterior, less prominent one over the ninth, tenth, and eleventh ribs in the line of the scapular angle ; in this the pulsation—synchronous with the heart-beats—was only apparent when the child lay on his right side. Thirty ounces of pus were evacuated, and the child made a complete recovery.

In the second case, a child, aged three years, there were all the signs of fluid in the left pleura and œdema of chest-wall. There were two distinct swellings—one over the præcordia, and the other over the eighth interspace in the mid-axillary line, which was red, glazed, and fluctuating. This latter

---

[1] The various experiments made by the writer in this direction have not been successful, perhaps for the reason given immediately as to its being sent into the portal vein.

swelling pulsated visibly, synchronous with the cardiac impulse and systolic in time. Twenty-five ounces of pus were evacuated. Subsequently persistent vomiting set in, and death occurred a fortnight later. Post-mortem there was evidence of right pleurisy and recent general peritonitis. No tubercle. Complete collapse of left lung.

The third case was a man, aged twenty, admitted with signs of large, left pleural effusion. Had been tapped a few weeks previously. Over the left fourth and fifth ribs, about one inch within the nipple line, was a glossy fluctuating and pulsating swelling. Eighty ounces of sweet pus were slowly evacuated, but the patient died soon after the operation. Post-mortem the left lung was completely collapsed and much compressed. The pericardium was adherent to the left pleura, and contained eight ounces of clear fluid. No tubercle.

All three cases presented the usual signs of pulsating empyema (pulsating empyema necessitatis). The production of pulsations necessitates a concourse of circumstances which are not commonly found in the same patient. The empyema represents a vast cavity, closed in all parts and full of fluid, which possesses a certain tension, compressing and displacing the heart to the right of the middle line of the sternum. The heart in contracting reacts against this compression, pushing back more or less strongly that part of the pleura which corresponds to the ventricular mass, and which is adherent intimately to the pericardium. The pleural sac of a left-sided effusion is in connection with the left ventricle, whereas a right-sided effusion would have its pleural sac more in connection with the right auricle and base of the right ventricle; hence, perhaps, one of the causes of the greater frequency of left-sided pulsating empyemata.

Further, the liquid effusion must possess a certain tension and exercise a compression on the heart itself, for the evacuation of a certain quantity of fluid in diminishing the tension of the effusion weakens, and even entirely suppresses, the pulsation. In order that the impulse communicated to the whole surface of the empyema may become appreciable to the exterior, it is necessary that there should exist a point of least resistance such as is afforded by the walls of external abscesses.

The condition is usually met with in empyemas of chronic character, hence the prognosis is less favorable than in cases recognized early, as chronicity is always a serious element in prognosis.—*Lancet*, 1891, No. 3552.

CRISES OF THE DIGESTIVE TRACT IN GRAVES'S DISEASE.

MR. A. MANDE (Westerham) directs attention to the diarrhœa and vomiting of this malady. Both are common symptoms. Four out of nine cases under his care in 1890–91 presented crises in a typical form. The diarrhœa is paroxysmal, and has been likened by Charcot to the gastric crises of tabes dorsalis. It sets in at any time, usually in the morning, without any warning. The patient has an urgent call to the closet, and passes a huge liquid motion without any pain or colic. The stools are serous, and generally light-colored. After a few days the attack ceases suddenly, to recur after an interval of days, weeks, or months. In one case the attacks were accompanied by pyrexia, and one of the attacks which occurred away from home was pronounced to be typhoid fever. No definite relation could be established in any of the cases between the diarrhœa and the pyrexia of Graves's disease. Ordinary treatment appeared to avail little or nothing.—*Practitioner*, 1891, No. 279.

SUPPURATING HYDATID OF THE LIVER SIMULATING GALL-STONES; RUPTURE THROUGH THE LUNG.

DR. C. H. CATTLE (Nottingham) records the following case: A married woman, aged fifty-six, was suddenly seized with vomiting, which was followed by an attack of jaundice. Previous health had been fair. She did not recover her usual health after this, and a month later the left lobe of the liver was found considerably enlarged downward, and subsequently a gradual progressive extension of liver dulness both downward and upward was noted. About the eighth week a succession of attacks of severe pain in the hepatic region commenced, attended by rigors, vomiting, perspiration, moderate pyrexia, and transient jaundice. There was now dulness over the right lung behind, as high as the middle of the scapula. About the thirteenth week the patient began to expectorate pus, which gradually became offensive, and a few days later physical signs of excavation were present below the right nipple. The lung was incised, and several ounces of thin pus with numerous grape-like cysts containing hooklets were evacuated. The patient only survived two days, and no post-mortem was made. In the writer's opinion a more successful result might have followed bold and timely resort to surgical measures.—*Lancet*, 1891, No. 3554.

SYPHILIS AND GASTRIC ULCER.

DR J. KESER (London) records the case of a barmaid, aged nineteen, who was admitted to hospital with symptoms of gastric ulcer, with frequent slight hæmatemesis. For the first ten weeks all treatment appeared to be of little or no avail. At this period definite evidence of syphilis—condylomata and mucous patches on the tonsils—was obtained, and the patient discovered to be four months pregnant. Under mercury the gastric symptoms speedily improved, and the sickness and hæmatemesis shortly ceased. The patient miscarried a few weeks later, and made a complete recovery.—*British Medical Journal*, 1891, No. 1604.

HYSTERIA IN A CHILD, SIX YEARS OLD, AFTER INFLUENZA.

The patient was under the care of DR. T. C. BAILTON, of Manchester. Personal and family history both good. She had influenza severely in May, with predominance of nervous symptoms, followed by protracted convalescence. She had neither walked nor spoken since the onset of the disease (five weeks). On admission she was apathetic, but conscious. No signs of visceral disease. No motor paralysis, but wavy, clonic spasm of arms when extended. Whines continually, but never speaks. Four days later she was made to sit up in bed. Moves head from side to side, and looks idiotic. There is complete analgesia to pin-pricks of all parts of the body. When lifted out of bed she holds the legs rigid at right angles to the trunk. Under treament by cold baths and faradization she made a perfect recovery in less than two months.—*Lancet*, 1891, No. 3554.

INTRA-VENOUS INOCULATION OF THE BACILLUS OF TYPHOID FEVER.

WELCH (*Bulletin of the Johns Hopkins Hospital*, ii. 15, 1891) has recorded an observation in which a rabbit that survived an injection into a vein of the ear of a bouillon culture of the bacillus of typhoid fever, died one hundred and twenty-eight days subsequently, in less than eighteen hours after a subcutaneous inoculation of a culture of the bacillus of swine-plague. At the autopsy, bacilli of swine-plague were found in the blood and organs. The gall-bladder, however, was small and contracted; its walls were grayish-white, opaque, and thickened; its contents being a turbid-gray, rather creamy fluid, in which no bile-pigment could be found. The walls of the common bile-duct were also thickened and contained turbid-gray matter. Microscopical examination of cover-glass preparations made with the fluid found in the gall-bladder and bile-duct disclosed the presence of the bacilli of typhoid fever, the identity of which was established by cultures.

THE HISTOLOGICAL CHANGES IN EXPERIMENTAL DIPHTHERIA.

WELCH (*Bulletin of the Johns Hopkins Hospital*, ii. 15, 1891) records the histological changes found in the organs of guinea-pigs, rabbits, and kittens that died at periods of from thirty-eight hours to eight and one-half days after receiving subcutaneous inoculations of pure cultures of the Klebs-Löffler bacillus obtained from undoubted cases of primary diphtheria. At the seat of inoculation a grayish, necrotic, pseudo-membranous focus developed, which was surrounded by a red zone of varying size; the subjacent muscle was greatly congested; the adjacent subcutaneous connective tissue was œdematous, and presented a gelatinous appearance; neighboring lymph-glands were enlarged. The peritoneal cavity contained an excess of fluid; the layers of the peritoneum were injected, and in some cases were the seats of ecchymoses. The liver was congested, in some cases fatty. In some cases the spleen was enlarged. The kidneys were moist and hyperæmie. The adrenals were congested, and in many instances hemorrhagic. The agminated glands of the intestine were abnormally prominent, and exhibited a number of whitish spots imbedded in a grayish material. In many cases the pleural cavity contained an excess of fluid. The mediastinal and bronchial glands were swollen and reddened. The heart appeared normal, while the lungs sometimes presented areas of congestion or of consolidation. The deep cervical glands were commonly reddened. The thyroid was uniformly congested, sometimes hemorrhagic. Bacilli of diphtheria were found at the seat of inoculation, both free and within leucocytes. Many of the leucocytes presented fragmentation of their nuclei. The local action of the bacilli is most intense. Not only the leucocytes, but the fixed cells and the nuclei of connective tissue and of muscle also suffer. There were hemorrhages beneath the capsules and into the substance of the affected lymph-glands. The bloodvessels contained a greatly increased number of leucocytes. The number, character, size, stain, ing capacity, and configuration of the nuclei of the cells of the glands were greatly altered, principally in the lymph-follicles, in less degree in the lymph-cords and lymph-sinuses. Similar alterations were found throughout the lymphatic structures of the body: in the spleen, mesenteric, retro-peritoneal,

bronchial, mediastinal, and cervical glands, and intestinal lymphatic apparatus (Peyer's patches, solitary follicles and diffused lymphatic tissue). Degenerative changes were found in the liver. Hemorrhages under the capsule
and in the subjacent lobules were common. The intra-lobular hemorrhages
resulted from breaches in the continuity of the walls of the central veins,
which had become hyaline. Fatty changes were found in the epithelium of
the tubes and glomeruli of the kidneys. Hyaline alterations were present in
the smaller vessels. There were hemorrhages beneath the pleura and into
the alveoli, with an exudation of leucocytes and fibrin into some. The heart
was the seat of varying degrees of fatty degeneration. Cultures made from
the blood, liver, kidney, and spleen were negative.

THE SPECIFIC GRAVITY OF THE BLOOD IN HEALTH AND IN DISEASE.

As a result of a series of fifty-four observations in conditions of great
diversity, SIEGL (*Wiener klin. Wochenschr.*, iv. 33, 1891) has arrived at the
following conclusions :

1. The specific gravity of the blood is dependent upon the proportion or
hæmoglobin and is independent of the number of blood-cells.

2. Diseases, acute as well as chronic, only affect the specific gravity of the
blood when they have led to gradual prostration. Rapid loss of strength, on
the contrary, appears to exert but little influence. In the course of diseases
in which the blood is contaminated by the products of pathological tissue-
metamorphosis, or in which the blood is deficient in its normal chemical constituents, there is, in addition to an absolute change in the specific gravity, a
disproportion between the specific gravity and the percentage of hæmoglobin.
In hepatogenous jaundice, in diseases of the lungs or of the heart attended
with cyanosis, in diseases atttended with loss of bodily fluids, the specific
gravity is (relatively to the percentage of hæmoglobin) raised. When the
blood is deprived of albumin as a result of albuminuria, and probably of
long-continued suppurative processes, the specific gravity is lowered. In
renal disease the quantity of urine and the degree of albuminuria will in
each case indicate how far hydræmia or hypalbuminosis is responsible for the
abnormal specific gravity.

3. In cases of anæmia, in which there is no organic disease that exerts an
influence upon the specific gravity of the blood, this constitutes an index of
improvement or of progression as regards the anæmia.

THE TOXICITY OF THE URINE.

Prompted by the view that various toxic products are eliminated in the
urine in acute infectious diseases, SEMMOLA (*La Union Méd.*, xlv. 95, 1891),
before the Académie de Médecine expressed the thought that, by the injection
of such urine in rabbits and guinea-pigs, the symptoms of the original disease
would be reproduced. Such a procedure would constitute a valuable diagnostic
aid. Thus, for instance, in a case of influenza-pneumonia, complicated by
tetanic and eclamptic attacks, the injection of the urine should reproduce
the symptoms in animals, and meningitis could be excluded.

Purulent Pleurisy.

Courtois-Suffit has made a study of the subject of purulent pleurisy, and presents certain facts of practical importance. Bacteriological research has revealed the existence of several varieties of purulent pleurisy, the etiology, symptoms, course, prognosis, and treatment of which differ with the active infectious agent. Three main groups may be recognized : 1, pleurisy due to the pneumonia-coccus of Fränkel; 2, that due to streptococci; 3, that due to the bacillus tuberculosis. In addition, there may be the following mixed forms: 1, pleurisy due to pneumonia-cocci and streptococci; 2, that due to streptococci and staphylococci; 3, that due to the bacilli of tuberculosis and streptococci; 4, putrid and gangrenous empyemata, caused by the microbes of suppuration associated with certain saprogenic organisms. There are, besides, rare forms of purulent pleurisy due to the bacillus of Friedländer, to the staphylococcus pyogenes, and to the bacillus of Eberth. In the pleurisy due to pneumonia-cocci—metapneumonic pleurisy—the pus is thick, greenish, creamy, without odor; the pleura is covered with false membrane, shreds of which may float in the effusion; the pleurisy has a tendency to become encysted; it often terminates in a vomica, and rarely becomes chronic; it may be primary, associated or not with other pathological conditions due to the pneumonia-coccus, in which case its onset is sudden; or it may appear insidiously in the course of a pneumonia or suddenly during defervescence; the temperature is that of a continued fever, without oscillations or irregularities; the effusion is copious in the acute primary form, moderate in the latent; the pleurisy terminates by absorption or by the formation of an encysted vomica; the prognosis is favorable; the mortality does not exceed five or ten per cent.; in this form, especially, is simple puncture justifiable. Purulent pleurisy due to streptococci may develop in the course of a constitutional affection caused by the same organisms as puerperal fever; in connection with other pathological conditions arising from infection by streptococci, as broncho-pneumonia and peritonitis, and secondarily to remote affections, as an otitis or a phlegmon: the pus is thin, yellowish, without odor, flocculent, and shows no tendency to become encysted. Occurring in the course of another affection the pleurisy is latent and insidious; appearing at the termination it may be acute, frank, and painful; its evolution is slower than in the case of pleurisy due to pneumonia-cocci; the temperature is that of suppuration due to streptococci, with decided remissions and exacerbations; the effusion, usually moderate in degree, never yields to simple puncture; it shows no tendency to absorption or spontaneous evacuation, and only exceptionally gives rise to vomicæ; death may occur from septicæmia or purulent infection; the duration is long; the mortality about twenty-five per cent. ; early and radical operative interference is necessary. The bacillus tuberculosis alone may occasion a purulent pleurisy, comparable to a cold abscess; the pus is thin, yellowish, opaque, without odor and flakes of fibrin ; the pleura is thickened by many layers of superimposed plastic exudate, containing tuberculous nodules; the pleurisy may set in frankly and acutely, or may be insidious and latent, the patient sometimes remaining unconscious of the presence of the effusion, though this be abundant; during the active stage the general health may be preserved, febrile reaction may be absent, and the fluid slowly but persistently reaccumulates; a fatal result occurs sooner or later, according to the course of the pulmonary disease; repeated puncture is necessary. In the purulent pleurisies due to mixed infection the condition assumes the gravity occasioned by the most virulent microbe. The association of streptococci and staphylococci gives rise to a pleurisy of grave type, insidious onset, irregular course, with the signs of pyæmia and wide range of temperature; early and energetic treatment by means of incision and lavage is required. Pleurisy from streptococci may be a complication of. pulmonary tuberculosis; although curable it may prove a serious complication, necessitating, perhaps, the operation for empyema. The pleurisy occasioned by the microbes of suppuration is especially grave when pulmonary cavities exist; the prognosis is then almost fatal. The putrid and gangrenous pleurisy rapidly gives rise to the grave general manifestations of sapræmia, it necessitates speedy and energetic intervention.—*Gazette Méd. de Paris*, No. 12, 1891.

DEFECTIVE INTER-VENTRICULAR SEPTUM WITHOUT CYANOSIS.

WILBOUSCHEWITCH (*Bulletins de la Soc. Anat. de Paris*, 1891, No. 2) reports the case of a seamstress, twenty-five years of age, with a tuberculous family history. The patient had been uninterruptedly at work, when suddenly a copious hæmoptysis took place. She was pale and thin. The chest was small and flat; the vertebral column kyphotic. The percussion note was dull and the respiratory murmur feeble over the upper third of the left lung. Râles and friction-sounds were heard, in greater number on the right. There was little cough and expectoration. At the apex of the heart both a presystolic and a systolic murmur were heard and a purring tremor felt. Duplication of the second sound was heard at the base. A second copious hæmoptysis in the course of a few days, was followed by death. At the autopsy pleural adhesions were found, and the lungs contained many tubercles and some cavities. The heart was relatively large; the vessels were given off normally; the mitral orifice admitted two fingers. The inter-ventricular septum was defective at its upper part, and by the foramen thus formed the ventricles communicated; the opening was oval, slightly elongated transversely, and about as large as a two-franc piece; the lower portion of the septum was thickened, its upper free border was smooth; a thin band of muscular tissue intervened between the abnormal opening and the aorta; the mitral and tricuspid leaflets came in contact; a tendon of a leaflet of the tricuspid valve was inserted into the free border of the opening, before which the left trienspid leaflet was stretched like a curtain. The pulmonary artery was dilated; the vessel bifurcated just above the valve; its branches in the lung were also dilated. Upon the endocardium of the right side of the heart and of the branches of the pulmonary artery were numerous patches and lines, probably the evidences of a fœtal endocarditis. During the ventricular systole the defect in the septum had apparently been partially closed by the tricuspid valve, preventing the admixture of venous and arterial blood and the production of cyanosis.

SURGERY.

UNDER THE CHARGE OF

J. WILLIAM WHITE, M.D.,

PROFESSOR OF CLINICAL SURGERY IN THE UNIVERSITY OF PENNSYLVANIA; SURGEON TO THE UNIVERSITY AND GERMAN HOSPITALS;

ASSISTED BY

EDWARD MARTIN, M.D.,

CLINICAL PROFESSOR OF GENITO-URINARY SURGERY IN THE UNIVERSITY OF PENNSYLVANIA; SURGEON TO THE HOWARD HOSPITAL AND ASSISTANT SURGEON TO THE UNIVERSITY HOSPITAL.

SKEWER AMPUTATION OF THE ENTIRE UPPER EXTREMITY.

McLEOD (*Lancet*, No. 3, vol. ii., 1891) reports a case in which a very large tumor was successfully removed, the hemorrhage being checked by a combination of skewers and an elastic cord. The patient on whom the operation was performed was suffering from a large globular tumor of three months' standing, placed beneath the right deltoid muscle, which was tightly stretched over it. The circumference of the limb at the shoulder was nineteen inches. The acromion process could not be felt. The entire axillary space was filled. The scapula was evidently implicated, and no movement existed at the shoulder-joint, the scapula and clavicle moving with the tumor. The outer end of the clavicle was lost in the mass. The overlying skin was not infiltrated or broken. This growth was evidently a sarcoma.

After chloroforming the patient, two punctures were made, one in the floor of the axilla, and the other a little above and behind the top of the shoulder. A stout packing-needle, about eighteen inches long, was passed from below upward through the cavity of the axilla, behind the vessels and nerves, within the girdle of the shoulder bones, and, finally, was made to emerge through the second puncture. A second needle of the same size was entered at the lower puncture, directed transversely beneath the scapula, and made to emerge behind the posterior or vertebral border of the bone. A strong India-rubber cord was wound, figure-of-8 fashion, around the projecting ends of these needles, encircling the part with a tight elastic loop, which was held in position by these skewers. A circular incision was now made about two inches to the distal aspect of these loops. The clavicle was divided at the junction of the middle and outer third, thus exposing the plexus and vessels; the latter were isolated, and a clamp forceps was put on them for additional security. The attachments of the scapula were then rapidly divided and the extremity was removed. The axillary artery was then secured, the elastic cord gradually loosened, and the vessels as they spurted were secured. The patient was severely shocked, but made a prompt recovery.

THE TECHNIQUE OF GASTROSTOMY.

WITZEL (*Centralblatt f. Chirur.*, No. 32, 1891) has devised an ingenious method of gastrostomy, for the purpose of preventing the escape of gastric

contents and the attendant inconveniences.   Trial upon two cases has given
good results.

His procedure consists in forming a canal passing obliquely from left to
right, by means of sewing together the free borders of two parallel folds
of the stomach-wall.   This canal leads to a small opening in the stomach,
which allows the tube to enter the cavity of the latter viscus in very much
the same way that a ureter enters the bladder.   To perform this operation
a sufficient portion of the stomach-wall is drawn out of the abdominal
wound.   This is always readily accomplished by steady, gentle traction.   Two
folds of the stomach are made, parallel to each other, running obliquely from
left to right.   Lembert sutures are now inserted passing through the crests
of the two folds and over a rubber tube about as large as a lead-pencil.   An
opening just large enough to introduce the tube is made at the extremity of
the furrow, the Lembert sutures are drawn tight, converting this furrow into
a canal.   The stomach-wall is secured to the parietal wound in the ordinary
manner, and the tube is brought through the external opening.

One and a half inches is sufficient length for the canal made by suturing
together the double folds of the stomach.   The fistula thus made is readily
kept closed by a small tampon, and in the two instances in which this operation was performed by the reporter there was never any leakage of the stomach
contents.

REMOVAL OF AN EXTENSIVE EPITHELIOMA.

TERRIER (*Bull. de l'Acad.*, 3e sér., tome xxvi.) operated upon a case presenting a tumefaction of the frontal region.   Sarcoma was suspected and
exploratory puncture showed the malignant nature of the growth.   The
greater portion of the frontal bone was involved, together with the dura mater
underlying it.   The superior longitudinal sinus was ligated in two places,
and resected between the ligatures.   The left frontal sinus was also invaded
by the malignant growth.   All the diseased tissue was removed, and to avoid
infection of the entire wound from the mucous cavity this part of the wound
was packed with iodoform gauze.   This packing was not removed until the
remainder of the wound was completely healed.   Cure was complete.

Microscopic examination showed that the tumor was an epithelioma.

SUCCESSFUL TREATMENT OF A PUNCTURED ORBITAL WOUND OF THE BRAIN.

Punctured wounds of the brain through the orbit are attended with such a
large mortality that the report of a successful case is always of interest.
POLAILLON (*Bull. de l'Acad. de Méd.*, 3e sér., tome xxxvi.) had brought into
his ward a man into whose left orbit the point of an umbrella was driven so
firmly that it was with some difficulty extracted.   The patient entered supporting the umbrella with his hands.   As it was drawn out by the assistant
the crackling of bones was distinctly perceived.   Its extremity had penetrated
to the depth of two inches, passing upward and outward toward the roof of
the orbit.   Shortly coma, stertorous respiration, and a weak, intermittent
pulse developed.

A large plate of the frontal bone was removed about the size of a silver dollar. The frontal sinus, which was very feebly developed, was not opened. The dura bulged through into this opening, so that the finger could not be entered for the purpose of exploring. The dura was incised, allowing some blood and cerebro-spinal fluid to escape. By means of the finger the opening into the roof of the orbit was readily found. This was placed far back near the lesser wing of the sphenoid. Five splinters of bone were removed, together with a certain quantity of cerebral matter, and a spouting cerebral artery was secured. The remains of the punctured eye were enucleated, the orbit was thoroughly cleaned out, and a drainage-tube was carried from the trephine opening through the supra-orbital plate and out at the orbit.

In a few hours following the operation the patient regained consciousness, and dangerous symptoms disappeared. The next day the drainage-tube traversing the punctured wound was replaced by two tubes, one passed through the trephine opening, the other through the orbit.

On the eighth day the frontal drain was removed, on the twelfth the orbital drain. The patient completely recovered.

TREATMENT OF SURGICAL TUBERCULOSIS BY INJECTIONS OF CHLORIDE
OF ZINC.

LANNELONGUE (*Journ. de Chir.*, tome xlii., 15 cah.), upon the observed fact that chloride of zinc injected into peri-tubercular tissues produces sclerosis and thereby renders such tissues unfit for the development of tubercle bacilli, advises the injection of this medicament into tissues immediately surrounding tubercular neoplasms, particularly in the regions through which pass the bloodvessels supplying the tubercular tissue. He ordinarily employs a 10 per cent. solution of chloride of zinc. This solution should not be injected into the cavity of an articulation, but rather into those regions from which the diseased synovia receives vascular supply—that is, immediately beneath the periosteum in the regions of synovial reflection. The fungosities found growing along the course of the ligaments should also receive attention. It is better to avoid the arteries, though in two cases where these were entered no bad effect seemed to follow. The injection should not be made immediately beneath the skin, but rather in the most superficial layer of the fungosity, and by preference at the points of reflection. The points of election for the injection are upon the bones, the ligaments, and the tendons. With a 10 per cent. solution there is violent local reaction, but if the injections are made sufficiently deep destruction of the skin is rare. Even should this occur it does not seriously compromise the case. Tubercular adenitis is amenable to this treatment. Where there are no foci of caseation injections in the periphery of the ganglia and upon the surface of these tumors produce a prompt diminution in the swelling. When caseation has taken place the treatment causes abscess, in which case there should be a free opening, abundant washing with sterilized water, and peripheral injections of chloride of zinc. It is best to inject small quantities—two drops, for example—and to make multiple injections.

Of 22 cases treated by zinc injection all have shown great improvement. In some this is so marked that they can be considered cured. Absolute cure depends upon the disappearance of the bacillus; that this takes place is not yet proven; but even should this microörganism persist, isolation by fibrous tissue would tend to render it harmless.

LAPAROTOMY FOR CONTUSION OF THE ABDOMEN.

LANE (*Medical Press*, No. 2728), from an experience of three cases, concludes that in cases of extensive rupture of the spleen or enlarged mesenteric vessels a fatal quantity of blood is lost within a very short time, probably within ten minutes, and that after this very little blood escapes, unless stimulants are used. From this it is obvious that surgical interference, even though adopted as early as possible, is not likely to be successful unless transfusion of blood be performed at the same time. His first case was injured by being pinned against a wall by the pole of a wagon striking against the abdomen. The patient was collapsed and suffered great pain in the abdomen, which was tender and rigid. No blood was vomited. The operation was performed in two hours. Blood and fluid feces escaped from the abdominal cavity, and a loop of small intestine was found perforated in two places, about eighteen inches apart. The mesentery corresponding to the loop presented at its attachment to the spine a hole so large that four fingers could be passed through it.

Two feet of intestines were resected. In a further search for damage the patient was eviscerated. Proximal and distal ends of the bowel were then brought together with Senn's approximation plates. The patient died the second day, apparently from exhaustion. The second and third cases were run over. In each instance the spleen was torn and the abdominal cavity was filled with blood. Death followed very shortly after operation.

MENTAL SYMPTOMS AFTER SURGICAL OPERATIONS.

KIERNAN (*The Medical Standard*, vol. x., No. 3) cites a formidable list of authorities from Ambrose Paré to Horatio Wood, showing the profound nervous effect produced by operation. He has found 186 cases of profound mental change following operation; 35 cases after operation for cataract; 65 following gynecological operations, and the remainder resulting from plastic operations, amputations, manipulations, etc. In 15 cases there was larvated epilepsy precedent to the operation; in 10 hysteria major was present; in 30 cases a neurotic element existed; in 35 cases the patients had arrived at periods of involution when instability of the nervous system usually results. In 10 cases only was the influence of blood-poisoning demonstrated.

The acute types of mental affection following operation are aptly designated as " acute confusional insanity." In the larvated epileptic cases, the neurotic, and the hysterical, the prognosis is good. In some of the cases occurring at periods of involution senile degenerations are precipitated. The majority of blood-poisoning cases died. Typho-mania is sometimes observed.

The moral treatment of the patient precedent to the operation is the best prophylaxis. If to the dread of the operation be added dread of the operator the nervous perturbation will necessarily be far greater. Sedatives and other measures tending to calm agitation are necessary. Quinine is strongly indicated. Opium and not chloral hydrate or the bromides will, as a rule, be found a most valuable aid in most of the cases. In many of the hysterical cases salix nigra and monobromate of camphor give good results.

RESECTION OF THE SECOND AND THIRD DIVISIONS OF THE FIFTH NERVE AT THE FORAMEN ROTUNDUM AND FORAMEN OVALE.

In reporting two cases of resection of the fifth nerve at the foramen rotundum and foramen ovale, MIXTER (*Boston Medical and Surgical Journal*, vol. cxxv., No. 7) makes some pertinent remarks in regard to the best method of reaching these nerve-trunks at their points of exit from the skull.

The first step in the operation consists in turning down a flap with the temporal muscle, zygoma, and pterygoid. The hemorrhage is always severe, and is only controlled by packing with sponges, and by compression with spatulæ. When the external pterygoid plate is reached, the soft parts are pushed back with the finger or blunt instruments. As a general rule, there is a sufficient space to admit the end of the index finger between the posterior border of the internal pterygoid plate and the spinous process. Between these bony points there is sometimes a bridge of osseous tissue replacing the ligamentous structure which normally lies here. If, on reaching the external pterygoid plate, the space between it and the spinous process is very small; or there is a bony bridge between these points, it is necessary either to use a chisel and cut through the obstruction, or to break it away with a blunt instrument until the finger passes readily to the foramen ovale, which is recognized by touch. By separating the attachment of the external pterygoid muscle from the external plate until the pterygo-maxillary fissure is reached the internal maxillary artery is exposed and may be readily tied. Then, in most cases, the second branch of the fifth pair can be drawn out as it emerges from the foramen rotundum by means of a blunt hook, when it may be seized with strong hæmostatic forceps and divided by means of a curved tenotome at its exit from the foramen. By means of the hæmostatic forceps the branches of the nerve are twisted out. In some cases a marked projection at the anterior end of the pterygoid ridge prevents easy access to the spheno-maxillary fossa; in this case the projection should be removed by means of a chisel. The three cases reported all made prompt recovery.

SPINAL SURGERY.

In the address on this subject delivered before the American Surgical Association, at the Congress of American Physicians and Surgeons, held in Washington in September (*Therapeutic Gazette*, October, 1891), DR. J. WILLIAM WHITE limited his discussion of the surgery of the spine to the conditions requiring operative interference, or to those in which operation may reasonably be considered, and excluded lateral curvature, the so-called "railway spine," etc., since some of these conditions belong to the province of the orthopædist, others to that of the neurologist.

He classifies those remaining as follows:

    A. Congenital deformities.

    B. Tuberculosis of the spine.

    C. Neoplasms.

    D. Traumatisms.

A. Under the first heading, spina bifida is the only condition which is at once of sufficient frequency and sufficient importance to demand special consideration. After reviewing the general subject, Dr. White expresses himself as in accord with the conclusion arrived at by the committee of the Clinical Society of London, and held by the majority of surgeons at the present day. This is, that while various successes have been reported by other methods, such as simple tapping and drainage, and more recently in a limited number of cases by excision of the sac, yet, on the whole, the method of injection of the sac offers the best prospect of ultimate recovery with the least immediate danger.

B. In the second group of cases, which includes the various forms of tuberculosis of the spine, the indications for operative interference may be: 1, the evacuation of pus; 2, the removal of a sequestrum or of the focus of carious bone; 3, the relief of the cord from pressure by pus, bone, or, more commouly, by the products of a simple or tuberculous external pachymeningitis. These indications may coexist or may be quite distinct.

In disease of the bodies of the vertebræ, the most accessible region is without doubt the lumbar, and the now well-known operative procedure of Treves may be adopted as the best. It makes the body of the twelfth dorsal vertebra safely accessible. The existence of a psoas abscess, whether its vertebral origin is proved or not, is sufficient warrant for the lumbar operation, affording the best drainage and at the same time permitting the removal of a sequestrum or the curetting of a patch of superficial caries, if either of these conditions should be discovered by the finger or the probe.

Where the disease is associated with caries of one or more ribs the processes are more likely to be affected, and are in all probability the portions reached by the finger and the curette of the surgeon. Dr. White states that Dr. Agnew and he have had one such case, in which caries of the vertebral extremity of the third rib was the cause of an enormous cold abscess occupying the whole of the right scapular region. They curetted the process, *not* the body of the corresponding vertebra.

Three principal objections have been made to attempts to reach the focus of bone disease in these cases of spinal abscess:

1. It is said that operative methods practicable upon the cadaver cannot be employed in the presence of the angular deformity of Pott's disease, in which the last rib may be in actual contact with the ilium. These cases, however, are rare, and in them there is little indication for surgical interference, as the bodies of many vertebræ are deeply affected. The favorable cases are those of superficial caries, in which there is a curve of very large radius, or those in which there is disease of but a single vertebra and a very slight angular projection. In these two classes of cases the costo-iliac space is but little reduced.

2. It is said that the solidity of the spine is affected by operation. This, of course, cannot apply to cases in which curetting is employed. It is scarcely possible that the removal of a sequestrum could materially affect the integrity of the spine; and indeed this has not occurred even after very extensive removal of portions of vertebræ.

3. Operation is said to be useless. As a matter of fact, we have now the records of fourteen operations upon the bodies of vertebræ, with eight cures,

five cases improved, and one death, which had no relation to the operation itself.

As to the third indication in tuberculosis of the spine, viz., the relief of cord-pressure in Pott's paralysis, there is some encouragement to operation held out in the clinical facts—

1. That there are very many examples of the relief of paralysis in spinal caries after the pointing of a psoas or an iliac abscess, or after the evacuation of pus by the side of the spine.

2. That the disease of the dura mater in Pott's disease is limited to the site of the diseased vertebræ. The change from an inflammatory to a normal area is an abrupt one.

The analysis of forty cases of this operation for Pott's paralysis, which are all the author was able to bring together, shows that in twenty-two there was either improvement or absolute cure. The unsuccessful cases which recovered from the operation were in some instances the subject of secondary disease. The deaths were twelve in number, showing a mortality of 30 per cent., and were due to various causes, such as shock, or extensive renal and pulmonry disease. In others death was directly due to the gravity of the disease of the cord.

In coming to a conclusion as to the indications for operative interference in Pott's paralysis, the age of the patient is of great importance, the proportion of cures and of improvements being much greater in children and in adolescents than in adults.

The seat and extent of the osseous lesion are also important, the prognosis being unfavorable in direct proportion to the height of the caries—above all, when respiratory complications exist previous to the operation. All the patients who died had an upper dorsal or a cervical lesion except one, in which case the equally fatal condition of tuberculosis of a large number of vertebral bodies existed.

The effect of suspension in the treatment of Pott's paralysis has been so favorable in a number of cases that it should occupy a prominent position in the consideration of our therapeutic resources, and should be always tried, or, at least, carefully discussed, before operative measures are thought of.

The evidence at present available in relation to the operative treatment of spinal tuberculosis with symptoms of pressure upon the cord appears to justify the following conclusions:

1. The paralysis in Pott's disease is not, as a rule, due to a transverse myelitis, or a hopeless degeneration, and is not usually due to the pressure of the carious or displaced vertebræ, but is, in the majority of cases, the result of an external pachymeningitis, which results in the formation of an extra-dural connective-tissue tumor.

2. Speaking generally, a favorable prognosis is to be given, especially in children, in cases of Pott's paralysis in which the abscess, if any exists, can be evacuated; the treatment by extension and with a plaster jacket can be employed, and the patient can be put under the most favorable hygienic conditions.

3. In cases in which all this has been tried unsuccessfully, or in those in which the disease is slowly but steadily progressing to an unfavorable termination; when with more or less complete loss of motion and sensation

below the level of the lesion there are incontinence of urine and feces and the development of bedsores, and especially when acute symptoms threaten life, resection becomes entirely justifiable.

4. Operation having been decided upon for any or all of the above reasons, the prognosis will be favorable in direct proportion to the youth and strength of the patient, the absence of generalized tuberculosis, and the nearness of the lesion to the base of the spine.

5. When the tuberculous process affects the arches and there is paraplegia, we may sometimes operate, hoping not only to free the cord, but to remove, at the same time, the focus of disease. This double indication may also be fulfilled in those cases where, without bony disease, there is posterior pachymeningitis or a tuberculoma occupying the canal. Here again, however, time and careful attention to hygiene, including change to sea or mountain air, often works wonders.

6. If the lesion of the bodies of the vertebræ is in the lumbar region at a point where these bodies are accessible, it might be possible in certain cases to expose the cord from the back, by removal of the laminæ, with the object not only of removing pressure, but of reaching and taking away the diseased bone and tubercular granulation.

7. In tuberculosis of the body of a vertebra and compression of the cord by anterior pachymeningitis we can fulfil one indication—liberate the cord from pressure. We should operate only in grave cases where acute compression, the appearance of respiratory complications, the rapid development of degenerative processes, force us to interfere, or where the course of a chronic case is steadly toward a fatal termination, although no advanced visceral tuberculous lesions are present.

As to the third division of the subject, viz., neoplasms, Dr. White concludes that every case of focal spinal lesion thought to depend on a tumor, and not distinctly a malignant and generalized disease, should be regarded as amenable to operative interference, no matter how marked or how long continued the symptoms of pressure may be.

The fourth division, that of traumatism, is first considered historically, a summary of all recorded cases of operation for fracture being given. Dr. White then adds that in reviewing the statistics of these operative cases it seems proper that those belonging to the pre-antiseptic period should be omitted, or should be considered in a category by themselves. This would leave thirty-seven operations for fracture, with six complete recoveries, six recoveries from the operation with benefit, eleven recoveries unimproved, and fourteen deaths—a mortality of 38 per cent.

The chief strength of the opponents of operation lies in the argument that the operation *per se* is of great danger, or in itself materially diminishes the patient's chances. If, as Dr. White believes to be the case, it can be fairly claimed that rapid reunion of all the soft structures down to the dura mater itself can be confidently expected; if it can be shown, as it has been, that extensive resections of the laminæ do not greatly or permanently weaken the spine; if under antiseptic methods the risk of consecutive inflammation of cord or membrane is practically *nil;* if hemorrhage is not to be feared, and if loss of cerebro-spinal fluid is unimportant; if it happens not so very infrequently that the cord is directly compressed by fragments of the laminæ themselves, or, if not, that by removal of the arches relief from anterior pressure *may* be afforded—if these are facts or even reasonably strong probabilities, it is evident that the operation is one which should no longer be rejected on the sole remaining ground that we cannot be certain in any given case as to the exact .amount of damage which has been done to the tissues of the cord. The argument that, if such damage were irreparable, operative interference would be useless, while if the cord retained the power of recovering itself the operation would only add another complication, has lost nearly all its force. It would seem rather to be the duty of the surgeon, after a reasonable and not very protracted delay, to endeavor to relieve any possible pressure, to remove any fragments or spiculæ of bone, to drain thoroughly the canal, or even the subdural space, if there be any oozing, and to do so with the consciousness that, if he met with none of these conditions, he is at any rate not performing a necessarily fatal operation.

In conclusion, the opinions arrived at after consideration of this last branch of the subject are summarized as follows:

1. Some objections urged against operative interference in spinal traumatisms—*i. e.*, hemorrhage, frequency of absolute destruction of the cord, pressure from inaccessible fragments of bone, etc.—have been shown to be unsupported by clinical facts; others were largely due to a well-founded dread of (*a*) the shock in those cases operated on in pre-anæsthetic times, and (*b*) consecutive inflammation, suppuration, and pyæmia in pre-antiseptic periods.

2. The results of recent operative interference in properly selected cases of fractures of the spine are encouraging, and should lead to the more frequent employment of resection of the posterior arches and laminæ: (*a*) in all cases in which depression of those portions, either from fracture or from dislocation, is obvious; (*b*) in some cases in which after fracture rapidly progressive degenerative changes manifest themselves; (*c*) in all cases in which there is compression of the cauda equina from any cause, whether from anterior or posterior fracture or from cicatricial tissue; (*d*) in the presence of characteristic symptoms of spinal hemorrhage, intra- or extra-medullary.

3. Operation is contra-indicated by a history of such severe crushing force as would be likely to cause disorganization of the cord. The question which will remain in doubt previous to operation will usually be, that of the extent of damage done to the cord and the possibility of its taking on reparative action. As to this, the safest rule is that which has been formulated by Lauenstein, namely, that if after the lapse of six or ten weeks there is incontinence of urine with cystitis, or incontinence of feces, and especially if there are also the development and spreading of bedsores, but little is to be hoped for from the unaided efforts of Nature. If, however, these symptoms be absent, and if there be the least improvement in either sensation or motion, it will be proper for the surgeon to delay operative interference still longer.

DISEASES OF THE LARYNX AND CONTIGUOUS STRUCTURES.

UNDER THE CHARGE OF

J. SOLIS-COHEN, M.D.,
OF PHILADELPHIA.

A New Form of Mirror.

DR. TH. HARKE, of Hamburg, describes (*Deutsche med. Wochenschr.*, No. 28, 1891) a new form of adjustable mirror, readily affixable to a double-stemmed handle, pressure upon the expanded extremities of which will, during its use, slant the mirror to any desired angle from 100 to 180 degrees.

Anomaly of the Larynx.

DR. WILHELM ANTON, of Prague, reports (*Prager med. Wochenschr.*, No. 27, 1891) a case in which a congenital pair of folds exist, above and apart from the normal ary-epiglottic folds, extending from each border of the epiglottis to the corresponding supra-arytenoid cartilage.

Anomaly of the Trachea.

DR. H. CHIARI describes (*Prager med. Wochenschr.*, No. 25, 1891) a new form of triple division of the trachea. The body of a male infant, sixteen days of age, from the clinic of Professor Epstein, was found to contain anomalies in the trachea, in the heart and aorta, and in the abdominal cavity, among the latter an overlapping of the hepato-duodenal ligament and an absence of the spleen. Just above the bifurcation of the trachea a third tracheal bronchus, three millimetres wide, was given off on the left side and was distributed to the upper lobe of the tri-lobed left lung. It differed from any of the eleven hitherto described instances of triple bronchus referred to in the paper.

Purpura of the Mouth, Pharynx, and Larynx.

DR. AUDUBERT, of Luchon, reports (*Ann. de la Polyclinique de Bordeaux*, No. 5, 1891) the case of a cooper, fifty years of age, whose health had been running down for several years with bronchitis, cough, pains in the shoulders, and slight modification of the voice. He was found to have extensive ulcerative tuberculous laryngitis. Two months later, Dr. Moure detected one day a number of purpuric spots disseminated in the palate, tongue, gums, and right ventricular band. They were not painful to the touch, and did not produce any functional disturbance. These spots had nearly disappeared ten days later, while fresh patches had appeared on the internal face of the left cheek, on the gums, and on the posterior wall of the pharynx, which supported a large ecchymotic patch, irregularly rounded, and from three to four centimetres in diameter. The nasal mucous membrane was healthy. There were no similar lesions upon any part of the cutaneous surface.

FRACTURE OF THE LARYNX.

PROFESSOR E. v. HOFMANN, of Vienna, reports (*Wiener klin. Wochenschr.*, No. 36, 1891) a number of instances of indirect fracture of the upper cornua of the thyroid larynx, the result of falls upon the head. They were all associated with serious lesions of the cranium or vertebra. The practical point illustrated is the medico-legal aspect of the subject in cases in which other lesions are not distinctive; it being the general opinion that fractures of this kind are due to strangulation, or to other direct injury to the neck.

SYPHILIS OF THE LARYNX.

DR. R. BEAUSOLEIL reports (*Annales de la Polyclinique de Bordeaux*, No. 5, 1891) a case of tardy hereditary syphilis in a lad, ten years of age, with gumma of the right ventricle, stenosis of the glottis, and ulceration of the pharynx.

MORBID GROWTHS OF THE LARYNX.

DR. J. GAREL, of Lyon, reports (*Ann. des Mal. de l' Oreille, du Larynx, etc.*, No. 6, 1891) an instance of spontaneous disappearance of a papilloma in a female infant, four years of age, after tracheotomy. The growth had occurred in sequence of an attack of influenza. It had occupied the entire left vocal band and the inter-arytenoid commissure.

FIBROUS TUMORS OF THE PREËPIGLOTTIC REGION.

DR. LAURENT, of Brussels, reports (*Rev. de Lar., etc.*, No. 12, 1891) the case of a woman, forty-seven years of age, who began to cough from time to time in March, 1890, and finally quite continuously for a period of six weeks, during which she had become very much emaciated. The voice was very hoarse. The larynx was normal, but three small tumors were seen in front of the epiglottis, the largest one the size of a nut. They were smooth, of fibrous consistence, and of the color of the surrounding mucous membrane. The epiglottis was sometimes pushed backward by the growths. The growths were extirpated with cutting-forceps under digital guidance. The voice immediately improved. The histological character of the masses was rather vague. There was considerable fibrous tissue, with some connective cells and vessels. The fibrous tissue circumscribed in places some very small spaces, which were not distinctly cellular.

EVULSION OF MORBID GROWTHS OF THE LARYNX.

An improved antero-posterior forceps for the evulsion of morbid growths is described by DR. SUAREZ DE MENDOZA, of Angers (*Rev. de Lar., etc.*, No. 15, 1891). The laryngeal branches are fenestrated with slits three millimetres broad and twelve and a half centimetres in length, well up to the curve of the instrument, and one branch fits into its companion when the instrument is closed. The mechanism is rather complex, and hardly to be understood without diagrams. The advantage is that the field of operation can be kept in view through the fenestra, and thus injury be avoided to the healthy tissues.

LARYNGECTOMY.

A case of unilateral laryngectomy for stricture in a boy, three years of age, is reported by MR. THOMAS F. CHAVASSE, of Birmingham (*Lancet*, 1891, No. 3547). The stricture was attributed to ulceration from an intubation tube which had been introduced nine months previously for laryngeal dyspnœa. The tube had to be reintroduced seven times in eight days, and was finally coughed up, swallowed, and voided per anum. When the tube was lost, tracheotomy was hurriedly performed to prevent asphyxia. The laryngectomy was performed practically without hemorrhage after the vertical cutaneous incision. The thyroid cartilage being divided in the middle line, the two sides were separated, disclosing complete occlusion of the larynx with cicatricial tissue. The soft parts were dissected from the right wing of the thyroid cartilage, which was then separated from its connection with the cricoid, and removed; and subsequently the right half of the cricoid had to be exsected by prolonging the incision down to the tracheal wound. The fibrous tissues were removed with scalpel and sharp spoon. Recovery was prompt. A chimney canula was then introduced, and was subsequently fitted with a phonal reed, with which the boy can speak clearly and distinctly in a monotone audible to a considerable distance.

[The compiler presumes that this operation was performed under the belief that mere extirpation of the cicatricial tissue in so small a larynx, without sacrifice of the cartilaginous framework, would have been followed by impermeable reconstruction.—ED.]

DOUBLE INNERVATION OF THE LARYNGEAL MUSCLES.

It is well known that EXNER has demonstrated that in animals the superior nerve participates in the innervation of those muscles of the larynx hitherto believed to be innervated by the inferior laryngeal only. It has even been supposed that spastic constriction of the glottis in certain instances of organic paralysis of the inferior laryngeal nerve might be explained on the theory that the superior laryngeal subserves the same functions in man that Exner claims for it in animals, and that its unimpeded influence when the recurrent is paralyzed produces the constriction, inasmuch as its distribution in animals predominates in the constrictor muscles. Two cases are reported by DR. NEWMAN, of Budapest (*Berliner klin. Woch.*, February 9, 1891), as negativing the idea that this double innervation exists in the human subject.

I. A man, thirty-five years of age, had complete bilateral paralysis of both recurrent nerves. His vocal bands were in the cadaveric position with incurvation of the edges anterior to the projecting posterior vocal processes. Secondary carcinomatous neoplasms, evident externally, compressed each recurrent nerve. When the patient succumbed from exhaustion to his carcinomatous disease, the larynx was subjected to the most rigid examination. Both recurrents were imbedded in masses of degenerated carcinomatous glands, where they were so thoroughly disorganized as to leave no traces, while they represented but an atrophic strand of connective tissue thence onward to the larynx. The superior laryngeals were fully intact; and hence the inference that in this individual at least they could not have innervated the muscles in question. The muscles innervated by the inferior laryngeal were atrophied, especially the posterior crico-arytenoids, which were practically completely atrophied; the lateral crico-arytenoids were less atrophied, and the transverse and thyro-arytenoids least of all: confirmative of the theories of Semon and Rosenbach that the abductor fibres degenerate earlier than the adductors. The crico-thyroid muscle, on the other hand, innervated by the superior laryngeal was practically intact. Hence the inference that its action in stretching the vocal bands must be preceded by fixation of the arytenoid cartilage under innervation from the recurrent.

II. This was a case of attempted suicide in which the hyo-thyroid membrane on the right side and the trunk of the upper laryngeal nerve had been severed. Examined after closure of the wound, the pharyngeal and laryngeal mucous membrane was found in a condition of catarrhal inflammation, the epiglottis especially being deeply injected. There was right-sided paralysis of the soft palate. The interior of the larynx was filled with saliva. The epiglottis maintained its usual position in phonation. The right vocal band was not distended as much as the left in phonation, appeared somewhat smaller, and maintained a slightly higher level. The patient was hoarse, not from the catarrhal condition, but from the relaxed activity of the affected vocal band. This case shows that the superior laryngeal nerve simply stretches the vocal bands in virtue of its supply of motor filaments to the crico-thyroid muscle.

THE ACTION OF THE GLOTTIS IN SINGING.

Notwithstanding the immense number of photographs taken by DR. THOMAS R. FRENCH, of Brooklyn, that enthusiastic student of the mechanism of singing refrains from formulating any theory, so constantly is the camera revealing to him new surprises in the action of the vocal bands in every part of the scale (*New York Medical Journal*, January 31, 1891). Dr. French's paper, read at the Tenth International Medical Congress, is illustrated by thirty-nine reproductions from his extensive photographic collection. A most interesting series is given from the larynx of a well-trained soprano possessing a range of four octaves. Dr. French has not been able to determine that the action of the glottis is affected by training the voice. Like conditions are occasionally seen in the larynges of trained and untrained singers while singing the same notes in the same register, and the difference in the action of the glottis in trained singers are as great as between the trained and the untrained.

Dr. French's conclusions regarding the voice of the female are as follows: 1. The larynx may act in a variety of ways in production of the same tone in different singers. 2. The rule (which, however, has many exceptions) is that the vocal bands are short and wide, and the ligamentous and cartilaginous portions of the glottis are open during the production of the lower tones; the vocal bands increasing in length and decreasing in width as the voice ascends the scale, the aperture between the posterior portions of the bands increasing and the capitula Santorini tilting more and more forward, while the epiglottis rises until a tone is reached in the neighborhood of E, treble clef first line. Then the cartilaginous glottis is closed, the glottic chink becomes much narrower and linear, the capitula Santorini are tilted backward, and the epiglottis is depressed. Shortening of the vocal bands in the change at the lower break in the voice is mainly due to closure of the cartilaginous portion of the glottis. As the voice ascends from the lower break the vocal bands increase in length and diminish in width, the posterior portion of the glottis chink opens more and more, the capitula Santorini are tilted forward and the epiglottis rises, until in the neighborhood of E, treble clef fourth space, another change occurs. The glottis is then reduced to a very narrow slit—in some subjects extending the whole length of the glottis, in others closing in front or behind, or both front and behind. Not only is the cartilaginous glottis always closed, but the ligamentous glottis is, Dr. French believes, invariably shortened. The arytenoid cartilages are tilted backward, and the epiglottis is depressed. As the voice ascends in the head register the cavity of the larynx is reduced in size, the arytenoid cartilages are tilted forward and brought closer together, the epiglottis is depressed, and the vocal bands decrease in length and breadth. If the posterior part of the ligamentous portion of the glottis is not closed in the lower, it is likely to become closed in the upper tones of the head register.

Paralysis of the Larynx.

Dr. A. Cartaz reports (*Arch. Internat. de Lar.*, etc., 1891, No. 4) a case of bilateral paralysis of the posterior crico-arytenoid muscles in a case of aneurism of the aorta.

Suppurative Phlegmon of the Epiglottis.

Dr. O. Chiari reports (*Wien. med. Woch.*, No. 13, 1891) an interesting case of suddenly developed suppurative inflammation of the epiglottis. Incisions into the epiglottis gave exit to fetid pus, but the symptoms increased so intensely as to require tracheotomy. The neck was so short that the trachea could not be exposed although the external incision extended to the sternal notch; so the thyroid gland was detached and the incision was made through the conoid ligament and the cricoid cartilage. Despite the desperate character of the case of the case, and considerable trouble with canulas owing to the anatomical relations of the larynx and trachea, the patient made a satisfactory recovery. It was supposed that infection had been produced by injury from a fishbone, although there was no positive evidence of traumatism; and the question is raised whether infectious phlegmon of the pharynx is not sometimes attributable to a similar cause though there be no direct evidence of its occurrence.

Œdema of the Larynx.

A case of œdema of the glottis in which tracheotomy seemed almost imperative was cured by M. Suarez de Mendoza, of Angers (*Arch. Internat. de Lar.*, etc., No. 3, 1891) by hypodermatic injections of pilocarpine. Three injections containing twenty-five milligrames were made at intervals of about twenty minutes. Marked relief followed the first one, and all danger had been passed fifteen minutes after the third. The same measure had been successfully resorted to by the same practitioner in two previous instances.

[The compiler can endorse this treatment from similar results in his own hands some years ago.—Ed.]

OBSTETRICS.

UNDER THE CHARGE OF

EDWARD P. DAVIS, A.M., M.D.,

PROFESSOR OF OBSTETRICS AND DISEASES OF CHILDREN IN THE PHILADELPHIA POLYCLINIC;
CLINICAL LECTURER ON OBSTETRICS IN THE JEFFERSON MEDICAL COLLEGE;
VISITING OBSTETRICIAN TO THE PHILADELPHIA HOSPITAL, ETC.

THE SURGICAL TREATMENT OF LABOR.

The recent literature of the surgical treatment of parturition contains among others the following papers of value:

In the *British Medical Journal*, 1891, No. 1606, page 789, DORAN describes a case of tubal abortion with double hæmato-salpinx. The patient had given evidences of disease of the left appendages for several years. Following a delay in menstruation of three weeks, the patient was seized with violent pain in the hypogastrium. Such attacks of pain recurred at intervals, after one of which it was decided to perform laparotomy. The peritoneal cavity was found full of clot; the left tube was lacerated near the ovary; the right tube was uniformly distended with blood; its fimbriated extremity was patulous. Much of the great omentum had to be removed, as it was strongly adherent. Irrigation with hot water was practised, and a drainage-tube used. Recovery was complicated by an attack of nephritis at the end of the second week, and by rigors and fever, for which no explanation could be found, on the eighteenth day. The passage of mucous stools occurred at the same time. Upon examining the specimens, chorionic villi were found in the right tube; in the left tube the pathological appearances of acute catarrhal salpingitis were observed, but no ovum.

THE DIAGNOSIS OF EARLY EXTRA-UTERINE GESTATION.

This is the subject of a paper by J. HALLIDAY CROOM (*Edinburgh Medical Journal*, October, 1891). His first case was that of a multipara, in whom the classic symptoms of ruptured ectopic gestation were present. On opening the abdomen, it was found filled with fresh blood and enormous clots. The ovaries were enlarged and cystic; the tubes unruptured; no gestation sac could be found. The abdomen was closed, the hemorrhage continued unabated, and the patient died. No post-mortem examination was possible.

In the second case, a large hæmato-salpinx was removed, every symptom of ruptured tubal pregnancy being present except the discharge of decidua.

In a third case, a diagnosis of ectopic gestation was made from an enlarged heavy uterus at the left and posterior side of the pelvis; a cystic mass upon the right side which was tense, elastic, and very tender to the touch. When the abdomen was opened, an ectopic gestation of about two months was found, the mass being very adherent to the surrounding tissues. Croom concludes that the following points are of value for diagnosis:

1. The general signs of pregnancy.
2. Displacement of the uterus to one side by a tumor which gradually grows.
3. Passage of decidua with hemorrhage.
4. Paroxysmal pain upon one side.

THE DIAGNOSIS OF PREGNANCY IN THE BROAD LIGAMENT.

An elaborate description of this form of ectopic gestation, with drawings illustrating its anatomy, is given by SCHAUTA (*Präger medicinische Wochenschrift*, Nos. 37 and 38, 1891). He describes the case of a patient who presented an abdominal tumor upon the right side reaching to the umbilicus; a second smaller tumor seemed connected with the first; these tumors were of varying consistence, and in the larger, fœtal parts could be plainly discerned. The smaller tumor was found to be the enlarged empty uterus. The tumor containing the child extended toward the right and behind the uterus, deep into the pelvis. It was not movable. A diagnosis was made of ectopic gestation upon the right side, the fœtus developing between the folds of the broad ligament. Upon opening the abdomen, the diagnosis being correct, the fœtal sac was removed, leaving a large cavity; the folds of the broad ligament were sutured to the peritoneum and fixed at the lower angle of the wound, and the aperture between the folds of the broad ligament was filled by a tampon. Recovery followed the operation.

PORRO'S OPERATION.

A Porro's operation for contracted pelvis is reported by GODSON (*British Medical Journal*, 1891, No. 1606, page 793). Labor had proceeded for some time, and instrumental interference had been attempted. The usual uterine amputation was performed, the stump being fixed by Koeberlé's *serre-nœud* with one long pin. Death ensued sixty hours after operation, from general peritonitis. The patient was greatly debilitated when first seen; the intestines escaped from the abdomen during the operation.

He also operated upon a patient with rhachitic pelvis, who came under his care at the beginning of labor, before the membranes had ruptured or interference had been practised. A similar operation was performed, and resulted successfully. The peritoneum of the pedicle in its upper part was carefully stitched to the edges of the peritoneum in the abdominal incision, to shut off the communication with the peritoneal cavity. The patient had recovered in four weeks after the operation. Godson believes that the Porro operation should supplant craniotomy in many cases, and that where it is undertaken very early in labor the prognosis is favorable.

TWO CASES OF AMPUTATION OF THE UTERUS DURING LABOR.

These are reported by MURPHY (*British Medical Journal*, 1891, No. 1606). One was a case of cancer of the cervix, in which no life was found in the fœtus when the abdomen was opened. The uterus was drawn out of the abdomen, the broad ligaments tied with silk, the bladder separated from the vagina, and the uterus was removed entire. A small aperture was made during the operation in the anterior wall of the vagina, and a drainage-tube was passed through this into the abdominal cavity. The patient died of exhaustion about thirty-six hours after the operation. On post-mortem no evidences of peritonitis were found in the abdomen, and the cancer had been entirely removed in removing the uterus. Murphy also operated by Tait's method of amputation in a patient who had contracted pelvis, and was in the beginning of labor. The patient made a good recovery. He urges the abandoning of craniotomy for uterine amputation, and states that he has never consented to be present at the performance of craniotomy upon the living child.

REMOVAL OF A LARGE MYOMA AND THE PREGNANT UTERUS.

In a series of four cases of removal of myomata by abdominal section, Ross (*American Journal of Obstetrics*, No. 165, 1891) describes a case of œdematous myoma accompanied by pregnancy. At an operation, a large myoma weighing thirty-five pounds was found at the back of the left broad ligament. A pedicle was made of the cervix uteri, and after tightening a rope clamp over the tumor and the pregnant uterus, both were cut away. A wire clamp was then applied, pins inserted, with antiseptic dressing. Recovery was complicated by obstinate vomiting, caused by traction upon the stump. The clamp was removed on the nineteenth day, and the patient made a good recovery.

REPEATED CÆSAREAN SECTION.

ROSENBERG reports three cases of repeated Cæsarean section by Leopold, at Dresden (*American Journal of Obstetrics*, No. 166, 1891). The operations were successful. Leopold has found that in the repeated operation separation of the recti muscles is often observed. The uterus is also frequently adherent to the abdominal walls. Atony of the uterus is sometimes observed. Leopold determines the position of the placenta by observing that when the major portion of the uterus is anterior to the insertions of the tubes, which in most cases can easily be felt, the placenta is anterior, and *vice versâ*. It is well to avoid the placenta in these cases, and also when inserting a bougie to induce labor. Silver wire is the least desirable material for uterine suture, and when stitches are found in the uterus in the line of the incision; it is well to dissect them out. Silk is most universally employed and gives good results. A table of thirty-six cases of the repeated operation is appended; ten of these ended fatally. The number of sections made upon a single patient varied from two to five.

THE TECHNIQUE OF CÆSAREAN SECTION.

POTEN (*Archiv für Gynäkologie*, Band xl. Heft 3) reports three cases of Cæsarean section for rhachitic pelves with good results, in which no special caution was taken to suture the peritoneum over the uterus separately. The needle was passed through the peritoneum and muscular substance at one time, and care was taken not to pass the suture through the decidua.

INTRODUCTION A L'ÉTUDE CLINIQUE ET A LA PRATIQUE DES
ACCOUCHEMENTS.
(MANUAL OF OBSTETRIC DEMONSTRATIONS.)

Under this title FARABEUF and VARNIER have prepared an elaborate manual adapted to illustrate a course of demonstrations of operative obstetrics given to the students of the Maternities of Paris. The book is a large volume of more than 400 pages, in large, clear type, with 362 illustrations. These are the best of their kind which we have seen. The mother's tissues are heavily shaded, the fœtus is in heavy outline only. Normal and abnormal presentations, the anatomy of the pelvis, the mechanism of labor, and version and the forceps are clearly represented, with the multiplicity of detail characteristic of French obstetric science.

At present the simple conception of labor and its mechanism prevalent in German teaching is being adopted by Americans, and, we think, greatly to their advantage. Aside from the complicated text with its minute detail, the illustrations make the book valuable to all who demonstrate obstetrics. We shall expect to meet some of these illustrations in the pages of future text-books.

———

DIE STERBLICHKEIT DER KINDER IM ERSTEN LEBENSJAHRE.
(INFANT MORTALITY.)

Under this title BERNHEIM has written a pamphlet, giving his studies in the causation of infant mortality at Würzburg. His conclusions are good for cities in the same latitude, and advance several points of practical interest. Finding infant mortality 37 per cent., among the chief causes are given failure to nurse and illegitimate birth. As a general endeavor to prevent the action of these causes, those agencies which lessen pauperism, drunkenness, and prostitution are to be encouraged. The mortality curve rises highest in July, and dry heat is most fatal. Hence the endeavor should be to provide air-spaces in cities and to sprinkle city streets freely. The use of sterilized milk and cold bathing are also urged.

———

MILK AND ITS CONTAMINATION.
(DIE MILCH, IHRE HÄUFIGEREN ZERSETZUNGEN, ETC.)

SCHOLL, of the Institute of Hygiene of Prague, writes an excellent pamphlet of 130 pages on this subject. His statements on milk contamination by germs and its conveyance to human subjects are especially interesting, and lead him to the emphatic conclusion: " Raw milk should not be used under any circumstances ; all milk should be sterilized before it is sold."

He quite agrees with the precaution taken by obstetricians in prohibiting an infected mother from nursing. ———

PYÆMIA FOLLOWING RUPTURE OF THE UMBILICAL CORD.

A case remarkable for the manner in which septic infection, originating at the umbilicus, became diffuse is described by DEICHMANN in the *Deutsche medicinische Wochenschrift*, No. 37, 1891. When first seen, the child, nine months old, was suffering from severe septic infection. The right half of the body, from beneath the axilla to the crest of the ilium, showed an œdematous swelling deeply injected, and especially prominent over the liver. Fluctuation could be felt near the mammary region. The entire swelling was painful, but no superficial lesion at which it originated was observed.

It was ascertained that the child's birth had been normal, and that when the cord separated hemorrhage occurred from the umbilical ring, which was checked by a midwife by the application of cotton and a bandage. This cotton was not removed for three days after its application. A discharge of serum, followed by pus, occurred after the removal of the bandage, and this discharge persisted from the umbilical ring for six months. After two months' treatment by the application of a powder, the secretion gradually ceased, but redness of the skin, with considerable swelling, ensued. On examination, it was evident that extensive suppuration in the deeper layers of the skin existed. Points of fluctuation were freely opened, undermined tissues were thoroughly douched with bichloride solution, and the dressings were frequently changed. At the end of the second week metastatic abscesses formed in various portions of the right half of the body. They were opened in turn, and the child finally made a complete recovery.

An Epidemic of Pneumonia in Infants, occasioned by Infected Straw.

It is the custom in the obstetric clinic at Heidelberg to use straw beds, which are emptied after each patient is convalescent, the tick thoroughly washed, and filled with fresh straw. GARTNER (*Centralblatt für Gynäkologie*, No. 27, 1891) noticed an odor from the straw in some of the beds, and observed that the patients in these beds had slight elevation of temperature, and that several of the children became ill with pneumonia. He made a bacteriological examination of the straw, of the dust about the bed, and found streptococci and staphylococci, beside other microörganisms. He then examined the lochia of the patients, finding the same germs there present, and also identified these germs in the secretions of the nose and mouth of the infants. In post-mortems upon five cases lobular pneumonia was present, caused by an abundance of streptococci and staphylococci. Control inoculations upon animals demonstrated infective power of these bacilli.

Gonorrhœa of the Mucous Membrane of the Mouth in the Newborn.

Five cases of gonorrhœal infection of the mouth in infants are reported by ROSINSKI in the *Zeitschrift für Geburtshülfe und Gynäkologie*, Band xxii., Heft 1, 1891. In most of the cases the maternal source of infection was clearly demonstrated. The lesion was an infiltration of the tissues upon the tongue and hard palate, with a characteristic yellowish mass composed of gonococci and pus-cells. The general health of the children was not especially disturbed, and very little pain or distress was observed. In some instances, gonorrhœal ophthalmia was also present. The children recovered under appropriate treatment. Those who had ophthalmia were sickest, and suffered considerably.

VAGINAL INJECTIONS UNNECESSARY IN NORMAL LABORS, ESPECIALLY WHERE EXTERNAL EXAMINATIONS ONLY ARE PRACTISED.

The belief already advanced by MERMANN, that injections and internal examinations could be dispensed with to advantage, finds support in a paper by LEOPOLD and GOLDBERG (Archiv für Gynäkologie, Band xl., Heft 3, 1891). Their material for comparison embraces 1358 cases, of which 1073 received no injections; 269 were not examined internally. A comparison of the percentage of infection during a series of years showed that only five-ninths as many cases occurred when no injections were given, as when they formed a routine treatment. In normal cases their employment has been abandoned. From the fact that the absolute disinfection of the hands is exceedingly difficult, it is argued that internal examinations should be as infrequent as possible, and especially in view of the present cultivation of the method of diagnosis by external examination.

[The recent researches of WELCH, described in his article on "Wound Infection," in the November number of the JOURNAL, bear directly upon the question of the disinfection of the hands. He found the ordinary method of using soap and water, and sublimate solutions, quite inefficient, and suggests the employment of a solution of permanganate of potassium, followed by dilute oxalic acid. He isolated a bacterium which seemed to have its especial habitat in the skin, and which is not destroyed by the ordinary disinfection with sublimate.—ED.]

LEUKÆMIA AND PREGNANCY.

In contrast to some recent writings upon the blood in pregnancy, which seemed to show that anæmia is not peculiar to the pregnant condition, is the paper by LAUBENBURG in the Archiv für Gynäkologie, Band xl , Heft 3, 1891. His study of the subject has led him to conclude that oftentimes lukæmia results from pregnancy, parturition, or the puerperal state. Pregnancy may even be interrupted by leukæmia, which exerts an unfavorable influence upon this condition. The prognosis of these cases may become seriously complicated by this disorder ; in such cases the early induction of labor is not only justifiable, but is the duty of the physician.

GYNECOLOGY.

UNDER THE CHARGE OF

HENRY C. COE, M.D., M.R.C.S.,

OF NEW YORK.

INTRA-VENOUS INFUSION OF SALT SOLUTION IN ACUTE ANÆMIA.

THOMSON (Deutscher med. Wochenschrift, 1891, No. 19) reports twelve cases of acute anæmia from hemorrhage (nine following labor and three surgical operations) which were treated by infusions of salt solution (one-half of one per cent.), eight being intra-venous, two intra-peritoneal, and two both intra-venous and intra-peritoneal. Four patients were saved. He prefers the intra-venous method, as it is simpler, can be rapidly practised, and is devoid of danger. Subcutaneous injections.of the same solution act too slowly, and when the heart is weak it is unable to carry the fluid into the general circulation. If the median vein cannot be found the vena saphena may be utilized. Intra-peritoneal infusion should be employed only after laparotomy. Other solutions have been recommended, but they possess no advantage over the saline.

STÄHLE (*Deutscher med. Wochenschrift*, 1891, No. 22) reports a case of postpartum hemorrhage in which the patient had become almost pulseless. A litre of Landerer's sugar and salt solution were injected in the course of an hour, with a successful result. He adds the caution that the proper time for the injection is when the pulse has improved a little, showing that the heart is able to carry the solution into the circulation.

CASTRATION IN OSTEOMALACIA.

THOM (*Centralblatt für Genäkologie*, 1891, No. 41) reports the following successful case: The patient, aged thirty-two years, had had three children. Her symptoms dated from the birth of the second child. She had severe pains in the pelvic bones, with marked deformity, was unable to walk, and showed progressive emaciation and œdema. The uterus was retroflexed and fixed. The adnexa were removed and the adhesions separated. It was noted that all the pelvic tissues were unusually softened and congested. The patient improved rapidly after the operation, the pains in her bones disappeared, and she was soon able to walk. A year after the operation she was perfectly well.

The writer accepts Fehling's theory that the disease is a reflex trophoneurosis of the bones dependent upon ovarian activity.

ARTIFICIAL PYO- AND HYDRO-SALPINX IN ANIMALS.

WOSKRESSENSKY (*Centralblatt für Gynäkologie*, 1891, No. 42), after a series of experiments upon rabbits, arrives at these conclusions:

1. In the Fallopian tube of the adult rabbit there is a secretion which in from four to six weeks forms a large hydrosalpinx, if both ends of the tube are ligated.

2, This secretion is most abundant at the abdominal end of the tube, so that a hydrosalpinx will be formed if the abdominal end alone is tied.

3. If croton oil, or a fluid containing the streptococcus aureus, is injected into the uterine cavity or tube, there results a localized exudation which neither tends to extend to the peritoneum nor does it cause any general disturbance.

THE ULTIMATE RESULTS OF REMOVAL OF THE ADNEXA.

In view of the general interest recently exhibited in this subject, the following statements by TAIT, made at the recent French Surgical Congress, are important. He divides these cases into three classes—those in which the adnexa are removed for the cure of myomata or metrostaxis, for disease of the tubes and ovaries, and for nervous disturbances. His mortality in 271 cases of myoma was 2.2 per cent. All but eight of the cases were successful. In patients under forty 70 per cent. of the tumors disappeared; in those between forty and fifty it diminished in size from one-sixth to one-third. There were transient climacteric disturbances, but only one case of permanent psychosis, in a patient who showed evidences of mental derangement before the operation. In 5 per cent. of the operations for diseased adnexa a suppurating sinus remained. It is necessary, he thinks, to wait longer for a cure in this class of cases than in the former. Persistent pain, exaggerated every month, is common, but it seldom lasts longer than a year after the operation. In only 4 cases was it necessary to perform a second laparotomy on account of cystic enlargement of the stumps. The writer has found that coitus is less painful after the operation, and that sexual desire is usually present.

He has seldom operated simply for the cure of neuroses, and always at the urgent desire of the patient, although he believes that the operation has a future. In the two cases in which a sufficient time had elapsed to judge of the result it was entirely satisfactory.

SEROUS RETRO-PERITONEAL CYSTS.

OBALINSKI (*Wiener klin. Wochenschrift*, 1891, No. 39) concludes an article on this subject with the following *résumé :* These cysts, though rare, occur more frequently than is usually supposed, and are found in the male, as well as in the female. As they develop slowly, they seldom attain a large size or give rise to symptoms. They are usually situated near the kidneys, and probably spring from the Wolffian bodies. As their walls are firm, though thin, and they are not adherent to the peritoneum (from which they are separated by loose connective tissue) their removal is not difficult. Their contents consists of an aqueous fluid, which may not reaccumulate after puncture; however, extirpation is preferable to puncture, as it can be accomplished easily and without danger.

PUBLIC HEALTH.

UNDER THE CHARGE OF
EDWARD F. WILLOUGHBY, M.D.,
OF LONDON.

SEVENTH INTERNATIONAL CONGRESS OF HYGIENE AND DEMOGRAPHY— LONDON, AUGUST, 1891.

The full text of all the papers sent in, whether read or not, will appear in the *Transactions* presented to every member. I propose, therefore, in this report to give brief notices of such only as contained something new or of special practical or scientific value, as I have hitherto done with the papers published in the English and foreign journals devoted to Public Health.

DIPHTHERIA.—Dr. Schrevens, of Tournai, from an analysis of the distribution of enteric fever and diphtheria in Belgium, and the relatively greater incidence of the latter in rural districts, concludes that, though both are fecal or filth diseases, pollution of the surface is more conducive to the development of Löffler's bacillus (diphtheria), as that of the subsoil to Eberth's enteric. Personal contact contributes greatly to its propagation, but Dr. Schrevens believes that poultry are susceptible to, and play an important part in creating foci of the disease.

At the annual congress of the British Medical Association, in 1883, I maintained this view of the etiology of diphtheria in opposition to Drs. C. Kelly, Slade King, Hubert Airey, and others, who connected its prevalence in rural districts with exposure to cold and wet, rather than with a specific cause. I asked: " Where does one meet, in close proximity to houses, with foul dunghills, pigstys, etc., saturating the surface soil with putrescent matters, more frequently than in villages and rural homesteads?" and, after quoting Soyka on the relative distribution of enteric fever and diphtheria in Munich, I said: " In fact it would appear that surface accumulations of filth are more likely to generate diphtheria, and pent-up putrid gases to produce enteric fever."

MATERNITY HOSPITALS.—Dr. Priestly, in an exhaustive review of these hospitals throughout Europe, showed that the saving of life effected within the last ten years amounted to over 3000 annually, which he attributed mainly to the general adoption of antiseptic measures.

MALARIA AND ENTERIC FEVER IN AFRICA.—Dr. Felkin observed that the comparative immunity of the natives from malaria was, to a great extent, due to acclimatization, for when moved from one area to another they suffered almost as much as Europeans. Enteric fever was endemic in all parts of Central Africa, and phthisis was by no means unknown ; but, so far as he knew, it occurred only in elevated areas where malaria was rare or altogether absent. In malarious districts he had never seen a case of phthisis. He did not believe in *typho-malarial* fever as a separate disease, but was convinced that the fever so called was merely enteric, occurring in an individual saturated with the malarial poison.

FILARIA SANGUINIS HOMINIS DIURNA AND PERSTANS.—Dr. Patrick Manson discussed the mutual relations of the *Filaria s. h.*, negro lethargy or the sleeping-sickness of the West Coast of Africa and the Congo, and the papulo-vesicular disease known as Craw-craw, peculiar to the same regions. He considered the *F. loa* to be the parental form of *F. s. h. diurna*, and the mangrove fly its intermediary host. The life history of *F. s. h.* was at present wrapped in obscurity, but from the analogy between it and the very similar *F. medinensis*, he believed the intermediary host of *F. s. h. perstans* to be a fresh-water animal, probably a cyclops or other entomostracon.

THE HÆMATOZOÖN OF MALARIA.—Dr. Laveran described the several forms of the *Plasmodium*, spherical, flagelliform, cruciform, and rosette-shaped, and the conditions under which each was assumed. He was satisfied as to the essential connection of the plasmodium with paludism, though he could not define the precise nature of this connection as cause, concomitant, or effect, and he admitted that hæmatozoa very similar morphologically were met with in the blood of other animals, even birds and reptiles, under circumstances precluding all suggestion of paludism. There were, however, differences quite sufficient to indicate that these were specifically distinct.

FERMENTATIONS EXCITED BY SPECIFIC MICROÖRGANISMS.—Dr. Percy Frankland had succeeded in isolating the bacillus of nitrification, or that which, present in the soil, has the power of oxidizing organic nitrogen and converting ammonia into nitrous and nitric acids. It had no action on gelatin plates. In his experiments nitrous acid only, not nitric, was formed. He had also isolated one which he called *B. ethaceticus*, which, when grown in any of the carbohydrates (except dulcite) produced ethyl alcohol and acetic acid, also formic and traces of succinic acid. By its means he split glycerin into an optically active form on which it had no effect, and an inactive one which it broke up by fermentation. The action of the pneumococcus of Friedländer on carbohydrates he found to be, as Brieger had already shown, identical with that of his *B. ethaceticus*.

IMMUNITY.—Mr. Hankin, Fellow of St. John's College, Cambridge, discussed the nature and action of defensive proteids, which he divided into *sozins* present in normally, and *phylaxins* in artificially, immune animals. Each was further divisible into myco- and toxo-sozins or phylaxins, according as they acted by killing the bacteria, or by destroying the toxins produced by them. The action of phylaxins was limited to one disease, while that of sozins extended to several species of bacillus and their products.

Conditions inducing susceptibility in animals otherwise immune, were found to be attended by a diminution in the amount of the defensive proteid previously present in the serum. This theory in no way excluded that of phagocytosis, since it was by means of these proteids that the phagocytes acted on the bacilli.

Dr. Armand Ruffer described a number of experiments with the *B. Chauveaui*, with somewhat paradoxical results, but proving, among other things, that the number of microörganisms introduced, and the inflammatory reaction, or rather the migration of leucocytes toward the point of inoculation, were in inverse proportion; that the leucocytes were attracted thither by a chemical poison; that they absorbed the bacilli while these were still living; that in acute infectious diseases the leucocytes did not emigrate, but were nevertheless active, and that if they were by any means prevented from reaching the virus, the disease ended fatally, even in animals naturally or artificially immune.

BACTERIOLOGICAL EXAMINATION OF WATER. — Dr. Percy Frankland insisted on the necessity for conducting such examinations immediately, since even in distilled water the multiplication of colonies was so rapid as to falsify all conclusions as to the purity of any sample.

MEAT INFECTION, OR FOOD POISONING.—Dr. Ballard gave the results of an inquiry conducted by him on behalf of the Local Government Board into numerous instances of poisoning by cooked meat, especially pork, during the last twelve years. The principal conclusions were: (1) The effects were usually gastro-enteric irritation, but in one case true pneumonia. (2) The immediate cause was a toxin generated by bacilli, either in the food itself or in the body of the consumer. (3) That the decision of this question rested chiefly on the interval elapsing between the ingestion of the food and the development of the symptoms. (4) The poison usually appeared to have been formed after the meat had become cold, and had been kept some time at the ordinary temperature ; while the greater frequency of such phenomena in pork seemed to be connected with the larger percentage of gelatin in it than in other flesh foods.

SCHOOL HYGIENE.—An exhaustive scheme for inquiry into the physical and psychical characters and antecedents of children of feeble intellect was submitted by Drs. Strumpell, F. L. A. Koch, Emil Schmidt, and Ernest Hasse, than which it would be difficult to devise a better.

Prof. Leo Burgerstein, the well-known school physician of Vienna, described an experiment designed to test the degree of brain fatigue consequent on continuous application, which consisted in engaging four classes of children, grouped according to sex and age, in ordinary arithmetic, for four consecutive periods of ten minutes separated by intervals of five minutes, and comparing the number of figures worked and errors made in each period. The errors increased in the second and notably in the third period far in excess of the increase in the number of figures worked ; though contrary to what might have been expected, there was some improvement in the fourth period. The idea is a good one and deserves to be further developed.

Mr. Arbuthnot Lane read a paper of great scientific interest to the surgeon, and to those in medical charge of the young, in which he insisted on the remarkable adaptation of structure in joints consequent on certain manual and mechanical employments, especially when commenced before growth and ossification were complete. In the light of these observations he explained the origination of spinal curvature and faulty attitudes, the true nature and causation of which were, he maintained, generally misapprehended, effects being taken for causes.

COPPER POISONING.—Prof. Lehmann, of Würzburg, while deprecating on every ground the addition of copper salts to preserved fruits and vegetables, and to flour in bread-making, saw no reason to condemn the use of copper for culinary utensils, provided common care and cleanliness were observed. It was only when strongly acid liquids were allowed to stand long and to cool in copper vessels, that any appreciable solution of the metal took place, and even then the amount could scarcely reach the 3 grains per head among the consumers required to set up symptoms of gastro-enteritis. Since there were no recorded cases of acute copper poisoning through " greened " preserves, but many from the use of copper utensils, he was strongly inclined to doubt the correctness of the latter, which he believed were really due to ptomaines and to toxalbumins, the copper having been assumed as the cause, since no definite poison has been detected—that is, none answering to the ordinary chemical tests.

SANITARY ENGINEERING.—The recorded instances of the occurrence of outbreaks of enteric fever following the specific pollution of wells or of reservoirs, as at Croydon, in England, and Plymouth, in America, are so numerous as to leave no doubt as to the propagation of that disease, as of cholera, by means of public water supplies. But it is certainly remarkable that until quite recently no indisputable case of such a result consequent on the entrance of the fecal discharges of enteric fever into large rivers at points above the in-takes of water companies could be appealed to. Almost the only classical example was that of the outbreak at Gloucester, following three or four weeks after the epidemic at Kidderminster, some twenty miles higher up the Severn. It is not unreasonable to attribute the immunity attending the use of running streams at points some miles below the point of such sewage discharge, to the fatal action of light on the bacillus of Eberth, in marked contrast to its inertness on cultures of those of cholera (Koch's) or of diphtheria (Löffler's).

But an instance at least as palpable as that of Gloucester was described by Mr. Kummel, of Altona, as having occurred in that town in February of the present year.

Hamburg and Altona both draw their water from the Elbe, the former without, the latter with careful filtration; but while Hamburg has its in-takes at some distance above the city, Altona pumps its below, *i. e.*, after it has received the sewage of half a million persons; and three or four weeks before the appearance of the disease the number of bacteria suddenly rose from 50 or 80 to 1500 in the cubic centimetre, falling again to the normal synchronously with the subsidence of the epidemic. As enteric fever was almost entirely absent from Hamburg at the time, Mr. Kummel suggests that the filter-beds themselves may have acted as culture fields.

Mr. Oesten, engineer to the Berlin Water-works, described an unexpected accident, viz.: the entrance of impurities (in this case, sand) into water mains under considerable internal pressure. Ordinarily, the tendency under such circumstances would be leakage outward, but if the fissure formed an acute angle with the direction of the flow in the mains, so soon as a certain velocity was attained a "suction action" was set up, drawing inward, notwithstanding the pressure, the ground-water and any impurities contained in the surrounding soil. ·

In a paper on the water-supply of maritime towns, including those on the tidal reaches of rivers, I approached the question from what was, so far as I could learn, an entirely new standpoint, viz.: that while *inland* towns—if, as I maintain they always would, they disposed of their sewage by irrigation —returned to the land the whole of the water they had taken, whether from rivers or wells, *maritime* towns discharged it directly or indirectly into the sea, leaving the land so much the poorer for the loss. In the case of London, the general lowering of the water in wells, and the drying-up of the smaller streams in the surrounding districts, showed that the demand already exceeded the available portion of the rainfall, and that no extension of the supply could be sought in the basin of the Thames without serious detriment to the agricultural interest.

Maritime towns, if of considerable size, must, therefore, have recourse to areas where the rainfall is in excess of the local requirements, as moorlands and lakes in mountainous districts, or to a source hitherto ignored by engineers, viz.: underground waters which find their way to the sea without giving rise to rivers, in other words run to waste. Such is the source of the Brighton supply, great part of the drainage of the Weald finding its way under the chalk of the South Downs to the sea; and I believe, on geological and hydrological grounds, a like waste would take place along the north coast of Kent, and in many other localities where ranges of hills run parallel to the coast, the dip of their beds inclining seaward.

In a warm discussion on burial reform, the advocates and opponents of cremation, represented by Sir Henry Thompson and Mr. Seymour Haden, were as one in condemning the use of strong imperishable coffins. The effect of thick elm or oak in preventing the natural disintegration of the body was strikingly illustrated, as Dr. Gibbons related, during the excavation of part of St. Andrew's Churchyard, where corpses interred two hundred years ago were found in nearly the same state as those buried within twenty years, being imbedded in layers of crushed and compressed wood.

SECTION OF DEMOGRAPHY.—Dr. Ogle showed the comparative mortality of men between twenty-five and sixty-five years of age, in a number of ocenpations selected as representative. This method was preferable to taking the mean age at death, since, after the age of sixty-five few continue in active pursuits. The clergy were set down as the standard of one hundred, and the several factors determining the proportion of disease and death given as—
(1) Working in cramped attitudes, especially such as impede respiration.
(2) Over-work, especially sudden muscular efforts and strains. (3) Dealing with noxious substances, as lead, mercury, infected hides, etc. (4) Working in ill-ventilated and over-heated rooms. (5) Alcoholic excess. (6) Liability to accident. (7) Exposure to inhalation of dust.

The influence of alcoholic indulgence was conspicuous in the comparative mortality of innkeepers, 274; and their male servants, 397, the highest figure of all; and scarcely less so among cab and omnibus drivers, 267; and costermongers, street-hawkers, etc., 338. Temperance advocates are guilty of a fallacy in ignoring foul air and long and late hours, from which barmen and barmaids, were they even total abstainers, would suffer still more than drapers, tailors, and printers.

The factor of good or bad ventilation in mines, where other things were fairly equal, was seen in the mortality of coal and iron miners, 160, and of the Cornish miners, 331, or more than twice that of those in the north.

That life in the open air should be attended by freedom from phthisis is what one would expect, yet men exposed to all vicissitudes of weather are no less exempt from other diseases of the respiratory organs.

Here fishermen are taken as the standard, having the lowest mortality from pulmonary diseases :

Occupation.	Mortality from :		
	Phthisis.	Other respiratory diseases.	Phthisis and other respiratory diseases.
Fishermen	55	45	100
Agricultural laborers	62	79	141
Grocers	84	59	143
Drapers	152	65	217
Tailors	144	94	238
Printers	233	84	317

The influence of dust is very marked, but in order to eliminate the fallacy involved in comparing occupations followed by men of very different physique and strength of constitution, I have selected four strictly comparable, and reduced them to the standard of the healthiest.

Occupation.	Mortality from :		
	Phthisis.	Other respiratory diseases.	Phthisis and other respiratory diseases.
Coal miners	38	62	100
Masons and bricklayers	76	62	138
Quarrymen	93	83	176
Cornish miners	210	140	350

In the case of the Cornish miners, the cause of the high mortality is, however, the absence of ventilation in the deep tin mines, rather than any excess of dust.

Taking in like manner four dusty occupations not necessarily confined to men of robust constitution, and reducing them to the standard of the least unhealthy, Dr. Ogle's figures would appear as follows:

Occupation.	Mortality from		
	Phthisis.	Other respiratory diseases.	Phthisis and other respiratory diseases.
Bakers	53	47	100
Cotton-mill hands	110	110	220
Cutlers	150	158	308
Earthenware-makers	192	260	452

Note to Contributors.—All contributions intended for insertion in the Original Department of this Journal are only received *with the distinct understanding that they are contributed exclusively to this Journal.*

Contributions from the Continent of Europe and written in the French, German or Italian language, if on examination they are found desirable for this Journal, will be translated at its expense.

Liberal compensation is made for articles used. A limited number of extra copies in pamphlet form, if desired, will be furnished to authors in lieu of compensation, *provided the request for them be written on the manuscript.*

All communications should be addressed to

Dr. EDWARD P. DAVIS,
250 South 21st Street, Philadelphia.

INDEX.

Lightning Source UK Ltd.
Milton Keynes UK
UKHW012346041218
333472UK00010B/330/P